NURSING RESEARCH

A Qualitative Perspective
Fourth Edition

Patricia L. Munhall, EdD, ARNP, PsyA, FAAN

President
International Institute of Human Understanding
Miami, Florida

JONES AND BARTLETT PUBLISHERS

Sudbury, Massachusetts

BOSTON   TORONTO   LONDON   SINGAPORE

World Headquarters

Jones and Bartlett Publishers
40 Tall Pine Drive
Sudbury, MA 01776
978-443-5000
info@jbpub.com
www.jbpub.com

Jones and Bartlett Publishers
Canada
6339 Ormindale Way
Mississauga, Ontario L5V 1J2
CANADA

Jones and Bartlett Publishers
International
Barb House, Barb Mews
London W6 7PA
UK

Jones and Bartlett's books and products are available through most bookstores and online booksellers. To contact Jones and Bartlett Publishers directly, call 800-832-0034, fax 978-443-8000, or visit our website, www.jbpub.com.

Substantial discounts on bulk quantities of Jones and Bartlett's publications are available to corporations, professional associations, and other qualified organizations. For details and specific discount information, contact the special sales department at Jones and Bartlett via the above contact information or send an email to specialsales@jbpub.com.

The authors, editor, and publisher have made every effort to provide accurate information. However, they are not responsible for errors, omissions, or for any outcomes related to the use of the contents of this book and take no responsibility for the use of the products and procedures described. Treatments and side effects described in this book may not be applicable to all people; likewise, some people may require a dose or experience a side effect that is not described herein. Drugs and medical devices are discussed that may have limited availability controlled by the Food and Drug Administration (FDA) for use only in a research study or clinical trial. Research, clinical practice, and government regulations often change the accepted standard in this field. When consideration is being given to use of any drug in the clinical setting, the health care provider or reader is responsible for determining FDA status of the drug, reading the package insert, and reviewing prescribing information for the most up-to-date recommendations on dose, precautions, and contraindications, and determining the appropriate usage for the product. This is especially important in the case of drugs that are new or seldom used.

Library of Congress Cataloging-in-Publication Data
Nursing research : a qualitative perspective / [edited by] Patricia L.
   Munhall.—4th ed.
      p. ; cm.
   Includes bibliographical references and index.
   ISBN-13: 978-0-7637-3864-8
   ISBN-10: 0-7637-3864-6
   1. Nursing—Research.   I. Munhall, Patricia L.
   [DNLM: 1. Nursing Research—methods.   WY 20.5 N9735 2007]
RT81.5.N866 2007
10.73072—dc22
                                                        2006010564

6048

Production Credits
Executive Editor: Kevin Sullivan
Associate Editor: Amy Sibley
Production Director: Amy Rose
Associate Production Editor: Kate Hennessy
Senior Marketing Manager: Emily Ekle
Composition: ATLIS Graphics

Manufacturing and Inventory Coordinator:
   Amy Bacus
Cover Design: Kristin E. Ohlin
Printing and Binding: Malloy, Inc.

Printed in the United States of America
10 09 08 07   10 9 8 7 6 5 4 3 2

CONTENTS

21 ETHICAL CONSIDERATIONS AND QUALITATIVE RESEARCH   501

Patricia L. Munhall

22 INSTITUTIONAL REVIEW OF QUALITATIVE RESEARCH PROPOSALS: A TASK OF NO SMALL CONSEQUENCE   515

Patricia L. Munhall

23 STRATEGIES OF INTRAPROJECT SAMPLING   529

Janice Morse

CONTRIBUTORS

EDITOR AND CONTRIBUTING AUTHOR

Patricia L. Munhall, EdD, ARNP, NCPsyA, CNLP, FAAN
President
International Institute of Human Understanding
Miami, Florida

CONTRIBUTING AUTHORS

Lioness Ayers, PhD, RN
Assistant Professor
University of Iowa
College of Nursing
Iowa City, Iowa

Terry A. Badger, PhD, ARNP, BC, FAAN
Professor
College of Nursing
The University of Arizona
Tucson, Arizona

Cheryl Tatano Beck, DNSc, CNM, FAAN
Professor
School of Nursing
University of Connecticut
Storrs, Connecticut

David M. Callejo Pérez, EdD
Assistant Professor of Curriculum Studies
Doctoral Program Coordinator
Department of Curriculum and Instruction/Literacy Studies
College of Human Resources and Education
West Virginia University
Morgantown, West Virginia

Ronald J. Chenail, PhD
Vice President
Office of Research, Planning, and Governmental Affairs
Professor
Department of Family Therapy
Nova Southeastern University
Fort Lauderdale-Davie, Florida

Roberta Cricco-Lizza, RN, PhD, MPH
Adjunct Assistant Professor
Center for Health Disparities Research
University of Pennsylvania School of Nursing
Philadelphia, Pennsylvania

Marcia Dombro, RN, PhD
Adjunct Professor
School of Nursing
University of Miami
Miami, Florida

Maureen Duffy, PhD
Professor and Chair
Department of Counseling
Barry University
Miami Shores, Florida

Lynne Dunphy, PhD, FNP
Assistant Dean, Graduate Program
Christine E. Lynn College of Nursing
Florida Atlantic University
Boca Raton, Florida

M. Louise Fitzpatrick, EdD, RN, FAAN
Connelly Endowed Dean and Professor
College of Nursing
Villanova University
Villanova, Pennsylvania

Edward Freeman, PhD, ARNP, BC
President, Primary Care Associates of South Beach, LLC
Director of Clinical Cardiology Research
Miami Beach, Florida

Patricia Becker Hentz, EdD, CS, PMH, NP-BC
Associate Professor
University of Southern Maine
College of Nursing and Health Professions
Portland, Maine

Sarah Steen Lauterbach, RN, MN, MSPH, EdD
Associate Professor
College of Nursing
Valdosta State University
Valdosta, Georgia

Joy Longo, MS, RNC
Doctoral Student
Christine E. Lynn College of Nursing
Florida Atlantic University,
Boca Raton, Florida

Marlene C. Mackey, PhD, RN, FAAN
Associate Professor
College of Nursing
University of South Carolina
Columbia, South Carolina

Janice Morse, PhD (nurse), PhD (anthro), DNurs (hon.), FAAN
Scientific Director
International Institute for Qualitative Methodology
Professor
Faculty of Nursing
University of Alberta
Edmonton, Alberta
Canada

Linda Niehaus
Project Director
International Institute for
Qualitative Methodology
Professor
Faculty of Nursing
University of Alberta
Edmonton, Alberta
Canada

Sally St. George, PhD
Associate Professor
Family Therapy Program
Kent School of Social Work
University of Louisville
Louisville, Kentucky

Barbra Mann Wall, PhD, RN
Associate Professor
School of Nursing
University of Pennsylvania
Philadelphia, Pennsylvania

Zane Robinson Wolf, PhD, RN, FAAN
Dean and Professor
School of Nursing and Health
Sciences
La Salle University
Philadelphia, Pennsylvania

Judith Wuest, RN, PhD
*Professor & Canadian Institutes
of Health Research/UNB
Investigator*
University of New Brunswick
Faculty of Nursing
Fredericton, New Brunswick
Canada

Dan Wulff, PhD
Associate Professor
Family Therapy Program
Kent School of Social Work
University of Louisville
Louisville, Kentucky

Patti R. Zuzelo, EdD, APRN-BC, CNS
*Associate Professor and CNS
Track Coordinator*
School of Nursing and Health
Sciences
La Salle University
Philadelphia, Pennsylvania
Associate Director of Nursing
for Research
Albert Einstein Healthcare
Network
Philadelphia, Pennsylvania

PROLOGUE

This edition, like the preceding ones, is written with an overwhelming concern for the subjective experience of individuals, groups, and/or culture. The concern is grounded in human compassion and caring. I believe through the lens of the philosophical underpinnings of qualitative research that qualitative nurse researchers contribute in a meaningful way to a very humanistic form of nursing practice. We use our different *ways of seeing* to uncover and discover *understanding*, which is the essential core, from my perspective, to authentic compassion and caring.

Qualitative researchers have a different worldview, paradigm, and research traditions than our quantitative colleagues. Given the proper encouragement, freedom, and resources to grow and develop in their methods, these researchers can provide the nursing profession understanding, description, theory, interpretation, and direction encompassing the intricacies and interconnectedness of being in this world—a world that is not one but many, made of multiple realities emerging from multiple perceptions. Qualitative researchers search for the differences not only between cultures but also within cultures. In so doing, they challenge stereotypes, presuppositions, and assumptions.

Inherent, then, in qualitative methods is the potential for liberation and emancipation from the constraints of outdated beliefs, myths, and theories. The sands of nursing science must keep shifting to breathe new life into the ever-changing and evolving world around us, as well as the worlds of those we serve.

Qualitative researchers break new ground by revealing what had been concealed. They look beyond appearance. They provide the reconstruction that time demands of us as these sands shift and knowledge changes. In their quest for discovery, qualitative researchers legitimize the existence of others in their differences. Conformity and generalizability are not the aims of our research: we know that a universal concept of meaning in experience is not possible and doubt that it would even be desirable. I believe we are attuned to our place in the universe, and while we may appear similar from a distance, we must move beyond appearances to embrace and celebrate the nuances of existence, and to understand the subtle and not-so-subtle differences between you and me and all members of the human race.

Because qualitative research has the power to liberate us from biases and prejudices that oppress people, research studies can expose the dark side, where a need for change is illuminated and a call for action results. Part of the intrigue of our work is understanding a "newness," a very different negotiation of meaning. I sometimes think of our studies as "awakenings," and very significant ones. The newness of or about some thing or experience awakens and expands our consciousness of others and self. The results from qualitative research raise our consciousness to what was not known; the unbeknownst becomes understood, the concealed becomes seen, the silence given voice.

ABOUT THIS EDITION

The first edition of this book was actually written in 1986, and as I write that date down, I think it has encompassed much of my professional life. It is almost 20 years! If you were to see the first edition, which right now is on my lap, you would not believe its size. First of all, it is in hardcover, reflecting the economics of the time, and it is composed of about 280 pages. Qualitative research in nursing at that time was emerging as a "home" for many nurse researchers for reasons discussed in Chapter 1 of this volume. Looking at the authors in that edition, however, one sees accomplished qualitative researchers and leaders in what really was a "movement" in nursing research.

The second and third editions followed the format of that text, as does this edition. The text is divided into three sections. Part I attempts to provide the essential foundational content to understanding the qualitative research perspective. As in the last edition, there are chapters on language, epistemology, and philosophy. In this edition, however, Part I has three new chapters. The first provides what is called the landscape of qualitative research in nursing and I hope you will actually get the *feel* for where qualitative research came from, where it has been, and where it can continue on its most worthwhile and wonderful journey. This chapter presents the situated context, and you will read lots about the situated context throughout this text because it is so essential to our understanding. The next new chapter by Marcia Dombro is a historical and philosophical background of qualitative research (some of this is also discussed in Chapter 1). I do not believe I have ever seen this in nursing literature, such a complete history of ideas and the attending philosophers with their particular ideas and constructs. It helps put into perspective the evolution of the philosophy that guides us in doing qualitative research.

The following chapter by Lynn Dunphy and Joy Longo is also new, and I thought it important to place in the foundation part the contemporary philosophies which are a part of many qualitative studies and discussions. In fact, each could be a method chapter on its own, but because of page limitations, certain decisions need to be made. However, I think it is essential to understand our postmodern world, critical social theory, and also feminist approaches. Either chapter can be used separately, but we see them here girding the method and exemplar chapters.

Part II is different in this edition. This section presents the more prevalent methods, and with each chapter an exemplar of the method follows. The exemplar might not follow exactly the method chapter because interpretation of methods can be different. So, this format remains the same, with the exception of the historical method chapter (the proposed author, unfortunately, had to deal with Hurricane Katrina, which is an example of the situated context); all chapters are by new authors and so the chapters are new and the approaches different. In every edition, the exemplar chapter changed. In this edition I thought it would be interesting to have new contributing authors for the method chapters.

Now this is important. Though there are new chapters on methods by different authors, I want to encourage you to also go back to the second and third editions and read those method chapters as well. There are a few different methods, but most important is that those authors are excellent, as are the new ones, and you do not want to miss reading their approaches to the same method. This is especially true if you are going to use a particular method. This principle also applies to the exemplar chapters. Go back and read some of the earlier editions to augment reading the ones in this edition. Such additional readings from all editions could be combined into one large volume, and you would be carrying around one of those back-breaking books like the ones you used to in medical-surgical nursing!

Part III has expanded with six new authors and actually, including my chapters, now has eight chapters that introduce and discuss more considerations essential to conducting qualitative research. These new authors enrich this section and provide wonderful discourses. You will find this section very helpful; actually I like the word *essential* better.

The world has changed dramatically since 1986, and some of the largest influences are, of course, the Internet and the use of personal computers. I remember a colleague who was one of the first to master the computer when most of us feared it and hoped it would go away, who encouraged me to at least try to learn to use it. Thinking back, I was being resistant, and my contributions to that edition were handwritten on my treasured yellow legal pads, which I placed on a chessboard I had given to my late father as a gift, and I got lots written in the early morning hours while in bed.

Today, I sit in front of the screen to write. Because there were three powerful hurricanes last year, I experienced what it was like *not* to have the use of the computer when there was no power, sometimes for weeks. So frustrating. I share this with you because there is a parallel to qualitative research in nursing. The hurricanes also serve as an example of the effects of the situated context.

One more thought about the computer: the computer is wonderful, the Internet amazing; however I caution you that when you conduct qualitative research not to have the software do too much of the classification of your material. Some software may be helpful, but remember the real "tool" for qualitative research is *your thinking, your dwelling, your insights*. For organizing your material, you might find such software helpful but the interpretation belongs to you and your participants.

To paraphrase Husserl, remember to the people themselves, to the experiences themselves. Stay close to your participants, to their descriptions, to their interpretations, and to their subjective perspective of their reality.

I often think of qualitative research, because of our closeness with individuals, with reverence and awe. As researchers, we are given permission to enter the experience of others as they openly share with us their pain and joy. So, it is not the research per se that prompts my reverence and awe: it is the generosity and courage of our participants, who allow us to accompany them and who share with us themselves. It is to these people to whom this book is dedicated.

Patricia L. Munhall

ACKNOWLEDGMENTS

The experiential component of intertwining all the various aims and goals of this edition through philosophy, methods, exemplars, and other qualitative research considerations reflects my extraordinary good fortune to have as friends and contributing authors a most talented, generous, and scholarly group of individuals. This is not hyperbole, *I could not be more privileged* than to have in one volume the amount of scholarship that is present here. To each one of these wonderful authors I wish to express my sincerest gratitude.

Each in different ways contributed not only chapters but also shared suggestions for this the fourth edition of *Nursing Research: A Qualitative Perspective.* In the temporal life world (a qualitative concept explained in this volume!) I would like to thank Sarah (Selen) Lauterbach for encouraging me to do a fourth edition in the first place: she obviously was very convincing. Selen, thank you for your support and unwavering encouragement. What seemed to follow after that was a qualitative research conference in Utrecht, where Sarah and Patricia Becker Heinz discussed with me suggestions for this volume and also individuals they thought would be excellent contributors. Our discussions during that conference stimulated much thought and I am indebted to them for their interest and contributions. *Thank you Sarah and Patricia* for devoting your time and contributing your ideas during that conference, sometimes over coffee, sometimes while riding a train past Dutch windmills, and one day in the most beautiful tulip garden! During these times, ideas and suggestions emerged; a form perhaps of aesthetic influence on academic thought.

Jan Morse who has been involved in every edition of this text was also part of this conference (most likely in charge!) and was so very helpful in suggesting individuals for various chapters. *Jan, thank you* for all your contributions over the years to this text, as well as this one. I am always impressed by the amount and quality of your work. Readers need to know that Jan is probably one of the biggest advocates of qualitative research in nursing in the world! Thank you Jan for your two chapters as well, one of which was co-authored with Linda Niehaus.

Bringing in different scholars for our method chapters provides the reader with the opportunity to read different interpretations and presentation styles. So in this edition I want to welcome the new method authors and thank them as well, for their outstanding contributions. In this edition we have *Judith Wuest, Zane Robinson Wolf* (doing a method chapter in this edition, she wrote an exemplar in the last edition), *Patricia Becker Heinz, Maureen Duffy, and Ron Chenail* with co-authors *Sally St. George and Dan Wulff.*

How grateful I always am to the contributing authors who comprise the new exemplar chapters. As is traditional all new research comprises the exemplars and complements in this edition all new method chapters! I want to thank so very much, Sarah Steen Lauterbach, who has been in all the editions with all new studies which demonstrate a scholarly progression of her phenomenological research and insights; Cheryl Tantano Beck who also has developed a outstanding scholarly record of qualitative research; Roberta Cricco-Lizza, who is doing a post-doctorate right now presenting an insightful and scholarly study; and Terry A. Badger, another highly esteemed qualitative research scholar, as are Barbra Mann Wall, Lioness Ayres, and Edward Freeman. Each author is held in the highest regard for their research in nursing. *For this I personally thank Sarah, Cheryl, Roberta, Terry, Barbra, Lioness, and my dear friend Edward.*

Additionally, the talent pool of research scholars within this text keeps growing in my acknowledgements and gratitude to them. There are new contributing authors in the Part I, Marcia Dunbro and Lynne Dunphy. Marcia has written a one-of-a-kind historical and philosophical chapter for qualitative research and Lynne Dunphy, who has written for other editions on historical research, has contributed to this edition a most insightful analysis of contemporary philosophy which situates qualitative research in the world of today. Lynne's chapter is co-authored by Joy Longo. *Thank you Marcia, Lynne and Joy* for your outstanding contributions.

Moving to Part III, I want to express my deepest appreciation for all new chapters, demonstrating wisdom, insight, and analysis in their chapters, to authors Patti R. Zuzelo, Janice Morse, Linda Niehaus, Marlene Mackey, Ron Chenail and Maureen Duffy, and David M. Callego Perez.

It is indeed a moving experience to write acknowledgements, when the volume is going into production and I look at the caliber of contributors, while also expressing gratitude for the trailblazers! I have written six chapters in this edition: three chapters in Part I, one chapter in Part II, and two chapters in Part III, and I am very grateful for that opportunity. This leads me to thank the editors at Jones and Bartlett: Kevin Sullivan, for giving me that opportunity, and Amy Sibley and Kate Hennessy for supporting and organizing all the activities that went into publishing this book. *Kevin, Amy, and Kate, thank you* for all your talent, support, patience, and professionalism.

An opportunity to write and also to be so privileged as to have a cadre of contributors who are so exemplary in scholarship is a very humbling experience. In the last edition I mentioned our interconnectedness: readers, authors, former students, friends and now perhaps you, a new reader coming to form an intertwined circle of discovery, understanding, meaning, and interpretations, ever-changing as our multistoried world keeps changing. As qualitative researchers in nursing, the profession depends on us to provide the authentic, inter-subjective, polyperceptual, and contextual studies which will enlighten and inform compassionate, expert, and caring nursing practice from the perception of those we serve. What qualitative research has to offer our profession is discussed throughout this text, but one thing is clear—it would not be possible without our participants. So to them goes the ultimate gratitude.

Patricia L. Munhall

PART I

The Qualitative Perspective

In Part I of this edition of *Nursing Research: A Qualitative Perspective*, I invite you to contemplate the emergence of qualitative research in nursing, from the past to this most exciting time in our history, where there seems to be a heightened search for meaning and understanding within the context of being. Today, more than ever, we see how meaning and understanding are fundamental to the caring and compassionate practice of nursing. In this section, the "why" of this will become explicit to you.

The chapters in this section provide you with the essential philosophical, epistemological, and contextual foundations critical *to the doing* of qualitative research. From the first chapter, which is a brush stroke of the landscape of qualitative research, to the last chapter of this section, which discusses contemporary philosophical thought, you should become grounded in the historical, the linguistic, the "how we come to know things" of epistemology and the philosophical underpinnings that comprise the qualitative research perspective. In the beginning of this section, you might encounter a newness of perception that might require you to reread different parts to gain a better understanding. Qualitative research does require *a shift in perception* from the positivist perspective. I think you will find it a most freeing and humanistic shift!

I hope you well immerse yourself in these five chapters to the extent that you can actually feel what it means to *be coming from* a qualitative perspective. When you hear or perhaps *you say*, "I am coming from a qualitative perspective," you will understand the meanings underpinning this very profound way of seeing and understanding *being* and *experience*.

The Landscape of Qualitative Research in Nursing

Patricia L. Munhall

I want to welcome you the student to the landscape of qualitative research in nursing, as well as the faculty member who is guiding this study. Oftentimes when reading a text such as this the first question one might legitimately want to ask is, *"What is qualitative research?"* In this volume you will find many definitions, perhaps each differing in some ways, reflecting the many ways of defining or perceiving qualitative research. In fact each method included in this book will have a definition for the specific method. However, character-istics of qualitative research, or tenets, if you like, follow through all qualita-tive methods. I like this way of perceiving qualitative research because I have long supported the proposition that *definitions limit possibilities*. Definitions can box people into *a* formula, which is the antithesis of qualitative research.

What I hope to do as I describe the landscape of qualitative research as I perceive it to be lived today is to include in this discussion the various com-ponents, beliefs, values, and characteristics that comprise qualitative re-search. So there will not be a one-sentence definition but instead an evolving sense of what qualitative research is, demonstrated throughout this chapter. When I write something that is not from a qualitative perspective, I will call your attention to it as distinct and probably belonging to the quantitative methods of research. Otherwise, this chapter is a reflection of the qualitative perspective, which *thus shows itself* through the content.

My intention in this chapter is to provide a holistic description and explanation—*to the extent* that one chapter can permit—of the qualitative research perspective in nursing and relate the discussion to your own world. I encourage you to begin thinking from a qualitative perspective as you read because this will help you understand the following chapters. Try to incorporate the concept of being discussed in your thinking to other instances of a particular idea or activity.

For example, have you noticed that the first person "I" is being used? Qualitative research is known for giving voice to people, to hearing people's own personal narrative and using the language of our participants in research. Often, this is distinct from quantitative research, where, for example, a questionnaire might be derived from a theory developed by a researcher (for example, the Myers-Briggs Type Indicator). So, in this class, if that is the case, or while reading this text, give yourself voice by using *I: I* see the world this way and *I* interpret the experience this way. Give your subjective experience voice. In this way you will also learn to give your research participants their voice, encouraging them to use their *Is*, and seeing through their eyes.

This chapter includes many cross-references to other chapters that explain specific concepts in greater depth. I want to reassure you that ideas discussed in Chapter 1 are further elaborated upon throughout the entire book. So, in reading this introductory chapter, please know that concepts that may seem puzzling now are covered in later chapters.

THE IRREDUCIBLE YOU

In this chapter and throughout the book, I hope you find the landscape you are traveling across interesting and stimulating, the methods challenging, and the exemplars revealing as well as quite meaningful. But let's begin with you, a place where thinking qualitatively is a natural place to start.

This might be your second or third course in nursing research, and you may have been introduced to qualitative research methods in your first course, which I *assume* was an overview. Here, I would like to emphasize one of the most important characteristics of qualitative research: *do not make assumptions!* To demonstrate how assumptions made at the very beginning of a study could lead to erroneous findings, let's examine what might be wrong with this paragraph.

First, I do not know how many courses in research you have already had, if any! A second erroneous assumption I make is that you may have had an overview of qualitative research. Preparing this chapter, I found many fundamentals of nursing research textbooks that did not address in any way qualitative research (which, of course, I find very distressful for many reasons, the most important of which is that it deprives you of the possibilities, pleasures, authenticity, and meaningfulness that comes from qualitative research).

I suggest that not making assumptions is a very good idea for any endeavor in which you are involved. The practice of not making assumptions indicates that qualitative research is very close to *real* life experiences, not ones that are assumed, which often means not based on anything but conjecture. Sometimes assumptions can reflect prejudice, biases, and stereotypes that, when acted upon, can be very unjust, unfair, and lead to all sorts of poor judgments. That is the downside of assumptions. Sometimes people make positive assumptions. Be wary of these, too.

Many introductory courses emphasize the scientific method, sometimes referred to as quantitative methods. You might remember discussion of independent variables and dependent variables, sampling techniques, statistical methods of analyzing data, and rules for reliability and validity, among other essentials of the scientific method.

Can you remember the difference between an independent variable and a dependent variable? For some reason, students find this distinction troublesome, perhaps because it does not actually follow *real* life experiences. Experience is so multifaceted that breaking it down into parts, such as independent and dependent variables, does little to contribute to understanding the whole. David Bohm (1985), who calls this the implicate order of organisms, states: "The word implicate means to enfold, in Latin, to fold inward. In the implicate order, everything is folded into everything" (p. 12).

Another critical component of qualitative research is its emphasis on holism and what Bohm calls the constraining grip of objectivity as a myth. Not only is an individual a holistic system, but he or she is much more than that: the individual is engaged in the world of others, in interacting worlds of experience. We come to see that qualitative research *does not practice reductionism*, does not reduce human beings or experiences to parts that require separate investigation. That we leave to quantitative researchers, who *do* remember the difference between independent and dependent variables! Variables are parts that, in the strict scientific worldview, influence other parts and are reduced from the whole. An example might be when we ask, "Is there a relationship between exercise and obesity?" A simple quantitative research project would distinguish two variables. Objectivity would play an important part in choosing the sample population so it is homogeneous and results can be generalized, meaning they can be applied to other *like* individuals.

In contrast, a qualitative researcher might even call this project the experience of obesity and view obesity as a holistic phenomenon of not only embodiment, the unity of body and mind, but also the unity of self with others and the environment. What is very interesting and very distinctive is the focus of qualitative research on subjectivity and intersubjectivity. Stolorow and Atwood (2002) describe this as: "the subjective world of the individual as its central theoretical concept, envisioning the world as evolving organically from the person's encounter with critical experiences that constitute his unique life history . . . the perspective toward being" (p. 2). What does this mean? We know what it means because we subconciously think this way and our life unfolds this way. We just may not have reflected on subjectivity before (go to page 147, Chapter 6). As individuals we each have a perspective of ourselves and the world. This is the reason why we might agree or disagree with others, because others also have a perspective, or a subjective world, their own subjective perspective. Other words to describe this perspective might be *worldview* or *paradigm* (discussed in Chapters 2, 3, and 6).

Our own subjective world evolves from all our previous experiences: our experiences as a child; our relationship with parents, siblings, and friends; the culture we grew up in or are currently a part of; the time in history we are situated in; the country, state, and town we are living in; our age; and the list goes on. The subjective perspective is the result of our experiences and forms the context of where we are at present. This is sometimes called the *situated context*, another critical consideration in qualitative research. Taking into consideration the situated context of participants in a study is imperative. Who they are is taken very seriously. More than just demographics, they are people who differ because of their subjective perspective, which evolved from their experiences. Considering the situated context demonstrates respect for these individuals by acknowledging their uniqueness and taking into consideration their personal narratives of their lives (an illustration of two subjective worlds can be found in Chapter 6).

THE SITUATED CONTEXT

I would like to demonstrate a situated context that might apply to you and your colleagues. Let us begin with the personal and your probable context, the place you find yourself right now. Most likely, part of your context is that you are studying at the master's or doctoral level of nursing. I acknowledge here all the assumptions I am making, and this is not how I would conduct qualitative research, *I would instead want to know the authentic situated context of the participants in my study.* Actually, authors make all sorts of assumptions about readers (like I am doing); in fact, it is essential to ensuring that a book will be useful to its audience. Paradoxically, though, it does not always work out correctly because readers most often have had different experiences, *even if* they have been classmates for the past three years. *Most important, students are different from one another, learn differently, and remember what they value most, which varies from individual to individual.* I emphasize this more when we discuss right-sided and left-sided brain dominance; more and more brain research seems to bear out very different characteristics of each side of the brain.

In Chapter 6 on the phenomenological method, I argue that one needs to "be" phenomenological to conduct that kind of research. But as you can see, one might "be" qualitative in perspective when writing, speaking, and most importantly delivering nursing care, whether as faculty, administrator, or practitioner. Thinking qualitatively is thinking of holistic beings that cannot be understood by reducing them to parts; each has a distinct situated context that will influence the individual's subjective world, perspective, and use of language. Perhaps this stance can be summed up by Bohm (1985) as he discusses enfoldment: "Language is implicit in feelings and thoughts . . . and words . . . move towards mutual enfoldment. *Thoughts and feelings also enfold intentions*" (italics added, p. 16).

For instance, it was not my "intention" to digress from considering your situated context, but obviously I kept writing words and using language that was *in the moment* reflecting thoughts and feelings that led to an intention to discuss "thinking qualitatively" which I thought was important. Now I return to your situated context!

Your Situated Context

When you first started your undergraduate education, I imagine you were not aware that nurses conduct research. I wonder how many of you went into nursing to do research! If you had a sister or friend, you may have had advance knowledge, but for the most part you did not enter the profession of nursing to become a researcher. And here you are, most likely in a class studying research and perhaps preparing now to do research.

Surprise! Congratulations! Research is so exciting and rewarding when you contemplate the wondrous idea that something not known is going to be found out by you or by the group you are working with. You are actually going to be creating and contributing knowledge to the discipline of nursing. You have the opportunity to improve the quality of life for others, to prevent hardship, to liberate people, to further understanding of life's mysteries of experience . . . indeed these are tasks of no small consequence.

If you had entered a field such as physics or chemistry, you would have known at the outset that you were going to become a scientist and indeed that would have been your dream. You would have already developed a propensity for logic and the rationality of the scientific method. You would have had visions of yourself in a white lab coat with microscopes and measuring tools around you. This would have been a focused choice for you: a vision of yourself more grounded in the expectations of your chosen field. Yes, you might also teach as a scientist, but you also knew you would be doing research. This is a field you could enter if you wanted or indeed were excited about doing research.

How different, then, for you and your colleagues in nursing. You enter the nursing profession with visions very different from our physics and chemistry friends. For the most part, you're not aware that nurses do research, and when you happen to hear that you are required to take nursing research courses, you could not imagine what nurses research. So, the initial socialization of nurses, from the perception of others (guidance counselors, peers, parents), is that nursing usually does not include research.

In your class ask how many of your colleagues, when they said, "I am going to be a nurse," heard, "Oh, that is wonderful—perhaps you will become a nurse researcher!" What most incoming nursing students envision is caring for people in need. It is not trite to say that the reason I went into nursing is that *I wanted to help people.* I think most students picture a more hands-on profession, perhaps encouraged by the media. I don't recall any episodes of hospital dramas showing nurses going off to do research, or nurses announcing that they are ready to start a research project. Way back when I was younger, there was a book series about a nurse, Cherry Ames . . . she was many things, but never Cherry Ames: Nurse Researcher!

At the undergraduate level, when you were introduced to the reality of research in nursing, the standard research textbooks, which are larger than this one, included *perhaps* 1 chapter out of 30 on qualitative research.

A situated context had been created for you in which entering nursing students do not have awareness that research is a part of the nursing role. And then, when the research role is introduced, the scientific method of the natural sciences seems to be the method of choice for research. You have probably found that the most prevalent worldview, paradigm, or model for research in nursing is the scientific method.

A FLUKE

Now another fluke that makes nursing students different in regard to research is that most will not make a career in research, unlike the aforementioned physics and chemistry students. Few will ever be solely nurse researchers, and those who do research will share their time between other responsibilities, such as being a faculty member. Because of these differences, your educational preparation does not include the inherent faculty–student expectation of research mentorship, where research is often the primary goal of education, as it is in the natural sciences. This is also part of your situated context.

Yet, research has become one of the many goals of your nursing education. Nurse educators expect you to read, critique, and utilize nursing research, and indeed the quality and effectiveness of your practice depend on keeping abreast of the new knowledge in the field.

However, is it realistic to think that graduates of undergraduate schools can understand and critique research? Especially if it is presented in an advanced mathematical format, which the student has little preparation to understand? One course in research at the undergraduate level, not to mention statistics, usually conjures up confusing memories for most graduates. This I have observed many times, so it is not an assumption, so to speak! However, it does not apply to everyone (another point about assumptions, even if they appear well grounded).

You now find yourself in graduate school. You are finding research discussed and focused on in much greater depth. You are told that you are the future nurse researchers and are the ones who will make the changes necessary to address the critical problems that individuals at all developmental stages and throughout the health care delivery system present.

In this textbook, you will be introduced in much greater depth and detail to qualitative research, the philosophical underpinnings, methods, outcomes, and how critical this perspective of research is to our understanding of human experience. This book represents a continuing conversation on qualitative research, which started before 1987, the year in which the first edition of this book was published. The interest, growth, and recognition of the value of qualitative methods for nursing research are evident in the enlarging conversation, which has grown from an original 288 pages of the first edition to the 628 pages of this fourth edition. Today we have journals, conferences, and classes specifically focusing on qualitative research. The acceptance of qualitative research as legitimate in the discipline of nursing was not an easy task to accomplish, and even today some nurse researchers, journals, and granting agencies still place paramount importance on the scientific method and its worldview, even though I have argued often that they are not congruent with our philosophy (see Chapters 2 and 3). However, I do believe that the Scientific Method, with capital letters, has its place in nursing research, as I do believe Qualitative Research Methods have. They lead us to different places, ask different kinds of questions, and *together can provide a multifaceted view of human experience.*

BROADENING THE LANDSCAPE

You might wonder what characteristics of qualitative research are different from the scientific method (from this point on, the capital letters are removed to indicate it is just one more method to be used, not *the* method). We have mentioned a few, such as *not making assumptions, the concept of holism, the critical importance of the situated context,* and *the all-important worlds of subjectivity and intersubjectivity.*

The qualitative research perspective recognizes the influences of a dynamic reality rather than a static one with the following five points, as articulated by Beneloiel (1984). These five points will help you differentiate between the scientific method approach and qualitative approaches:

♦ Social life is the shared creativity of individuals and *their perceptions.*
♦ The character of the social world is *dynamic* and *changing.*
♦ There are *multiple realities* and frameworks for viewing the world: the world is *not* independent of humankind and *objectively identifiable.*
♦ Human beings are active agents who *construct their own realities.*
♦ *No response sets* are highly predictable. (italics added, p. 4)

Furthermore, in distinguishing between the two paradigms, it is important to understand that nursing is a human science. According to Dilthey (1926), the human sciences are to be distinguished from the natural sciences because of critical and fundamental differences in attitude toward their respective phenomena of research. Stated simply, the natural sciences investigate objects *from the outside to the inside,* whereas the human sciences depend on a perspective from *the inside to the outside.* The most important concern in the human sciences is that of *meaning.* Meaning exists within human subjectivity rather than in material nature. Thus, the aims of the two sciences are different. The natural sciences seek *causal explanation, prediction,* and *control.* The human sciences seek *understanding, interpretation,* and *meaning.*

Remember, this chapter is an introduction, and all these ideas are discussed in much greater detail as you go through the various chapters. In other words, if some of this sounds a bit foreign as far as research is concerned, it will be further clarified. However, for most of you, the preceding five characteristics will sound familiar because this is often how human beings are conceptualized in nursing philosophies and theories. You might wonder why it does not always follow into nursing research. It does, in qualitative nursing research, making much of nursing philosophy, theory, and research, philosophically and linguistically congruent.

So much difference goes unacknowledged as we try earnestly to create human laboratory systems untainted by the outside world. Then the human being must eventually return to the outside world, to the entire context and all the contingencies of his or her life. These are the concerns of the qualitative researcher:

♦ The meanings within context
♦ The interpretation of the individual person
♦ How a person narrates his or her own story
♦ How a self is socially constructed
♦ How truth is an interpretation

Truth arrived at by numbers is often held suspect by qualitative researchers because they worry about all the variables that were not factored into the equations. They also worry about how individual people interpret words differently and assign different values to numbers. Qualitative researchers have a different propensity and different worldview. Given the freedom to grow and develop in their methods, they can provide to the profession understanding, description, theory, interpretation, and direction concerned with the intricacy and interconnectedness of being in this world that is not one but many in perception; a world that is not one but many in language. One language has many languages within that language, as does one culture. Qualitative researchers search for the differences not only between cultures but also within cultures. They challenge stereotypes, presuppositions, and assumptions.

Qualitative researchers break new ground by *revealing what had been concealed* because they look beyond appearance. They provide the reconstruction that time demands of us, as the sands shift and the known is no longer valid. In their quest for discovery, qualitative researchers legitimate the existence of others in their differences. Conformity is not the object; we know that a universal concept of meaning is not possible and doubt that it is desirable.

Since publication of the first edition of this book (a relatively short period of time), nursing research has burgeoned. Doctoral programs for nursing, research journals, research conferences, and courses continue to expand. Research and the concomitant dissemination of results are required of faculty and are essential for promotion and tenure. You, as a graduate student, might write a research proposal; some of you will complete a master's theses; and, of course, a dissertation must be completed for the doctoral degree. A profession that was once housed in 3-year diploma schools affiliated with hospitals is now, 45 years later, ensconced in the university setting and has responsibly taken on the values of an academic profession.

One of the most important values in the academy is the search for truth. Broadly speaking, this search for truth is a search for new knowledge for the profession. One of the most remarkable changes since 1987 is what is sometimes called "the knowledge explosion," which is concurrent with the explosion of technology. Technology has enabled advances in the health sciences, changes in the health care system, and the rapid communication of knowledge moment to moment.

Today when we embark on a research project, we see a change more in how we believe something than in what we believe. There are shifts in belief about belief, questioning the idea of absolute truth and acknowledging the possibility of many truths (Anderson, 1995). Before the introduction of qualitative methods of research in nursing, the profession embraced the scientific method as the paradigm for nursing research. The reasons for this are discussed in Chapters 2 and 3 of this text. However, some nurse researchers had a bent, so to speak, to look for other ways of coming to know.

Other Disciplines' Methods

Other disciplines, other than the natural sciences, had methods that interested nurse researchers. For those pioneers of qualitative research in nursing, the rationale for their use was as strong and compelling as the use of a natural science method. As with most new ideas—and we need to remember that the pursuit of qualitative research was a new idea for nursing research—some conflict ensued. Professional legitimacy was seen as affiliation with the "hard" sciences. Linear progress, absolute truths, and rationality were all thought to be ideals for a science. Before nursing entered the academy, it was popular to say that nursing was an art and a science, but, once in the academy, the art component was subsumed and the science component was elevated for reasons that were socially constructed within the situated context. This social construction is explained in the beginning chapters of this book.

The Sands of Science

The sands of science itself are shifting as more and more scientists, including nurse scientists, realize that science cannot be a field of absolute and final truth but is an endeavor focused on illuminating an ever-changing body of ideas. For many, though, this focus is still not accepted and is considered a grievous loss; others find the shifting sands exhilarating and liberating. In 1987, few dissertations and publications indicated an acceptance of qualitative methods of inquiry in nursing. Ironically and unfortunately, in the year 2006, qualitative nurse researchers and quantitative nurse researchers, who often call themselves nurse scientists, do not garner the same prizes. In 2001, the National Institute of Nursing Research, a branch of the National Institutes of Health, mostly rewarded quantitative/scientific research proposals. Colleges of nursing pride themselves on establishing centers for nursing science or the science of nursing. Of course, a Center for Nursing Research would be more embracing, at least in name, of various approaches to the pursuit of knowledge. As you will read in this text, the situated context in which we live influences what we want to be "like" and how we wish to "appear" in the academic or medical setting. Qualitative research methods are indeed scientific in that they have their own paradigmatic philosophical underpinnings consistent with the qualitative worldview and methods that stay true to these beliefs and values. The evaluation strategies for qualitative research are real-world oriented, rather than mathematically determined, and are as rigorous as any for the scientific method.

From this perspective, qualitative methods are as scientific as quantitative methods; however, the capital S seems to belong to the Scientific Method. Qualitative researchers are indeed doing scientific research as the word *science* is generally understood.

I have yet to meet a qualitative nurse researcher who believes his or her method of doing research is the "only" and the most legitimate way of coming to know and advancing knowledge. I suppose this belief itself is reflective of the philosophical underpinnings of qualitative research methods so that it should not come as a surprise that here we see the difference about "how" we believe. Following are more concepts that characterize qualitative research:

♦ Multiplicity
♦ Simultaneity
♦ Perspectivity
♦ Polyvocality
♦ Multiple realities
♦ Individual and cultural social construction of reality

All lend themselves to a broader acceptance of the many and different ways of being in the world and, in this case, nursing research.

The Multistoried World

It would certainly be unfair to portray all nursing scientists based in the natural science method as unreceptive to qualitative nurse researchers, but it would also be unfair to have you as a student of nursing research not be aware of the dichotomy that persists within the field. I am very encouraged that, in spite of what some may view as the superiority of the scientific method, more and more nurse researchers change their whole view of research once they become acquainted with this alternative paradigm. Some have said that they have come home. They have found a home in *this world* of research.

Hence, the conversation enlarges and now includes you and your class.

Within the dialogue and within this text are many reasons to consider just how critical qualitative research methods are for a human science field, a profession dedicated to alleviating suffering and promoting well-being. The need for the scientific method is not in dispute here. In fact, it is celebrated for specific problems and questions. However, it is inappropriate for seeking answers and solutions to other problems and questions of equal if not greater significance to a human science.

Transitioning within a Postmodern World

Consider the world that we human beings inhabit at present. We have the breakdown of the "Enlightenment Period," discussed in Chapter 4, where there was the belief that there were rational explanations for all phenomena. Inherent in that belief is the idea that only one possible answer exists to any question or problem. In today's world, we are acknowledging the real influence of the local, the subjective, the meaning, the heterogeneity, the myriad of perceptions, the polyvocality, and the fact that we are overwhelmingly pluralistic and living multiple realities of experience, as mentioned earlier.

Science, with a capital S, fascinated us and was and still is an interesting story, *but it is only one story* to describe you and me and the world we inhabit. It is interesting to note that we discuss science in a somewhat dispassionate discourse, a statement of a discovery, a theory proved, a theory refuted, so to speak. And, though sometimes dispassionate, there are moments of passion when a cure for some terrible condition arrives and quality of life is improved. Ironically, many of these scientific discoveries are found by accident; while something else is being searched for, a serendipitous discovery is made. Thomas Kuhn (1970) in *The Structure of Scientific Revolutions* speaks of many discoveries as anomalies that lead to a new way of looking at a phenomenon. I think it is critical to read this work of Kuhn's, if you have not as yet. You will really understand the nature of science as a process, a changing one, and a changing one that is not always rational!

As nurses, though, we have much to contribute to understanding the multistoried world, the diversity and the plurality of the people who we serve through other methods of science, through qualitative methods. I have seen the excitement of students when they come upon these methods. A body of students reflects this multistoried world within their own individual situated contexts.

I would like to emphasize we are all blessedly pluralistic: students, faculty, patients, family, and the community. There is not one best answer and there is not one best way of doing research. For instance, because incoming nursing students are often not aware of the research component, when it is introduced students might separate into groups in which some seem mathematically inclined and the others seem linguistically inclined. It is imperative to sort that out, for ourselves and for our students.

Toward that end, our research endeavors become enlarged as we help to develop a multitalented group of students in their specific propensities. Because we have both the mathematically logic–minded and the linguistically/philosophically interpretive–inclined student, our potential is *magnified*, as is our field of understanding. Those who are linguistically, interpretive, and philosophically inclined need our encouragement to develop their talents and propensities in their research endeavors. No one way is superior to another. Students and faculty alike might have noticed that many students develop a dislike for research. Perhaps this dislike is because only one language is spoken and those students need to hear and learn the other languages of discovery.

There is growing support for the idea that the left or right side of an individual's brain is dominant. We need both sides to function in this world, just like we need a science to indicate the hard sciences associated with strict adherence to the scientific method, and we need a science associated with qualitative methods, which are indeed scientific but more multidimensional.

The Problem with Generalizations

In our practice we are exposed to languages, semiotics, and beliefs of different cultures. We need to have nurses and nurse researchers who hear the differences and who question generalizations. These are additional characteristics of qualitative research. We need to have researchers who will assist people in interpreting the meaning of different realities, personal subjective realities, so that we can approach individuals with the respect they deserve regarding their individual perceptions and how they are viewing what is occurring and not employ preconceived protocols that provide a general way to proceed, *even* if you do not know a person.

Let us distinguish again between someone who thinks from a quantitative paradigm and one who thinks from a qualitative paradigm in relation to the idea of a protocol. A protocol for patients with a specific condition is a prescription for action and process. As stated earlier, you may not know the patient, but you have the protocol with which to treat the person based on his or her diagnosis.

For most qualitative nurse researchers, the idea of a protocol without the emphasis on individual differences characteristic of qualitative research can be daunting. That is because qualitative researchers do not claim to generalize their findings—how could they when there is such emphasis on individual interpretation and subjectivity? Simply stated: one size or explanation cannot fit all! So protocols attempt to be a one-size or one-way approach to very complex conditions.

Sometimes following a protocol works; often it does not. When it does not, *instead of questioning* the protocol, often we assume there is something different about the patient and the result then *becomes a complication*. Of course, there is something *different*; generalizations made, for example, for wound healing cannot possibly take into account all the different variables in process for a particular person. Often it is said we cannot afford individualized care, so there must be protocols and procedures. I believe with the cost of complications that we cannot afford *not* to have individualized care. It is from the philosophical underpinnings of qualitative research and subsequent research that we come to see there are many truths and limitless possibilities to meet the differences that occur among our patients. We respect the person, and we respect that there are many truths and limitless possibilities.

Today there is an emphasis on *evidence-based practice*. We must realize that approximately every 5 years, new phrases call for the same response, have the same purpose, and mean very much the same. We have lived through an emphasis on theory-based practice, and this may be a good question for you to address with your class. What is the difference between theory-based practice and evidence-based practice? With theory-based practice, there was also a focus on developing taxonomies, nursing diagnoses, and interventions based on the diagnoses. The interventions came from accepted scientific practice or newly developed protocols based on the newest research. Whatever system you are using—today it is evidence-based practice—as an advanced practice nurse, faculty member, administrator, or researcher, you need to be particularly focused on meaning: meaning of what a person may be experiencing, how a person might behave, what meaning a person gives to health, and even "meaningless" information. If a person believes that your evidence-based practice is meaningless to him or her, that belief should become meaningful to you. It changes your approach to the person. A current example is what some believe to be occurring in the United States, and that is an obesity epidemic. We focus on all age groups but, for the sake of this example, consider do we have evidence-based practice means to reduce obesity in specifically adolescents? Without finding the *meaning* and *motivation* for why some adolescents may overeat, we may never understand this behavior and be able to design a means to change it.

A critical component that differentiates quantitative, scientific method–driven research from qualitative (scientific) methods is the unequivocal focus on meaning. Without knowing the meaning of a patient's behavior, the evidence-based intervention that in some samples did change behaviors in certain circumstances will undoubtedly be meaningless for others.

This happens in hospitals and other health care settings. If the patient does not follow the practice or intervention, then the patient is labeled noncompliant, a negative judgment against the patient. Measures will be taken against such noncompliance, and they also will be doomed until a qualitative approach into the meaning of events or behavior of the patient is carried out. And this qualitative approach is done to acknowledge the plurality, the diversity, and the different ways of being that most nursing philosophies subscribe to in their descriptions of a human being.

PERCEPTIONS

The patient undoubtedly has different perceptions of reality from those of the inventor of the intervention or what might have been deemed as evidence-based practice. I think I better say here that evidence-based practice is a great idea; how it is different from quality control, applying theory, diagnosis with interventions I am less clear about, but I certainly do not think that any practice should be performed without solid evidence. What I am saying is that *even with* solid evidence, one cannot expect it to be successful — if it is based on generalizations made from highly controlled research. This is a personal intuition that the evidence-based approach will be successful some of the time, hopefully most of the time, if we learn to *contextualize people's experiences* and *incorporate their individual perceptions* in its implementation.

Most of our practices in fact come from the perceptions of the *reality of the professional,* which is far removed from the interior of the experience and the interior meanings of the patients' behavior. This is where the qualitative researcher is at home. He or she, in whatever qualitative method used, is interested in the subjective experience and perception of the person.

Transition from an Information Age to a Conceptual Age

According to Pink (2005), we are currently moving from an information age to a conceptual age. The title of his book reflects the qualitative concept of holism: *A Whole New Mind: Moving from the Information Age to the*

Conceptual Age. His major thesis is the differences between left- and right-sided brain dominance for this coming conceptual age.

I think you might agree that as mentioned earlier some of us are more mathematically, logically inclined and others of us seem more linguistically inclined, perceptive, and more open to uncertainty than our math and hard science friends, who search for proof and certainty. Meanwhile, those who are inclined to look for meaning in perceptions and subjectivity learn early the meaning of uncertainty. The first looks for facts and truths, the latter looks for understanding and variation of truth or "what works" for whom.

Perhaps you might think the following quote is too simplistic. I agree, but let it stand for the sake of simplicity in explanation. In Pink's (2005) own words: "The left hemisphere is sequential, logical and analytical. . . . The right side of the brain is nonlinear, intuitive and holistic" (p. 3).

Pink reassures us that we are using both sides of the brain, and that this is presented as a metaphor. Yet the demands of the information age require left-sided brain work, in which some of us are more gifted. And if it is the case that we are moving away from the information age to a conceptual age, we are going to need to use our right-sided brain capacities to a much greater extent.

One can posit from the greater descriptions in Pink's thesis (which is not unlike Goleman's *Emotional Intelligence* [1997]) that there is bound to be greater recognition and demand for qualitative research in nursing, *if holism, intuition, and nonlinear thinking are at the forefront in the creation of new knowledge and ways of being.* We are moving away from a society built solely on logical, linear, and computer-like capabilities to one that will also incorporate *creators, empathizers, pattern recognizers,* and *perhaps most important of all "meaning makers."*

I would like to list a few of Pink's ideas to perhaps whet your appetite to read his book if you have not already. Additionally, these ideas are foundational to the need for qualitative research and inherent in the methods as well. You will find these ideas in many chapters of this book. I include them here because Pink never mentions once in his book that we need more qualitative research because his is not a research-promoting book. However, his predictions lead to that path and make qualitative research essential to this conceptual age.

A whole new mind: moving from the information age to the conceptual age (following are just a few of Pink's observations peppered with my own):

♦ The last few decades have belonged to number crunchers, contract people, rules-based medicine, and the future will depend on creators and empathizers, pattern recognizers, and meaning makers.

♦ We are moving away from a society built on the logical, linear, and computer-like capabilities of the information age to one that is inventive, empathic, and has big-picture capabilities . . . the conceptual age.

♦ For more than a century, society has been dominated by thought that is mostly narrowly reductive and deeply analytical . . . the knowledge worker, manipulator of information.

♦ We are moving to high concept and high touch . . . crafting a satisfying narrative, combine seemingly unrelated ideas into something new, and pursuing purpose and meaning.

♦ The left side of brain: sequential, logical, and analytical, whereas the right side is nonlinear, intuitive, holistic, and can interpret things simultaneously such as faces and words, specializes in context such as how something is said, can comprehend metaphors, synthesizes and is particularly good at putting isolated elements together to perceive things as a whole: a Gestalt perception.

♦ The left hemisphere knows how to handle logic, and the right hemisphere knows about the world. Put the two together and one gets a powerful thinking machine. Use either on its own, and the result can be bizarre or absurd (p. 18).

♦ Right-directed thinking: simultaneous, metaphorical, aesthetic, contextual and capable of synthesis; exemplified by *caregivers* and most often *neglected in schools* (italics added).

In Chapter 3 of Pink's book is something very important to our task: In 2000, Paul Ray and Sherry Ruth Anderson identified a subculture of 50 million Americans that they dubbed "cultural creatives." Right-directed thinking cultural creatives "insist on seeing the big picture." They are good at synthesizing. They "see women's ways of knowing as valid: feeling empathy and sympathy for others, taking the viewpoint of the one who speaks, seeing personal experiences and first-person stories as important ways of learning and embracing an ethic of caring." (Ray and Anderson)

Patients tell their signs and symptoms in narratives. We need to listen to the patient's story from the patient's point of view in order to understand the context and the patient's meaning. We need to hear and feel:

♦ Multiple realities—symphony, creativity

♦ The big picture, integrating relationships, the embeddedness of context, appreciating the unfolding of experience

♦ Empathy—the ability to imagine yourself in someone else's position and to intuit what that person is feeling. Feeling *with* someone while understanding the importance of context

This is not to say, of course, that our left-brain colleagues—and you might be one of them—do not have enough to keep you busy in research but it is to say that perhaps now more than ever we need to honor and respect those individuals whose right brain dominance, which in science, has been not celebrated in our society and yet is capable of providing meaning just when a society seems to be *starving for meaning*. The meaning they will seek, for the purpose of this book, will be human understanding, and include the meaning of perceptions and experience, the living of meaning in specific cultures and subcultures, creating meaning by giving individuals a role in research thereby emancipating some from the dominance of the researcher, meaning that will help us create grounded theories, and theories from the experience, not of the researcher, thus creating a person-oriented narrative, one of holism and not of parts (still necessary, though, for natural science research).

To do qualitative research well, you need the capacity to see some of the world as confusing, not orderly, and that which cannot be forced into order. You must be able to be intuitive and to interpret many variables simultaneously in your head (using the computer that is there, not the one on your desk)!

Talking with people and listening to people sound so simple, yet they are the critical domains of the qualitative researcher. However, listening is an art, and qualitative researchers have their own rules for listening and collecting material for research. We listen "unknowingly," as described in Chapter 6, in our approach, and let individuals tell us their interpretation, the meaning they ascribe to an experience, culture, or research activity. We need to listen with empathy, comprehend metaphors, synthesize material, and place all within specific contexts.

To use the previous example of an obesity study, imagine taking away food from a lonely child who eats for comfort. What might happen next? Without qualitative research methods to contextualize what might not work, we cannot devise other alternatives specific to all the variations that occur in individual lives. From a health care professional's perspective, a person with diabetes who is not taking the prescribed medication is simply not cooperating. However, there could be many reasons for a patient's so-called noncooperation. I have often found the word noncompliant ascribed to the uncooperative patient as offensive. It is a *punitive*, mechanistic term that does not go further to explore the possible reasons that patients may have for not "following orders." Once labeled as such, there is closure.

Some might argue we cannot do research for such individuals. Ethically, I find that argument unacceptable. I believe one of the most urgent areas for qualitative research is to listen to the narratives of individuals who actually *may be in despair, who may have given up, or who do not have access,* or a synthesis of all three.

OUR BRAINS LIGHT UP!

I wonder what you are thinking right now. Perhaps you might be thinking I am dichotomizing. I must interpret this and explain that I am simplifying. I do want you to know that I believe that the left and right hemispheres of our brains, although they might light up to differing degrees on brain scans when engaging in these kinds of thinking patterns, work together and compose an integrated, whole, complete brain. We are fortunate to have access to this whole, and both hemispheres are essential.

I would like to go back to an earlier point, when I suggested that the traits associated with the left side of the brain have dominated research and education. I do think, however, that university curricula need to acknowledge the bent or even exclusivity of left-brain training in the sciences, including nursing, so that qualitative researchers who have the contrasting right-sided brain dominant traits can then be given the education and knowledge they need.

Is it not true for most of you, especially if you are doctoral students, that you are required to take courses that support quantitative research? You do need to be exposed to the tenants of quantitative research so that you will understand its merits and shortcomings. A graduate course in quantitative methods for those interested in qualitative research is still essential. But does it have to be in such detail, as though you are going to carry out scientific method research in your career? Add to that at least two statistics courses at the graduate level, after you most likely had one at the undergraduate level. How much do you retain from these courses if you don't practice using quantitative methods? These courses consume credits that you must pay for and use up your study time instead of the very critical courses you need if you are to pursue a qualitative research trajectory. Let me suggest the courses that you need.

My belief goes back to where your orientation and talents lie, whether you appear to be more left-sided or right-sided brain dominant. Does everyone entering graduate school need a brain scan? They might need their heads examined but not a brain scan! (Humor is right-sided and not to be dismissed, which will be discussed shortly.) Actually, students can self-identify their talents quite accurately. What I find sad is that those who are not left-sided brain dominant, because of our cultural values, criticize themselves, "I am not good at math," "I am not good at test taking," and so forth. I have yet to hear left-sided brain dominant people saying, "I am not good at empathy," "I lack a sense of humor," and so on.

No, you do not need a brain scan; you already know your propensities. Math, linear thinking, positivism, rationality, statistical models, objectivity, and a clear method to follow—if that is you, you clearly have a left brain dominance and may have been favored in the current culture of academia.

In this book, I hope you gain greater awareness after reading Pink's (2005) descriptions of how left-sided individuals gain and keep power and how they have the decided advantage in our current culture. I hope that Pink's forecast that we are moving from an information age to a conceptual age does come to be because it will be a great equalizer.

Now if you have a propensity for creativity, nonlinear thinking, seeing that life is not easily explainable through all things measurable (in fact some things cannot be measured) and you value subjectivity and intersubjectivity, appreciate the characteristics mentioned regarding postmodernism, are more linguistically inclined, and appreciate the value of a story or narrative, *your academic curriculum most likely fell short in developing these characteristics of yours*. However, if you do have these propensities, qualitative research is for you.

This is especially true in all areas of nursing. There has always been a "no margin for error" ethos in nursing, which indeed would favor the scientific method and evidence-based nursing. However, some have pointed out that actually the results of these studies apply only to a majority of people (and then the sample of people have to be hammered into similarities). So a margin for error always exists, and it might be a lot larger than we care to acknowledge. Today, in a hospital, most of us are alarmed at the errors committed there, and there are most likely many more errors because many vulnerable people are fending for themselves and errors often go unreported. How many of us have heard "a hospital is a dangerous place to go" and the advice that patients should bring a friend or advocate, write everything down, and question everything (which, if you do, labels you as "difficult"). The "no margin for error" ethos used to support quantitative research cannot really be substantiated.

THE LANDSCAPE NEEDS A CURRICULUM CHANGE; UNTIL THEN . . .

We are free to develop a research curriculum specifically designed for the qualitative researcher. First, an overview class such as the one you might be taking with this textbook is required. Then there would be a philosophical course that speaks to meaning, today's postmodern context in thinking about the world, and a course on interviewing, listening, attending to cues, and understanding human beings in situations who are part of a qualitative study. Following would be a course in interpretation and narrative: whose interpretation to use, how does one interpret, what is interpretation based on, and how does one write a qualitative narrative. Statistics may be the definitive approach of quantitative research, but words and narrative are the definitive means to communicate in qualitative research.

I think Max van Manen, who has devoted much of his academic life to qualitative research, has done more than any other qualitative researcher to emphasize the critical component of writing. His latest book *Writing in the Dark* (van Manen, 2002) includes 10 researcher examples of excellent phenomenological writing. van Manen himself provides the reader with a heartfelt intimate understanding of the difficulties and challenges of writing. Writing in this particular manner would definitely be another course.

I include this here because I believe it is critical. Qualitative nurse researchers are shortchanged when it comes to conducting their research. Until there is a curriculum change, reading a book or taking a course just does not do it (more on this in Chapter 6). I recommend, if you are about to pursue qualitative research, that you read philosophy books pertaining to meaning, subjectivity, phenomenology (even if that is not your particular method, most methods depend critically on understanding this philosophy), existentialism, interviewing within the qualitative domain, interpretation (hermeneutics), and I also urge you to "become" phenomenological, become "qualitative," "be" phenomenological, because it is a way of being and even if the contributing authors in this text might not think of themselves in this way, it comes through in their wonderful writings. The search for understanding and meaning undergirds all qualitative methods. Some qualitative methods do have different aims, yet understanding and meaning assist them in meeting those aims.

What I am suggesting to you if this is to be your path is to prepare yourself intellectually for a new way of thinking, a new "how" you think. Sitting quietly and thinking without an agenda can lead to striking insights. You will need such time. You will also need patience. Unlike statistics, with the computer programs today, that can give you almost instant answers, you need patience to be still with your qualitative material (data) so that there is a "sense"-making and "meaning"-making period of conscious and unconscious thinking. Often, writing in a free-form way without concern for sentence structure or grammar can assist in this activity.

A CAUTIONARY TALE

Many activities we see in qualitative research studies actually evolve from the quest to appear scientific with the capital S. Usually, they can be quickly identified, such as lists of themes with frequencies and lists of words used with frequencies. The caution here is not that these activities are not part of the process, but they must be accompanied with the variation of meanings. For example, when I say I have experienced anxiety over an event and someone else says she has as well, there is no way for a researcher to know anything more than that two people *used the same word in a description*. A qualitative researcher must explore the meaning and manifestations of what the perception of anxiety was to a particular person. Sometimes, for the sake of efficiency in communicating results, tables accomplish that; I certainly use tables when writing space is limited. But qualitative researchers should be careful that their reports are not numerical (can be part of the overall results) but are interpretive and written mostly as narrative.

THE POWER AND SIGNIFICANCE OF QUALITATIVE RESEARCH

Qualitative research has not been long accepted in nursing, as has been discussed; however, the progress has been astounding. Science always seemed to be the goal, and it has been a long road for most nurse scholars to recognize the importance of qualitative research, which is also scientific in that there are as many, if not more, qualifications and characteristics to ascertain in effective and well-done qualitative research.

When qualitative research was first introduced into the field of nursing, many students erroneously thought that doing qualitative research might be easier and more manageable, especially for those who were more right-sided brain dominant. And for them, it would be easier only because they had the capacities. However, those who wanted "to finish as soon as possible" and mistakenly decided to do a qualitative study would think quite differently in retrospect. It is definitely not a contest in difficulty but should be a choice of *intellectual fit*. The difficulty of one or the other research method has more to do with one's propensity for the different ways of being, and those ways need to be considered paramount to choice.

Some of those unfortunate students who wanted to finish as soon as possible found themselves in the world of uncertainty, multiple interpretations, and mountains of interview notes or transcripts. Today, reflecting on your own best talents is the way to choose your method, and I hope that more faculty will develop the curriculum you need.

We used to say, and perhaps still do, that your method should be determined by your question. From more than 24 years of working with students on dissertations, I can see how some students seem natural doing either quantitative or qualitative research. The latest brain research supports why this is so. Today I would advise you to start your research project with reflection on where your talents lie and capacities are at their best. Your research interests can be studied from many perspectives, so choose the one that flows from the "how" you think, your worldview, your propensities, that is, what you do best!

Those who know they are definitely going be *quantitative* researchers need to understand this alternative worldview and how their qualitative colleagues will approach objectivity and subjectivity, for instance. It makes for rich conversations and understanding of one another's work because both worldviews are equally essential to nursing research.

Earlier I mentioned how the conversation on qualitative research expands with each new edition. One critical question I want to discuss here (and in Chapter 6) is the question of the significance of qualitative research. (Morse [2004a] also brings up this concept in an editorial.)

Let me digress with a short but true story. In 1996, Michael Crotty (1996), a professor from Australia, now deceased, wrote a book entitled *Phenomenology and Nursing Research*. His major contention after reviewing 30 pieces of published nursing research was that North American nurse researchers were missing the intent, in this case, of phenomenological research. In fact, if they wanted to continue in the direction they were going he believed, they should call their work the "new" phenomenology because it certainly did not follow, from his perspective, the original intention of phenomenology.

I, like most nurse researchers at first, thought it was an unnecessarily harsh indictment of a safe group to critique (after all they were half way around the world), and my first reaction was one of defensiveness. After all, who is he? Does he realize how early we are in our development? Does he realize how phenomenology made it through the academy? As discussed in Chapters 2 and 3, nurses were following methods mostly developed by psychologists, who were trying their best to "fit" phenomenology into the rigorous scientific model. Perhaps it was not the best way, but it accomplished their goals, and we have these psychologists to thank for bringing us to this point.

After the dust settled and I went back and studied Crotty's argument more closely, I *began to understand* that his critique could assist us in furthering our endeavors. This, of course, is what a good critique does (though I still believe he was overly harsh, and I cannot tell you how thankful I was that he had not reviewed one of my studies)! Perhaps because I did not feel personally attacked, it was easier for me to take in a very critical element that we were not including in our phenomenological studies, which has to do with his assertion: "The goal of phenomenological inquiry goes beyond identifying, appreciating and explaining current and shared meanings. It seeks to *critique* these meanings" (p. 5, italics added).

He goes on to quote Halton's claim that pragmatism "speaks to the contemporary hunger for *significance*" (p. 13, italics added). I don't think it is necessary in this context to discuss the merits or demerits of pragmatism other than that our work, within this definition, *should indeed have significance.* It is absolutely essential, it is self-evident. In quite simple terms, the litmus test for all our research, *quantitative* or *qualitative*, is the answer to the question, "So what?"

In nursing, a profession concerned with the well-being of humankind, the question of "So what?" should be of utmost concern in our research. In nursing, a profession in which we want to improve the quality of life of individuals, this same question is essential to ask about the outcome of our research.

Part of Crotty's (1996) critique influenced my attempts of planning to do phenomenology. Originally, I called the last part of the study "Writing a Narrative on the Meaning of Your Study," where, among other items, I asked the researcher to *"critique this interpretation with implications and recommendations for political, social, cultural, health care, family, and other social systems"* (Munhall, 2001, p. 133). This was what Crotty said was missing from many of our studies. Simply describing the meaning of experience fails to call it into question, and he went on to say: "it perpetuates traditional meanings and reinforces current understandings" (Crotty, 1996, p. 7).

I found it interesting and relevant to all qualitative and quantitative studies. The research reports "what is" and "not what might be." Whichever method one chooses to use, the preceding italicized component should be included. In many of our research studies today we do point the way for future research on the phenomenon, but perhaps we could go farther and suggest what might be done within the significance of our own study.

For a long time in qualitative research existed a belief among many researchers that interpreting and telling the story of experience were enough. If you read a research report that demonstrated an obvious need for change, it was not necessarily the researcher's obligation to suggest the change. If the researcher began to suggest changes, he or she enters a different territory. So much of qualitative research was considered the *report of understanding what was going on* with the belief that once that was known, action would be taken. Perhaps that has validity. For example, media reports describing and interpreting natural disasters in a journalistic way accomplish just that: report the disaster, and human and financial resources *should* flow to the area.

Some qualitative researchers might say after completing a research report, "Need I say more?" For instance, Sylvie Tourigny's 1998 article "Some New Dying Trick" on African American youths in Detroit revealed that in certain desperate circumstances adolescents are intentionally and deliberately contracting acquired immune deficiency syndrome (AIDS). After reading the research report, I must admit I saw no reason for Dr. Tourigny to then write a critique of the breakdown of our social system—I thought the research or health care system spoke for itself. However, research has always had as a benchmark significance. It is fairly easy in quantitative research: either you achieve statistical significance or you do not.

I think it is essential, as Crotty suggests, that we heed the initial aim of phenomenology, which is a *social critique* with an imperative for improving the social fabric of human life. Let's return to the main idea of a critique following, in this instance, Tourigny's research. What is the responsibility of the researcher when he or she discovers such critical findings with implications that should be heeded immediately. Writing as critique can take the form of articles or reports specifically addressed to those that can make change. This same kind of research resulted in a film (by nonnurses), which is to be discussed later in this chapter.

Often our studies remain in our own nursing domain instead of being communicated to the wider public domain. The critique then may not necessarily be one of the breakdown of the social order, as was previously mentioned; it might take the form of making sure that such important findings find their way into the hands of policymakers and the public. The question of this responsibility is the next subject to be discussed. Responsibility might be different for qualitative researchers than quantitative researchers for different studies.

THE QUESTION OF DISSEMINATION

Returning to the idea that when most of us entered nursing we were not aware that nurses did research, we can safely assume that the public was not aware that part of nursing is to conduct research. Nursing research is to this day a largely underground activity where nurses report their research to other nurses. While this is critical, it is not enough to fully realize the power of qualitative research.

Among the public are policymakers in health care, politicians that influence health care practices and spending, health care institution administrators who may not be nurses, other health care practitioners such as physicians, nutritionists, physical therapists, and occupational therapists. The public also includes the entire population, which has health care needs, including needs for information and education, problem solving, and questions answered.

Some nursing research has gone beyond the field of nursing and has reached policymakers and the public's attention. Sometimes, when I am reading the *New York Times*, I come across a research report that mentions research by Dr. so-and-so of New York University, and I remember her from graduate school when we were both studying for our master's degrees in nursing. Although this is good for the public that our findings are being disseminated, many readers will think the researcher is a medical doctor. Placing the *Dr.* in front of names often infers to the public, "MD", especially because the public is largely unaware that nurses do research. One way to avoid this is for nurse researchers to request that the credential *Nurse Researcher* be inserted after their names. *The most important issue here is that we are not communicating our research to the public.*

Qualitative research narratives and reports are very readable, if done well and directed to the audience. They can generate interest in the subject matter of human experience, culture, ways to emancipate oneself, and ways to know about different ways of being.

The September 25, 2005, *New York Times Sunday Magazine* (Dideon, 2005a) featured a piece on Joan Dideon's response to finding her husband collapsed at their dining room table and shortly thereafter transported to a nearby hospital. A few Sundays later came a review of her book *The Year of Magical Thinking* (Dideon, 2005b). The writing is stunning; her introspection and interpretation of her experience are brilliantly described—and all from a qualitative perspective, from the subject's perspective with her own authentic perceptions of the experience of grief.

Nurses assist individuals in the experience of grief. This is a critical area where qualitative nurses could conduct research (and they actually have) *and also* present the outcome of their studies to the public. They could write articles for lay magazines. They could write books for the public. From my perspective, these activities are critical components of critique that Crotti (1996) was discussing, also critical components of what our research should be most concerned about: improving the quality of life of human beings. In the Dideon example, many people have commented on her piece, expressing how the article resonated with their own experience of grief. *They felt understood.* This bears repeating. *They felt understood.* Feeling understood seems to be so much more important than most people realize, and in fact it may be one of the most important desires and wants of human beings, the need to be understood by others.

Qualitative research's focus on human understanding of experience, culture, illness, birth, and death highlights another difference from quantitative research in nursing. Many quantitative research findings are also important to the public and policymakers and need to be communicated when appropriate. However, much of quantitative research in nursing belongs in nursing journals, especially when it has to do with providing evidence for nursing practice or has implications for changing procedures or protocols for patients. In other words, when quantitative studies appear in journals, the communication is most often to the right audience: the nursing community and the nurses who are policymakers can implement the called-for changes once the studies have been replicated to ensure the findings are valid, reliable, and needed.

On the other hand, qualitative research findings often belong not only to nurses but to a wider audience. The implications of qualitative studies must be broadly disseminated to the public, physicians, educators, public health policymakers, and the media. And it cannot wait.

DIFFERENT ROADS TO DISSEMINATION

Recently, this announcement came to me from a psychoanalytic message service:

> **SEX & DEATH IN THE AGE OF AIDS: A Screening of "The Gift,"** a Documentary Film by Louise Hogarth and a Discussion with Dr. Mark Blechner, Dr. Jack Drescher, and Dr. Perry Halkitis
>
> As many men in the community become condom weary, and some even consciously desire HIV infection, disturbing new trends of risky behavior have pushed the rate of new infections back into a rapid rise, all to the mantra of "Don't Ask, Don't Tell." Using Internet sites for promotion and connection, a community of barebackers (those who have sex without a condom) is flourishing. This includes bug chasers who host conversion parties where men actively seek the gift of HIV infection.
>
> Doug, a central character of the film, is a bright, articulate young man who moved from the Midwest to San Francisco in search of a gay community. He became a bug chaser and actively sought the gift of HIV infection. When Doug became infected with the virus, he felt a sense of belonging to a community. He is now dealing with the unexpected severity of his illness.
>
> Also featured in the documentary is noted psychoanalyst and community activist Walt Odets, MD, author of *In the Shadow of the Epidemic*. Dr. Odets examines the loss, grief and anxiety experienced by HIV negative men living with the AIDS epidemic, and he speaks out about why prevention has failed and what needs to be done.
>
> It is the filmmakers' hope that *The Gift* will create dialogue within the community and raise awareness of the issues of isolation and

division in the gay community around HIV status, thereby leading to a renewed prevention effort.

So the question now becomes, "How come this is not happening, this dissemination to the public and beyond, with qualitative research findings from nursing?" I include the preceding announcement as an example of what could have resulted from Tourigny's study, discussed earlier. It could have become, and should have become, a documentary or a report to the press. Many qualitative nurse researchers are very talented writers of the experiential nature of being alive and what the experiences of living are all about. We must take it the next step: dissemination, publications, and documentaries to the public.

Here is the hitch, though. Most of nursing research today is being done by nursing faculty. This situation can be likened to the situated context or contingencies of a person's life, which are discussed in many chapters in this book. Nursing faculty do research, many because they love research, and because it is required for promotion, retention, and tenure. In the quantitative way of thinking or the left-brain dominance of the academy, candidates for promotion, retention, and tenure are evaluated on the number of research articles published in peer-reviewed journals. There is a *discounting of articles published in lay magazines*, which are often considered unworthy for tenure consideration.

Ironically, other fields of science are happy to report research findings on diet, health, exercise, various diseases, and so forth to the reading public. The reading public is a critical audience to reach if researchers want their research to make a difference in understanding various subjects. Hopefully, this valuing of only peer-reviewed journals will come in step with valuing what the public reads. Also what the public reads is not always presented in a scholarly fashion, and so is dismissed as unscholarly. Does *unscholarly* mean that people are able to read it comfortably without a dictionary next to them and understand the message?

My intent in this introductory chapter is to present an overview of qualitative research in nursing in language that the beginning qualitative research student can understand. A second intention correlates with qualitative research and is inherent to qualitative methods, the situated context. Qualitative researchers observe the complexity of the world and pay attention to the influences of the time, place, and contingencies in the environment and do not reduce the environment to variables that are proposed to be measurable and not contaminated by—what else can I call it?—the "situation" the person finds himself or herself in. They find themselves in a "situation" that needs changing, and they need to publicize it.

Changing Rules for Publication and Presentation

In addition to changing the research curriculum for qualitative researchers, the rules for publication need to be scrutinized. Perhaps all nursing research, but in particular qualitative research, needs to be rewarded and counted equally whether it is published in lay publications or scientific journals.

Tenure review committees are aware of the gold standard journals, but in all fairness because some are published only four times a year, space is limited and it is very difficult to be published in the gold standard journals. Furthermore, you could debate some of the practices of the gold standard journals, especially when it comes to publishing qualitative research reports. Having been on many editorial review boards, I can recall hearing remarks similar to the following, "We need at least one qualitative research report in each issue," said not because the board valued such research but rather so the journal will not be accused of bias toward qualitative research.

In 2006, the qualitative research narrative continues, and we have much to discuss and understand. Most of all, we have potential, the potential to truly humanize the profession of nursing and increase the well-being of people and the spirit of caring. Specifically, this is our time to understand our patients and the public.

Today, many different approaches are available for nurse researchers who use qualitative research methods. Today, there is a much greater acceptance of qualitative research in nursing than there was 25 years ago, when the scientific method was the only one used. However, the quantitative paradigm for research is still paramount to many nurse researchers and educators. Recently, I picked up a fifth edition of an introductory research textbook for nurses published in 2004 and did not find even *one* chapter on qualitative research, nor was there an entry in the index for qualitative research. It is a good quality textbook, but without further study the reader would graduate not knowing about an alternative worldview to positivism and perhaps without an essential respect for subjectivity. *Embracing another's subjectivity is the critical activity for compassionate nursing practice.*

This type of conceptualizing, where the scientific method assumes superiority or is "the only way" of doing research, perpetuates an unnecessary dichotomy. Nurse researchers to this day still delineate nursing research in a way that places them in opposition rather than in a complementary position. The *combination* of qualitative and quantitative research methods, the use of both paradigms, is very powerful. We have all these methods available to us, and we should celebrate not the methods, but good research that comes from either paradigm or both. Good research with significance for human beings is our aim, not claiming that good research with significance can come from only one paradigm.

Let us encourage and reward those researchers who are more linguistically inclined. There are those of us who believe that language constitutes reality, instead of reflecting reality. How important it is, then, to ensure that these researchers are rewarded in their search to seek knowledge of others in their worlds and in their language and to understand how others negotiate their own meanings.

Part of the intrigue of qualitative research is understanding a "newness," a very different negotiation of meaning. What I value about qualitative research is that I am constantly amazed about and awakened to new ways of being. I find that through the beginning stance of qualitative research, the "unknowing" stance, often what I "knew" cannot be substantiated, that preconceptions are often biased, that assumptions have nothing but myth or prejudice upholding them, and that practice thought scientific is just ordinary tradition without evidence to support the practice.

Qualitative research methods have the potential to free us from erroneous preconceptions, raise our consciousness, encourage emancipation, and even lift us from oppression. How can I communicate how critical qualitative research is when it has all this potential? Here, my own language fails me. A paradigm that searches for meaning from the perspective of the individual or searches for what can give meaning to an experience sometimes defies description. It is almost ethereal, while maintaining the rigor of science.

Qualitative nurse researchers return the following through their research to practice, among many other things:

- ✦ Caring for the individual
- ✦ Legitimization
- ✦ Understanding of experience
- ✦ Acceptance
- ✦ Change
- ✦ Emancipation
- ✦ Compassion
- ✦ Understanding of meaning, whether experiential or spiritual
- ✦ Empathy

Qualitative nurse researchers want to provide the following to the knowledge base of nursing, among other things:

- ✦ Discovery
- ✦ Description

- ◆ Explanation
- ◆ Interpretation
- ◆ Critique
- ◆ Understanding
- ◆ Sensitization
- ◆ The meaning of being within and among various cultures, genders, and religions
- ◆ Grounded theory
- ◆ Direction toward improving the quality of life for all people

The work of qualitative nurse researchers offers to us, through the interpretation of meaning and experience, as well as the critique of the researcher's own methods, an expanding and wakeful consciousness of others and the self.

I would suggest to you, that after you read each exemplar of a specific method in this text, as well as other qualitative research reports, you ask yourself, "What did this qualitative study result in?" Here, I do not mean for you to specify the specific results, but to decide whether there was an increase in understanding, a different way of perceiving an experience unknown to you prior to reading the study, a critique of an accepted practice, and/or an interpretation of experience otherwise not known to you.

READING THIS BOOK

I would like to assist you in understanding the format of this book and also how you might return to earlier editions for additional exemplars and interpretations of various methods. My primary wish is that you will *actually enjoy* this book. You will find the studies fascinating. The content-oriented chapters you will find informative and understandable. Since the advent of qualitative research, the 5 or 6 most common qualitative methods have expanded to probably 15 different variations.

This text is primarily a qualitative research text and therefore presents the most accepted and used methods within the field of qualitative research. The expanded methods often are variations of these fundamental methods. As with all learning, understanding the foundations is critical to any expanded conceptualization of a method.

This text is divided into three major sections. Part I is incredibly important to read and to understand because it explains what may be for many of you a brand new worldview or paradigm. The chapters in this section present the situated context of qualitative research. This introductory chapter attempts to situate qualitative research in nursing in its current place in the nursing research world. It touches on many topics discussed later in this text and also at conferences and in nursing research periodicals.

Chapter 2, "Language and Nursing Research: The Evolution," introduces you to the journey that nurse researchers have traveled to arrive at the embrace of qualitative research. The chapter presents essential content to understand the differences between looking at the world from an objective, perhaps scientific method way of believing knowledge and the more subjective, perhaps philosophical perspectives associated with qualitative research. We also look at these two worldviews as they also occur in other disciplines.

Chapter 3 focuses on epistemology, furthering our growing knowledge of the philosophical underpinnings of qualitative research. I used Pink's (2005) recent book as an important reference. When I read Chapter 3 and see how closely Pink's six essential aptitudes necessary for the upcoming conceptual age are attuned to Paterson and Zderad's (1976) concepts identified as critical to nursing practice, I can see a full circle. In 1976, Paterson and Zderad focused on the following definition of nursing, which is so phenomenological: the act of nursing is "the intersubjective transactional relation, a dialogue experience, lived in concert between persons where comfort and nurturance produce mutual human unfolding" (p. 51). As Pink suggests, we then marched into the information age. Pink (2005) proposes six essential aptitudes we need to ensure success in the coming conceptual age: design, story, symphony, empathy, play, and meaning. Looking back, Paterson and Zderad placed great emphasis on comfort, nurturance, clinical presence, empathy, and all-at-once awareness (what Pink might call symphony).

Also within Paterson and Zderad's definition we see the emphasis on intersubjectivity as further emphasized in Chapter 6, and we also realize the importance that David Bohms (1985) discusses in *Unfolding Meaning*. These two women were certainly philosophically inclined, humanistic and futuristic. Nursing has many definitions, as you will read in Chapter 2. Paterson and Zderad is still my favorite!

Chapter 4, "Historical and Philosophical Foundations of Qualitative Research" by Marcia Dombro is a feat in its own right. Marcia goes back to Parmenides in 515 BC and researches the philosophical path from then until now. What has been missing in most research textbooks (including past editions of this text) is this kind of background description of idea progression. Often we hear people speak and write as though nothing came before them and their ideas! This is also accompanied by the idea that only the latest references have validity. From this perspective, this chapter is wonderful to read. It is not ponderous and enables us to experience the humility essential to knowing that we indeed stand on other's shoulders. Marcia also provides us the meanings of words we read or use regularly and often forget, such as *emic* and *etic*.

Marcia's chapter gives perspective to Chapter 5, "Reflections on Post-modernism, Critical Social Theory, and Feminist Approaches" by Lynne Dunphy and Joy Longo. Both Chapter 4 and Chapter 5 are new to this edition and provide a much-appreciated addition of depth and breadth to the philosophical understanding of qualitative research methods. Lynne and Joy chose these three schools of thought to add to our understanding of what other kinds of influences are in process within our qualitative research endeavors. Today's period is often referred to as the postmodern period, or is sometimes called postpositivist or poststructualist. It is critical to understand what beliefs and values this period represents as our situated context. Discussion moves to critical social theory, which can be used as a method on its own, can be an underpinning of some types of action research methods, and/or can spur us to a critical introspective look at specific ideologies. It is important to qualitative research in that it also values subjectivity and rejects restricting ideologies that could potentially limit freedom. The chapter ends with a section on how feminist approaches are a part of our situated context, or the postmodern period. We learn here about the "social construction of roles," a critical idea for almost all of our social behavior, beliefs, and values. We can ask where our attitudes, beliefs, and values come from and answer from our socialization. But that is not enough. What is critical to understand is that so much of it is *socially constructed*, usually to benefit someone or some group.

Part I of this volume in essence provides the history, the situated context, the language, the rationale, the philosophies, the epistemologies, and some of the theories that will assist you in understanding Part II, the section comprising qualitative methods and exemplars.

Having a firm grasp on Part I will enable you to understand the various processes of methods and also the actual research in Part II. Part III provides you with information and descriptions that you must either do or take into consideration for your research to be ethical and meet evaluation criteria. Part III also includes the resources (Chapter 26) that are available on the Internet.

Again, *welcome* to a new way of thinking, seeing, conceptualizing, imagining, and creating. One of the most wonderful components of qualitative research is the human activity of meeting and talking with participants, becoming acquainted, often in an intimate way, with people and worlds that are foreign or unknown to us. We come to understand what we would have never known and have the wonderful opportunity to make lives better for others. To me doing qualitative research is a privilege, a privilege that others allow for us, and for that, I am always humbled and appreciative. Qualitative research does indeed incorporate the *human* in *human science*.

Postscript

Remember what was written in the Preface, and go back to other editions of this text for different interpretations of methods and different exemplars. It is so very interesting!

REFERENCES

Anderson, W. (1995). *The truth about truth*. New York: Putnam.

Beneloiel, J. (1984, March). Advancing nursing science: Qualitative approaches. *Western Journal of Nursing Research in Nursing and Health, 7*, 1–8.

Bohm, D. (1985). *Unfolding meaning*. New York: Routledge.

Crotty, M. (1996). *Phenomenology and nursing research*. South Melbourne, Australia: Churchill Livingstone.

Didion, J. (2005a, September 25). After life. *New York Times Magazine*.

Didion, J. (2005b). *The year of magical thinking*. New York: Knopf.

Dilthey, W. (1926). *Meaning in history*. London: Allen and Unwin.

Goleman, D. (1997). *Emotional intelligence: Why it can matter more than IQ*. New York: Bantam.

Kuhn, T. S. (1970). *The structure of scientific revolutions*. Chicago: University of Chicago Press.

Morse, J. (2004a). Editorial: Qualitative significance. *Qualitative Health Research, 14*(2), 151–152.

Paterson, J. A., & Zderad, L. J. (1976, reissued 1988). *Humanistic nursing*. New York: National League for Nursing.

Pink, D. (2005). *A whole new mind: Moving from the information age to the conceptual age*. New York: Riverhead Books.

Ray, P., & Anderson, S. (2000). *The cultural creatives: How 50 million people are changing the world*. New York: Three Rivers Press.

Stolorow, R., & Atwood, G. (2002). *Contexts of being: The intersubjective foundations of psychological life*. Hillsdale, NJ: Analytic Press.

Tourigny, S. (1998). Some new dying trick: African American youths "choosing" HIV/AIDS. *Qualitative Health Research, 8*(2), 149–167.

van Manen, M. (2002). *Writing in the dark: Phenomenological studies in interpretive inquiry*. Ontario, Canada: Althouse Press.

ADDITIONAL REFERENCES

Bohm, D. (1998). *On creativity*. New York: Routledge.

Morse, J. (2004b). Editorial: Using the right tool for the job. *Qualitative Health Research, 14*(8), 1029–1031.

Watson, J. (1999). *Postmodern nursing and beyond*. New York: Churchill Livingstone.

2

Language and Nursing Research: The Evolution

Patricia L. Munhall

Discussing or talking is the way in which we articulate significantly the intelligibility of Being-in-the-world. The way in which discourse gets expressed is Language.

—M. Heidegger, *Being and Time*

So the main function of a language symbol is not to stand for or represent an object to which it corresponds. Rather, it initiates a total movement of memory, imagery, ideas, feelings, and reflexes, which serves to order attention to and direct action in a new mode that is not possible without the use of such symbols.

—D. Bohm, *On Creativity*

Being in the world, for those nurse researchers who embark on the path of discovery through qualitative research designs or methods, has many challenges. One of these challenges has to do with the limits and power of language. Our world is narrated and organized through language. The use of language is one way in which we communicate meaning. We also experience moments when we cannot find the language to express a feeling, an emotion, or a response. So our language at once allows expression and also constrains expression. In the very way that we narrate with language, the particulars of our context, personal, social, and cultural agendas are set. So too in our research language: values, beliefs, and aims are communicated from which varying meanings of being in the world will evolve.

For many years, nurse researchers and theorists have engaged in a lively and enlightening dialogue of various paradigms, the two most common being the logical positivist or empirical-analytic paradigm and the contrasting one, phenomenology. This dialogue was prompted by many nurse researchers who initiated what was to become an "interpretive turn" in nursing research (Munhall, 1989). These nurse theorists and researchers began to raise these questions:

- ◆ Was nursing a natural science, like that of chemistry and biology, and therefore based on similar linguistic assumptions?
- ◆ Was nursing a human science based on differing linguistic assumptions?
- ◆ Was nursing research ready for a poststructuralist perspective? (Dzurec, 1989)

The purpose of this chapter is to illustrate the words and perspectives that gave rise to these discussions and the evolution of nursing research. You will most likely see that much of the same language is relevant in today's historical context. Nursing language is both concealing and revealing of the stances and perspective that we pose to nursing as we interact with the phenomenon of concern. For some nurse researchers, this discussion will be historical because they have chosen one paradigm over another for various reasons. For other nurse researchers, it will also be historical because they see a postmodern perspective of multiple research paradigms as not only acceptable but essential. At this point in time, many nurse researchers are encouraging moving beyond what they see as an unruly dualism between what in the early 1980s was structured as a debate. The debate was centered on two different research paradigms, the quantitative and the qualitative. These two research paradigms were often compared and contrasted, elucidating their different philosophical underpinnings. However, it remains extremely important to students studying qualitative research at the outset to become familiar with some of the fundamental and basic assumptions, beliefs, and outcomes of these two paradigms. Using the concreteness of placing paradigms in stark relief to one another should be of assistance to our beginning understanding of various worldviews.

In this chapter, we will see, in the form of contrasting systems of language, competing articulations in other fields as well as our own that are characteristic of various philosophical orientations. This particular focus on philosophical analysis is further elucidated in Chapters 3, 4, and 5.

Research in nursing is at the center of this linguistic exploration. Methods of doing research are still divided into two purportedly ideological (and thus far considered conflicting) schools of thought with two distinct language systems. These schools of thought have been categorized as the qualitative and quantitative approaches to research. By quantitative methods of research we mean the traditional scientific methods as presented in most of the contemporary nursing research textbooks. These methods are characterized by deductive reasoning, objectivity, quasi-experiments, statistical techniques, and control. In contrast, the qualitative methods, many of which are described within this text, are characterized by inductive reasoning, subjectivity, discovery, description, and process orienting (Reichardt & Cook, 1979). The outcome, depending on the method, can be derived from description, interpretation, and analysis (Ashworth, 1997).

This chapter explores this qualitative-quantitative dichotomy and perhaps will appear culpable of unnecessary polarization. This is done for the pedagogical advantage of clearly revealing the possible differences between these two research traditions. I hope to absolve myself of this polarization as the third chapter of this book begins. In that chapter a cyclical continuum is suggested that finds its origins in qualitative research and its validation in quantitative research. Others have also suggested moving to postpositivism and reconciliation (Clark, 1998).

The present chapter begins with a discussion of the living aspect of language and then progresses to a contextual analysis of nursing research so that we may ferret out the meanings of our linguistic expressions, their origins, and subsequent propulsions. This motion of transition from our earliest identification with medicine represents a broad worldview transition or paradigmatic shift. Nursing research and the quest for nursing theory development are discussed from the perspective of language development and language usage as we seek out the pattern and process of our articulation of meaning and experience. Before we begin our exploration, see if you can hear the words of encouragement from David Allen (1995).

> The emphasis on language, and particularly the insistence that individuals inherit and are constituted by their language, is a helpful corrective to the solipsistic and individualist models that continue to plague our theory and research about practice. (p. 181)

LANGUAGE AND LIVED EXPERIENCE

Long before children speak actual words, they have learned effectively to express their physical, mental, and emotional states of being. Very early in our childhood we learn that laughing, crying, pouting, and looking quizzical stimulate a response from those who are "significant others." We are indeed beginning to learn the power of expressive language.

Eventually, we begin to develop a vocabulary and, interestingly, by the time we are 2 years of age or so, we have learned to treasure the word *no*. Individuation, assertiveness, posturing, and a continuing desire for power in our environment render this one of the most important words in any language. People have written entire books on how, when, and where to say *no* effectively.

Nursing as a profession, concomitantly with women as a social force, is still very much involved in those processes of individuation, assertiveness, posturing, and claiming power in our environment. Like the significance of the word *no*, our language and the use of specific sets of words simultaneously reveal and conceal who we are, both to ourselves and to the world at large.

Thus, in our quest for individuation and, we should mention, our autonomy *(auto-no-my)*, we are in the process of developing a language system that defines our particular role with our clients. This focus on autonomy correlates well with the point of the revelatory and concealing power of language and the exemplary word *no*. Nursing has claimed the power to say *no* through the Greek word *autonomous*, meaning self-ruling. Thus, we see language alive in a word that says, "I have a right to be self-determined." The living of autonomy expresses the position of a profession and, in nursing, has called attention to our transition from the physician's handmaiden (just look at that word!) to an independent self-ruling practitioner. This posturing of ourselves is consistently illustrated in our transition from the primary usage of medical language to our concerted efforts to develop a nursing language, taxonomy, nomenclature, and nursing diagnostic system.[1]

The moment-to-moment language that we choose defines the posture or stance that we assume in the space that we believe is ours in the health care _____ (fill in the blank):

1. system
2. arena
3. delivery system
4. field

---

[1] There is considerable ambivalence within the profession about the usage of the term *nursing diagnosis* and developing taxonomies. Many view these systems as reductionistic, acontextual, and a continued imitation of medicine.

For example, in the preceding multiple-choice option, we find it most interesting to study such words in their starkness for their literal or metaphorical meaning. Is health care "delivered"? Is there a "system" of health care? The word *arena*, which is frequently used with health care, is a word that is often associated with a circus or sports. (The temptation is too great to resist pointing out how that word, with its noted association, may be the most apt description of the present so-called health care system.) The word *sports* is also associated with the word *field*, where many games are played, with winners and losers. So, of these words, which one or two or perhaps one not mentioned would characterize, for you the reader, the state of health care today?

As noted, nursing language, like that of other professions, is revelatory of the stance and perspective that we suppose as we interact with the phenomena of our experience. The symbols that we choose as expressions either implicitly or explicitly lay open our assertions, propositions, assumptions, beliefs, values, and priorities. The significance of such expressions is centered in our emergence: our expressions bring us into existence. The noumenal, or "thing in itself," depends on the phenomenal for its expression.

DeVries (1983) succinctly and humorously illustrated the noumenal emerging from felt obscurity into shared, understood experience in the following passage:

> In the beginning was the word. Once terms like identity doubts and midlife crisis become current, the reported cases of them increase by leaps and bounds, affecting people unaware there is anything wrong with them until they have got a load of the coinages. You too may have an acquaintance or even a relative with a block about paper hanging or dog grooming, a high flown form of stagnation trickled down from writers and artists. Once my poor dear mother confided to me in a hollow whisper, "I have an identity crisis." I says, "How do you mean?" and she says, "I no longer understand your father." Now we have burnout, and having heard tell of it on television or read about it in a magazine, your plumber doubts he can any longer hack it as a pipefitter, while a glossary adopted by his wife has turned him overnight into . . . a male chauvinist pig, something she would never have suspected before. (p. 4)

We can identify readily in the foregoing what is referred to as concept development, though satirized. The "thing itself" (the noumenon) existed, was felt; yet we needed the description and language of shared experience to connect us within the world and provide a way of perceiving the phenomenon. We have developed other recent contemporary phenomena into abstractions of concrete events or, from some intuitive sense, into empirically expressed concepts and words that are commonly used to express our own or others' position/posture/stance in the world. Thus, we have codependency, women who love too much, deficit spending, premenstrual syndrome, and seven steps to obtain almost anything you would like—success, financial freedom, a good marriage, and more! The proliferation of support groups for various conditions of life as well as the many 12-step programs speak also to our need for shared language to connect us within the world with one another. The Internet has provided many ways of using language, ranging from informational purposes to once again allowing language to connect one human being to another. Blogs (Weblogs) help form virtual communities. We now can find groups of people who believe and speak the same language, spending hours a day, most of the time substantiating their common beliefs. See Chapter 26 for qualitative research sites and resources for nursing and other interdisciplines.

The various forms of language that we use, as with all disciplines, bring us into emergence. We need to recognize and articulate our points of contact in this pluralistic world, and we need language with the referent of nursing phenomena to have a recognized place in that world. Qualitative research is poised with its emphasis on language and meaning to assist us in understanding the meaning of our various places in experience.

For example, the word *undeveloped*, describing Third World countries, was judged to be a pejorative adjective and was discontinued. The word *emerging* was used instead to describe these countries and to express optimism. Our emergence, like that of children and emerging countries, will depend on our ability to express ourselves clearly within the context of this pluralistic world. Let us look at the lived experience of nursing through a contextual analysis of our language development.

THE CONTEXT OF NURSING RESEARCH

Stolorow and Atwood (2002) argue that there can be *no meaning* (italics added) without context, and they question the myth of the isolated mind. Allen (1995) encourages us to recognize the social, political, and historical location in the role of nursing research. The historical context in which individuals live places them in a world specific to that time and place, of contingencies that must be recognized and acknowledged if research or discourse is to be meaningful (Rorty, 1991). So it appears appropriate, especially in a text on qualitative research that readily acknowledges and embodies its search within the context of "things," that we begin this exploration of language in nursing research by attending to the context in which it has occurred and is continuing to evolve.

Context is defined as "that which leads up to and follows and often specifies the meaning of a particular expression" and "the circumstances in which a particular event occurs" (*American Heritage Dictionary*, 1992). I believe that within this definition of context the following three antecedents and their evolutionary concurrent factors should be acknowledged:

1. Research in nursing evolved predominantly when nursing education became a part of higher education and was seeking its own body of knowledge, different from that of medicine.
2. Nursing's first researchers were being prepared in fields other than nursing and have brought to nursing the various paradigms from those fields.
3. Derivation and/or deduction for nursing research was (is) being drawn from disciplines other than nursing. Each factor will be explored from the perspective of its contributions to our nursing research language.

TRANSITION IN WORLDVIEWS OF NURSING

During the 1950s, as an outgrowth of the development and acceptance of new theoretical approaches to understanding physical and human phenomena emerging from other fields (approaches such as systems perspectives, quantum physics, adaptation, and ecological views), nurse scholars began questioning the prevalent acceptance and alignment of the medical model as the basis for nursing practice. Nursing was also entering the university setting at that time. These two historical events converged, and the need for our own distinct body of knowledge, a benchmark of a profession and the research imperative of the university, spurred a revolution in nursing.

These two factors, the acknowledgment of a major scientific revolution in other disciplines as well as our own, and the desire to attain a level of professionalism at which we would base practice on a distinct body of nursing knowledge, led to a perceptual shift in the way that we spoke about nursing phenomena and simultaneously led to the scientific investigation of nursing phenomena.[2] It seemed, though, that the way in which we spoke

---

[2] For a more detailed explanation of the scientific revolution that eclipsed determinism and objectivism, the reader is referred to works on quantum physics, Heisenberg's principle of uncertainty, and Bohr's principle of complementarity. In Floyd Matson's *The Broken Image* (1964), a most readable discourse can be found, and Larry Dossey's *Space, Time and Medicine* (1982) is wonderfully explicit and enjoyable reading on this topic.

about nursing and the way in which we investigated nursing phenomena often reflected assumptions, propositions, beliefs, and priorities of two different worldviews, the first reflecting one worldview and the other reflecting a different worldview. We will see shortly that this is a characteristic of paradigmatic shift within a discipline.

The spoken language in nursing began to change, reflecting this perceptual shift from the medical, atomistic, causal model to a distinct nursing, holistic, interactive model. This represented a paradigmatic innovation for nursing. The way in which phenomena were viewed in nursing was changing in a way that was considered by some to be irrevocably conflictual in its basic premises and assumptions with the medical model.

This shift, which was well recognized in the discipline of physics, began to permeate the language of other fields as well as nursing. The change is representative of a transition from a mechanistic to an organismic perspective, from the reliance on objectivity to intersubjectivity, and from the received view to a nonreceived view (Watson, 1981). Today, Watson (1999) urges us farther "away from the reaction worldview, past the reciprocal and into the transformative-simultaneous" and urges nurses to create nursing's own postmodern paradigm. Many of the qualitative methods of research, before the language of postmodernism became commonplace, have as underpinnings many of the values and beliefs of postmodernism.

Illumination of the differences between and among these worldviews and/or paradigms can be demonstrated in the scrutiny of the respective language systems. It seems appropriate, though, to be clear at this point as to what a worldview or paradigm is. Patton (1978), in terms consistent with those of Kuhn (1970), defines a paradigm as follows: "A worldview, a general perspective, a way of breaking down the complexity of the real world. As such, paradigms are deeply embedded in the socialization of adherents and practitioners: paradigms tell them what is important, legitimate and reasonable" (p. 203).

If we accept the premise that things come into being through language, the language paradigm of a discipline will tell the practitioner what is important, legitimate, and reasonable. Kuhn (1970) suggests that a paradigm is a discipline's specific method of solving a puzzle, of viewing human experience, and of structuring reality. It is a worldview, a way of viewing phenomena in the world.

Laudan (1977), in a similar vein, uses the phrase "research tradition" to communicate the same theme: "A research tradition . . . is a set of assumptions about the basic kinds of entities in the world, assumptions about how these entities interact, assumptions about the proper methods to use for constructing and testing theories about these entities" (p. 97). Morgan (1983) calls our attention to the significance of these assumptions. He states: "Assumptions make messes researchable, often at the cost of great simplification, and in a way that is highly problematic" (p. 377).

This reference about assumptions becomes more powerful when, as Morgan suggests, *researchers choose their own assumptions* on which to base their studies. One could then say that this latitude enables the means for achieving what the researcher values. In the paradigms introduced in this chapter are assumptions about the world, believed in some way to be true, though they are actually the "taken for granted" views of human scientists. In a fundamental sense, then, researchers choose the values, "truths," and perspectives on which they base their research endeavors.

Another way of expressing this shift was the idea that nursing was a human science. Nursing seems to be philosophically expressed through language to be compatible with the ideas and concepts of a human science. German philosopher–historian Wilhelm Dilthey (1926; as translated in Atwood & Stolorow, 1984) held these critical assumptions about a human science:

> The supreme category of the human sciences is meaning. (p. 2)
>
> The natural sciences investigate objects from the outside whereas the human sciences rely on a perspective from the inside. (p. 2)
>
> The central emphasis in the natural sciences is upon causal explanation: The task of inquiry in the human sciences is interpretation and understanding. (p. 2)

Our transition in worldviews then seems to have moved from a narrowly defined type of science to a much broader connection of what constitutes science. However, in that broader view, there remain two very distinct sciences: natural science and human science. Some would even question the idea of a human science, if using the strict parochial rules of *science*. However, as the human sciences have evolved, there is little doubt that they have legitimated their place as a science, one with a different philosophy from the philosophy of natural science.

THE LANGUAGE OF WORLDVIEWS

What follows are expressions belonging to different ways of viewing phenomena (worldviews). The language reveals different assumptions, beliefs, and values concerning human and physical reality. In essence, the paradigm or research tradition is a philosophy: it conceptualizes fundamental beliefs. For this reason, the research paradigm as a puzzle-solving method should be congruent with the discipline's larger paradigm, that is, the paradigm of nursing or nursing's philosophy.

Although this idea of congruency is not held as essential by all researchers, the most sophisticated or reasonable response to any either-or discussion would be to choose a dialectic approach (Moccia, 1988; Morgan, 1983). This approach, as Morgan (1983) states, "also accepts the diversity of assumption and knowledge claims as an inevitable future of research and attempts to use the competing perspectives as a means of constructing new modes of understanding" (p. 379). A postmodern perspective would transcend *the either-or stalemate as an unnecessary obstacle* to understanding and would beg the question with an emphasis on plurality of perspectives, which would be context dependent.

To assist students in understanding the different language systems of various fields, the tables included in this chapter present language in stark relief. They are purposely presented to demonstrate the different meaning systems and are more for explicitness than for the subtleties that, of course, also can be discussed. Each of the five tables (Table 2–1 through Table 2–5) of paradigmatic-type language presents two contrasting belief systems. The language of the systems in the left-hand columns is often the same language or, if not literally the same, it is at least consistent in syntax and meaning, reflecting the underlying continuity of beliefs, values, and assumptions. The same continuity in language will be observed in the systems presented in the right-hand columns of the tables. The observations are important when we take into account that the paradigm preserves and perpetuates the disciplinary matrix of a field (Kuhn, 1970).

A major premise that this text suggests is that the language expressed in the left-hand columns and found within the paradigms of the mechanistic, the realists, the received view, behaviorism, and the medical model is consistent with the scientific method or quantitative research. In contrast, the language expressed in the right-hand columns reflects the paradigms of the organismic, the idealists, the nonreceived view, humanism, and many nursing models and is consistent with qualitative research methods.

We know well that there are more cultures than the two described by C. P. Snow (1959) in *The Two Cultures and the Scientific Revolution*. Today, there are hundreds, and there are disciplines and subdisciplines of those disciplines. Often, the subdisciplines of a discipline speak in foreign tongues to one another. For this reason, it is important to understand the overall fundamental differences so that we may intelligently see what Kirby (1983) calls "the points of contact in a plural world." Illustrating the plurality of worldviews, he optimistically states that "there could be an underlying unity . . . and thus a single earth-centered perspective from which all problems may be viewed" (p. 25). Twenty-one years later, which is just a blip on the time screen, we have yet to come to this perspective. The following tables and the language should illustrate the fundamental differences. Perhaps the reader can surmise possible points of contact and propose an alliance where all sorts of evidence will contribute to the richness of our comprehension and our ability to make sense of the world around us.

Paradigms in Psychology. It has been said that all contemporary psychological systems are derivative of either the mechanistic or the organismic paradigms (Table 2–1) (Looft, 1973). Many philosophers and psychologists argue that the assumptions of each are unbridgeable. Either humans are reactive organisms, as Skinner (1953) would have them, or individuals are active and thinking organisms, as Piaget (1970) would predicate. One lays before us a thesis; the other, an antithesis.

The reader is asked to contemplate the differences in meaning as expressed in the descriptive language of the mechanistic and the organismic paradigms of psychology (see Table 2–1).

Are the perspectives unbridgeable? With these paradigms, as well as the ones that follow, discussion about the bridgeability of these perspectives should prove lively and fruitful.

Paradigms in Philosophy. Filstead (1979, p. 34) states that at the core of the distinction between the quantitative and qualitative methods of research lies the classical argument in philosophy between the schools of realism and idealism and their subsequent derivatives (Table 2–2). The Baconian reality of "seeing is believing" led to believing in the "real" as the only reality about which one could be positive. Hence, those who ascribed to that belief system

TABLE 2–1 Paradigms in Psychology	
Mechanistic	Organismic
Human being reacts and responds to the environment	Human being acts on and creates the meaning of an experience
Predictable response sets from human beings can be determined	Understanding comes from individual human perspective—variable responses
Empirical reality	Social construction of reality
One reality—same rules	Dynamic reality—different responses
Human beings can be controlled	Human beings can be self-determined
Behavior—should be prescribed	Behavior—many possibilities acceptable and desirable

TABLE 2–2   Paradigms in Philosophy

Realism	Idealism
Static conception of world	Evolving conception of world
Seeing is believing	There is more than what meets the eye
Logical positivism	Dynamic, chaotic
Social world as given	Social world as created
Independent physical reality	Reality is mentally perceived— sense perception

were called "positivist." When reality could be held static, observations made, and experiments performed, science was done and the truth revealed. Those philosophers who questioned this positivist logic and method of science when it was applied to the understanding of human beings became known as "idealists" (Kneller, 1964). Today, the same questions asked by the idealists have been amplified by postmodernists. Science is no longer absolute or the final truth. Science is an ever-changing body of ideas, and we have daily shifts about beliefs. The whole concept of universality and generalizability is put into question. We have come to see that "being in the world" may be more aptly stated as *"beings-in-the-worlds."* There are multiple worlds, multiple realities, and multiple perspectives (Anderson, 1995).

Although the idealists acknowledged the existence of a physical reality, they argued that the mind was the creator and source of knowledge. In addition to the language expressed in Table 2–2 from the idealist school, the following short Zen parable is indicative of idealists' ideas and the place of human perception (*Zen Buddhism*, 1959):

> One windy day two monks were arguing about the flapping banner. The first said, "I say the banner is moving, not the wind." The second said, "I say the wind is moving, not the banner." A third monk passed by and said, "The wind is not moving. The banner is not moving. Your minds are moving." (p. 52)

Although briefly presented, inherent here is the great debate between the objective and subjective means of knowing. We are about to see now how research methods as worldviews are an inherent outgrowth of a philosophical worldview that precedes it and establishes its epistemological ways of coming to know about the world.

Subsequent Paradigms in Epistemology.   Flowing from the paradigms of philosophy should be congruent paradigms or research traditions for the way

TABLE 2–3   Paradigms in Epistemology

Received View	Nonreceived View
Logical positivism	Uncertainty
Materialism	Mental perception
Reductionism	Holism
Laws—quantification	Patterns—qualification
Predictions	Interpretations
Objectivity	Subjectivity
Neutrality	Human values
Operationalization	Context integration
Knowing something	Understanding meaning

in which each school of thought establishes how it comes to know about its particular account of the world. Epistemology is the branch of philosophy that concerns itself with the nature of knowledge. Each school of philosophy will have an epistemology. In other words, each belief system will have a congruent belief system about coming to know about the world and the nature of knowledge.

For our purposes, the realist philosophy is connected with the epistemological paradigm of the received view, and the idealist is connected with the nonreceived view (Table 2–3). I must acknowledge at this point or perhaps call attention to this very simplified version of what is most complex to philosophers. We are examining the gist of language differences, yet I strongly recommend further study in this area for those who are interested in greater in-depth knowledge. (Chapters 3 and 4 provide a further base to this aspect of the discussion.)

The expressions of the received view are those of the positivists and/or realists (Suppe, 1977; Watson, 1981). They are consistent with the scientific method[3] and are representative of expressions found most often in our present nursing research texts. The nonreceived view of coming to know about nursing phenomena is emerging, and those expressions are found in the language of qualitative epistemology as well as most nursing philosophies.

Paradigms in Education.   The mechanistic and organismic paradigms are reflected in the field of education as behaviorism and humanism (Table 2–4). Learning theories emerging from these two paradigms are distinctively

---

[3] As defined in the traditional sense. All the methods presented in this text are considered scientific methods of research.

TABLE 2–4   Paradigms in Education

Behaviorism	Humanism
Homogeneous group	Heterogeneous group
Human reactiveness	Human activeness
Human malleability	Self-determination
Human passiveness	Unique interpretation of reality
Human objectivity	Subjectivity
Shaping concrete behavior	Changes in consciousness
Measurable outcomes	Hoped-for outcomes—variable
Preparation for specific roles	Preparation for world at large

different because they are reflective of differing beliefs, values, and assumptions about the world and the nature of human beings. You may find it interesting here to reflect on which paradigm is more prevalent in nursing education and discuss the relative merits of each and, again, the bridgeability or points of contact (Munhall, 1992).

Paradigms in the Health Professions.   Table 2–5 seems to reflect nursing's congruity with the preceding paradigms of the organismic, the idealists, the nonreceived view, and humanism. In contrast, the language of medicine seems to be congruent with the mechanistic, the realists, the received view, and behaviorism. It seems important to note, then, that our language system is congruent with some paradigms and not logically consistent with other paradigms. This is particularly relevant when we acknowledge that each paradigm should have a compatible research paradigm or method. The relevance is demonstrated in the philosophical paradigms of the realistic and idealistic and in the concomitant epistemological paradigms of the received view and nonreceived view, respectively. The languages of the medical model and most nursing models are readily distinguishable as to their perspectives, worldviews, tradition, or paradigms.

It is important to return here to our first consideration: "Research in nursing evolved predominantly when nursing was in transition between broad philosophic worldviews." The language presented in Table 2–5 as the language of medicine was for a long time that of nursing. When the worldview for nursing began changing, as reflected in proposed nursing models, the activity of nursing research concomitantly was under way. Ironically, the research activities that occurred in a parallel fashion often were not congruent with the premises of the nursing model. However, this incongruity is quite understandable when we review the second consideration in our language

TABLE 2–5   Paradigms in Health Professions

Medicine	Nursing
Reductionism—treating the part; treating the symptom	Holism—coming to the whole care for the whole person, whether "sick" or well
Reactive human being—reacts as prescribed	Active human being—transformative
Physical symptomatology	Integrated human being
Linear causality—cause and effect	Multiple interaction—self, others, environment, cosmos
Closed system	Open system
Steady state	Dynamic
Objective	Subjective
Manipulation	Self-determination
Control	Choice
Paternalism	Advocacy

development: Researchers in nursing were being prepared in fields other than nursing.

EARLY PREPARATION OF NURSE RESEARCHERS

It is so commonplace today that our nurse scholars and researchers have doctorate degrees in nursing that we need to reflect on the influence of the earlier doctoral preparation of nurses. Before the opening of specific nursing doctoral programs in the United States, nurse faculty and others sought this degree in other disciplines that seemed to relate to nursing. On completing these degrees, many of those doctorally prepared nurses began to think of developing nursing's own degree, a doctoral degree in nursing. Because our doctoral education evolved in this way, we will proceed to examine its influence rather than discuss the merits and limitations of such evolution.

The outcome was the development of a community of nurse researchers who were educated in the better-established disciplines and who subsequently developed a commitment to that discipline's research method (Chinn, 1983; Corbin, 1999). Although this development offered nursing a wide array of methods from which to choose, it soon appeared evident that the scientific method, with its own language, was adopted to such an extent that, Watson (1981) reported, "The scientific method is considered the one and only process for scientific discovery, experimental quantitative research methodology and design" (p. 414). Swanson and Chenitz (1982) state: "While nursing exists almost exclusively in the empirical social world, the profession uses the laboratory method of the basic sciences in its research design" (p. 241).

Norris (1982) attributes this supremacy of the scientific method in part to nursing's "desperate attempt" to become a legitimate science by embracing the experimental research model as the way to proceed. Indeed, *science* and *scientific* cannot be considered neutral words (if there are such words). In today's world, they are extensively value laden as expressing truth, goodness, worthwhileness, and legitimacy. Kaplan (1964) emphasizes this legitimacy point: "There are behavioral scientists who in their desperate search for scientific status give the impression that they don't much care what they do if only they do it right: substance gives way to form" (p. 406).

However, as Norris (1982) points out in a discussion of nursing's leap to experimental research, many nurse researchers are hampered by the lack of concept clarification, theory development, and descriptive methods of research, all of which are linked to qualitative research methods. Norris (1982) observes that, during the period from 1958 to 1975, nursing scholars made a concerted effort to develop a body of nursing knowledge without the necessary training in the methods of concept clarification, which are prerequisite to experimental research. This "scientific" influence continues to exercise its exclusivity, as is evidenced in the following scenario (Tinkle & Beaton, 1983):

> It was her first dissertation committee meeting. The topic of discussion was the proposed research methodology. Two of the committee members (well-known for their "hard" research) began to dialogue about the "softness" of the approach in the proposal before them—the lack of control, the lack of quantitative measurement, and the lack of manipulation of variables. Before long, the committee was in accord about the relatively low scientific merit of this type of research methodology as opposed to an experimental approach. The student found herself agreeing to shift her methodology to one involving experimental manipulation. (p. 27)

What makes this anecdote relevant 21 years later is that, in some colleges of nursing, this belief system has become *even more prominent*. The status and sometimes the requirement to attain National Institute of Nursing Research (NINR) or National Institutes of Health funding to advance, obtain a position, and even earn tenure demonstrate how fundamental to the research enterprise this commitment to "hard" science is.

Downs (1982), in response to a similar theme, observes: "This distorted value system rode in on the coattails of the idea that scientific method was equivalent to experimental research" (p. 4). Bronowski (1965), with a broader conception of science, surpasses this narrow view of the scientific method and enlarges the aperture. Science, he says, is: "Nothing else than the search to discover unity in the world variety of nature or . . . in the variety of our experiences. Poetry, painting, the arts are the same search." (p. vi)

In a cogent argument for a poststructural perspective, Dzurec (1989) comments on the tenacity of logical positivist methodology in nursing:

> The period beginning in the 1960s and stretching to today is perhaps the first in which the power relations in nursing and in human sciences in general have allowed the recognition of logical positivism as a single philosophy of science rather than as science itself. (p. 74)

However, we do know that our worldview has opened to allow for other methods of research. Coming to know and coming to discover rather than verify have become acknowledged as essential to the base of nursing knowledge.

Watson (1981) attributes this increased acknowledgment to the same processes of scientific development that have taken place in other sciences. She states that our commonality with other fields lies in the process of first adopting the received-view idea and then undergoing processes of rejection of that particular paradigm. We would not advocate the abandonment of all the characteristics of the received view or the scientific method, but two important points need to be made about the early preparation of nurse researchers (and, to a large extent, the present preparation of nurse researchers). These points, as first addressed in the introduction, are still discussed today and will lead us into the next contextual consideration (Ashworth, 1997; Clark, 1998; Watson, 1999). They are as follows:

1. Nurse researchers predominantly use the scientific method of inquiry and that language system.
2. The scientific method is used in nursing research prior to the description and understanding of the phenomenon within the nurse–patient context. In other words, we take leaps to a step without the necessary conditions for that step. Often we take those leaps within the context of deduction and derivation from theories from other disciplines and from nursing theories representing a totality paradigm (whose assumptions are congruent with those of natural science research).

A third possible point here is that some of nursing research is research done by nurses but is not research in nursing. An example of this is nurses participating in medical research studies.

DEDUCTION AND DERIVATION FROM THEORIES: FROM THEN TO NOW

In this section I attempt to provide for you our origins in nursing research and theory development. Some trained in nursing research say they were spoon-fed these first pioneers. It is always critical to know the origins and history of your field, lest someone bring up old information as a new discovery!

Walker and Avant (1983) define theory derivation as "the process of using analogy to obtain explanations or predictions in another field" (p. 163). These authors make a good distinction between theory derivation and borrowing theory (p. 163), but, for our purpose here, we are speaking about a process in which the description and explanation of phenomena for the development of nursing theory evolved from a discipline or field of knowledge other than nursing. Therefore, the language originates from a world other than the nurse–patient world. Nursing researchers identifying similarities from other fields believe a specific theory to be appropriate to a nursing or patient situation and proceed to generate deductions and/or hypotheses from that theory. This theory derivation is asserted to be useful when there are no available data or when the phenomenon is poorly understood (Walker & Avant, 1983). Thus, we had almost 25 years of nursing research based on theoretical frameworks that did not originate within a nursing or patient context.

One point that should be considered is that many borrowed and derived theories in nursing are based first on the natural and behavioral sciences and, with that, a mechanistic paradigm. Subsequently, the hypothesis deduced from such theories originated from how physical matter behaves, how people respond to forced-choice questions, and, probably all too often, how college students respond to questionnaires and various experiments.

It is amazing to realize with a simple perusal of psychology texts that one experiment after another, leading to the development of theory, has been performed on college students. In these many instances, theories evolved from a very specific age sample and then were generalized to the population at large. The very specific sample has been for researchers of human behavior a real convenience sample, that is, their 19-year-old sophomore students.

Another potential problem with theory derivation and language development from other fields is the male bias inherent in many of our developmental theories (Belenky, Clinchy, Goldberg, & Taub, 1986; Chinn, 1985; Gilligan, 1978). Pinch (1981) proposes that we should critically examine theories of development generated by Freud, Piaget, Erickson, and Kohlberg to recognize how we have accepted worldviews as developed and evolved from a male perspective (this topic is further discussed in Chapter 5). When we apply a hypothesis derived from such theory to individuals who may be ill—whether the derivation is from a male perspective, a college student's perspective, a well person's perspective, and so on—we will always have problems of authenticity, validity, and, most important, contextual meaning.

In our history of knowledge development, Dickoff and James (1968) propose a schema of four levels of theory: factor-isolating theories, factor-relating theories, situation-relating theories, and situation-producing theories. This schema dominated the development of nursing theory. We now need to evaluate how well we have proceeded with each of the four levels of theory. Often, when borrowing or deriving from theories from other fields, we proceed directly to situation-producing theories, sacrificing meaning and true significance to expedience. As far back as 1968, Dickoff and James cited this lack of attention to the beginning levels of theory development as being detrimental to the development of nursing theory. Wald and Leonard (1964) suggest that nurses develop their own concepts for nursing theory from inductive analysis of nursing experience rather than from deductive analysis from others' experiences. Perusal of many of the nursing research articles published today still indicates dependence on deducting hypotheses from unrelated contexts or unrelated populations.

Diers (1979), in a context correlative to the work of Dickoff and James, provides us with another classification of levels of theory (Table 2–6). Wolf (see Chapter 10 of this book) demonstrates how the qualitative method of ethnography fits into the factor-searching level of inquiry proposed by Diers (1979, p. 54) and shown in Table 2–6.

Indeed, all the qualitative methods of research presented herein seem essential to the beginning steps of theory development. In the first and second levels of inquiry, the questions "What is this?" and "What's happening here?" are answered within our own nurse–patient context. With qualitative research methods, theory is not derived, borrowed, or modified from other fields but rather springs from observation of and participation in an actual phenomenon. Norris (1982) believes that the phenomena with which nurses have the social prerogative and mandate to manage concern human health, illness, and comfort. Newman (1983, 1999) identifies additional patient–nursing phenomena, such as reciprocities, patterns, configurations, rhythms, and composition, and emphasizes context dependency, recognizing the simultaneity of our human-environmental processes.

The Social Policy Statement of the American Nurses Association (1995) specifies that the phenomena of concern to nurses are human responses to actual or potential health problems. All are phenomena researchable through qualitative methods and in the end may well stimulate the development of knowledge grounded in the experience of the patient, in complex

TABLE 2–6   Levels of Inquiry and Study Design

Level of Inquiry	Kind of Question	Study Design	Kind of Answer (Theory)	Study Design
1	What is this?	Factor-searching	Factor-isolating (naming)	Exploratory Formulative Descriptive Situational
2	What's happening here?	Relation-searching	Factor-relating (situation-depicting, situation-describing)	Exploratory Descriptive
3	What will happen if . . .?	Association-searching	Situation-relating (predictive)	Correlational Survey design Nonexperi-mental Natural experiment Experimental Explanatory Predictive
4	How can I make . . . happen?	Prescription-testing	Situation-producing (prescriptive)	

Source: From *Research in Nursing Practice* (p. 54), by D. Diers, 1979, Philadelphia: Lippincott.

interactions, and situated in an individual life-world. In the last edition, I had voiced hope that these discussions and debates of a socially constructed dichotomy would be a historical curiosity. Although some literature speaks to moving beyond this debate (Clark, 1998), Watson (1999) offers a strikingly contemporary worldview for nursing in which the old traditions largely dominate. What might influence the dominance of one paradigm over another or one theory over another is the importance placed today on interdisciplinary, multidisciplinary, or intradisciplinary theory and development. With the example of intradisciplinary theory, especially in nursing, we can actually come to see the benefit of combining or bringing together various theories, where there are philosophical consistencies or where one theory may be applicable to a particular experience and another theory better able to explain another area of experience.

Here is a place for human understanding in that nurse theorists who have devoted their life careers to development of their own theories are reluctant to let any part go or combine with another theorist. This is often unspoken, but for the sake of knowing, we need to be aware of this dynamic.

Intradisciplinary and interdisciplinary theory development and research could also come about with the six or so different specialty areas of nursing working together, which is so very complementary to the concepts of holism and the situated context.

Multidisciplinary theory development and research are also compatible with the ideas and tenets of qualitative research. Working with other human science disciplines enriches our understanding and broadens the possibilities by incorporating the many facets of being human. A suggestion, though, if you are to embark on multidisciplinary work, is to think of the following two considerations. First, is your project multidisciplinary because a granting agency is calling for that? If so, are you committed to a multidisciplinary approach beyond that requirement? Second, it is very helpful to work with an established or experienced researcher who has done multidisciplinary research previously. This can also be said for mixed-method research, which is discussed in Chapter 24.

A TRANSITION: NURSING WORLDVIEWS, NURSING RESEARCHERS, AND THEORY DEVELOPMENT

One of the purposes of this chapter is to explore nursing's coinages (language), its situatedness in this world, and how we choose to express ourselves. The foregoing discussion is an attempt to place in context our present posture in nursing research and to suggest the origin and evolution of how we have come to express ourselves and the language that we use to bring nursing phenomena into being. I suggest that this and other texts on qualitative research methods are a natural outgrowth of this context. It is contemporary, evolutionary, and congruent with changing worldviews. Expanding research horizons, acquiring new languages, and bringing phenomena into view constitute a reconstructing process.

Transitions in worldviews or paradigms are a gradual process wherein beliefs, values, and practices of the old and the new overlap (Kuhn, 1970). This continues to be a time when there is often conflict, incongruity, and confusion. However, these times are good times for self-reflection, self-consciousness, and clarification. Thesis, antithesis, and paradigmatic shifting are all parts of scientific revolutions or, in Laudan's (1977) terminology, the evolution of research traditions. They are the history and essence of science.

Returning now to the three identified factors that seem to influence the context of nursing research most, let us consider them from the perspective of Kuhn's language in an application to nursing research. Kuhn (1970) observes:

> During the transition period [of worldviews] there will be a large but never complete overlap between the problems that can be solved by the old and by the new paradigm. But there will also be a decisive difference in the modes of solution. When the transition is complete, the profession will have changed its view of the field, its methods and goals. (p. 84)

Evidently, we have not reached this stage, with two paradigms ironically being taught, in some cases simultaneously: the totality paradigm and the simultaneity paradigm. Each of these paradigms indicates a method of research. The former yields best to the scientific method and the latter to qualitative methods of research.

Chapter 3 discusses epistemology in nursing and the qualitative and quantitative methods of knowing, but let us see here the role of transition.

Nursing Worldviews

Nursing has attempted to abandon the language of the medical model and, concomitantly, to reject the mechanistic paradigm expressed by that language. To a lesser extent, medicine itself appears to be in transition from its own medical model to one that seems more aligned with some of the beliefs that we have most recently been espousing. There is within that field an emerging language that focuses on holism, psychosomatic phenomena, and the influence of environmental factors.

Even though nursing has attempted to develop nursing language, it often continues to retain the philosophical foundations of the medical model for research and to express its significance and importance in the symbols and practices that traditionally belong to medicine. Perhaps readers will consider some of these nonverbal symbolic forms of language that nursing continues to use and even seeks to acquire from the perspective of paradigmatic transition (Roberts, 1973).

In view of Kuhn's suggestion (1970, p. 84) that when "the transition is complete, the profession will have changed . . . its methods," let me repeat a question I asked a while back (Munhall, 1982a): "Could it be that when nursing abandoned the medical model and the language of that discipline, it retained the research paradigm that perpetuated what nursing was seeking to dissociate from?" (p. 68). Today I would ask the question, not so much regarding an abandonment of the medical model but the hard scientific research model, vis-à-vis logical positivism/scientific method. Is that what we are invested in because of the academic scientific community of the natural sciences and not the human sciences?

Because transitions are gradual and because of the aforementioned contextual variables, I am inclined to view this question as characteristic of a trajectory of transition in worldviews. Things do not change at once; Kuhn's (1970) words were: "When the transition is complete, the profession will have changed . . . its *methods*" (italics added). Our transition is far from complete. However, many nurse researchers and scholars are catalyzing the progress and process of this transition.

Nurse Researchers and Scholars

Many of our nurse researchers and scholars, many of whom were socialized in the scientific method, are emerging strongly from that orientation (often meaning experimental research) and are contributing now to the logical shift in research paradigms that would be congruent with the shift in the larger philosophical worldview and new perspective of viewing phenomena. What seems to have occurred is that questions and problems of the profession with its new and unique nursing perspective, that is, holism versus reductionism and/or simultaneity versus totality, cannot be answered or solved by the old methods, at least not at first.

Laudan (1977) reassures us with the following observation: "But there are times when two or more research traditions, far from mutually undermining one another, can be amalgamated, producing a synthesis which is progressive with respect to both the former research traditions" (p. 103).

Although we have moved from what Norris (1982, p. 6) identifies as "the occasional nurse who used the podium or the literature to support a descriptive route to knowledge [as] a 'voice crying in the wilderness'" to regular publication of the merits of qualitative research, the need for qualitative methods, research programs highlighting qualitative research, and in general the recognition of the advantages of a broadened repertoire of research methods, we seem now to have divided ourselves into two different schools. When we first debated the various methods, it was as though we were seeking a place for each method for a specific purpose. Now we see conferences, journals, and particular programs specializing in either quantitative or qualitative methods. It is an interesting evolution, and we need to be cognizant of the need to hear one another's voices, regardless of the orientation. Hardly hidden in the agendas of various schools or organizations is a strong bias toward one orientation, and, unfortunately, there may even appear to be suspicion of or disrespect for the other. Such suspicion or disrespect is so very counterproductive, and just as tolerance for individual differences is part of our nursing philosophy, it needs to extend to differences in research orientations; these differences need to enrich us and assist us in ultimately meeting the needs of our patients.

At this point it might be helpful to analyze not only the syntactical parallelism but also the contextual congruency of our larger philosophical paradigm with our most prevalent research method. The language that we use in the expression of the two demonstrates the emergence of the new worldview and the residual of the old worldview.

The expressions in Table 2–7 are provided to demonstrate the transitional nature of our worldviews and research paradigms. Table 2–7 illustrates the expressions of competing paradigms and Kuhn's overlap as we examine the contextual parallelism for logical syntax. This overlap has stimulated for many nurse researchers the proliferation of competing views, debates about methods, and discontent over the effect of nursing research on practice. Kuhn (1970) believes such debates are symptomatic of a "transition from normal to extraordinary research," but, as just mentioned, we should beware of splintering. The wholeness and the interaction that we propose in nursing models should be reflected in our own community of nurse researchers.

For the sake of conceptual clarity, the various paradigms have been presented in a dichotomized way; however, the practice is used more for its illustrative purposes. The goal here is to build bridges rather than erect walls. The bridge may well represent a transcendence of the two competing worldviews with the emergence of a research paradigm that either utilizes the two views or goes beyond them.

Theory Development

The transition from one paradigm to another paradigm or to the inclusion of another paradigm will be reflected, as has been suggested, in our language and expressions. We previously mentioned the borrowed theoretical frameworks that are used so prevalently in nursing research. We borrow freely from physics, biology, physiology, psychology, and sociology. We seem, as was mentioned, to also have two different nursing paradigms: the totality and the simultaneity. These practices often lead to fuzzy language and, in this context, the discovery of unique knowledge for nursing. Although the benefits of interdisciplinary work must be acknowledged and recognized, it still remains essential for each discipline to develop its own essence, its own substance, its own reason for being, and its own meaning.

TABLE 2–7   Expressions in Nursing Philosophy and Research Paradigms, and Contextual Parallelism

Expressions of Contemporary Nursing Philosophy

Humanism	Uniqueness
Individualism	Relativism
Self-determination	Autonomy
Active organism	Advocacy
Open system	Organismic
Holism	Situated context
Life-worlds	Simultaneity
Multiple realities	Multiplicity
Self-interpretive	

Expressions of the Scientific Method

Reductionism	Theory for the average
Objectivity–positivism	Categorization
Delimited problems	Prediction
Reality reduced to the measurable	Control
Human and environmental passivity	Mechanistic
Manipulation	Totality

Conceptual Parallelism

Nursing Philosophy	**Nursing Research Based on the Scientific Method**
Individualism	Commonalities
Uniqueness	Generalizations
Relativism	Categorization
Open system	Closed system
Holism	Reductionism
Individual interpretations	Statistical analysis
Active organism	Reactive organism
Organismic	Mechanistic
Self-determination	Control
Simultaneous interaction	Totality
Situated context	Acontextual
Multiple realities	Objective reality
Subjective perceptions	Objectivity

TABLE 2–8   The Quintessence of Nursing

Acceptance	Give and Take
Authenticity	Laughing–crying
Awareness	Loneliness
Becoming	Openness
Caring	Patience
Charge	Readiness
Choice	Response
Commitment	Responsibility
Confirmation	Self-recognition
Confrontation	Sustaining
Dedication	Touching
Dying and death	Trust
Fold—its meaning	Understanding
Freedom	Waiting
Frustration	

Source: Reprinted with permission from "The Tortuous Way Toward Nursing Theory," in *Theory Development: What, Why and How?* (p. 65), by J. Paterson, New York: National League for Nursing, 1978.

Paterson (1978) compiled a list of nursing phenomena (Table 2–8) selected by practicing nurses as being essential to nursing. We ask you to compare these expressions with the expressions found in many of our contemporary research titles. It bears repeating that we must recognize just how pioneering Paterson (1978) and Zderad (Paterson & Zderad, 1976) were. To pay tribute to them, their jointly written book, *Humanistic Nursing,* was reissued in 1988 as being contemporary and relevant for the present after its first publication in 1976. Read, think about, and respond to these words in Table 2–8 as perhaps the quintessence of nursing. Could any of us argue that they do not constitute nursing phenomena?[4] Would we not want them to? Are these not the words that express caring in experience? To those who wonder why there is not adequate description of such experiences in nursing literature, I believe the answer lies in the arguments for qualitative research. Qualitative researchers eagerly await the extraordinary research that Kuhn promises as the outcome of scientific revolutions.

---

[4] Additional phenomena are discussed in Chapter 3.

LANGUAGE AND COMPREHENSIBILITY

The existential-ontological foundation of languages is discourse or talk. (Heidegger, 1962, p. 203)

Discourse is existentially language, because that entity whose disclosedness it articulates according to significations, has, as its kind of being, being-the-world and being which has been thrown and submitted to the world. (Heidegger, 1962, p. 204)

For in conversation, as in research, we meet ourselves. Both are forms of social interaction in which our choice of words and actions return to confront us in terms of the kind of discourse or knowledge we help to generate. (Morgan, 1983, p. 406)

And where does a nurse researcher thrown into and submitted to the world learn to speak? In the pedagogical world of research, a new language is learned. We noted earlier that this language is sometimes chosen freely, sometimes encouraged in one or another direction, and sometimes "raised" to such high levels of abstraction that it becomes incomprehensible. From a qualitative perspective, language and the ability to express oneself to others is the only way in which we can bring experience into a form that creates in discourse a conversational relation (van Manen, 1990).

Before this chapter ends, it seems essential to mention an obvious inherent component of language: listening. Discourse and conversing include keeping silent and hearing. The openness that is required for new ideas to penetrate into a belief system requires silence and hearing. Additionally, when considering language, many people silence themselves, they do not give voice to their experience, and what may be meaningful in the "said" may even be more meaningful in the "unsaid."

The language of human science or phenomenology may at first sound strange to people who are steeped in a natural-science language (see Table 2–9). Paterson and Zderad's (1976) first attempts to introduce this language into nursing were often met with firm preconceptions and assumptions about being in the world that were dramatically different.

As I suggest in Chapter 1, one key idea is to lay groundwork in many curricula to assist students in the language of understanding the meaning of both being human in our different perspectives and understanding those differences in nursing and nursing research. The symbols, signs, and words that we use have inherent meaning. They are signifiers of who we are, what we are, and what is meaningful to us.

TABLE 2–9 Expressions of Qualitative Research Methods	
Subjective experience	Closeness to the data
Intuition	Process orientation
Variability	Dynamic reality
Communication	Open system
Individual perceptions	Time and space considerations
Shared language	Patterns
Interrelatedness	Configurations
Lived experience	Context dependence
Holism	Complementarity
Naturalism	Human development
Nonmanipulated observation	Life-worlds
Self-interpretation	Contingencies
Multiple perspectives	Multiple realities
Intersubjectivity	Narratives/stories
Existential meaning	

SUMMARY

The intent of this chapter can be summarized by borrowing Paterson's (1978) words: "For responsible, effective existence the professional requires *language* to relate authentically the purposes, beliefs, concerns, and events experienced continually to the nursing world" (p. 51, emphasis added). A mystery exists in those phenomena listed by practicing nurses, but each seems to be a "thing in itself," something waiting for description to bring it into our everyday awareness and to give it significance. It is as though we need to assert these events as belonging to nursing, to articulate our authentic experience with patients, and to claim what we and our patients believe to be essential to health and to our quality of existence. We then assign language to what is uniquely the abstract and the concrete, the enduring and the relevant meanings of shared human experience between patient and nurse. It is indeed a privilege and a calling to assist a patient in finding meaning in experience.

Qualitative research methods have much to offer as a research paradigm that is congruent with nursing's larger worldview, paradigm, or model. These methods offer ways to approach individuals in experiences, to encourage them to give voice to their experiencing, and to care enough to search for meaning within the experience. We refer again to Table 2–9 as an illustration of the language of the qualitative research methods and leave you to draw your own conclusions.

REFERENCES

Allen, D. (1995). Hermeneutics: Philosophy, traditions, and nursing practice research. *Nursing Science Quarterly, 8*(4), 175–181.

American Heritage Dictionary. (1992). New York: American Heritage.

American Nurses Association. (1995). *Nursing: A social policy statement.* Washington, DC: Author.

Anderson, W. (1995). *The truth about truth.* New York: Putnam.

Ashworth, P. D. (1997). The variety of qualitative research (Part 2: Non-positivist approaches). *Nurse Education Today, 17*(3), 219–224.

Atwood, G., & Stolorow, R. (1984). Structures of subjectivity: Explorations in pyschoanalytic phenomenology. Hillsdale, NJ: Analytic Press.

Belenky, M., Clinchy, B., Goldberg, N., & Taub, J. (1986). *Women's ways of knowing: The development of self, voice and mind.* New York: Basic Books.

Bronowski, J. (1965). *Science and human values* (rev. ed.). New York: Harper & Row.

Bohm, D. (1998). *On Creativity.* New York: Routledge.

Chinn, P. (1983). Editorial. *Advances in Nursing Science, 5*(2), ix.

Chinn, P. (1985). Debunking myths in nursing theory and research. *Image: The Journal of Nursing Scholarship, 17*(2), 45–49.

Clark, A. M. (1998). The qualitative-quantitative debate: Moving from positivism and confrontation to post-positivism and reconciliation. *Journal of Advanced Nursing, 27,* 1242–1249.

Corbin, V. (1999). Misusing phenomenology in nursing research: Identifying the basic issues. *Nurse Researcher, 6*(3), 52–65.

DeVries, P. (1983). *Slouching towards Kalamazoo.* Boston: Little, Brown.

Dickoff, J., & James, P. (1968). A theory of theories: A position paper. *Nursing Research, 17,* 197–203.

Diers, D. (1979). *Research in nursing practice.* Philadelphia: Lippincott.

Dossey, L. (1982). *Space, time and medicine.* Boulder, CO: Shambhala.

Downs, F. (1982). It's a great idea but it won't work. *Nursing Research, 31*(1), 4.

Dzurec, L. (1989). The necessity for and evolution of multiple paradigms for nursing research: A poststructuralist perspective. *Advances in Nursing Science, 11*(4), 69–77.

Filstead, W. (1979). Qualitative methods: A needed perspective in evaluation research. In C. Reichardt & T. Cook (Eds.), *Qualitative and quantitative methods to evaluation research.* Beverly Hills, CA: Sage.

Gilligan, C. (1978). In a different voice: Women's conception of self and of morality. *Harvard Education Review, 47,* 481–517.

Heidegger, M. (1962). *Being and time* (J. Macprairie & E. Robinson, Trans.). New York: Harper & Row.

Kaplan, A. (1964). *The conduct of inquiry.* Scranton, PA: Chandler.

Kirby, D. (1983). Seeing the points of contact in a plural world. *Chronicle of Higher Education, 26*(7), 25.

Kneller, G. (1964). *Introduction to the philosophy of education.* New York: Wiley.

Kuhn, T. S. (Ed.). (1970). *The structure of scientific revolutions.* Chicago: University of Chicago Press.

Laudan, L. (1977). *Progress and its problems: Toward a theory of scientific growth.* Berkeley: University of California Press.

Looft, W. (1973). Socialization and personality throughout the life span: An examination of contemporary psychological approaches. In P. Baltes & K. Schaie (Eds.), *Life-span developmental psychology.* New York: Academic Press.

Matson, F. (1964). *The broken image.* New York: George Brazillier.

Moccia, P. (1988). A critique of compromise: Beyond the methods debate. *Advances in Nursing Science, 10*(4), 1–9.

Morgan, G. (1983). *Beyond method: Strategies for social research* (pp. 377–382). Newbury Park, CA: Sage.

Munhall, P. (1982a). Ethical juxtaposition in nursing research. *Topics in Clinical Nursing, 4*(1), 66–73.

Munhall, P. (1982b). Nursing philosophy and nursing research: In apposition or opposition? *Nursing Research, 31*(3), 176–177, 181.

Munhall, P. (1989). Philosophical pondering on qualitative research methods in nursing. *Nursing Science Quarterly, 2,* 20–28.

Munhall, P. (1992). A new ageism: Beyond a toxic apple. *Nursing and Health Care, 13*(7), 370–375.

Newman, M. A. (1983). Editorial. *Advances in Nursing Science, 5*(2), x–xi.

Newman, M. A. (1999). The rhythm of relating in a paradigm of wholeness. *Image: Journal of Nursing Scholarship, 31*(3), 227–230.

Norris, C. (1982). *Concept clarification in nursing.* Rockville, MD: Aspen.

Paterson, J. (1978). The tortuous way toward nursing theory. In *Theory development: What, why and how?* New York: National League for Nursing.

Paterson, J. A., & Zderad, L. J. (1976, reissued 1988). *Humanistic nursing.* New York: National League for Nursing.

Patton, M. Q. (1978). *Utilization focused evaluation.* Beverly Hills, CA: Sage.

Piaget, J. (1970). *Structuralism.* New York: Basic Books.

Pinch, W. (1981). Feminine attributes in a masculine world. *Nursing Outlook, 12,* 29–36.

Reichardt, C., & Cook, T. (Eds.). (1979). *Qualitative and quantitative methods in evaluation research.* Beverly Hills, CA: Sage.

Roberts, S. (1973). Oppressed group behavior: Implications for nursing. *Advances in Nursing Science, 5*(4), 21–30.

Rorty, R. (1991). *Essays on Heidegger and others.* New York: Cambridge University Press.

Skinner, B. (1953). *Science and human behavior.* New York: Appleton-Century-Crofts.

Snow, C. P. (1959). *The two cultures and the scientific revolution.* Cambridge, England: Cambridge University Press.

Stolorow, R., & Atwood, G. (2002). Contexts of being: The intersubjective foundations of psychological life. Hillsdale, NJ: Analytic Press.

Suppe, F. (Ed.). (1977). *The structure of scientific theories* (2nd ed.). Champaign: University of Illinois Press.

Swanson, J., & Chenitz, C. (1982). Why qualitative research in nursing? *Nursing Outlook, 30*(4), 241–245.

Tinkle, M., & Beaton, J. (1983). Toward a new view of science: Implications for nursing research. *Advances in Nursing Science, 5*(2), 27–36.

van Manen, M. (1990). *Research lived experience: Human science for an action sensitive pedagogy.* New York: SUNY Press.

Wald, F., & Leonard, R. (1964). Towards development of nursing practice theory. *Nursing Research, 13,* 4–9.

Walker, L., & Avant, K. (1983). *Strategies for theory construction in nursing.* Norwalk, CT: Appleton-Century-Crofts.

Watson, J. (1981). Nursing's scientific quest. *Nursing Outlook, 29*(7), 413–416.

Watson, J. (1999). *Post modern nursing and beyond.* New York: Churchill Livingstone.

Zen Buddhism. (1959). Mount Vernon, NY: Peter Pauper Press.

ADDITIONAL REFERENCES

Allen, D., Benner, P., & Diekelmann, N. (1985). Three paradigms for nursing research: Methodological implications. In P. Chinn (Ed.), *Nursing research methodology issues and implementation.* Rockville, MD: Aspen.

Asp, M., & Fagerberg, I. (2005). Developing concepts in caring science based on a lifeworld perspective. *International Journal of Qualitative Methods, 4*(2), article 5. Retrieved December 14, 2005, from http://www.ualberta.ca/~ijqm/backissues/4_2/html/asp.htm.

Baer, E. (1979). Philosophy provides the rationale for nursing's multiple research directions. *Image, 2*(3), 72–74.

Barbour, R. S. (2000). The role of qualitative research in broadening the "evidence base" for clinical practice. *Journal of Evaluation in Clinical Practice, 6*(2), 155–163.

Benner, P. (Ed.). (1994). *Interpretive phenomenology: Embodiment, caring, and ethics in health and illness.* Thousand Oaks, CA: Sage.

Benoliel, J. (1984). Advancing nursing science: Qualitative approaches. *Western Journal of Nursing Research, 6*(3), 1–8.

Byrne, M. M. (2001). Linking philosophy, methodology and methods in qualitative research. *AORN, 73*(1), 207–210.

Cheek, J. (2002). Advancing what? Qualitative research, scholarship and the research imperative. *Qualitative Health Research, 12*(8), 1130–1140.

Chenetz, W. C., & Swanson, J. M. (1986). *From practice to grounded theory: Qualitative research in nursing.* Menlo Park, CA: Addison-Wesley.

Clark, C. L., & Wilcockson, J. (2002). Seeing need and developing care: Exploring knowledge for and from practice. *International Journal of Nursing Studies, 39*(4), 397–406.

Creswell, J. (2003). *Research design: Qualitative, quantitative and mixed methods approaches.* Thousand Oaks, CA: Sage.

Davies, D., & Dodd, J. (2002). Qualitative research and the question of rigor. *Qualitative Health Research, 12*(2), 279–289.

Fawcett, J. (1983). Hallmarks of success in nursing theory development. In P. Chinn (Ed.), *Advances in nursing theory development* (chap. 1). Rockville, MD: Aspen.

Field, P., & Morse, J. (1985). *Nursing research: The application of qualitative approaches.* Rockville, MD: Aspen.

Foucault, M. (1977). *Language, counter memory, practice: Selected essays and interviews.* Ithaca, NY: Cornell University Press.

Gaita, R. (2002). *A common humanity: Thinking about love and truth and justice.* London: Routledge.

Gorenberg, B. (1983). The research tradition of nursing: An emerging issue. *Nursing Research, 32,* 347–349.

Harden, J. (2000). Language, discourse and the chronotope: Applying literary theory to the narratives in health care. *Journal of Advanced Nursing, 31,* 506–512.

Jacobs-Kramer, M. K., & Chinn, P. L. (1988). Perspectives on knowing: A model of nursing knowledge. *Scholarly Inquiry for Nursing Practice: An International Journal, 2*(2), 129–139.

Johnson, J. (1991). Nursing science: Basic applied or practical implications for the art of nursing. *Nursing Research, 14,* 7–15.

Leininger, M. (1985). *Qualitative research methods in nursing.* New York: Grune & Stratton.

Light, R., & Pillemer, D. (1982). Numbers and narrative: Combining their strengths in research reviews. *Harvard Education Review, 51*(1), 1–23.

Lock, L. F., Silverman, S. J., & Spirduso W. W. (2004). *Reading and understanding research* (2nd ed.). Thousand Oaks, CA: Sage.

Ludemann, R. (1979). The paradoxical nature of nursing research. *Image, 2,* 2–8.

MacPherson, K. I. (1983). Feminists methods: A new paradigm for nursing research. *Advances in Nursing Science, 5,* 17–25.

Maggs-Rapport, F. (2001). "Best research practice": In pursuit of methodological rigour. *Journal of Advanced Nursing, 35*(3), 373–383.

Meleis, A. (1985). *Theoretical nursing: Development and progress.* Philadelphia: Lippincott.

Meshier, E. (1979). Meaning in context: Is there any other kind? *Harvard Education Review, 49*(1), 1–19.

Moccia, P. (Ed.). (1986). *New approaches in theory development.* New York: National League for Nursing.

Morse, J. M. (1999). Qualitative methods: The state of the art. *Qualitative Health Research, 9,* 393–406.

Morse, J. M. (2002). Enhancing the usefulness of qualitative inquiry: Gaps, direction, and responsibilities. *Qualitative Health Research, 12*(10), 1419–1426.

Morse, J. M. (2003). Toward holism: The significance of methodological Pluralism. *International Journal of Qualitative Methods, 2*(3), Article 2.

Morse, J. M. (2004). Constructing qualitatively derived theory: Concept construction and concept typologies. *Qualitative Health Research, 14*(10), 1387–1395.

Munhall, P. (1986). Methodological issues in nursing: Beyond a wax apple. *Advances in Nursing Science, 8*(3), 1–5.

Munhall, P. (1992). Holding the Mississippi River in place and other implications for qualitative research. *Nursing Outlook, 10*(6), 257–262.

Munhall, P. (1993). Toward a fifth pattern of knowing: Unknowing. *Nursing Outlook, 41,* 125–128.

Munhall, P. (1994). *Qualitative research: Proposals and reports.* New York: National League for Nursing.

Munhall, P. (1997). De ja vu, parroting, buy-ins, and opening. In J. Fawcett & I. King (Eds.), *The language of nursing theory and metatheory.* Indianapolis, IN: Sigma Theta Tau International.

Newman, M. A. (1979). *Theory development in nursing.* Philadelphia: Davis.

Newman, M. A. (1986). *Health as expanding consciousness.* St. Louis, MO: Mosby.

Oiler, C. (1982). The phenomenological approach in nursing research. *Nursing Research, 31*(3), 178–181.

Oiler, C. (1986). Qualitative methods: Phenomenology. In P. Moccia (Ed.), *New approaches to theory development.* New York: National League for Nursing.

Omery, A. (1983). Phenomenology: A method for nursing research. *Advances in Nursing Science, 5*(2), 49–64.

Patterson, D., & Brogden, L. M. (2004). Living spaces for talk with/in the academy. *International Journal of Qualitative Methods, 3*(3), Article 2.

Reeder, J. (1987). The phenomenological movement. *Image, 19,* 150–152.

Sandelowski, M. (2004). Using qualitative research. *Qualitative Health Research, 14*(10), 1366–1386.

Sandelowski, M., & Barosso, J. (2002). Reading qualitative studies. *International Journal of Qualitative Methods, 1*(1), Article 2.

Sarter, B. (1988). Philosophical sources of nursing theory. *Nursing Science Quarterly, 1,* 52–59.

Silva, M. C. (1977). Philosophy, science, theory: Interrelationships and implications for nursing research. *Image, 9*(5), 59–63.

Stolorow, R., & Atwood, G. (2002). *Contexts of being: The intersubjective foundations of psychological life.* Hillsdale, NJ: Analytic Press.

Thorne, S., Joachim, G., Paterson, B., & Canam, C. (2002). Influence of the research frame on qualitatively derived health science knowledge. *International Journal of Qualitative Methods, 1*(1), Article 1.

Walters, A. J. (1996). Nursing research methodology: Transcending Cartesianism. *Nursing Inquiry, 3*(2), 91–100.

Watson, J. (1985). *Nursing: Human science and human care and theory of nursing.* Norwalk, CT: Appleton-Century-Crofts.

West, M. (1983). *The world is made of glass.* New York: Morrow.

3

Epistemology in Nursing

Patricia L. Munhall

Since we have come to the understanding that science is not a description of "reality" but a metaphorical ordering of experiences, the new science does not impugn the old. It is not a question of which view is "true" in some ultimate sense. Rather, it is a matter of which picture is more useful in guiding human affairs.
—Willis Harman, *Symposium and Consciousness*

I qualified in the preceding chapter that perhaps I might appear culpable of unnecessary polarization of worldviews; so I hope you will understand that this indulgence is for ease in conceptual clarity and pedagogical purposes. Furthermore, I could not agree more with Gould (1984) when he observed,

Dichotomy is the usual pathway to vulgarization. We take a complex web of arguments and divide it into two polarized positions—them against us. We then portray 'them' as a foolish caricature of extremes in order to put 'us' in a better light. (p. 7)

However, complex webs are starker when placed in contrasting systems; the differences between the systems become more focused. Our intention is not to see one system as the truth, but to see each as different. As Harman (1977) states, "It is not a question of which view is true [but which] is more useful in guiding human affairs." This is our connectedness with the subject. In this chapter, I propose an epistemology for nursing research that, as a whole, incorporates the qualitative and quantitative methods of research. This does not represent a conciliatory effort at compromise but rather a belief in a cyclical continuum that begins with discovery and moves toward verification. These activities represent, respectively, the first- and second-order activities of science. We believe there are appropriate research methods for different questions, and errors occur when a method is used prematurely or acontextually to answer a specific question or solve a problem. As was suggested in Chapter 2, there are times when many research traditions are amalgamated to produce a synthesis that is progressive to both traditions (Laudan, 1977). Perhaps at this time in our development we are witnessing a search for ontological and epistemological authenticity in which we recognize the multiplicity of perspectives and perception of reality and in which postmodernism "is an intellectual movement (and as such) challenges the ideas of a single correct approach to knowledge development, of a single truth, and has a single meaning of reality, rejecting the ideal that there is one true story about reality" (Uris, 1993, p. 95).

In this chapter, there will be an overview discussion of paths to knowledge, the purpose of science, research paradigms, and research traditions. I will attempt to answer the questions "Knowing about what?" and "How do we get to know?" as well as "Toward what end?" and will then propose a qualitative-quantitative cyclical continuum for knowing. Emphasis throughout is on qualitative research methods as beginning points. Too often we engage in experimental research before the variables significant to that research have been determined, or we conduct quantitative studies based on *our* knowledge of the world and not the knowledge of experiencers of phenomena. Currently, because of the situated context of the necessity of grant funding, we are witnessing once again the dominance of the scientific method for funding purposes. Following is from an e-mail message I received, not one word changed:

> I am putting together my tenure portfolio and feel great trepidation. There is such an emphasis on grants and, as you know, qualitative research does not receive much funding of note. Someone told me that without an NIH grant I am not going to get tenured. In the criteria for tenure, it does mention "evidence of external funding," and I did get a small grant from Sigma Theta Tau, but supposedly that does not count or measure up. I have actually received awards for my research but the secret message seems to be that the gold standard is the NIH grant. It's as though a wall is closing in on me, and I worry if I don't comply with doing quantitative research, which is the paradigm rewarded, I am not going to make it. Perhaps I should ask for an extension and quickly send in a grant proposal for a quantitative study, though it compromises who I am as a researcher. No. I believe in my work.
>
> —Sandy

This qualitative researcher in nursing recognizes and fears that what she wants to do, which should be the essence of academic freedom, is being corrupted by outside influences, one of which is the return of the dominance of quantitative research or the scientific method. Some nurse researchers argue this approach is essential to evidence-based practice. (This chapter as well as Chapters 1, 2, and 20 discusses how essential qualitative research is to evidence-based practice.)

From the preceding we also can ascertain the writer's concern for what she believes are the central values in nursing: caring and compassion. Indeed, even if you did not think they were central, most of us would agree that caring and compassion are high on the list of our aspirations.

Ironically, for any research enterprise to be authentic, we *must begin* with qualitative inquiry as a foundation from which we can identify variables, understand the context of experiences, and develop instrumentation. That is exactly the kind of research the preceding nurse researcher wants to do, and from my perspective we need to encourage and support this work if we are actually going to have research that is applicable. In this chapter, a theme as articulated by Morgan (1983) will guide us: "To steer clear of the delusion that it is possible to know in an absolute sense of 'being right' and devote our energies to the more constructive process of *dealing with the implication of our different ways of knowing*" (p. 18). I also envision a postmodern perspective where the necessity for and evolution of multiple paradigms for nursing research will create new possibilities of coming to understand and develop the knowledge that is necessary to nursing practice par excellence. This is the study of nursing epistemology, that branch of philosophy that deals with knowledge and how we come to know about the world as we experience it. P.S. Sandy received tenure *AND* special recognition for her research! "Times they are a changing."

PATHS TO KNOWLEDGE

Knowledge for nursing, about nursing, in nursing—where does this knowledge come from? In Chapter 2, I mentioned knowledge (theory) borrowed from related disciplines. Other disciplines are indeed sources of knowledge, perhaps more accurately called "shared knowledge" (Stevens 1979, p. 85): because disciplines have indistinct boundaries, there are areas "where the inquiries and answers of one field overlay those of another." At the turn of the 21st century, we have almost abandoned the term *borrowed theory*, recognizing the interconnectedness of various disciplines, and so today interdisciplinary research is encouraged by nurse researchers and sometimes is a requirement for funding. Wilson (1998) states this so clearly:

Most of the issues that vex humanity daily, ethnic conflict, arms escalation, overpopulation, abortion, environment, endemic poverty to cite several most persis-tently before us cannot be solved without integrating knowledge from the natural sciences with that of the social sciences and humanities." (p. 13)

However, caution must be used when integrating similarities from other disciplines and then utilizing those respective theoretical frameworks to derive hypotheses for nursing. We need to understand that if the first- and second-order activities are not from the same world or discipline, there is a risk that the inquiry will not be logically consistent or experientially valid. For example, if the first-order activities of coming to know, discovering, and understanding come from another discipline and from that discipline's perspective and the second-order activities of validation and verification are then performed within the nursing discipline and apply nursing's particular perspective, you can see the risk. Before we go further, however, let us in a foundational manner consider where knowledge generally comes from and some of the structures of knowing. In a pedantic fashion, philosophers who study the way that we come to know (epistemologists) have identified specific sources of knowledge, generally acceptable as structures of knowing. Among them are the following (Kneller, 1971):

1. **Revealed knowledge** — knowledge that God has disclosed. Revelations of truth are found in the Bible, the Koran, and the Bhagavad-Gita. In the past decade, we have seen a growth of research on spirituality — for example, religion as a source of comfort and inspiration; belief as having curative power; and so on. We do know that from revealed knowledge comes the imperative to care for and about one another.
2. **Intuitive knowledge** — knowledge within a person, in the form of insight that becomes present in consciousness; an idea or thought produced by a long process of unconscious work. This process of discovery is nurtured through experience with the world.
3. **Rational knowledge** — knowledge from the exercise of reason. This knowledge takes the form of abstract reasoning and is exemplified in the principles of formal logic and mathematics.
4. **Empirical knowledge** — knowledge formed in accordance with observed or sensed facts and associated with scientific hypotheses that are tested by observation or experiments.
5. **Authoritative knowledge** — knowledge accepted on faith because it is vouched for by authorities in the field.

In the foregoing brief description of the sources of knowledge, the one least attended to, but the one holding much potential for nursing, is intuitive knowledge, which for the purpose of this text will be experiential knowledge. The repudiation of intuition as a source of knowledge was one of the major themes when nursing moved toward establishing itself as a science. Intuition was unscientific; it was associated with women, who themselves were thought to be unscientific. More confident today, women of science—including nurses—recognize the vitalness of intuition and have come to trust and value this important source of knowledge.

Belenky, Clinchy, Goldberg, and Taub (1986), in describing the different ways in which women come to know, have legitimized to a great extent the place of intuition, personal meanings, and the connection to ideas as means of knowing. Rather than focusing on proof, these women scientists seek understanding. The work of Gilligan (1982), Belenky et al. (1986), and Freiri (1971) challenges us all to rethink our concepts about epistemology—underlying assumptions and the critical consequences. Critical theory (discussed in Chapter 5) is one way to analyze the underlying structural and power relations inherent in the sanctioned ways of knowing (Allen, 1991). Allen (1995) expands the importance of critique in his discussion of critical hermeneutics with great emphasis on the subjective reality that research can socially construct.

Carper's (1978) framework of four fundamental patterns of knowing, based on the work of Philip Phoenix, continues to this day to be a way in which nursing identifies its epistemological interests. These patterns of knowing are described as follows:

1. **Empirics**—the science of nursing; emphasis is on the generation of theory and of research that is systematic and controllable by factual evidence. Within this pattern of knowing, there is a need for emphasis on knowledge about the empirical world, knowledge that will be organized into general laws and theories for the purpose of describing, explaining, and predicting phenomena of concern to nursing.
2. **Esthetics**—the art of nursing; emphasis is on expressiveness, subjective acquaintance, individual perceptions, and empathy. Rather than uniformity and general laws, there is recognition of alternative modes of perceiving reality, which then clearly asks for a "many different ways" approach to designing and participating in nursing care.
3. **Personal knowledge**—the focus is on the importance of the interpersonal process and the "therapeutic use of self"; on knowing the self, knowing the other as a subject, and striving toward authentic personal relations.
4. **Ethics**—the focus is on matters of obligation or what ought to be done. Knowledge within this domain requires an understanding of

ethical theories, conditions of society, conflicts between different value systems, and ethical principles.

All of the foregoing patterns are rich and essential sources of nursing knowledge that can be studied from various perspectives of science.

I have suggested a fifth pattern of knowing, while at the same time questioning the categorization of knowledge in this way (Munhall, 1993). The fifth pattern is one of "unknowing." "Knowing," in contrast with "unknowing," leads to a form of confidence that has the potential of a state of closure to alternatives and differences. Unknowing, from an epistemological perspective, is a condition of openness and seems essential to the understanding of intersubjectivity and perspectivity (discussed further in Chapter 6). Kurtz (1989) states: "Knowledge screens the sound the third ear hears, so we hear only what we know" (p. 6). We can become limited by our own belief systems. Often, once we believe something or think we know something, we cease further exploration or explanation. Many practitioners in all fields will continue to hold the body of knowledge that they attained in their formal education. The impractibility and danger of continuing to do so in an unsurpassed age of knowledge explosion are apparent.

Only by unlearning comes wisdom.

—James Russell Lowell

Although the patterns of knowledge are presented for historical and pedantic reasons, they are organized as categories; I think we can see them as mutually interdependent, not mutually exclusive. Intuiting in the empirical world while using one's personal knowledge embedded in an ethical context or founded on a philosophical perspective is a holistic approach to theory development.

We move now from general structures of knowing to the purpose of exploring those structures. Because nursing has identified itself as a science, let us review the purpose of science or science in general. How does nursing conceptualize itself as a science?

PURPOSE OF SCIENCE

Laudan (1977), a philosopher, simply states that the purpose of science is to solve problems, and theory tells us how to do so. He further proposes that the rationality and progressiveness of a theory are not linked with its confirmation or its falsification but instead with its problem-solving effectiveness. This conception of science opens the windows and doors in the hallowed halls of science to include important nonempirical and even nonscientific knowing in the traditional sense. This provides a broader perspective that Laudan suggests is necessary to the rational development of science. Insight, spontaneity, accidental findings, mutability, vicissitude, and fortune all play a role in science.

On the basis of this conception of science and theory, it seems that all sources of knowledge and patterns of knowing are essential sources for problem solving. Nursing research, in its earliest years, began its quest to become a legitimate science with an almost unilateral pattern of knowing that can be categorized as empirics, logical empiricism, logical positivism, or, as described in most nursing research textbooks, the scientific method.

Laudan (1977) sets forth—in contrast or in explanation—a philosophy of science of historicism that incorporates the human elements of science; the study of scientific knowledge is often fostered by illogical and nonrational decision making. The following two quotations may illuminate this point:

> That no major scientist ever has proceeded in his work along either Baconian or Cartesian lines has not prevented the *consecration of method* by these two powerful minds from exacting a dismal toll. (Nesbitt, 1976, p. 14, italics added)

> Insight announces itself in mental images. Newton's conception of gravity and Einstein's notion of the constant speed of light came to them as perceptions, as images, not a hypothesis or conclusions drawn from logical deduction. Formal logic is secondary to insight via images, and is never the source of new knowledge. (Bohm, cited in Smith, 1981, p. 444)

van Manen (1990), in contrast with Laudan's emphasis on problem solving, summarizes what a phenomenological human science cannot do: "Phenomenology does not problem solve" (p. 23). van Manen believed, from a research perspective, that phenomenological questions are meaning questions. However, as addressed in Chapter 1, if we did understand the meaning of specific phenomena, might we not have the basis for problem solving? In fact, do we not have a responsibility to attempt to problem solve as Crotty (1996) maintained? Furthermore, might we also have understanding that could significantly contribute to the promotion of health and well-being? However, van Manen does not include problem solving when he states:

> Natural science studies objects of nature, 'things,' 'natural events' and the way that objects behave. Human science, in contrast, studies 'persons' or beings that have 'consciousness' and that act purposefully in and on the world by creating objects of 'meaning' and that are expressions of how human beings exist in the world. (p. 4)

Allen (1995) argues further that meaning, understanding, and interpretation gleaned from *acontextual research* will lead us back to foundationalism. He describes foundationalism as referring "to the claim that there is a way to anchor knowledge by referring to ahistorical, nonsocial, non-contextual criteria" (p. 175). This adds to Laudan's science of historicism, of not only incorporating the vicissitudes of the scientist, and so forth, but also to enlarge; what is necessary to knowing something is the essential nature of also knowing what is going on in the contingencies of history and life-worlds when that knowing something occurs (see Chapter 6 for further discussion). We return to the postmodern idea that truth is not immutable and is indeed an ever-changing body of ideas and meaning contingent on multiple factors.

These ideas are not necessarily contradictory; rather, they seem to be woven together as a whole. In addition, discussions about sciences and methods of sciences often seem to lead us away from concrete, lived experiences unless that lived experience is the discussion of sciences. Researchers, I believe, need to be well grounded in the pedantic and philosophical underpinnings of the research enterprise but not for conformity, which can sacrifice creativity. We suggest to students that it is far more scientific to find a phenomenon that interests them, piques their curiosity, and perhaps even fills them with passion than it is to become befuddled by method.[1] Substance should lead the way to form. Interest in some thing or experience should light many sparks of imagination and light the path to method.

However, it is essential to understand the influence and power of research paradigms and traditions in interweaving the ways of knowing and shaping them into a body of knowledge. They can be restricting or liberating, depending on their own ontology and supporting constituencies. Qualitative research methods seek to be of the liberating, illuminating, and emancipatory kind. The critical nature embedded in research paradigms and traditions is found in the circumstance that they are rarely questioned in the study of a discipline. It is a rare undergraduate or graduate student in any field who questions the research methods prevalent in that field. If most of us find guidelines helpful and a research tradition provides us with those guidelines—and if success within the field will be determined by how well one follows those guidelines—the importance of those guidelines can hardly be overstated! The next section describes the nature of research paradigms and traditions connected with our discussion of paths to knowledge and the purpose of science. It is paradoxical to hear the purpose of education to be one of liberation and then to hear students cite the common wisdom of "just do

---

[1] van Manen's (1990) interpretation of why Gadamer's (1975) book *Truth and Method* became popular in North America is relevant and recommended to readers.

what they tell you to do," subsuming to the unfair power structure that we often encounter in our educational settings.

PARADIGMS AND RESEARCH TRADITIONS

Kuhn (1970) believes that a paradigm structures the questions to be asked within a discipline and systematically eliminates those kinds of questions that cannot be stated within the concepts and tools supplied by the paradigm. This function then is enormously powerful. A paradigm can actually prevent questions from being answered!

Laudan (1977), elaborating on his definition of a research tradition, writes: "A research tradition is a set of general assumptions about the entities and processes in a domain of study, and about the appropriate methods to be used for investigating the problems and constructing the theories in that domain" (p. 81).

In both these ways, as suggested by Kuhn and by Laudan, the research paradigm and tradition will specify the domain of study, the legitimate modes, and the methods of inquiry open to a researcher within a discipline. This directedness is seldom questioned; in fact, complicity is usually required as well as rewarded.

Why one proceeds in this fashion is explained by Laudan's idea that we need to explore the scientists' work and their reasoning processes. Laudan suggests that scientific knowledge is often developed by illogical and nonrational decision making. Let us now tie together that idea with nursing's historical acceptance of the logical empiricist's worldview or, as stated, the large reliance on logic and empirics as our primary paths to theory development.[2]

The preparation of many nurse researchers in fields in which the research tradition was one of logical empiricism was considered in Chapter 2. Let us look for evidence that supports the further use of this tradition and that may exemplify the nonrational or illogical side of science. This evidence is not always negative, but let us reflect on nursing research and on the subtle and not so subtle ways in which this paradigm or tradition has been perpetuated and still prevails today.

The answers to the following questions, which were asked in the first edition of this book (1986), demonstrate how the values of scientists and their practices influence the general account of human nature. I believe it is quite significant that the same questions are relevant 20 years later. I attempted to

---

[2] Silva and Rothbart (1984) have written a most readable and highly recommended work synthesizing this material. Dzurec (1989), presenting a poststructural perspective, should also be considered.

explain the reason for their relevance in a discussion of life-world fittingness (Munhall, 1992):

♦ If you were to request a research grant from the Division of Nursing of the Department of Health and Human Services or the National Institute of Nursing Research (NINR)–National Institutes of Health (NIH), which research method do you believe would be viewed most favorably?

♦ If you wanted guidelines for doing research and consulted the most prevalent nursing research textbooks, which research method would seemingly be the only one available? What is the research method most taught in research classes?

♦ If you wish to submit an abstract of research for a research conference, which research method is represented in the format for the abstract?

♦ If you wanted to critique a research study, which method is most represented under criteria for evaluation?

Now in the fourth edition of this book, I might ask you to consider additional questions:

♦ If you are enrolled in a PhD program, which method do your required courses support and prepare you for? (There are exceptions!) We looked at this problem in Chapter 1.

♦ If you are seeking a faculty position, how will you get the evidence of extramural funding that is required to be demonstrated?

♦ Peruse the list of recent NINR grants and ask: Which paradigm is most rewarded?

For those nurse researchers who have been questioning the general acceptance of the answers to these questions, I suggest we enlarge our lens, broaden our scope, and widen our perspective. Furthermore, the answers to these questions demonstrate the subjectivity of the entire research enterprise. Human beings determine which paths to explore. We need to explore all the paths to knowledge and all the patterns of knowing because we would then be researching the whole of the human condition, both the subjective and objective worlds of our research endeavors.

Capra (1982) stated our need almost two decades ago:

What we need, then, is a new vision of reality—a fundamental change in our thoughts, perceptions and values. The beginnings of this change, of the shift from the mechanistic to the holistic conception of reality, are already visible in all fields and are likely to dominate the entire decade. (p. ix)

My endeavor here, built upon the works of many nursing scholars, among them the contributors to this book, is to encourage this vision, to incorporate the qualitative and quantitative methods of research as representative of an epistemology of wholeness, and to respect and reward all patterns of knowing. Despite the answers to the preceding questions, the processes and rewards of doing qualitative research certainly have continued to grow, and we have become more sophisticated and savvy. In fact, many NINR grants today require a qualitative section! That is progress. Yet, it still seems we qualitative researchers have to defend our work to a much greater extent. A friend said to me recently, "It is like they tolerate us." How unfortunate because I fear we will be left behind. When so many scholars are calling for this consilience, we need to heed their wisdom. Reread Wilson's quote in the section titled "Paths to Knowledge" and the preceding quote by Capra.

It has been said that your research question should determine your research method. Today I am not sure that is the best way to think about choosing a research method. Over many years, I have seen that students have specific leanings toward one or another way of thinking, as was discussed in Chapter 1. I believe these leanings reflect a natural attitude toward the world at large, and students—just as we acknowledge students have different ways of learning material—have different philosophical orientations toward questioning and how one answers those questions. I believe most of my colleagues respect these innate tendencies. Actually recognizing individuals as being more left-sided brain dominant and others as more right-sided brain dominant should make the whole research enterprise holistic, more consistent with the times in which we live, and contribute to a much greater depth and breadth of knowing and understanding. Our differences enrich us and inspire us to see the new.

Let us move now to a consideration of two epistemological questions: What is it that we want to know about? and What is it that we wish to understand?

EPISTEMOLOGICAL INTERESTS OF NURSING

As stated earlier, one of the purposes of science is to solve problems, and the subsequent theory development involves the solution of problems (Laudan, 1977). Qualitative researchers can qualify that purpose with the caveat that, before you can solve a problem, you need to understand the many facets of a problem. In this section, we explore schemata that have been developed by nurses in an effort to focus nursing research on nursing phenomena.

Six nursing perspectives are summarized in an effort to identify our epistemological interests. They are presented chronologically and may demonstrate consistency, overlap, complementarity, and/or much variation. Also they are presented here as a demonstration of our historical evolution. I begin with Paterson and Zderad, out of great respect for their major groundbreaking work of 1976, in which they were the first nurses to actually use the language and the method of phenomenology. It is important to understand these different perspectives so that one can debate the merits or lack of merit of the various perspectives. Each provides varying answers to the question, "What do nurses study?" We will also reexamine the ideas of Donaldson and Crowley (1978), the American Nurses Association's Social Policy Statement (1995), Fawcett's (1984) metaparadigm for nursing, and the emphasis on care (Newman, Sime, & Corcoran-Perry, 1991; Watson, 1985). We conclude with Watson's (1999) ideas of what nurses should be studying at the beginning of this new century. This summary does not do justice to the field of theory development, nor does it intend to; the intent of this section is to consider exemplars and a historical perspective. Undoubtedly, if you are reading this book, you probably are very knowledgeable about theory and can ask, "What does a particular theorist think we should 'know' and 'how' should we research particular phenomena?" These questions could provide a good seminar discussion.

Paterson and Zderad (1976), to the question "What do nurses study?" (or "What should nurses study?"), might reply in this manner. Because the act of nursing is "the intersubjective transactional relation, a dialogue experience, lived in concert between persons where comfort and nurturance produce mutual human unfolding," nurses would do well to study the following situations (Paterson, 1978, p. 51):

♦ Comfort—persons being all that they can be in particular life situations
♦ Nurturance—promoting growth through relating
♦ Clinical—presence in the health situation, reflected and acted upon
♦ Empathy—imaginative moving toward oneness with another, sharing his or her being in a situation, resulting in an insightful knowledge of another's perspective
♦ All-at-once awareness—awareness of living many concepts, emotions, desires, and beliefs in a particular instance

From these situations, the phenomenon of concern to nurses is the need for quality nursing descriptions of those experiences inherent in the preceding situations and suggested in Table 2–7 in Chapter 2. Paterson and Zderad (1976) call our attention to existential, humanistic, phenomenological phenomena that should be our epistemological interests. This they did in 1976, and you can see how future oriented they were. I urge students of current theory to read through their pioneering book, which was reissued in 1988.

Widely cited and more traditional, yet showing promises of a new world-view, were Donaldson and Crowley (1978), who identified three major themes of nursing:

1. Concern with the principles and laws that govern the life processes, well-being, and optimal functioning of human beings, sick or well.
2. Concern with the patterning of human behavior in interaction with the environment in critical life situations.
3. Concern with the processes by which positive changes in health status are affected.

Concepts within the nurse–client world that relate to the preceding themes need to be discovered, and the methods of the first order of scientific activity, the qualitative methods of science, are essential to this process. Within this book, an effort is made to demonstrate this basic activity of discovering what is there, naming it, understanding it, and explaining it. We can then give examples of what is meant and what is the potential within the scope of these themes.

Our own professional organization, the American Nurses Association, has consistently revised its definition of nursing according to society's needs and has focused nurse researchers' perspectives on human responses within the following context: "Nursing is the diagnosis and treatment of human responses to actual or potential health problems" (American Nurses Association, 1995). Possible phenomena that bear investigation from this perspective of nursing are further suggested, including the following:

♦ Self-care limitations
♦ Impaired functioning—physiological needs
♦ Pain and discomfort
♦ Emotional problems, such as anxiety, loss, loneliness, and grief
♦ Distortion of symbolic functions
♦ Deficiencies in decision making
♦ Self-image changes
♦ Dysfunctional perceptual orientations
♦ Strains related to life processes
♦ Problematic affiliative relations

Readers familiar with the works of Rogers (1970), Roy (1976), Johnson (1980), Orem (1980), King (1981), Watson (1985), and other nursing theorists can readily see the influence of these theorists on the various phenomena that would constitute human responses.

Fawcett (1984) identifies in her earlier works a metaparadigm for nursing in pursuit of establishing boundaries within which the purview of nursing can be delineated. She proposes that the metaparadigm comprises the central concepts and themes that represent the phenomena of interest to the discipline. Paradigms, then, are the conceptual models that provide "distinctive contexts for the metaparadigm concepts and themes" (p. 2).

The metaparadigm of nursing that has evolved, according to Fawcett (1984, p. 2), consists of four major concepts: person, environment, health, and nursing. These central concepts are defined as follows:

1. Person—the recipient of care
2. Environment—significant others and the surroundings of the recipient of care; the setting in which nursing care takes place
3. Health—the wellness or illness state of the recipient at the time when nursing occurs
4. Nursing—actions taken by nurses on behalf of or in conjunction with the recipient of care

Fawcett (1984) adds the themes explicated by Donaldson and Crowley, presented earlier, to the metaparadigm of nursing by indicating the central concepts and the themes that should represent the phenomena of interest to nurse investigators. She then suggests that the four patterns of knowledge, as discussed by Carper (1978) and in this chapter, link the concepts and themes. With these varying perspectives have come articles that call for a focus of the discipline of nursing. Newman et al. (1991) point out that nursing's domain of inquiry distinguishes it as a discipline. As is readily apparent in the foregoing paragraph, nursing has a rather large domain of inquiry. Newman et al. (1991) suggest that nursing should have a focus statement. They point out that, from the time of Florence Nightingale to the present era of Leininger (1984), Watson (1988), and Benner and Wrubel (1989), health and caring have been linked. Incorporating Pender's (1987) use of the term *health experience*, Newman's focus statement at the time was this: "Nursing is the study of caring in the human health experience" (p. 3).

Nursing's domain of inquiry was then stated as "caring in the human health experience" (p. 3). Present-day perspectives in nursing research and theory seem to have evolved from this eclecticism of thought. This eclecticism is philosophically congruent with the world at large. Today the prefixes *multi* and *poly* are frequently used to reflect the shift from foundationalism to hermeneutics, or interpretation of phenomena. Newman (1986) and Watson (1999) are among the many nursing scholars who have expanded the worldview of nursing and the domains for nursing inquiry. Postmodern in their perspectives, they recognize that whatever is studied must be viewed within the context and possibility of multiple realities. The idea that individuals, families, cultures, and societies construct their own realities is readily evident in a world that all of a sudden has found itself so interconnected — that what we hear is polyvocality, what we see is individually perspectival, and what we read is contextually interpreted. Multiple realities are recognized as being based on subjective experience; so multiplicity and multimind emerge. Qualitative researchers are most synchronous with these conditions of uncertainty, flux, discontinuity, and indeterminacy. Qualitative researchers have long recognized the social construction of reality, contingencies, and the situated context as critical parts of their research efforts. This topic will be further considered in the next section, but, for our purposes here, whatever domains or phenomena nurses want to research, it is most important for them to take into account the situatedness of a person in a multi-world of endless variations.

We should enjoy the complexity of our profession because it affords us an opportunity to study and research an almost infinite variety of human and environmental phenomena. Some could say we are "all over the place"; and, in actuality, nurses themselves are all over the place, in every developmental phase of an individual's life, in health and in crisis, in private practice, in schools, in hospitals, in foreign countries, and in the homes of patients. They are practitioners, educators, administrators, writers, researchers, and politicians. With all this complexity, it is quite understandable why nurses would need a variety of research methods or approaches from which to choose.

EPISTEMOLOGICAL COMMITMENTS TO QUALITATIVE RESEARCH

In the foregoing discussion, I present different perspectives on what nurses might investigate. The broad scope reflects the expansiveness of the profession of nursing. Discussions among theorists and researchers often revolve around narrowing this scope, perhaps by adopting one model or accepting, for equally good reasons, a multiple-perspective approach. I do not think we have any choice but to be representative of the world, and, being in the world, that demands a multiperspectival epistemological commitment. In Chapter 2, I defined quantitative methods of research as ". . . the traditional scientific methods as presented in most of the contemporary nursing research textbooks. These methods are characterized by deductive reasoning, objectivity, quasi-experiments, statistical techniques, and control." In contrast, I defined the qualitative methods, many of which are described in this text, as "characterized by inductive reasoning, period, subjectivity, discovery, description, and process orienting." Benoliel (1984) enhances that description in this observation: "Qualitative approaches in science are distinct modes of inquiry oriented toward understanding the unique nature of human thoughts, behaviors, negotiations and institutions under different sets of historical and environmental circumstances" (p. 7).

We should view these two approaches from a historical perspective. During the 17th century, empiricism, as the scientific method, reigned supreme. That form of empiricism proceeds through sense knowledge, and that which connects with our senses is matter. This often is the origin of conceived objectivity, in which the physical world can be seen, touched, or measured. The hold that matter (materialism) has on us is connected with the simple fact that we think we can get hold of matter and control it. Thus, we have the controlled experiment with validation, significance, and the premises of confidence and prediction. As has been suggested, nursing research has, to a large extent, aligned itself with this positivistic and materialistic view of science. In the 1993 edition of this book, I discussed the postpositivistic perspective articulated by Polkinghorne (1983), who cited recognition and acceptance of the following factors as enlarging the scope of science:

♦ Different language systems reflect different perceptions of the same reality (as was illustrated in Chapter 2).
♦ The essential study of complex wholes is through system theory, and human beings are complex wholes.
♦ The ideas of purposive and intentional activity explain human action.
♦ *All knowledge, instead of being truth, is an expression of interpretation.* (italics added)

Such beliefs and assumptions have contributed to the acceptance of the worthiness and credibility of methods of knowing other than the positivistic worldview. Additionally, there has been growing acceptance and recognition of the differences between the material and the experiential nature of human behavior and relationships. Benoliel (1984) cites some of these differences as follows:

♦ Social life is the shared creativity of individuals and their *perceptions.* (emphasis added)
♦ The character of the social world is *dynamic* and *changing.* (emphasis added)
♦ There are *multiple realities* and frameworks for viewing the world: the world is not independent of humankind and objectively identifiable. (emphasis added)

- ◆ Human beings are active agents who *construct their own realities.* (emphasis added)
- ◆ There are not any response sets that are highly predictable. (p. 4)

Since that earlier edition, one can easily see how these ideas have come to expression in most contemporary philosophies of nursing. Because the emergent nursing philosophies reflect, whether stated or not, poststructualist or postmodern perspectives, the stated beliefs and values about the individual are congruent with the research methods presented in this text. We are involved in an emergent shift from the modern characteristics of science to a postmodern perspective of science. This shift is not a negation of science but recognition of a "more." Science expands its boundaries from strict materialism and recognizes the need for accommodating a dynamic reality and describing individual situatedness to be essential to good research.

The shifts that are most prevalent in the qualitative domain are the focus on meaning of experience; understanding what it means to be in this world, or that world; listening to others to provide us with this material; and interpretation by both the research participant and the researcher. Contrary to the traditional scientific method, where the problem is stated at the outset of the research project by the researcher, the qualitative researcher usually begins with a phenomenon or an experience. Going to the people who are involved in the phenomenon or experience, the qualitative researcher engages with the participant and the environment and lets both speak to her or him. The narratives, semiotics, and interaction allow for the development of coming to understand some "thing." Problems may emerge as part of the wholeness of the experience, but the identification of a problem comes from the source, the individual in experience.

This involvement calls for the nurse researcher to have many characteristics. It is important for qualitative researchers to grasp the complexity of experience, of its wholeness. Rather than compartmentalizing experience into two or three different variables, which may be necessary in experimental research, experience needs to be met with openness by the researcher. In addition to being open, *the researcher needs to be the one who is unknowing.* The participant is the expert who is imparting to the researcher existential material that should be *co-interpreted and then interpreted for its implications* for nursing practice.

Before specific questions for research are formulated, overarching questions and commitments should guide researchers in choosing a research method. What is it that interests you? Do you think of yourself as more concrete and more comfortable with structure? Do you like discovering relations, correlations, and possible solutions to problems? Do you find beauty in a perfect scientific design with complex statistical analysis? If you have these propensities, then what we are calling quantitative designs are probably what you will enjoy doing and be successful at, as well as contributing to nursing's body of knowledge.

Those considering qualitative research methods need to be more comfortable with uncertainty and unpredictability. The primary focus is on meaning, and the aims of inquiry are found in understanding and interpretation. A critical commitment is to faithfully, without your own presuppositions or judgments, represent another's experience, meaning, and interpretation. There needs to be an authentic caring about how another person perceives his or her world, and there needs to be authentic respect for many differences, as was discussed in Chapter 1.

These considerations do not in any way imply that a nurse researcher cannot combine these commitments. Indeed many hold all these commitments toward research. Yet, in the years of my own experience, students and researchers seem to show different ways of being in the world, and one should reflect on and recognize one's leanings before embarking on learning a specific method, which is its own commitment.

And that brings us to considering the last commitment in this section. This text is an overview, as are many textbooks. If you are interested and excited about a specific method, this is your first step: read the particular chapter on that method and the following exemplar. The real commitment is to further in-depth study of the particular method; its philosophical, ontological, theoretical, and conceptual underpinnings; and the human requirements, abilities, and characteristics needed to implement the method well. With more and more reading and practice, you will evolve, change, have your own insights, and truly understand what you are doing in a way that becomes a part of you. The first meaning, understanding, and interpretation are those of the experience itself, those of grasping the wholeness and complexity of the method.

An Epistemological Circle

Questions are often asked about the relatedness of quantitative and qualitative methods, if there is a relation at all. Chapter 24 addresses this question. The following epistemological circle is offered as one perspective. This conceptualization is one of process and demonstrates how theory evolves, is revised by a nuance, and is first discovered through qualitative inquiry and validated in some way by quantitative inquiry. Quantitative inquiry in a human science, I believe, should always have its origins in qualitative inquiry. Otherwise, the researcher is the knower of the experience and the phenomenon, and therefore, whatever instrument is developed or intervention tested, it is grounded in the life-world of the researcher rather than in the life-world of those experiencing knowers who can inform, through their sharing with us, the descriptions and interpretations necessary for congruency grounded in specific contexts.

My own dissertation was an example of not following this sequence. Using an instrument, which was derived and tested on an all-male population, Kohlberg (1976) derived a theory on moral development. Unknowingly, I used this instrument on women, an instrument based on his theory, and the women participants performed much "lower" in scores than the norms. The norms, I did not realize, were based on only males, and only males were utilized to develop and evaluate the instrument. After Carol Gilligan's (1982) groundbreaking work, *In a Different Voice,* I came to realize why my own sample of nurses did not seem to fare so well.

I wrote an article critiquing my own study and illustrating that using a theory and instrument derived from another population is a serious epistemological error. The article was rejected by a nursing research journal on the grounds "that the last thing we need in nursing research is criticizing ourselves." The manuscript did find a home (Munhall, 1982), and I do hope it called attention to the need for this epistemological circle and the thorough thinking through of any method, as well *as the critical need for self-critique of one's research.*

In this nonlinear schema, qualitative descriptions, interpretations, and understandings lead to quantitative analysis (when that is appropriate), and from that analysis, nuances, or what Kuhn (1970) terms anomalies, become sources of further qualitative inquiry. For example, many studies statistically support the proposition that preoperative teaching reduces anxiety for the majority of preoperative patients. Such teaching increases anxiety in some patients, however. This is a nuance and calls us back to a qualitative study: "What about those patients?" We need to discriminate further within our populations. Theories always need reevaluating, and the nuances or the exceptions often alert us to alternative or evolving ways of viewing phenomena. Thus, the qualitative-quantitative cyclical continuum represents the dynamic and changing life-worlds. The linkages of the qualitative and quantitative methods are circular, as shown in Figure 3–1. *This circularity does not have to be the outcome of all qualitative research.* The findings of qualitative research can stand on their own merit with implications for nursing practice found in the descriptions, interpretations, and narratives by the researcher. However, for congruency in arriving at a hypothesis, a qualitative base line from the same situated context—that is, people, place, time, culture, sex, and other characteristics—should be the origin of good quantitative research. Perhaps Campbell (1975) summarizes this point best when he says:

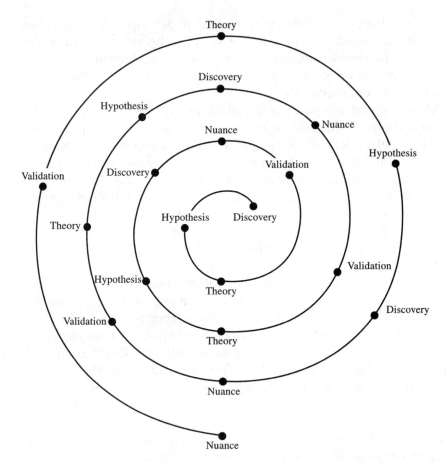

FIGURE 3–1 Qualitative-quantitative cyclical continuum. A nuance is defined here as a variation or a subtle aspect or quality.

After all, man in his ordinary way is a very competent knower, and qualitative common sense is not replaced by quantitative knowing. Rather quantitative knowing has to trust and build on the qualitative, including ordinary perception. We methodologists must achieve an applied epistemology which integrates both. (p. 191)

SUMMARY

I hope that you hold with me a belief in the rich potential that qualitative methods of research have to offer to our practice and our understanding of ourselves, our patients, the multiworlds in which we live, and what it means to be human at this time in history. I think we have come to understand the importance of the subjective experience of the one who experiences to the development of nursing theory. In Chapters 2 and 3, I have attempted to provide the background necessary for you to understand the differences in language, the philosophical perspectives, and the contexts in which nursing research first developed and continues to grow and evolve. Additionally, an effort has been made to explicate patterns of knowing, the purpose of science, what it is we want to know about, how we go about knowing, and what commitments are needed to engage in qualitative research.

REFERENCES

Allen, D. (1991). Applying critical social theory to nursing education. In N. Greenleaf (Ed.), *Curriculum revolution: Redefining the student–teacher relationship.* New York: National League for Nursing.

Allen, D. (1995). Hermeneutics: Philosophy, traditions, and nursing practice research. *Nursing Science Quarterly, 8*(4), 175–181.

American Nurses Association. (1995). *Nursing: A social policy statement.* Kansas City, MO: Author.

Belenky, M., Clinchy, B., Goldberg, N., & Taub, J. (1986). *Women's ways of knowing.* New York: Basic Books.

Benner, P., & Wrubel, J. (1989). *The primacy of caring.* Menlo Park, CA: Addison-Wesley.

Benoliel, J. (1984, March). Advancing nursing science: Qualitative approaches. *Western Journal of Nursing Research in Nursing and Health, 7,* 1–8.

Campbell, D. J. (1975). Degrees of freedom and the case study. *Comparative Political Studies, 8,* 178–193.

Capra, Z. (1982). Foreword. In L. Dossey (Ed.), *Space, time and medicine* (p. ix). Boulder, CO: Shambhala.

Carper, B. A. (1978, October). Fundamental patterns of knowing in nursing. *Advances in Nursing Science, 1,* 13–23.

Crotty, M. (1996). *Phenomenology and nursing research.* South Melbourne, Australia: Churchill Livingston.

Donaldson, S. K., & Crowley, D. M. (1978). The discipline of nursing. *Nursing Outlook, 26,* 113–120.

Dzurec, L. (1989). The necessity for and evolution of multiple paradigms for nursing research: A poststructural perspective. *Advances in Nursing Science, 11*(4), 69–77.

Fawcett, J. (1984, October). Hallmarks of success in nursing research. *Advances in Nursing Science, 7,* 1.

Freiri, P. (1971). *Pedagogy of the oppressed.* New York: Seaver.

Gadamer, G. H., Sheed & Ward, Ltd. (1975). *Truth and method.* New York: Crossroad.

Gilligan, C. (1982). *In a different voice: Psychological theory and women's development.* Cambridge, MA: Harvard University Press.

Gould, S. J. (1984, August 12). Review of the book *Science and gender*. *New York Times Book Review*.

Harman, W. (1977). *Symposium and consciousness*. New York: Penguin.

Johnson, D. E. (1980). The behavioral system model for nursing. In J. P. Riehl & C. Roy (Eds.), *Conceptual models for nursing practice* (2nd ed.). Norwalk, CT: Appleton-Century-Crofts.

King, I. M. (1981). *A theory for nursing: Systems, concepts, process*. New York: Wiley.

Kneller, G. (1971). *Introduction to the philosophy of education*. New York: Wiley.

Kohlberg, L. (1976). Moral stages and moralization. In T. Lickona (Ed.), *Moral development and behavior*. New York: Holt, Rinehart and Winston.

Kuhn, T. S. (Ed.). (1970). *The structure of scientific revolutions*. Chicago: University of Chicago Press.

Kurtz, S. (1989). *The art of unknowing*. Northvale, NJ: Aronson, Inc.

Laudan, L. (1977). *Progress and its problems: Toward a theory of scientific growth*. Berkeley: University of California Press.

Leininger, M. (Ed.). (1984). *Care: The essence of nursing and health*. Thorofare, NJ: Slack.

Morgan, G. (1983). *Beyond method*. Newbury Park, CA: Sage.

Munhall, P. (1982). Methodic fallacies: A critical self appraisal. *Advances in Nursing Science, 5*(4), 41–47.

Munhall, P. (1992). Holding the Mississippi River in place and other implications for qualitative research. *Nursing Outlook, 10*(6), 257–262.

Munhall, P. (1993). Toward a fifth pattern of knowing: Unknowing. *Nursing Outlook, 41*, 125–128.

Nesbitt, R. (1976). *Sociology as an art form*. New York: Oxford University Press.

Newman, M. (1983, January). Editorial. *Advances in Nursing Science, 5*(2), x–xi.

Newman, M. (1986). *Health as expanding consciousness*. St. Louis, MO: Mosby.

Newman, M., Sime, A., & Corcoran-Perry, S. (1991). The focus of the discipline of nursing. *Advances in Nursing Science, 14*, 1–5.

Orem, D. E. (1980). *Nursing: Concepts of practice* (2nd ed.). New York: McGraw-Hill.

Paterson, J. (1978). The tortuous way toward nursing theory. In *Theory development: What, why and how?* New York: National League for Nursing.

Paterson, J., & Zderad, L. (1976). *Humanistic nursing*. New York: Wiley.

Pender, N. J. (1987). *Health promotion in nursing practice*. Norwalk, CT: Appleton-Lange.

Polkinghorne, D. (1983). *Methodology for the human sciences*. Albany, NY: SUNY Press.

Rogers, M. E. (1970). *An introduction to the theoretical basis of nursing*. Philadelphia: Davis.

Roy, C., Sr. (1976). *Introduction to nursing: An adaptation model*. Englewood Cliffs, NJ: Prentice Hall.

Silva, M., & Rothbart, D. (1984, January). An analysis of changing trends in philosophies of science on nursing theory development and testing. *Advances in Nursing Science, 6*(2), 1–12.

Smith, H. (1981). Beyond the modern Western mind set. *Teachers College Record* (Columbia University), 82(3), 444.

Stevens, B. J. (1979). *Nursing theory: Analysis, application, evaluation*. Boston: Little, Brown.

Uris, P. (1993). Postmodern feminist emancipatory research. Unpublished doctoral dissertation, University of Colorado, Denver.

van Manen, M. (1990). *Research on lived experience: Human science for action-sensitive pedagogy*. New York: SUNY Press.

Watson, J. (1985). *Nursing: The philosophy and science of caring*. Boulder: Colorado Associated University Press.

Watson, J. (1988). New dimensions of human caring theory. *Nursing Science, 1*(4), 175–181.

Watson, J. (1999). *Post modern nursing and beyond*. New York: Churchill Livingstone.

Wilson, E. (1998). *Consilience*. New York: Knopf.

ADDITIONAL REFERENCES

Anderson, W. (1995). *The truth about truth*. New York: Putnam.

Appleton, J. V., & King, L. (1997). Constructivism: A naturalistic methodology for nursing inquiry. *Advances in Nursing Science, 20*(2), 13–22.

Arslanian, C. (1998). Taking the mystery out of research: Qualitative nursing research. *Orthopaedic Nursing, 17*, 31.

Ashworth, P. D. (1997). The variety of qualitative research (Part 2): Non-positivist approaches. *Nurse Education Today, 17*, 219–224.

Atkinson, P., Coffey, A., & Delamont, S. (2003). *Key themes in qualitative research: Continuities and changes*. New York: Rowman & Littlefield.

Bohm, D. (1998). *On creativity*. New York: Rutledge.

Bolster, A. (1983). Toward a more effective model of research on teaching. *Harvard Education Review, 53*(3), 294–308.

Boulton, M., & Fitzpatrick, R. (1994). Quality in qualitative research. *Critical Public Health, 5*(3), 19–26.

Brenner, P. (Ed.). (1994). *Interpretive phenomenology: Embodiment, caring, and ethics in health and illness*. Thousand Oaks, CA: Sage.

Bunkers, S. S., Petardi, L. A., Pilkington, F. B., & Walls, P. A. (1996). Challenging the myths surrounding qualitative research in nursing. *Nursing Science Quarterly, 9*, 33–37.

Byrne, M. M. (2001). Evaluating the findings of qualitative research. *AORN Journal, 73*(3), 703–706.

Carey, M. A., & Swanson, J. (2003). Funding for qualitative research. *Qualitative Health Research, 13*(6), 852–856.

Carnevale, F. A. (2002). Authentic qualitative research and the quest for methodological rigour. *Canadian Journal of Nursing Research, 34*(2), 121–128.

Charmaz, K. (2004). Premises, principles and practices in qualitative research: Revisiting the foundations. *Qualitative Health Research, 14*(7), 976–993.

Clark, A. M. (1998). The qualitative-quantitative debate: Moving from positivism and confrontation to post-positivism and reconciliation. *Journal of Advanced Nursing, 27*, 1242–1249.

Cook, S. D. N., & Brown, J. S. (1999). Bridging epistemologies: The generative dance between organizational knowledge and organizational knowing. *Organization Science,* 10(4), 381–400.

Coyle, J., & Williams, B. (2000). An exploration of the epistemological intricacies of using qualitative data to develop a quantitative measure of user views of health care. *Journal of Advanced Nursing, 31,* 1235–1243.

Cutliffe, J. R., & Mckenna, H. P. (2002). When do we know that we know? Considering the truth of research findings and the craft of qualitative research. *International Journal of Nursing Studies, 39*(6), 611–619.

Dahlberg, K., & Drew, N. (1997). A lifeworld paradigm for nursing research. *Journal of Holistic Nursing, 15,* 303–317.

Diers, D. (1979). *Research in nursing practice.* Philadelphia: Lippincott.

DiGiacomo, S. M. (1992). Metaphor as illness: Postmodern dilemmas in the representation of body, mind and disorder. *Medical Anthropology, 14,* 109–137.

Drew, N., & Dahlberg, K. (1995). Challenging a reductionistic paradigm as a foundation for nursing. *Journal of Holistic Nursing, 13,* 332–345.

Efinger, J., Maldonado, N., & McArdle, G. (2004). PhD students' perceptions of the relationship between philosophy and research: A qualitative investigation. *Qualitative Report, 9*(4), 732–759.

Estabrooks, C., Rutakumwa, W., O'Leary, K., Profetto-McGrath, J., Milner, M., Levers, M., & Scott-Findlay, S. (2005). Sources of practice knowledge among nurses. *Qualitative Health Research, 15*(4), 460–476.

Farrel, G. A., & Gritching, W. L. (1997). Social science at the crossroads: What direction mental health nurses? *Australian New Zealand Journal of Mental Health Nursing, 6,* 19–29.

Findlay, S. (2005). Sources of practice knowledge among nurses. *Qualitative Health Research, 15*(4), 460–476.

Forbes, D. A., King, K. M., Kushner, K. E., Letourneau, N. L., Myrick, A. F., & Profetto-McGrath, J. (1999). Warrantable evidence in nursing science. *Journal of Advanced Nursing, 29,* 373–379.

Frank, A. W. (2004). After methods, the story: From incongruity to truth in qualitative research. *Qualitative Health Research, 14*(3), 430–440.

French, P. (2002). What is the evidence on evidence-based nursing? An epistemological concern. *Journal of Advanced Nursing, 29*(1), 72–78.

Greene, G., & Freed, S. (2005). Research as improvisation: Dancing among perspectives. *Qualitative Report, 10*(2), 276–288.

Hall, E. O. C. (1996). Husserlian phenomenology and nursing in a unitary-transformative paradigm. *Vard-I-Norden Nursing Science and Research in the Nordic Countries,* 16(3), 4–8.

Holliday, A. (2001). *Doing and writing qualitative research.* London: Sage.

Hones, M. L. (2004). Application of systematic review methods to qualitative research: Practical issues. *Journal of Advanced Nursing, 48*(3), 271–278.

Irving, J., & Klenke, K. (2004). Telos, Chronos, and Hermeneia: The role of metanarrative in leadership effectiveness through the production of meaning. *International Journal of Qualitative Methods, 3*(3), Article 3.

Johnson, D. E. (1978). State of the art of theory development. In *Theory development: What, why, how?* (p. 9). New York: National League for Nursing.

Kearney, M. H. (2001). Levels and application of qualitative research evidence. *Research in Nursing and Health, 24*(2), 145–153.

Letourneau, N., & Allen, M. (1999). Post-positivistic critical multiplism: A beginning dialogue. *Journal of Advanced Nursing, 30,* 623–630.

Light, R., & Pillemer, D. (1982). Numbers and narrative: Combining their strengths in research reviews. *Harvard Education Review, 52,* 1–23.

Lincoln, Y., & Guba, E. (1985). *Naturalistic inquiry.* Newbury Park, CA: Sage.

Lutz, K. F., Jones, K. D., & Kendall, J. (1997). Expanding the praxis debate: Contributions to clinical inquiry. *Advances in Nursing Science, 20*(2), 23–31.

Madjar, I., Taylor, B., & Lawler, J. (2002). The role of qualitative research in evidence based practice. *Collegian, 9*(4), 7–9.

Mantzoukas, S. (2004). Issues of representation within qualitative inquiry. *Qualitative Health Research, 14*(7), 994–1007.

Marks, M. D. (1999). Network. Reconstructing nursing: Evidence, artistry and the curriculum . . . including commentary by L. Nyatanga & M. Johnson. *Nurse Education Today, 19,* 3–11.

McAllister, M., & Rowe, J. (2003). Blackbirds singing in the dead of night? Advancing the craft of teaching qualitative research. *Journal of Nursing Education, 42*(7), 296–303.

Monti, E. J., & Tingen, M. S. (1999). Multiple paradigms of nursing science. *Advances in Nursing Science, 21*(4), 64–80.

Morse, J. (2005). Decontextualized care. *Qualitative Health Research, 15*(2), 143–144.

Morse, J., & Chung, S. (2003). Toward holism: The significance of methodological pluralism. *International Journal of Qualitative Methods, 2*(3), Article 2.

Morse, J. M. (1999). Qualitative methods: The state of art. *Qualitative Health Research, 9,* 393–406.

Munhall, P. (1982a). Nursing philosophy and nursing research: In apposition or opposition? *Nursing Research, 31*(3), 176–177, 181.

Munhall, P. (1982b, April). Ethical juxtapositions in nursing research. *Topics in Clinical Nursing, 4,* 66–73.

Munhall, P. (1986). Methodological issues in nursing: Beyond a wax apple. *Advances in Nursing Science, 8*(3), 1–5.

Munhall, P. (1989). Philosophical pondering on qualitative research methods in nursing. *Nursing Science Quarterly, 2,* 20–28.

Munhall, P. (1992). A new ageism: Beyond a toxic apple. *Nursing and Health Care, 13,* 370–376.

Munhall, P. (1994a). *Qualitative research: Proposals and reports.* New York: National League for Nursing.

Munhall, P. (1994b). *Revisioning phenomenology: Nursing and health science research.* Sudbury, MA: Jones and Bartlett.

Munhall, P. (1997). Déjà vu, parroting, buy-ins, and opening. In J. Fawcett & I. King (Eds.), *The language of nursing theory and metatheory.* Indianapolis, IN: Sigma Theta Tau International.

Munhall, P. (1998). Qualitative designs. In P. Brink & M. Wood (Eds.), *Advanced designs in nursing research* (2nd ed.). Newbury Park, CA: Sage.

Munhall, P. (2000a). *Qualitative research reports and proposals: A guide.* Sudbury, MA: Jones and Bartlett.

Munhall, P. (2000b). Unknowing. In W. Kelly & V. Fitzsimons (Eds.), *Understanding cultural diversity.* Sudbury, MA: Jones and Bartlett.

Munhall, P., & Oiler, C. (1986). *Nursing research: A qualitative perspective.* Norwalk, CT: Appleton-Century-Crofts.

Munhall, P., & Oiler, C. (1993). *Nursing research: A qualitative perspective* (2nd ed.). Sudbury, MA: Jones and Bartlett.

National Institutes of Health. (2001). *Qualitative methods in health research: Opportunities and consideration in application and review* (NIH Publication No. 02-5046). Washington, DC: Author.

Norris, C. (1982). *Concept clarification in nursing.* Rockville, MD: Aspen.

Oakey, A. (2004). Qualitative research and scientific inquiry. *Australian and New Zealand Journal of Public Health, 28*(part 2), 106–108.

Plack, M. (2005). Human nature and research paradigms: Theory meets physical therapy practice. *Qualitative Report, 10*(2), 223–245.

Reichardt, C., & Cook, T. (Eds.). (1979). *Qualitative and quantitative methods in evaluation research* (pp. 33–48). Beverly Hills, CA: Sage.

Rorty, R. (1991). *Essays on Heidegger and others.* New York: Cambridge University Press.

Sandelowski, M. (1995). On the aesthetics of qualitative research: *Image: Journal of Nursing Scholarship, 27*(3), 205–209.

Sandelowski, M. (2002). Reembodying qualitative inquiry. *Qualitative Health Research, 12*(1), 104–115.

Sandelowski, M. (2004). Using qualitative research. *Qualitative Health Research, 14*(10), 1366–1386.

Sandelowski, M., & Barroso, J. (2002). Finding the findings in qualitative studies. *Journal of Nursing Scholarship, 34*(3), 213–219.

Schultz, P. R., & Meleis, A. I. (1988). Nursing epistemology: Traditions, insights, questions. *Image: Journal of Nursing Scholarship, 20*(4), 217–221.

Silva, M. C. (1997). Classic image. Philosophy, science, theory: Interrelationships and implications for nursing research. *Image: Journal of Nursing Scholarship, 29*(3), 210–215.

Thorne, S. E., Kirkham, S. R., & Henderson, A. (1999). Ideological implications of paradigm discourse. *Nursing Inquiry, 6*(2), 123–131.

Thorne, S., Jensen, L., Kearney, M., Noblit, G., & Sandelowski, M. (2004). Qualitative metasynthesis: Reflections on methodological orientation and ideological agenda. *Qualitative Health Research, 14*(10), 1342–1365.

Tobin, G. A., & Begley, C. M. (2004). Methodological rigour within a qualitative framework. *Journal of Advanced Nursing, 48*(4), 388–396.

Turner, D. S. (2003). Horizons revealed: From methodology to method. *International Journal of Qualitative Methods, 2*(1), Article 1.

Wainwright, S. P. (1997). A new paradigm for nursing: The potential realism. *Journal of Advanced Nursing, 26*, 1262–1271.

Waterman, H. (1998). Embracing ambiguities and valuing ourselves: Issues of validity in action research. *Journal of Advanced Nursing, 28*(1), 101–105.

Watson, J. (1995). Postmodernism and knowledge development in nursing. *Nursing Science Quarterly, 8*(2), 60–64.

Wilson, L., & Fitzpatrick, J. (1984, January). Dialectic thinking as a means of understanding systems in development: Relevance to Rogers' principles. *Advances in Nursing Science, 6*(2), 41.

4

Historical and Philosophical Foundations of Qualitative Research

Marcia Dombro

INTRODUCTION

Qualitative research is not a method; it is a philosophical approach that over-arches many different ways of collecting and analyzing data. Phenomenology, grounded theory, ethnography, case study, historical research, narrative inquiry, and action research are some examples. All of these are explained and exemplified in Part II of this book. This chapter is a genealogy of the philosophers who influenced what we know as the qualitative approach to research. According to Munhall (1989):

> The philosophical underpinnings of qualitative research methods reflect beliefs, values and assumptions about the nature of human beings, the nature of the environment and the interaction between the two. A nurse researcher doing qualitative research would perceive reality and assign meaning to his or her research efforts from the perspective of some of the following assumptions:
>
> ♦ Individuals are viewed within an open perspective in that they are active agents, interpreting their own experience and creating themselves by their inner existential choices.

♦ Individuals and specific groups of individuals have varying histories, varying here-and-nows, and varying perceptions of the future. The world and its people are constantly changing and evolving: this assumes a dynamic reality.

♦ "Truth" is an interpretation of some phenomenon; the more shared that interpretation is, the more factual it seems to be yet it remains temporal and cultural. Exploration may be partially "true" depending on certain variable conditions and then only "true" for specific individuals.

♦ Interacting with subjects does not mean the suspension of "objectivity." "Objectivity" is the simultaneous realization of as much reliability and validity as possible (Kirk & Miller, 1986, p. 20). Objectivity itself can be viewed as a subjective discovery, a perception of its own.

♦ The subjective experience of the individual and/or groups is valued and described. Meaning comes from the source and is not presumed, assumed, or assigned.

♦ Experience is imbued with meaning with linguistic, social and cultural patterning. (p. 22)

When a researcher chooses a qualitative approach, a philosophical position is taken about what is real (metaphysics), what is true (epistemology), and what is of value (axiology). These age-old questions are answered in different ways by different philosophers and schools of thought, creating *paradigms* or mental models of the world and how it works. This chapter surveys the tangled web of philosophers who grappled with these questions and influenced the qualitative approach to research.

Each generation of thinkers is influenced by previous philosophical thought and by world events that occur during a thinker's own lifetime. Thinkers are also strongly affected by their teachers, colleagues, and friends. Albert Einstein (1939) said:

There is . . . such a thing as a spirit of the times, an attitude of mind characteristic of a particular generation, which is passed on from individual to individual and gives a society its particular tone. Each of us has to do his little bit towards transforming this spirit of the times. (p. 14)

This transformation of knowledge is what nursing researchers are striving for and toward which they make their individual contributions.

THE LANGUAGE OF PHILOSOPHY: ISMs, ICs, AND OLOGIES

Quantitative and qualitative approaches to research have different methods of discovering and different ways of reporting the truth of those discoveries.

The quantitative approach uses mathematics and statistics as a universal language to express what is viewed as the truth. Preconceived ideas or hypotheses are a beginning point. Then collected data, symbols, and signs are converted via mathematics to higher levels of abstraction. The result of this kind of research is an aggregate of data, which does not represent the experience of any one individual.

Qualitative research, on the other hand, aims to allow the questions and the data to reveal themselves as they are in a natural system, which may be a "culture" or the "life-world" of an individual, to reveal and to understand that which may be hidden from everyday awareness. Language is viewed as the route to discovering essences, those ineffable qualities that cannot be expressed with numbers.

Some philosophers, such as Martin Heidegger, who influenced qualitative research, found that everyday language was inadequate and created new words (neologisms) and expressive systems. Just as one needs to learn mathematics and statistics to understand quantitative research, qualitative researchers must learn a new descriptive system and syntax.

Reading philosophical texts can be frustrating because of the many unfamiliar terms that are used to describe esoteric concepts, but discovering their meaning is mind-expanding. An "ism" is a doctrine, school, or theory; an "ist" is a person who follows an "ism." The art, science, or study of something has the suffix "-ics," for example, "hermeneutics." Another suffix standing for the study of something is "ology," for example, "psychology." Table 4–1 is a brief (and incomplete) list of definitions that can be used as a quick reference.

This chapter is a brush stroke of a very complex and fascinating history. Table 4–2 shows the philosophers who will be discussed. Each one was chosen because his ideas are interconnected and all eventually had an influence on the present-day approaches to qualitative research. The interested student is strongly encouraged to use the reference list to deepen understanding. Many of the older works are freely available in full text on the Internet.

The philosophers who will be discussed were most often trained in religion, philosophy, mathematics, or physics. They all faced questions of what is real (metaphysics), what is true (epistemology), and what is of value (axiology). (See Table 4–3.) The first metaphysical question (ontology) must have been about what it means to be alive or not alive. Beyond simply existing or not existing, it is clear that being and living are not the same from one individual to the next. Being is a state of reality. What constitutes reality for one person may not hold for another. Developing a personal understanding of what "being" means is of great importance to nurses who are constantly involved in the birth, growth, decline, and death of individuals. Ontological questions are often topics for qualitative research in nursing. Here are some

---

TABLE 4–1   Abbreviated Definitions of Philosophical Concepts

---

Apologia. Defense of one's opinions, positions, or actions.

A priori. Prior to, or independent of experience; contrasted with a posteriori (empirical). (Audi, 1999, p. 35)

Deduction. Logic that flows from the general to the specific.

Determinism. "The view that every event or state of affairs is brought about by antecedent events or states of affairs in accordance with universal causal laws that govern the world." (Audi, 1999, p. 228)

Dialectic. The art or practice of examining statements logically, as by question and answer, to establish validity, for example, Hegel's dialectic-thesis, antithesis, synthesis, opinions.

Dualism. The idea that there is an unbridgeable gap between mind and body as separate substances with different properties.

Emic perspective. Understanding social and cultural systems in the way that people themselves see them. The people native to a society have an emic understanding of its culture. (http://www.emic.biz/)

Emic/Etic. "Relate to the cultural specificity or universality of knowledge or truths. An emic refers to results or findings of studies that appear to differ across cultures; thus, an emic refers to culture-bound or culture-specific truths.

Etic perspective. "Refers to results and findings that seem to be consistent across cultures, and therefore refers to universal truths." (http://www.uri.edu/artsci/psy/harris/lab.htm)

Experimentalism. Use of empirical or experimental methods in determining the validity of ideas. (Funk & Wagnalls, 1976/1979)

Induction. Logic that flows from the specific to the general.

Linguistics. The scientific study of language.

Lived experience. The reciprocal relationship between the respondent and the environment as he or she sees it. "Qualitative research can take the researcher into the mind and life of the respondent." (McCracken, 1988, p. 54)

Materialism. The metaphysical view that only physical matter and its properties exist. Mind is considered to be part of and dependent upon matter.

Ontology. "The branch of metaphysics dealing with the philosophical theory of reality." (Funk & Wagnalls, 1976/1979, p. 457)

Rationalism. "The position that reason has precedence over other ways of acquiring knowledge." (Audi, 1999, p. 771)

Reductionism. Phenomena can be analyzed and understood by reducing them to their component parts, such as Cartesian reductionism: of the whole to its parts.

Reductionistic explanation. Explanation in terms of the simplest elements that constitute a given phenomenon.

TABLE 4–1   continued
Relativism. There are many "truths" and many correct views of reality.
Semantics. The study of the underlying meanings of words and word groups.
Syllogism. Pairs of propositions that, taken together, give a new conclusion. Aristotle describes it as "a discourse in which, certain things being stated, something other than what is stated follows of necessity from their being so." (Aristotle Book I, Part I, para 4)
Transcendentalism. Any of several doctrines holding that reality is essentially mental or spiritual in nature, and that knowledge of it can be attained by intuitive or a priori, rather than empirical principles. (Funk & Wagnalls, 1976/1979, p. 719)

examples: How does it feel to be a new mother with postpartum depression? What goes on in a family where there is a child who has a developmental disability? What is it like to be aware of one's own decline into Alzheimer's disease? What is the experience of student nurses who care for patients who are nearing death?

TABLE 4–2 The Philosophers	
(515–? BC) Parmenides	(1838–1917) Franz Brentano
(480?–411? BC) Protagoras	(1844–1900) Friedrich (Wilhelm)
(470–399 BC) Socrates	Nietzsche
(427–347 BC) Plato	(1857–1913) Ferdinand de Saussure
(384–322 BC) Aristotle	(1859–1938) Edmund Husserl
(AD 205–270) Plotinus	(1889–1951) Ludwig Josef Wittgenstein
(1561–1626) Francis Bacon	(1889–1976) Martin Heidegger
(1596–1650) René Descartes	(1900–2002) Hans-Georg Gadamer
(1724–1804) Immanuel Kant	(1905–1980) Jean-Paul Sartre
(1768–1834) Friedrich Schleiermacher	(1908–1961) Maurice Merleau-Ponty
(1770–1831) Georg Hegel	(1913–2005) Paul Ricoeur
(1813–1855) Soren Kierkegaard	(1926–1984) Michel Foucault
(1813–1911) Wilhelm Dilthey	(1929–) Jurgen Habermas
(1818–1883) Karl Marx	(1930–) Jacques Derrida

TABLE 4–3 Philosophies Influencing Qualitative Research

	Metaphysical Beliefs (What Is Real?) A world of:	Epistemological Beliefs (What Is True?) Truth as:	Axiological Beliefs (What Is of Value?)		Philosophers	
			Ethics	Aesthetics	Names	Influenced by:
Idealism	Mind	Idea	Imitation of the supreme being	Reflection of the ideal	Socrates, Plato, Aristotle, Kant, Hegel	Greeks
Rationalism	Knowledge coming from the ability to reason	A priori and self-evident	Universal truths, e.g., right and wrong	Human progress coming from reason	Plato	Socrates
Empiricism	Senses/experience, sole source of knowledge	What works	The public test	The public taste	Bacon, Locke, Berkeley, Hume, Mills	Aristotle St. Thomas Aquinus
Existentialism	Existing	Existential choice	The anguish of freedom	The revolt from the public norm	Kierkegaard, Sartre, Heidegger	Hegel
Structuralism	Mental structures	Language	Structures of society are reorganized	Parallels between art and language	Wittgenstein, Habermas	Vienna Circle
Causal interactionism	Mind/body interactions	Mind and body are mutually exclusive	The good as discerned by reason	The wonder of complexity	Descartes	Plato

Dialectical materialism	Senses/experience, which precede ideas	Thesis-antithesis-synthesis	Constant conflict between what is right and what is wrong	Logical consistency	Kant, Engels, Hegel	Greeks, Spinoza, Rousseau, Kant, Schelling, Holderlin
Functionalism	Systems interacting	What is useful, practical, pragmatic	Religious beliefs reinforce social solidarity	A smoothly functioning society	William James, Dewey, Durkheim	Charles Darwin Chicago School
Critical theory	Domination and authority in society	Undistorted ways of thinking	Human freedom	Pacify radical inclinations	Habermas, Adorno	Marx, Freud, Frankfurt School Derrida
Logical positivism	No "mentalistic" concepts	Experience and empirical knowledge	Philosophy adheres to the rigor of science	Meaningful statements are defined	Wittgenstein	Vienna Circle

ANCIENT PHILOSOPHERS

The qualitative approach to research is strongly rooted in both modern and ancient philosophies, with strands of thought that interlace, disappear, and then recur across the centuries. The ancient philosophies endure because they are basic to the human condition and are just as inspiring today as they were when they were first recorded more than 2,500 years ago. Many of the ancient philosophers were physicians and scientists with multiple interests. While they tried to discover how the world worked, they looked at what is real (metaphysics), what is true (epistemology), and what is of value (axiology). In their search for the nature of reality, they divided "being" into (1) a world of material existence and the perceptions of the senses (empiricism); and (2) a world of ideas and the perceptions of the mind (rationalism).

Greek Philosophers

Parmenides of Elea (ca. 515–450 BC) "was the first Greek thinker who can properly be called an ontologist or metaphysician" (Audi, 1999, p. 646). Solomon and Higgens (1996) report that Parmenides "argued [his bold claims], . . . attempted to demonstrate [them], and . . . expected, indeed, invited counter arguments in return" (p. 26). This pattern is still being repeated as other philosophers construct their ideas in response to what has gone before. Parmenides also said that "nothing can change, and that our sensory perceptions must therefore be unreliable. His contemporary, Heraclitis [of Ephesus (500 BC)], on the other hand, said that everything changes ('all things flow'), and that our sensory perceptions are reliable" (Gaarder, 1996, p. 35). This foundational argument is still being played out in our own time in the discussions about the truth-value of quantitative versus qualitative research. The quantitative approach says that only mathematics in the form of statistical measures represents "true" science and that perceptions are not scientific or reliable. The qualitative approach says that numbers cannot express the essence of the life-world and perceptions about it. The goals and aims of qualitative and quantitative research have different concepts of the word "truth."

Protagoras (490–420 BC) gives us the first traces of thought about the importance of language and subjectivity. He was a proponent of (1) agnosticism: we cannot know anything about the gods; (2) relativism: "Man is the measure of all things," in other words, knowledge is relative to the knower; and (3) orthoepeia: the study of the correct use of words. "He emphasized how human subjectivity determines the way we understand, or even construct, our world, a position which is still an essential part of the modern philosophic tradition" (Poster, 2005, para. 1).

Socrates (470–399 BC) disagreed with what he viewed as the moral relativism of Protagoras. He began the search for transcendent (ideal) forms or knowledge, which could somehow anchor moral judgment. These ideals (axiological beliefs) define what is of value. They determine how we use our resources, and they constitute the yardstick by which we live our lives.

The dialogues of Socrates and his student Plato (429–347 BC) "applied the method of going back from current knowledge and belief of his time to the justification for every proposition" (Dilthey, 1988, p. 184). Socrates' opening position in every discussion was: "I know nothing except the fact of my ignorance" (Diogenes, AD 3/1959). He preferred talking to writing, so Plato was obliged to remember what Socrates said to preserve it for posterity. Plato's "The Meno" describes the dialectical method of Socrates, by which he demonstrates his contention that all knowledge exists in the mind "a priori" or independent of experience. It is the first recorded discussion of epistemology, which examines how we know what we know and its corollary, the nature of truth.

Socrates chose to lead a slave boy through the steps of a geometric proof, because geometry was considered to be the cutting edge of science at that time. The boy finds the right answer, which proves that he had the knowledge without being told. Socrates claimed that this knowledge came from a past life. "For Plato, the soul—or mind—obtained knowledge through recollection of [ideal forms]. By doing this the soul was simply returning to the state of knowledge which it had before birth" (Dennett, 2005, para. 3). He saw the mind as identical with the soul, as did Descartes in later centuries.

Plato's "Allegory of the Cave" illustrates his belief that we live our everyday lives "in bondage to superficialities, [and] to shadow rather than to substance. Truth is taken to be whatever is known by the senses. . . . We are unaware that we are living with illusion, superficial knowledge, and false and conflicting ideals" (Lavine, 1984, p. 29).

Aristotle (384–322 BC) was a student in Plato's school "the Academy of Athens" (385 BC–AD 529), which produced many and varied philosophers. Those who considered themselves Plato's followers were called "Platonists." Gaarder (1996) describes Aristotle as "Europe's first great biologist." He was preoccupied with nature's changes and processes. These were not of much concern to his teacher, Plato, which sparked many of Aristotle's thoughts on philosophy (p. 107). "Aristotle [an empiricist] pointed out [in contrast to Socrates and Plato] that nothing exists in consciousness that has not been first experienced by the senses. Plato [a rationalist] said that there is nothing in the natural world that has not first existed in the world of ideas" (Gaarder, 1996, p. 108). In his Nichomachean Ethics Aristotle (350 BC/2004) says: "To be conscious that we are perceiving or thinking is to be conscious of our own existence." This foreshadows Descartes' famous statement in his *Discourse on Method* (1867/1950) "I think, therefore, I am" *(Cogito ergo sum)*.

Aristotle was "a meticulous organizer who set out to clarify . . . concepts. . . . He demonstrated a number of laws governing conclusions or proofs that were valid" (Gaarder, 1996, p. 112). For example: If I first establish that "every nurse is a person who cares" (first premise), and then establish that "Kelly is a nurse" (second premise), I can then conclude, "Kelly is a person who cares" (final premise). He also proposed the concept that the earth was the center of the universe and consisted of four elements: earth, water, air, and fire. One can see how science has evolved and that what was long thought to be the truth can eventually be turned on its head. "The scientific knowledge of antiquity was systematized and organized by Aristotle, who created the scheme which was to be the basis of the Western view of the universe for [more than a thousand years]" (Capra, 1983, p. 21). He also laid the groundwork for the empiricism and inductive reasoning in the scientific method of Francis Bacon, discussed later.

NEOPLATONISM: AD 3RD CENTURY TO 20TH CENTURY

Interpretations of the ideas of Aristotle and Plato evolved over the centuries and were consolidated by a Roman philosopher Plotinus (AD 205–270) into what was called Neoplatonism. He disagreed with Plato's concept of ideas as the link between God and the material world. Plotinus believed in a kind of world intelligence called "nous" that flows from God and then into the souls of humans, animals, and material things. This divided humans into two worlds, one of pure intelligence and the other of the senses. He believed that union with God or "nous" could occur only by abandoning the world of the senses by meditation and purification.

The Neoplatonist Saint Augustine of Hippo (AD 354–430) was strongly inspired by a work of Plotinus called *The Enneads.* Saint Augustine combined Christian and Greco-Roman philosophies to influence profoundly the cosmology and epistemology of the Middle Ages. "He emphasized the role of belief as opposed to understanding, pointing out that we must believe many things that we cannot understand but also that belief is a necessary condition of understanding" (Mendelson, 2000, para. 11). Most of the populace could not read and depended on the Church for much of their information about the world. This is an excellent example of situated context or contingency, which is discussed in Chapter 6. Learning was concentrated in religious institutions where clerics had access to and could read Latin texts. These were copied by hand to preserve ancient knowledge. Part of this work was translation and analysis of Biblical texts to better understand their meaning, which was the beginning of what we now know as hermeneutics.

Books were not available to the general public until 1450 when the printing press was invented. By 1492, a Latin translation of *The Enneads* of Plotinus had been printed, which caused a renewed interest in Neoplatonism and in other Greek and Latin texts. The printing of *The Enneads* in 1492 and other Greek texts in 1580 challenged Christian doctrines and caused a "successful revival of Platonic philosophy" (O'Meara, 1993, p. 113).

MODERN PHILOSOPHERS: 16TH TO 20TH CENTURIES

The terms *modern, modernity,* and *modernism* refer to the rejection of traditional doctrines. During the Renaissance, there was an explosion of efforts to explain and explore the world in new ways.

> In every field of physical science, men were learning that nature's apparently chaotic processes had pattern and regularity and . . . could be controlled. . . . There was an effort to look for a pattern, an order within the apparent disorder of a changing world. (Blitzer, 1967, p. 13)

Frances Bacon (1561–1626) encouraged thinkers to break free of the constraints of the Church and of Aristotle's view of the world.

> To take the place of the established tradition . . . (scholasticism, humanism, and natural magic), he proposed a . . . new system based on empirical and inductive principles [from fact to axiom to law] . . . whose ultimate goal would be the production of practical knowledge for 'the use and benefit of men.' (Simpson, 2005, para. 1)

The famous quote "knowledge is power" comes from his essay "Religious Meditations, of Heresies" (1597).

René Descartes (1596–1650), in his very readable essay "Discourse on Method," stated that if he could conceive of anything clearly and distinctly, through deductive logic, then he could rely upon it as being true and build the rest of knowledge on it. Descartes gave four rules for reasoning: (1) accept nothing as true that is not self-evident; (2) divide problems into their simplest parts; (3) solve problems by proceeding from simple to complex; and (4) recheck the reasoning. His system of thought has defined science for centuries. His followers were called "Cartesians." "Throughout the 17th and 18th centuries, [philosophers like] Locke, Hume, Leibniz and even Kant felt compelled to [argue about the ideas of] this philosophical giant. For these reasons, Descartes is often called the 'father' of modern philosophy" (Burnham, 2005, para. 4).

ENLIGHTENMENT PERIOD—THE AGE OF REASON: END OF 17TH CENTURY TO END OF 18TH CENTURY

Immanuel Kant (1724–1804) and his fellow thinkers who called themselves "idealists" "wanted men to shake off the hand of authority in politics and religion and think for themselves. . . . Although they knew one another and corresponded, they did not always think alike. . . . They had in common, a critical attitude toward all orthodoxy" (Gay, 1966, p. 11). Kant made sweeping revisions in nearly all branches of philosophy. He is important to the qualitative approach to research because, as Jones and Wilson (1987) write: "he believed that the human mind . . . has an inherent structure through which we filter all experience and which imposes its own order on the world of phenomena (though not on the real/ideal world of 'things-in-themselves,' which is unknowable)" (p. 316). Today, the field of cognitive neuroscience is still looking for ways that human behavior is ordered.

ROMANTIC MOVEMENT—ENGLAND: 1798–1840

Romanticism or the "romantic revolution" was a reaction to the controlling rationalism of the Enlightenment. Romantics gave central importance to "the creative imagination as the only true source of order in the world, the poet, rather than the philosopher or the theologian, becomes the chief interpreter of reality. . . . Poets, Shelley affirmed, are the unacknowledged legislators of the world" (Johnston, 1999).

The following well-known poem by William Wordsworth (Wordsworth & Coleridge, 1798) captures the spirit of the Romantic movement (and perhaps how the reader of this text might feel about now):

The Tables Turned

Up! Up! My friend, and quit your books,
Or surely you'll grow double.
Up! Up! My friend, and clear your looks;
Why all this toil and trouble. . . .

Books! 'Tis a dull and endless strife:
Come, hear the woodland linnet,
How sweet his music! On my life,
There's more of wisdom in it. . . .

One impulse from a vernal wood
May teach you more of man,
Of moral evil and of good,
Than all the sages can.

Sweet is the lore which Nature brings;
Our meddling intellect
Misshapes the beauteous forms of things—
We murder to dissect.

Enough of Science and of Art,
Close up those barren leaves;
Come forth, and bring with you a heart
That watches and receives.

"We murder to dissect" has always been a powerful slogan against mechanical science (Johnston, 1999, para. 7).

HERMENEUTICS

Hermeneutics is a word from the Greek, meaning "to interpret or translate." The Bible was translated with a process of "exegesis," which involves critical interpretation to draw out the meaning of a given text. The word comes from the Latin verb *exigere*, meaning "to weigh or measure." Hermeneutics, as opposed to exegesis, is the theory, rather than the practice, of interpretation. The hermeneutic circle is the process of repeatedly returning to a text, or to the world, and finding a new interpretation of it each time we, or someone else, sees it.

Friedrich Schleiermacher (1768–1834) is considered to be the earliest developer of hermeneutics as a discipline of study. He was a Protestant theologian who studied the classic philosophers and translated Plato. He was a contemporary of other German philosophers such as Georg Hegel, Immanuel Kant, and Friedrich Von Schlegel.

His friend Von Schlegel (1772–1829) was a leading German Romantic philosopher who wrote about Greek and Roman antiquity. His work as a literary critic may have influenced Schleiermacher's conception of the hermeneutic circle. In later centuries, this also influenced the work of Dilthey, Gadamer, and Ricoeur.

Wilhelm Dilthey (1813–1911) was a philosopher and historian of philosophy. He was a great admirer of Friedrich Schleiermacher as "the father of scientific hermeneutics" (Dilthey, 1988, p. 27). He was in agreement with Schleiermacher that learning was being dominated by the "objective" natural sciences. His book *Introduction to the Human Sciences* was an effort to establish a "subjective" science of the humanities, which he called "Geisteswissenschaften," or the human sciences.

Georg Wilhelm Friedrich Hegel (1770–1831) was interested in the history of philosophy and in constructing a grand system that would explain everything. He admired and emulated Kant and was variously influenced by the Greek philosophers, by Spinoza, Rousseau, and his college friends, the poet Holderlin and the philosopher Schelling. His best-known work is *The Phenomenology of Spirit* (1807), in which he shows that history reveals a dialectical pattern. Appiah (2003) describes it this way: "A systematic theory [is developed] . . . called a 'thesis.' Then it is challenged . . . by . . . supporters [of] the antithesis; finally, a new view develops [taking] what is best of each to produce a new synthesis. . . . The new idea . . . 'transcends' the old debate, moving it to a higher level" (pp. 378–379). Hegel thought that this would then lead to new thesis-antithesis-synthesis discussions, which would take philosophy closer to absolute truth. Therefore, movement or progress is the result of the conflict of opposites. Although he wrote in a rather obscure style, and invented his own words, by the end of the 19th century, he had a significant following of "Hegelians." Jones and Wilson (1987) say: "They embraced, theoretically, the notion of Change, accepted Strife as essential to Progress, saw things as Parts of a Whole, and themselves as characters in the Unfolding of History" (p. 317). Lavine (1984/1989) calls Hegel "the principal historic, philosophic source of existentialism and phenomenology" (p. 397). Later, existentialists like Kierkegaard and Sartre conceived some of their ideas as refutations of Hegelianism. Phenomenology has been profoundly influenced by Hegel's ideas on consciousness, whose terminology later appeared in the work of Heidegger. For example: "the essential reality of that which has being-for-itself is not in an 'other' . . . [it] is self-existence. The Absolute is being in-and-for itself, and is thus an absolute negation of otherness" (Hegel, 1967, p. 86).

In 1859, Darwin's book *On the Origin of Species* sold out on its first day of publication. The new concept of evolution, as well as discoveries in psychology, archaeology, and ancient history required people to interpret history and religion in different ways. In the process of being freed from tradition, there grew up a general sense of insecurity and "anomie," where behavioral norms were confused, unclear, or not present.

> Meaning was lost at an escalating scale when . . . values were severed from their anchors in tradition with nothing to replace this former solid ground. Freedom was lost when reason started to objectify humans, making them cogs in rational, efficient human organizations. (Carspecken, 2004, p. 12)

This school of thought is critical to understanding an alternative way of viewing humans as subjective beings embedded in their own contexts.

Karl Marx (1818–1883) was one of the most influential thinkers of all time. He was a Hegelian and admired the dialectical method. He emphasized the importance of economics as an organizing factor in social systems and the struggle between rulers and oppressors. Marx and Engels (1845) wrote that

> the French Enlightenment of the eighteenth century, . . . was not only a struggle against the existing political institutions . . . religion and theology; it was a . . . struggle against the metaphysics of the seventeenth century, and against all metaphysics, in particular that of Descartes. Para. 3)

"[His] world of mathematical properties . . . could only be grasped by the intellect and . . . was entirely at odds with the false testimony of the senses" (Levi-Strauss, 1978, p. 4). Human needs and feelings did not enter into the equation. Marxist philosophy influenced Jean-Paul Sartre's existentialism and the development of critical theory of the Frankfurt School in the early 20th century.

Friedrich Nietzsche (1844–1900) was a philosopher and classical philologist (a student of religion, classical languages, and literature) who was an admirer of Kant. His primary concern was with a fundamental problem, which he viewed as "pervasive intellectual and cultural crisis. . . . [He called this the] 'death of God' and the advent of 'nihilism.' Traditional religious and metaphysical ways of thinking were on the wane, leaving a void that modern science could not fill and endangering the health of civilization" (Audi, 1999, p. 613). Nietzsche "believed in life, creativity, health, and the realities of the world we live in, rather than . . . the world beyond. Central . . . is the idea of 'life-affirmation,' which [questions] all doctrines, which drain life's energies, however socially prevalent those views, might be" (Wicks, 2004, para. 1). Nietzsche had many detractors, some of whom objected to his book *The Antichrist* (1926), in which he says:

> What is good? All that heightens the feeling of power in man, the will to power, power itself. What is bad? All that is born of weakness. What is happiness? The feeling that power is growing, that resistance is overcome." (Section 2)

"Nietzsche indisputably insisted upon the interpretive character of all human thought; and he called for 'new philosophers' who would follow him in engaging in more self-conscious and intellectually-responsive attempts to assess and improve upon prevailing interpretations of human life" (Audi, 1999, p. 615). He influenced existential writers such as Heidegger, Camus, and Sartre. His wide-ranging thoughts are often quoted.

PHENOMENOLOGY

Phenomenology, existentialism, and the people named along with them overlapped in time and were identified in both "movements." Many of the phenomenologists were also considered existentialists, although some did not want to be designated in this way.

Dreyfus (1999b) describes phenomenology as a "philosophical movement dedicated to describing the structures of experience as they present themselves to consciousness, without recourse to theory, deduction, or assumptions from other disciplines such as the natural sciences" (para. 1). van Manen (1990) says: "Phenomenology is the study of the lifeworld—the world as we immediately experience it pre-reflectively rather than as we conceptualize, categorize or reflect on it" (p. 9).

Franz Brentano (1838–1917), philosopher and psychologist, sought to establish "philosophy as a rigorous science . . . [He] is generally regarded as the philosopher who reintroduced [from its origins in Aristotle and Aquinus] the concept of 'intentionality' [which will be discussed in Chapter 6] into modern philosophy—a concept later characterized by Husserl as the principal subject of phenomenology" (Münch, 1997, pp. 71–75). (See also Siewert, 2003.) Brentano was a teacher of both Edmund Husserl and Sigmund Freud.

Edmund Husserl (1859–1938), in his book *Ideas: General Introduction to Pure Phenomenology* (1913), presented a rigorous program for the systematic investigation of things as they appear to consciousness. "Consciousness [is] important as the unique source of our knowledge, [but we must] transcend the . . . limitations of ordinary experience in order to fathom the . . . reality that underlies it. It was this version of phenomenology that most significantly influenced the philosophy of Martin Heidegger" (Deely, 1968, p. 293). It also gave rise to Gestalt psychology.

Max Scheler (1874–1928) was a student of Wilhelm Dilthey and was influenced by Franz Brentano and the followers of Edmund Husserl. Scheler's major work was *The Nature of Sympathy* (1970). Frings (2005) notes that

> Scheler criticized the well known positions held by Husserl, Kant, and the ideas of German Idealism. It is the human 'heart' or the seat of love, rather than a transcendental ego, reason, a will or sensibility, that accounts for the essence of human existence. (para. 4)

Cline (2005) notes: "Some of Scheler's ideas include the concept of the individual person not as an object or thing, but rather as a 'doer'—that which takes action and engages life" (para. 2). Scheler's ideas were greatly respected by his peers, who considered him to be an important force in philosophy during his lifetime.

EXISTENTIALISM

From 1813 to 1900, industrialization changed the quality of European life. Factories and control of production led to an increasing dehumanization of individuals who had moved to the cities. Marx, Nietzsche, and Kierkegaard lived through this time period. Although their philosophies diverged widely, they all perceived the Western world to be approaching a time of crisis. "They all address their philosophies to the coming crisis—they offer a diagnosis of their own time and a prescription for what ought to be done" (Lavine, 1989, p. 325).

Soren Kierkegaard (1813–1855) is viewed as the originator of existentialism, which evolved, in part, because of his antipathy to the prevailing philosophy of Hegelianism. His book *Concluding Unscientific Postscripts to Philosophical Fragments* (1992) documented his disagreement with Hegel's global and abstract philosophical system. He viewed it as impersonal and not sufficiently concerned with "being" as an individual, subjective experience. His other writings, such as *Either/Or*, read like literary works and express his thoughts about the meaning of subjectivity and the anguish of individual freedom of choice. Kierkegaard believed that "the individual must find his/her spiritual path, not through the comfortable dogmatic rituals of the established church or the pseudo-clarity of Hegelian dialectics, but through action, action that is conscious of religious conviction" (Jones, 2003b, para. 3).

Martin Heidegger (1889–1976) studied under Husserl and was influenced by many other philosophers, especially the presocratics. Important to him were Husserl, Kant, Nietzsche, and Kierkegaard. He was most interested in the "question of being." He believed that Western philosophy had been too concerned with the study of how we know. For Heidegger, knowing the world is not our primary way of being in the world. His most important book *Being and Time* (1927; English trans. 1962) united the philosophical approaches of Kierkegaard and Nietzsche.

In his later works, such as *On the Way to Language* (1971) and *Poetry, Language and Thought* (1975), Heidegger became more interested in language as a way to disclose or uncover the concealed nature of being. He uses neologisms (words of his own construction) to express many of his ideas and makes frequent allusions to ancient philosophers and myths. His writing is very dense and difficult to interpret. Although Heidegger claimed he was not an "existentialist," his influence on Sartre and the existentialist movement is unmistakable.

Hans-Georg Gadamer (1900–2002) was a pupil of Heidegger's, but disagreed with the obscure language of his writing. He "believed that philosophy was [useless] unless it could be understood. . . . In his magnum opus, *Truth and Method,* which contributed enormously to the field of hermeneutics, he argued that experience, culture, and prior understanding render the scientific ideal of objectivity impossible" (Gadamer, 2002, p. 47). Gadamer believed that "the meaning of any text is a function of the historical situations of both author and interpreter." Since each reading is grounded in its own context, no one reading offers a definitive or final interpretation of the text; the virtual dialogue continues indefinitely. "Gadamer's thinking began and always remained connected with Greek thought, especially that of Plato and Aristotle. . . . [This] was determinative of much of the character and philosophical direction of his thinking" (Malpas, 2005).

Jean-Paul Sartre (1905–1980) is, perhaps, the best-known existentialist, although he disliked being placed in that category. He was a philosopher, journalist, novelist, and political activist. He was a Marxist because he felt that human freedom had both political and personal dimensions. Many other thinkers, including Nietzsche, Husserl, and Hegel, influenced him. Heidegger's works inspired him with the fundamental question: Why should there be being at all, when there could be nothing? Sartre's best-known work is *Being and Nothingness: A Phenomenological Essay on Ontology* (1943).

Because Sartre was an atheist, he disagreed with Kierkegaard's position that God defines the essence of human nature. Sartre did not believe that there were any predefined "essences."

> Man . . . is conscious of [his] own existence. . . . A material thing is simply 'in itself' but mankind is 'for itself.' The being of mankind is therefore not the same as the being of things . . . man's existence takes priority over whatever he might otherwise be. (Gaarder, 1996, p. 456)

Therefore, Sartre says that existence precedes and rules essence.

If there is no God to define being, then Sartre (1984) felt that "man is condemned to be free. Condemned because he did not create himself, yet is nevertheless at liberty, and from the moment he is thrown into this world, he is responsible for everything he does." Although we cannot choose our gender, class, or country, we can choose what we make of them. These future-directed choices could create anguish and uncertainty.

Maurice Merleau-Ponty (1908–1961) cofounded with Jean-Paul Sartre the Paris journal *Les Temps Modernes*. He was an existential philosopher like Sartre, but disagreed with him about existential freedom. He claimed that freedom is never total, but is limited by our embodiment. In other words, it is through our bodies that we have access to the world, and it is through perception that we know both our interior and exterior worlds. The interior and the exterior cannot be separated. Merleau-Ponty's work is particularly important to the health sciences because of his investigations on the role of the body in perception and society. The influence of Husserl and Gestalt psychology is evident in his major work, *Phenomenology of Perception* (1945/1962). "[It is a] critique of cognitivism—the view that the working of the human mind can be understood in terms of rules or programs . . . and the existentialism of Jean-Paul Sartre" (Dreyfus, 1999a).

Albert Camus (1913–1960) was a journalist and Nobel Prize–winning novelist. He was influenced by Kierkegaard and Nietzsche, and like many thinkers before, revered the ancient philosophers. His dissertation, was a study of the influence of Plotinus and neo-Platonism on the thought and writings of Saint Augustine. [According to] "Camus's (1955) own judgment . . . his fictional works were . . . 'narratives' combining philosophical and psychological insights. . . . 'The great novelists are philosophical novelists'; that is, writers who eschew systematic explanation and create their discourse using 'images instead of arguments' " (p. 74). His books, such as *The Stranger, The Plague*, and *The Fall*, give rich insight into the nature of existentialism, which continues to exist as an important philosophy related to nursing. "Practitioners [of nursing] work with narrative knowledge [every day when they write nurses notes. Their research is also] concerned with people's stories; they work with case histories and use narrative explanations to understand why the people they work with behave the way they do" (Polkinghorne, 1988, p. x).

20TH-CENTURY PHILOSOPHERS

The following is an overview of contemporary philosophers who influence qualitative research; this is discussed in much greater detail in Chapter 5. From the turn of the 20th century on, there began to emerge a dizzying array of new approaches to philosophy. They were influenced by the ideas of Sigmund Freud (1856–1939) about the nature of the unconscious, Albert Einstein's theories about time and space, Marx's revolutionary philosophy about the economic bases of human problems, and many others. Many schools of thought existed simultaneously and sometimes seemed to blend into one another. Some of these were structuralism, deconstructionism, logical positivism, postmodernism, and critical theory. Needless to say, deciphering all of these terms complicates the process of understanding where we are today.

Structuralism

The ideas that began with structuralism have evolved and branched in many directions over the years. Its premises are (1) that the brain has an inherent structure that produces language; it is language that produces our reality; and (2) that

> the source of meaning is not . . . experience or being, but the sets
> of oppositions and operations, the signs and grammars that govern
> language. Meaning doesn't come from individuals, but from the
> system that governs what any individual can do within it. (Klages,
> 2004, para. 7)

The philosopher Charles Pierce (1839–1914) is credited with promoting acceptance of the theory of signs or "semiotics," which had been previously introduced by the philosopher John Locke.

Ferdinand de Saussure (1857–1913) was a linguist and philosopher whose book *Course in General Linguistics* (1916/1966) laid the foundations for structuralism. In it, he describes Pierce's semiology as "a science which studies the role of signs as part of social life. . . . It . . . investigate[s] the nature of signs and the laws governing them. . . . Linguistics is only [one branch] of this general science" (pp. 15–16). He was also interested in myth, ritual, and cultural patterns rooted in the basic structures of the mind as described by Hegel. Saussure's work has influenced anthropology, literary criticism, and the modern study of signs and symbols.

Claude Levi-Strauss (1908–   ) is an anthropologist and philosopher who looked for the existence of universal truths, especially in the basic structures of human relationships. He "was well-known for his development of structural anthropology. . . . His belief that the characteristics of man are everywhere identical was found after countless [visits to native] Indian tribes. . . . The method he used to study the social organization of these tribes is called structuralism" (Schmitt, 1999, para. 1). "Levi Strauss is also known for his structural analysis of mythology . . . [which] explains why myths from different cultures from around the globe seem so similar" (Schmitt, 1999, para. 6). Other thinkers interested in the significance of myths were Margaret Mead, Gregory Bateson, Carl Jung, and Joseph Campbell. The work of Levi-Strauss and other philosophers of anthropology provide foundational ideas for those doing ethnographic research. The difference between narrative inquiry and ethnography is that in narrative inquiry one studies a phenomenon and in ethnography one studies a culture.

Roland Barthes (1915–1980) was a "French social and literary critic, whose writings on semiotics made structuralism one of the leading intellectual movements of the 20th century" (Liukkonen, 2002, para. 1).

Poststructuralism/Deconstructionism

In the 1960s, philosophers in the French structuralist movement criticized it for being "too narrow, too ahistorical (Foucault) and too definitive (Derrida)" (Lemke, 2005). They synthesized the ideas of Marx, Freud, and de Saussure into what is now called "poststructuralism" or "deconstructionism." They disagreed with "existentialist claim[s] that each man is what he makes himself. [They believed that] the individual is shaped by sociological, psychological and linguistic structures over which he/she has no control, but which could be uncovered by using their methods of investigation" (Jones, 2003b, para. 2).

Marx, Freud, and de Saussure share with modern structuralists a conviction that

> surface events and phenomena [are] explained by structures, data, and phenomena below the surface. . . . [These] deep structures, unconscious motivations, and underlying causes . . . account for human actions at a more basic and profound level than do individual conscious decisions and . . . shape, influence, and structure these decisions. (DeGeorge & DeGeorge, 1972, p. xii)

Michel Foucault (1926–1984) was a philosopher who had an impact on many areas of the humanities and social sciences, such as history, medicine, nursing, literature, and philosophy. He opposed systems of authority, which are socially sanctioned definers of "truth," for example, medicine categorizing someone by sexual practices. He called this "biopower," held by medicine, law, and psychology. He said that claims to knowledge in medicine are actually claims to power. He was also interested in "capillary" modes of power that control individuals and their knowledge, the mechanisms by which power "reaches into the very grain of individuals, touches their bodies and inserts itself into their actions and attitudes, their discourses, learning processes and everyday lives" (Foucault, 1980, p. 30). Foucault helps us to see "through the rigorous examination of history, [that] things have not always been as they are now and can be changed even at the most mundane and seemingly insignificant levels so that they eventually become different tomorrow" (Allen, 2004, p. 21).

Jacques Lacan (1901–1981) "was a French psychoanalyst . . . [who] began in the 1950s to develop his own version of psychoanalysis. . . . [He] reinterprets Freud in light of structuralist and post-structuralist theories, turning psychoanalysis from an essentially humanist philosophy or theory into a post-structuralist one, [where he claimed that the unconscious is structured like a language]" (Klages, 1997, para. 2). He uses geometrical figures (topography) to symbolize patterns of relationships. For example:

> He uses the model of the Möbius strip as a vivid metaphor to describe how what is exterior to human subjectivity becomes not only interior but central. Exterior and interior are, as it were, in a continuum: what is interior can become exterior and vice versa. (Gurewich, 1998, p. 7)

"This emphasis on the symbolic organization of human experience staked out a radically new territory for psychoanalytic inquiry, one that Lacan claimed had been discovered by Freud but obscured by his followers" (Clarke, 1997, para. 5).

Paul Ricoeur (1913–2005) was a poststructuralist hermeneutic philosopher. "His constant preoccupation was with a hermeneutic of the self, fundamental to which is the need we have for our lives to be made intelligible to us" (Atkins, 2005, para. 1).

> Ricoeur refers to his hermeneutic method as a 'hermeneutics of suspicion' because discourse both reveals and conceals something about the nature of being. Unlike post-structuralists such as Foucault and Derrida, for whom subjectivity is nothing more than an effect of language, Ricoeur anchors subjectivity in the human body and the material world, of which language is a kind of second order articulation. In the face of the fragmentation and alienation of post-modernity, Ricoeur offers his narrative theory as the path to a unified and meaningful life. (Atkins, 2005, para. 4)

Ricoeur's philosophy has been used as a starting point for many published European nursing research projects, but few from the United States. Jacques Derrida (1930–2004)

> is a contemporary . . . philosopher. . . . Derrida's deconstruction was a complex response to a variety of twentieth century theoretical and philosophical movements including the phenomenology of Husserl, the structuralism of Saussure, and the psychoanalysis of Freud. [It] was also a critique and continuation of Nietzsche's negative reaction to all the above and Heidegger's deconstruction of philosophy and metaphysics. He was heavily influenced by Hegel's opposites. Therefore, Derrida explored meaning by 'tracing' back and forth, on the continuum line between two opposites. (Carrigan, 1996)

Logical Positivism

From the 1920s until the 1950s, logical positivism was the leading philosophy of science. It began with a group of philosophers in Austria, known as the Vienna Circle (1922–1936), who advanced what was called "logical positivism" (as discussed in Chapters 1–3), also known as "analytic and linguistic philosophy."

> Linguistic philosophers agree that the proper activity of philosophy is clarifying language, or, as some prefer, clarifying concepts. The aim of this activity is to settle philosophical disputes and resolve philosophical problems, which, it is argued, originate in linguistic confusion. (Baird, 1999, para. 1)

Ludwig Wittgenstein (1889–1951) was noted for his contribution to the movement. He was interested in the language games that people play; the "rules of the game" depend upon the context in which the game is played (as discussed in Chapter 1). In his book *Philosophical Investigations*, Wittgenstein (1968) writes, "Our investigation is a grammatical one. Such an investigation sheds light on our problem by clearing misunderstandings away . . . misunderstandings concerning the use of words" (sect. 90). He felt that if these misunderstandings were cleared up, the "knots" in communication would be untied. For Wittgenstein, the world was constituted and limited by language.

The "postpositivist" position was that there is no absolute truth, all observation is fallible and has error, and all theory is revisable. "Because all measurement is fallible, the post-positivist emphasizes the importance of multiple measures and observations, each of which may possess different types of error, and the need to use triangulation across these multiple errorful sources" (Trochim, 2002, para. 6).

Postmodern Critical Theory

"Postmodernism and Critical Theory are . . . intellectual movements rather than specific theories. . . . Postmodernism derives from Post-Structuralism and Deconstructionism, which were initially criticisms of the Structuralist movement of the 1960s" (Lemke, 2005, para 1). Postmodernism is a complicated set of ideas that has only emerged as an area of academic study since the mid-1980s.

> It is a general and wide-ranging term, which is applied to literature, art, philosophy, architecture, fiction, and cultural and literary criticism, among others. [It is] "a reaction to the assumed certainty of scientific, or objective, efforts to explain reality. . . . It is highly skeptical of explanations which claim to be valid for all groups, cultures, traditions, or races, focusing instead on the relative truths of each person. (no author, 2005)

Critical theory is a style of analysis and cultural criticism that centers on the Frankfurt School for Social Research (1923–1935) and at the New School for Social Research in New York (1939–1949). Critical theory has been applied primarily to linguistics, literature, and philosophy (Lemke, 2005, para. 1). "Intellectually, the Frankfurt School drew on diverse but related traditions of philosophy and social thought. Many of these can be traced back to Hegel's dialectical phenomenology, the leftist (or 'critical') Hegelianism of the 1840s, and Karl Marx's dialectical materialism" (Pecora, 1997, para. 5). "Karl Marx says, 'one must become conscious of how an ideology reflects and distorts . . . reality . . . and what factors . . . influence and sustain the false consciousness which it represents—especially [regarding] powers of domination' " (MacIsaac, 2005). Critical theory had its greatest social influence in the late 1960s and early 1970s.

Jurgen Habermas (1929–   ) is a philosopher and sociologist.

> His roots are in the tradition of German thought from Kant to Marx, and he has been associated with the Frankfurt School of critical theorists which pioneered in the study of the relationship of the ideas of Marx and Freud. (Mezirow, 1981)

SUMMARY

In this chapter, we have looked at the web of philosophical ideas that has brought us to our current understanding of the qualitative approach to research. We have barely scratched the surface of the body of work of each of these philosophers. Much more can be gained by looking at their original writings. Many of these works can be found in full-text format on the Internet, through Web sites such as http://www.gutenberg.org.

Research methodologies such as phenomenology, grounded theory, ethnography, case study, historical research, narrative inquiry, and action research have all grown out of this philosophical base. They are further elaborated in the chapters that follow.

The next chapter expands on the philosophical schools of thought and the contemporary philosophers, whose outgrowth includes postmodern thought, critical theory, and feminist theory, among others, and provides an analysis of the relationships to nursing and qualitative research. This chapter is one brief examination of the understanding of the temporal period we now occupy.

REFERENCES

(No author, 2005). Postmodernism. Retrieved September 5, 2005 from http://www.pbs.org/faithandreason/gengloss/decon-body.html.

Allen, D. (2004, June 2). Fishing for Foucault. *Nursing Standard*, 38(18), 20–21. Retrieved July 20, 2005, from http://www.foucault.qut.edu.au/allen.pdf.

Appiah, K. (2003). *Thinking it through: An introduction to contemporary philosophy.* New York: Oxford University Press.

Aristotle. (2004). *Nichomachean ethics.* (W. D. Ross, Trans.) Retrieved June 3, 2005, from http://etext.library.adelaide.edu.au/a/aristotle/nicomachean/. (Original work published in 350 BC)

Aristotle. (350 BCE) Prior Analytics (A. J. Jenkinson, Trans.) Retrieved May 1, 2005, from http://studentwebs.coloradocollege.edu/~j_torres/Prior%20Analytics.htm.

Atkins, K. (2005). Paul Ricoeur (1913–2005). Retrieved September 8, 2005, from University of Tennessee at Martin Web site, Internet Encyclopedia of Philosophy: http://www.iep.utm.edu/r/Life%20and%20Works.

Audi, R. (Ed.). (1999). *The Cambridge dictionary of philosophy*. New York: Cambridge University Press.

Blitzer, C. (1967). *The age of kings*. New York: Time.

Burnham, D. (2005). René Descartes (1596–1650). Retrieved April 15, 2005, from *The Internet encyclopedia of philosophy*. James Fieser (Ed.): http://www.iep.utm.edu/d/descarte.htm.

Camus, A. (1955). *The myth of Sisyphus and other essays* (Justin O'Brien, Trans.). New York: Vintage.

Capra, F. (1983). *The tao of physics*. Boston: New Science Library.

Carspecken, P. (2004). Quality, quantity and the human sciences: The qualitative research movement and its implicit philosophical and methodological issues. Retrieved August 1, 2005, from University of Michigan Web site: http://www.umich.edu/~qualnet/keynote2004.htm.

Clarke, Michael P. (1997). Lacan, Jacques. Retrieved August 20, 2005, from Johns Hopkins Guide to Literary Criticism Web site: http://www.press.jhu.edu/books/hopkins_guide_to_literary_theory/jacques_lacan.html.

Cline, A. (2005). Agnosticism/Atheism: Max Scheler. Retrieved August 30, 2005, from http://atheism.about.com/library/glossary/general/bldef_schelermax.htm.

Deely, J. (1968). The immateriality of the intentional as such. *New Scholasticism, 42,* 293–306. Retrieved June 5, 2005, from http://www.ditext.com/deely/deely.html

DeGeorge, F., & DeGeorge, R. (1972). *The structuralists from Marx to Levi-Strauss*. New York: Doubleday.

Dennett, D. (2005). *Philosophy of mind: Platonic dualism* (Gareth Southwell, Ed.). Retrieved May 18, 2005, from Philosophy Online Web site: http://www.philosophyonline.co.uk/pom/pom_platonism.htm.

Descartes, R. (1950). *Discourse on method* (L. J. Lafleur, Trans.). New York: Bobbs-Merrill. (Original work published 1867).

Dilthey, W. (1923/1988). *Introduction to the human sciences: An attempt to lay a foundation for the study of society and history* (R. Betanzos, Trans.). Detroit, MI: Wayne State University Press.

Diogenes Laertius. (1959). *Lives of eminent philosophers* (2 vols.) (R. D. Hicks, Trans.). Cambridge, MA: Harvard University Press. (Original work published AD 3).

Dreyfus, H. (1999a). Maurice Merleau-Ponty. *Microsoft Encarta 99* [Electronic media].

Dreyfus, H. (1999b). Phenomenology, 20th-century. *Microsoft Encarta 99* [Electronic media].

Einstein, A. (2000). *The world as I see it*. New York: Citadel Press. (Original work published 1939).

Foucault, M. (1980). *Power/knowledge: Selected interviews and other writings 1972–1977* (Colin Gordon, Ed.). New York: Pantheon. (Original work published 1972).

Frings, M. (2005). Max Scheler. Retrieved September 12, 2005, from http://www.maxscheler.com/scheler2.shtml#2-Synopsis.

Funk & Wagnalls (a)(1976/1979). Standard desk dictionary: Volume 1 A-M. New York: Funk & Wagnalls, Inc.

Funk & Wagnalls (b)(1976/1979). Standard desk dictionary: Volume 2 N-Z. New York: Funk & Wagnalls, Inc.

Gaarder, J. (1996). *Sophie's world: A novel about the history of philosophy*. New York: Berkley Publishing Group.

Gadamer, H. (2002, June). Obituary. *World Press Review, 49*(6), 46.

Gay, P. (Ed.). (1966). *Age of enlightenment*. New York: Time.

Gurewich, J. (1998). Who's afraid of Jacques Lacan? In J. F. Gurewich, M. Tort, & S. Fairfield (Eds.), *The Subject and the self: Lacan and American psychoanalysis*. Northvale, New Jersey and London: Jason Aronson.

Hegel, G. (1967). *The phenomenology of spirit*. (J. B. Baillie, Trans.). New York: Harper & Row. (Original work published 1807).

Heidegger, M. (1927). *Being and time*. (J. MacQuarie & E. Robinson, Trans.) New York: Harper & Row Publishers.

Heidegger, M. (1971). *On the way to language*. (P.D. Hertz, Trans.) New York: Harper & Row Publishers.

Heidegger, M. (1975). *Poetry, language, and thought*. (A. Hofstadler, Trans.) New York: Harper & Row Publishers.

Johnston, I. (1999). Romantic era in English poetry: Some reflections on the trends which produced romanticism. Retrieved August 15, 2005, from http://www.mala.bc.ca/~johnstoi/introser/romantic.htm.

Jones, J., & Wilson, W. (1987). *An incomplete education*. New York: Ballantine Books.

Jones, R. (2003b). Poststructuralism. Retrieved August 7, 2005, from http://www.philosopher.org.uk/poststr.htm.

Kierkegaard, S. (1992). *Concluding unscientific postscripts to philosophical fragments* (H. Hong & E. Hong, Trans.). Princeton, NJ: Princeton University Press. (Original work published 1846).

Kirk, J., & Miller, M. (1986). *Reliability and validity in qualitative research*. Beverly Hills, CA: Sage.

Klages, M. (1997). Jacques Lacan. Retrieved August 17, 2005, from University of Colorado Web site: http://www.colorado.edu/English/ENGL2012Klages/lacan.html.

Klages, M. (2004). Structuralism/poststructuralism. Retrieved August 20, 2005, from University of Colorado Web site: http://www.colorado.edu/English/ENGL2012Klages/1derrida.html.

Lavine, T. Z. (1984). *From Socrates to Sartre: The philosophic quest*. New York: Bantam Books. (1984–1989 7th printing).

Lemke, J. (2005). Postmodernism and critical theory. Retrieved September 8, 2005, from City University of New York Web site: http://academic.brooklyn.cuny.edu/education/jlemke/theories.htm, http://academic.brooklyn.cuny.edu/emke/copyrite.htm.

Levi-Strauss, C. (1978). *Myth and meaning*. London: Routledge.

Liukkonen, P. (2002). Roland Barthes: 1915–1980. Retrieved September 6, 2005, from http://www.kirjasto.sci.fi/rbarthes.htm.

MacIsaac, D. (2005). The critical theory of Jurgen Habermas. Retrieved June 30, 2005, from Buffalo State University Web site: http://physicsed.buffalostate.edu/danowner/habcritthy.html.

Malpas, J. (2005). Hans-Georg Gadamer. In E. N. Zalta (Ed.), *Stanford encyclopedia of philosophy*. Retrieved September 8, 2005 from http://plato.stanford.edu/archives/fall2005/entries/gadamer/.

Marx, K., & Engels, F. (1845). *The holy family* (chap. 6). Retrieved May 3, 2005, from http://www.marxists.org/archive/marx/works/1845/holy-family/ch06_3_d.htm

McCracken, G. (1988). *The long interview*. Beverly Hills, CA: Sage.

Mendelson, M. (2000). Saint Augustine: Psychology and Epistemology. The stanford encyclopedia of philosophy. Retrieved April 25, 2005 from http://plato.stanford.edu/entries/augustine/#4.

Merleau-Ponty, M. (1962). *Phenomenology of perception*. New York: Routledge and Kegan Paul. (Original work published 1945).

Mezirow, J. (1981). A critical theory of adult learning and education. *Adult Education, 32*, 3–24.

Münch, D. (1997). Franz Brentano and phenomenology. In L. Embree et al. (Eds.), *Encyclopedia of phenomenology* (pp. 71b–75b). Dordrecht: Kluwer.

Munhall, P. (1989). Philosophical ponderings on qualitative research methods in nursing. *Nursing Science Quarterly, 2*, 20–28.

Nietzsche, F. (1926). *The antichrist* (H. L. Mencken, Trans.). Retrieved May 2, 2005, from http://www.fns.org.uk/ac.htm (Original work published 1895).

O'Meara, D. J. (1993). *Plotinus: An introduction to the Enneads*. New York: Oxford University Press.

Pecora, V. (1997). Frankfurt school. Retrieved September 10, 2005, from *Johns Hopkins Guide to literary theory and criticism* (M. Groden & M. Krieswerth, Eds.): http://www.press.jhu.edu/books/hopkins_guide_to_literary_theory/frankfurt_school.html.

Plato. (1999). The meno (B. Jowett, Trans.) [Etext #1643]. Retrieved February 5, 2005, from http://www.gutenberg.org (Original work published 347 BC).

Polkinghorne, D. (1988). *Narrative knowing and the human sciences*. Albany: State University of New York Press.

Poster, C. (2005). Protagoras (490–c. 420 BC). Retrieved March 2, 2005, from *The Internet Encyclopedia of Philosophy* (J. Fieser, Ed.): http://www.iep.utm.edu/p/protagor.htm.

Sartre, J. (1943). *Being and nothingness: A phenomenological essay on ontology.* (H. E. Barnes, Trans.) New York: Editions Gallimard.

Sartre, J. (1984). *Existentialism and Human Emotions.* Sacramento, CA: Citadel Press. (Original work published 1967).

Saussure, F. de (1966). Course in general linguistics (C. Bally & A. Sechehaye in collaboration with A. Riedlinger, Eds., W. Baskin, Trans.). New York: McGraw-Hill. (Original work published 1916).

Scheler, M. (1970). *The nature of sympathy.* Hamden, CT: Archon Books. (Original work published 1913).

Schmitt, S. (1999). Claude Levi-Strauss, 1908. Retrieved September 1, 2005, from Minnesota State University at Mankato Web site: http://www.mnsu.edu/emuseum/information/biography/klmno/levi-strauss_claude.html.

Siewert, C. (2003). Consciousness and intentionality. In E. N. Zalta (Ed.), *The Stanford Encyclopedia of Philosophy*. Retrieved May 19, 2005 from http://plato.stanford.edu/archives/fall2003/entries/consciousness-intentionality/.

Simpson, D. (2005). Francis Bacon. Retrieved May 20, 2005, from *The Internet encyclopedia of philosophy*: http://www.iep.utm.edu/b/bacon.htm#SH2k.

Trochim, W. M. (2002). Positivism and post positivism. Retrieved May 16, 2005, from http://www.socialresearchmethods.net/kb/positvsm.htm.

van Manen, M. (1990). *Researching lived experience: Human science for an action sensitive pedagogy*. New York: State University of New York Press.

Wicks, R. (2004). Friedrich Nietzsche. In E. N. Zalta (Ed.), *The Stanford encyclopedia of philosophy*. Retrieved April 25, 2005, from http://plato.stanford.edu/archives/fall2004/entries/nietzsche/.

Wittgenstein, L. (1968). *Philosophical investigations*. Englewood Cliffs, NJ: Prentice Hall. (Original work published 1953).

Wordsworth, W., & Coleridge, S. (1798). *Lyrical ballads*. London: Biggs and Cottle for T. N. Longman, Paternoster-Row.

ADDITIONAL REFERENCES

Bacon, F., Ellis, R. L., & Heath, D. D. (Eds.). (1863). The works, Vol. VIII (J. Spedding, Trans.). Boston: Taggard and Thompson.

Baird, R. (1999). Analytic and linguistic philosophy. *Microsoft Encarta 99* [Electronic media].

Best, S., & Kellner, D. (1991). Postmodern theory, critical interrogations. Retrieved May 10, 2005, from http://www.uta.edu/huma/pomo_theory/ch1.html.

Carrigan, C. (1996). Deconstructionism and postmodernism. Retrieved September 9, 2005 from http://ontruth.com/derrida.html.

Jones, R. (2003a). Existentialism. Retrieved August 7, 2005, from http://www.philosopher.org.uk/existen.htm.

Lye, J. (1999). Structuralism. Retrieved June 14, 2005, from Brock University Department of English: http://www.brocku.ca/english/courses/4F70/struct.html.

Newton, I. (1985). Letter to Robert Hooke (1642–1727), English mathematician and physicist. In M. Kline, *Mathematics and the search for knowledge* (pp. 107, 121). New York: Oxford University Press. Retrieved September 5, 2005, from http://www.blupete.com/Literature/Biographies/Science/Newton.htm#fn20 (Original work published 1675).

Shawyer, L. (2005). Commentary on Wittgenstein's *Philosophical Investigations*. Retrieved September 9, 2005, from http://users.rcn.com/rathbone/lwtocc.htm.

Smith, D. (2003). Phenomenology. In E. N. Zalta (Ed.), *The Stanford encyclopedia of philosophy*. Retrieved June 23, 2005, from http://plato.stanford.edu/archives/win2003/entries/phenomenology/.

Smith, S. (1999). Frankfurt school. *Microsoft Encarta 99* [Electronic media].

Solomon, R., & Higgens, H. (1996). *A short history of philosophy*. New York: Oxford University Press.

5

Reflections on Postmodernism, Critical Social Theory, and Feminist Approaches: The Postmodern Mind

Lynne Dunphy
Joy Longo

We would posit that postmodernism is a state of mind. We write these words in the context of a post-9/11 world and surrounded by news of the devastation wreaked on the United States, specifically the states of Louisiana and Mississippi, by Hurricane Katrina in late August, early September of the year 2005, when all rational and centralized systems seemed to fail to respond in a meaningful way. An understanding of the term *postmodernism* must be preceded by a discussion of the concept of *modernism* and all that it implies. This chapter first outlines current understandings of *modernity* and its counterpart, *postmodernism*; it then proceeds to the historical emergence of *critical social theory* and its implications for research, in this case, specifically nursing research. We then examine *feminist* scholarship and its impact on the research enterprise, again specifically nursing research; and we conclude with a discussion of *postmodernism* and, by implication, the postmodern world.

MODERNITY

The term *modernity* refers, in common parlance, to the progressive, ratio-nalist endeavors of the West. Currently, the term is often popularly used as a contrast to what is seen as the primitive, irrational worldview of Islamic fun-damentalism. Beginning as a way of thinking that arose from the 17th-cen-tury scientific revolution, termed the Enlightenment, modernity is a set of beliefs that all aspects of nature, including human nature and society, are reg-ulated by universal laws, natural laws that can be uncovered through the ap-plication of "scientific thinking and deduction" (Jardine, 1999). The individual is seen as rational and self-interested. Historian Paul Johnson (1991) places "the Modern" as commencing around the end of the Napoleonic Wars. On the heels of the French and American Revolutions, Enlightenment idealists such as William Godwin and the Marquis de Con-dorcet held that humankind was infinitely improvable and that a golden age of social justice, political harmony, equity, abundance, brotherhood, happi-ness, and altruism loomed imminently. There were always critics of this Utopian view, such as Thomas Robert Malthus (1766–1834). Author of the famed (and in some circles, infamous) 1798 "An Essay on the Principle of Population as It Affects the Future Improvement of Society," Malthus postu-lated that population growth faced strict and inevitable natural limits, not a popular view. Indeed, the pejorative term *Malthusian* remains attached to any idea that suggests that human ingenuity cannot overcome any challenges posed by nature.

The 1800s saw the beginning of the great rise of industrialization, a hall-mark of modern society. Initially powered by wood, coal, and water, it was the discovery of oil and its many uses that fueled the modern age, replete with the magic of antibiotics, sports utility vehicles, and computers that support the foundation of our day-to-day lives.[1] We have put men on the moon. We have defeated microbes. We are entering a new, ever more modern age, coined the Information Age, allegedly an exciting sequel to the Age of Industrialization, which retrospectively is viewed by many as dirty, noisy, and unhealthy.

Modernity is seen as tied to democratic, political structures, supportive of individual freedoms and rights. The modern, scientific endeavor, it is thought, is best supported by progressive societies. Scientific and economic development requires "a stable government that reliably provides law and order, impartially protects private property and enforces contracts" (David-

---

[1] See James Kunstler, *The Long Emergency* (2005), which points out that "cheap oil" has per-mitted the human race to enjoy "an unprecedented orgy of nonrenewable condensed solar energy accumulated over eons of prehistory" (p. 7).

son & Rees-Mogg, 1993, p. 102). Our current American endeavor to democratize Iraq is predicated on such thinking.

William Butler Yeats in his poem "The Second Coming" describes an image of impending chaos on the eve of the Great Depression of the 1930s. The poet tells us that even before the collapse of the world economy had been registered in the cash markets, it was prefigured in the psyches of people. The dark side of progress has been a well-chronicled, integral part of the 20th century—World War I, World War II, the Holocaust, the atomic bomb, the AIDS pandemic. Modern art, with its abstractions, may be seen as a frightening foreshadowing of fragmentation. Philosophers at the end of the 19th century—Friedrich Nietzsche, Soren Kierkegaard—foresaw a crisis of faith. Great power (of all varieties) came with "fear and trembling."

POSTMODERNISM

The very term *postmodernism* implies that one is "beyond" the modern; that one has grasped the limitations of positivistic modes of knowledge acquisition and dissemination; that one recognizes multiple voices, multiple views, and multiple methods when analyzing any aspect of reality; and that one challenges the assumptions of modernist thought and reality. Disowning ideas of universal truths, postmodernism, as Cheek (2000) notes, "challenges the notion of a rationale and unified subject that is so central to modernist thought" (p. 6). Defined by what it comes after, postmodernism is a self-consciously transitional moment, "the boundary between the 'not yet' and the 'no longer' " (Lather, 1991, p. 87). The exhaustions of the paradigms of modernity create an affective space where we feel we cannot continue as we are. The modernist endeavor of control through knowledge has imploded. Lather (1991) describes the postmodern project as a "turning away from the enormous pretensions of positivism . . . to the development of a human science much more varied and reflexive about its limitations" (p. 102). Postmodern thought has infiltrated any number of disciplinary fields, most commonly since World War II. Initially influencing art and architecture, it spread rapidly to philosophy and literary studies in the 1950s and 1960s, and since then, it has influenced all fields, including health care, nursing, and feminism (Cheek, 2000, p. 18).

Method

According to Bauman (1992), postmodernism is an unstable concept, difficult to define. It does not represent a unified position or coherent school of thought; indeed, it is notable for its incoherence. Likewise, there is no one

TABLE 5–1   Postpositivist Inquiry

Predict	Understand	Emancipate	Deconstruct
Positivism	Interpretive	Naturalistic	Poststructural
	Naturalistic	Neo-Marxist	Postmodern
	Constructivist	Feminist	Postparadigmatic
	Phenomenological	Praxis-oriented	diaspora
	Hermeneutic	Educative	
		Freirian participatory	
		Action research	

Source: From Lather P. Getting Smart. Routledge, 1991.

postmodern "method." According to Foucault (1980), postmodern and post-structural approaches become "instruments of analyses" (p. 62) rather than rigid sets of rules. If one links positivism to prediction, postpositivist inquiry, encompassing postmodern and poststructural approaches, can be said to aim to understand, emancipate, and/or deconstruct. According to Lather (1991), each of these three postpositivist "paradigms" offers a different approach to generating and legitimating knowledge (p. 7). Table 5–1 lists the functions of postpositivist inquiry.

Postmodern thought argues that "knowledge is contextualized by its historical and cultural nature" (Agger, 1991, p. 117). Thus, researchers must expose rather than conceal (for instance, behind methodological frames) "their own investment in a particular view of the world" (Agger, 1991, p. 117). Personal values manifest themselves in the very research questions posed as well as the methods used to seek answers to those questions. It is a short leap from postmodern thought to critical social theory, and further to feminist approaches. They spring from similar soil and intermingle in ways that enrich the growth of each.

CRITICAL SOCIAL THEORY

Individual freedoms can be limited by existing sociopolitical and economic restraints. These limitations often are embedded within the structure of society and remain hidden, which allows a continuous oppressive presence. The recognition of these constrictions enables one to critically examine one's situation and to find a path to freedom or emancipation. The purpose of critical social theory is to provide a framework for examining and critiquing these socially constructed borders that are placed on human freedom (Kendall, 1992). Critical social theory originated as a German intellectual movement in the 1920s in response to an escalating concern with Fascism in post–World War I Germany as well as to the growing appeal of logical positivism in intellectual thought in Europe. Critical social theory presents a way to go beyond the economics of Marxist theory and the positivistic view that the social world can be viewed in the light and same culture as the methods of the natural sciences. Critical social theory posits that social science is influenced by human activity, which further affects large social structures (Ritzer & Goodman, 2004).

Critical social theory began at the Institute for Social Research in Frankfurt, Germany, and is often referred to as the Frankfurt School. The original group of scholars at the institute was interdisciplinary and included Max Horkheimer, a philosopher and social psychologist; Friedrich Pollock, an economist; Theodor Adorno, a philosopher and musicologist; Erich Fromm, a psychologist; Herbert Marcuse, a philosopher; and Leo Lowenthal, a popular theorist of culture and literature. In acknowledgment of its Marxist roots, the epistemology of critical social theory has been to dictate that knowledge should be used for emancipatory political aims with the goal to free one's perceptions from ideological constraints to allow one to evaluate the true situation. The consciousness of the masses is seen as heavily influenced by external forces, so there is no opportunity to develop a revolutionary consciousness. For critical theorists, these ideologies are the idea systems produced by the ruling elite that are often proved to be false (Ritzer & Goodman, 2004).

According to Weber (2005), the first generation of the Frankfurt School was characterized by the conceptual framework of deconstruction and "salvage operation" of Marxism/Hegelianism, but the second stage signaled a shift from this framework that refocused the thrust of social theory onto epistemological problems. This directed critical social theory away from the concentration on method and ontology, which dominated the first generation, and returned it to the intersubjectivity of social life. This second generation was introduced in the 1960s by German theorist Jürgen Habermas. Habermas wanted to return knowledge to that which was secured in the social sciences as originally intended by Marx, and to include the examination of power structures that create oppression in a social system. The task set forth by Habermas was to understand how people communicate and develop symbolic meanings. An understanding of this process would uncover the constraints that impede equal, free, and uncoerced participation in society. An understanding of the theory and the practice of interpretation is known as hermeneutics (van Manen, 1990). Bernstein (1983) describes Habermas's (1999) concern with communication and its relationship to human action as follows:

> Habermas, who discovered that hermeneutics not only helps to highlight the limitations of positivist modes of thought but that there is also an essential hermeneutic dimension in all social

knowledge, has been primarily concerned with the question of the foundation of a critical theory of society. From his perspective, neither the critique of ideology, as developed by Marx, nor the critical theory of the older Frankfurt thinkers is sufficient to provide a satisfactory answer to this foundational question. Habermas gradually came to realize more and more clearly the need to elaborate a comprehensive theory of rationality. (pp. 180–181)

What is imperative to critical social theory is that the human actions are not limited to the account of the individual or actor, but that knowledge is contextual so that standards of truth require interpretation in a social, historical, economic, and cultural perspective (Allen, 1986).

One of Habermas's interests was the relationship that existed between knowledge and human interests as a reflection of the broader dialectical relationship between subjective and objective factors. These could not be dealt with in isolation from one another. Habermas recognized that knowledge systems exist at the objective level, whereas human interests are a more subjective phenomenon. He defined three types of cognitive interests: (1) analytic science, in which technical prediction and control are applied to the environment, societies, and individuals; (2) humanistic knowledge, which is an understanding of the world today based on an understanding of the past; and (3) critical knowledge, which is the knowledge of human emancipation. It was hoped that the critical knowledge generated by Habermas and others would raise self-consciousness and lead to a social movement that would result in emancipation (Ritzer & Goodman, 2004).

Method

The application of critical social theory to research is the use of a conceptual framework in a manner that is consistent with the philosophy and beliefs of the approach. It is not a mechanistic application of a methodology for emancipatory insight. The purpose of the analysis of the issues is to emphasize the context and historicity to increase the emancipation of individuals and groups. The process is praxis, or the critical reflection, on the ends and means of activity for the purpose of transformation and is a means of consciousness raising in which theory and action become one. Research and analysis within a critical social theory framework promote a consciousness among persons who are impeded by oppressive constraints. It brings about conditions in which oppressive elements are brought forth to initiate a dialogue about action so that change occurs. This can only aid in the anticipation of strategic action but cannot compel action. If it were to compel this action, those doing the research and theorizing would be placed above those who are experiencing the phenomenon addressed by the theory, which itself creates a state of domination (Stevens, 1984).

Habermas contends that certain conditions have to be met to make research critical. These include (1) analysis and unveiling of hidden power sources, (2) commitment of the study to full and equal participation of the researcher and the observed, and (3) commitment of the study to a mutually agreed upon plan for change (Welch, 1999). Hedin (1986) outlines general steps to be used in applying a critical theoretical approach. After identifying an object of which the nature and meaning are in question, dialogue is used to gain data and explore interpretations of this object. These interpretations must go beyond usual methods of interpretation to bring the participants' interpretations out from behind oppressive contexts, and then the meanings should be explained by existing theory. There is no one method to be used in conducting research using a critical social theory framework. Methods can include qualitative methods in the historical/hermeneutic tradition and quantitative methods in the empirical/analytic tradition (Stevens, 1984).

In its application to nursing research, critical social theory promotes a consciousness among persons affected by oppressive constraints, illuminates oppressive elements, and initiates dialogue for action to occur. By offering challenges and identifying possible strategies for action, critical social research and theory can serve to interpret hypothetically the constellations of struggle for liberation and political change. Methods must not only recognize the condition but also the action that is to be taken. Freire (1970/2003) states:

> The pedagogy of the oppressed, as a humanist and libertarian pedagogy, has two distinct stages. In the first, the oppressed unveil the world of oppression and through the praxis commit themselves to its transformation. In the second stage, in which the reality of oppression has already been transformed, this pedagogy ceases to belong to the oppressed and becomes a pedagogy of all people in the process of permanent liberation. In both stages, it is always through action in depth that the culture of domination is culturally confronted. (p. 54)

Critical Social Theory and Nursing Science

The significance of critical social theory in nursing is the recognition of the perspective of subjectivity in individuals as well as the acknowledgment of the contextual constraints that may prohibit the delivery of health care and services to the population. It is theorized that critical social theory can impact the educational process and the practice of the nurse through reflection upon their circumstances and acknowledgment of boundaries that exist and prohibit freedom. Nurses work under conditions in which previously unacknowledged power relations anchored in race, gender, and class can be recognized. A critical view based on reflection, insight, and consciousness raising enables one to see forces that exist and influence an individual's growth. This helps in making power relations and modes of domination visible to the nurse (Thompson, 1987).

In the pursuit of scientific knowledge, objectivism is a goal of natural science, but to assist in developing new knowledge, no restricting ideologies that limit freedom must be present. The goal of science is to find the truth, and that which has been determined to be acceptable as evidence or knowledge must have been arrived at through rationality and must have been uncoerced. Two key values of this rationality are autonomy, which is being free from conscious or unconscious restraints, and responsibility, which is the creation of an environment in which others can speak freely (Allen, Benner, & Diekelmann, 1986). These two values enable the scientist to freely discover new information. One must use a critical lens in viewing how knowledge development is approached, and then envision emancipatory goals for nursing science. If there is no critique, there is a risk of maintaining the status quo (Browne, 2000). Oppression, then, is unchallenged, and the dominant group retains power over the oppressed group.

It has been theorized that nurses are an oppressed group as a result of their position in the medical hierarchy and because the majority of nurses are female (McCall, 1996; Roberts, 1983; Skillings, 1992). In this oppressive situation, the domination of the hierarchy suppresses the recognition of nurses and what nursing can bring to health care. Freire (1970/2003) states:

> As long as the oppressed remain unaware of the causes of their condition, they fatalistically "accept" their exploitation. Further, they are apt to react in a passive and alienated manner when confronted with the necessity to struggle for their freedom and self-affirmation. Little by little, however, they tend to try out forms of rebellious action. In working towards liberation, one must neither lose sight of this passivity nor overlook the moment of awakening. (p. 64)

By reflecting on the oppression that is present and taking actions against such boundaries, nursing science can move beyond the ideology of the dominant group. Not only the forces outside of nursing can represent a dominating culture, but also those forces within nursing. Nursing theory is often developed by the educated elite; therefore, this knowledge is removed from the domain of the bedside nurse. Ideally, theory should be applicable to the practice situation in which nurses engage and should reflect the lived experience of the nurse. According to Wuest (1994), nursing theories evolved from an "elite group" of nurse educator/academicians who often were far removed from the reality of the practice world and thereby endorsed a patriarchal structure. Professionalism is a patriarchal invention, and by its nature it alienates women. If one accepts the liberal tradition of knowledge development that is embodied in professionals, nurses have not appreciated their own knowledge acquired through caring (Wuest, 1994). In critical social theory, power is interpreted in terms of coercion and domination. It is extrapersonal so that an increase in one person's power must be compensated by a surrender of power by someone else. Relinquishing power is known as legitimization. *Empowerment* is a useful umbrella term to describe the elements of professional growth and development in the nursing profession. Empowerment signifies influence rather than striving to enhance one's power by taking it from others (Kuokkanen & Leino-Kilpi, 2000) where the acquisition of power would again create a structure of domination rather than equality.

Critical self-reflection that examines and challenges the liberal ideological basis of nursing knowledge, inquiry, theory development, and practice is imperative to this emancipation process and consciousness raising. In nursing and nursing education, a critical praxis, or reflection and action, helps one attain freedom and enables one to question what knowledge is, how we know, and who provides the evidence. The use of critical reflection patterns of communication and socialization enables nurses to analyze knowledge that is attained in an androcentric ideology that impedes health promotion and maintainence in a caring, contextual, and humanistic perspective (Wilson-Thomas, 1995). The emancipation that is facilitated by critical social theory enables freedom from oppressive systems and brings about an awareness of the patriarchal models that exist in hospitals and universities. The study of these models can help nurse researchers communicate what is going on in nursing practice and understand the theory–practice link. Critical social theory can reveal previously hidden sources of domination and power to show human suffering and suggest new emancipated modes of human action (Thompson, 1987).

Critical Social Theory and Health Care Delivery

One purpose of emancipating nurses from these ideologies is for nurses to gain a better understanding of the patient situation and what is needed to care for these patients. In contrast to a positivistic approach, in critical social theory the humanness of patients does not allow the application of all lab-tested and certified information based on the historical aspect of the patient. The patient must have the freedom to act and achieve health. Emancipatory nursing actions are those that increase the potential for an oppressed group to gain power. The patient can be oppressed by health care in that not all knowledge fits all patients. This understating enables one to treat a patient individually. Emancipatory actions include taking gender, race, and class considerations seriously and conceiving all social structures as containing an interplay of contradictory forces that require dialogic critique to understand social reality (Kendall, 1992). Critical social theory can be applied to a therapeutic nurse–patient relationship and can enable patients to be empowered based on mutual respect, trust, and equality of worth (Kuokkannen & Leino-Kilpi, 2000).

Critical Social Theory and Nursing Education

Another application of critical social theory to nursing is the understanding of the educational process and a shift from teaching-directed learning to an equal partnership between student and teacher. This type of system enables the student to partake actively in the educational process rather than to be a bystander. Several authors (Hedin, 1986; Ironside, 2001; Owen-Mills, 1995; and Wilson-Thomas, 1995) have applied this theory to nursing education. The use of critical social theory in nursing education permits a revisioning and restructuring of ideology by both the faculty and the students so that both groups can recognize that the ideology is potentially oppressive and cohesive. Traditional nursing education deemphasizes the subjective needs of the students. The ideal is to create an autonomous and socially responsible nurse, and this requires the provision of an unconstrained learning environment that seeks to uncover hidden meanings and nurture critique (Duchscher, 2000). It is imperative that students also learn to critique the environment to analyze the sources of their own interrelations, to question and resist predefined meaning that educators encourage them to adopt, and to develop tools to negotiate the world of nursing (Allen et al., 1986).

The application of critical social theory to nursing enables nurses to view the reality of the nurse or patient situation in regard to oppressive systems that exist in the health care structure and within society. Reflection on the situation allows these once hidden constraints to be brought to the surface, critiqued, and acted upon. This process must remain dominant-free so that the decisions and action are uncoerced. Any coercion feeds into the domination.

FEMINIST APPROACHES AS PART OF THE POSTMODERN ENTERPRISE

Feminist inquiry, as it relates to nursing, can be viewed from several perspectives. It can shed light on issues of gender that enable us to provide better care for our female patients, as well as their families and loved ones; and it can shed light on sources of our own oppression/experiences as nurses and/or as women. In a wonderful and not very widely available (in this country) book chapter entitled "Women and the Politics of Career Development: The Case of Nursing," Ellen Baer (1997), nurse historian, relates a quote from Ethel Manson Fenwick, the organizer of the British Nurses Association, editor of the *Nursing Record* (which later became the *British Journal of Nursing*), and a strong antagonist of her contemporary Florence Nightingale regarding the state registration of nurses. According to Baer, Fenwick aptly summed up the situation in 1887 when she said: "The Nurse question is the Women question, pure and simple. We have to run the gauntlet of those historic rotten eggs" (Fenwick quoted in Baer, 1997, pp. 256–257).

In the words of Lather (1991), to do feminist research is "to put the social construction of gender at the center of one's inquiry" (p. 71). Feminists see gender as a basic organizing principle that profoundly shapes and mediates the concrete conditions of our lives. Gender is viewed as central in the shaping of our ideas of the world, the skills we acquire, the institutions in which we reside and work, and the distribution of power and privilege. According to Callaway (1981), this entails the substantive task of making gender a fundamental category for our understanding of the social order, "to see the world from women's place in it" (p. 460). An overt ideological goal of feminist research in the human sciences, according to Lather (1991), is "to correct both the invisibility and distortion of female experience in ways relevant to ending women's unequal social position" (p. 71).

The relatively short history of feminism is often described in "waves." The first wave was the 19th- and early 20th-century women's rights movement that ultimately led to voting rights for women in Great Britain and the United States. The second wave commonly refers to the 1960s and early 1970s when women's "lib" (women's liberation) burst into the nation's consciousness along with the anti-war protests of the same era. There was the introduction of the birth control pill and the legalization of abortion (*Roe v. Wade*, 1973). The genie was out of the bottle; Pandora was out of the box. Women's studies formally entered the academy.

As a consequence of the methodological legacies that early feminist scholars inadvertently took from their teachers, feminist theory from the late 1960s to the mid-1980s tended to exhibit the problematic universalizing tendencies of academic scholarship in general. Additionally, its analyses tended to reflect the viewpoint of the largely privileged, white, middle-class women of North America and western Europe, who composed this group of early scholars. These women tended to reflect "liberal" feminist thought, which views women's oppression as stemming from a lack of equal civil rights and educational opportunities, which thus channels women into "traditional" roles.

This liberal perspective may account for some of the differences that existed between the early feminist movement of the 1970s and 1980s and nursing. Baer (1997) made this point, taking mainstream feminism to task. She argues that the "women as equal" perspective seemed to have greater resonance with feminists than did the "women as different" perspective. She notes that the equality perspective has had the

> effect of seeming not to comprehend or support the values and ideas of people who *choose* society's care-taking roles. In fact, such feminists seem to refuse to believe that women who engage in 'women's work' chose it, thoughtfully and happily, with full consideration of other possibilities, and were not merely following their biological destiny. (Baer, 1997, pp. 245–246)

This continuing disdain for "women's work," she points out, threatens the entire health care system, which relies heavily on nursing expertise, and recipients of care and their families.

Even more striking, according to Fraser and Nicholson (1990), these early scholars tended to repeat the specific types of universalizing found in the particular schools of thought to which their work was most closely allied. Fraser and Nicholson point to examples of Marxist-feminist scholarship, which suffered from the same faulty universalizations found in nonfeminist Marxist scholarship, and feminist developmental scholarship, which mimicked, early on, the mistakes present in developmental psychology. "The irony was that one of the most powerful arguments that feminist scholars were making was the limitation of scholarship which falsely universalized on the basis of limited perspectives" (Fraser & Nicholson, 1990, p. 1). Feminist scholars were becoming increasingly aware that the problem with much existing scholarship was that the voices of many other social groups were not represented. Clearly, new methods were necessary. The time was ripe for a fusion of postmodern perspectives and feminist approaches, each able to enrich the other.

Toward a Postmodern Feminism

Feminists, like postmodernists, have sought to develop new paradigms of social criticism that do not rely on traditional philosophical underpinnings. Both schools of thought have criticized modern epistemologies and universal and ahistorical "truths." There has been a "growing interest among feminists in modes of theorizing which are attentive to differences and to cultural and historical specificity" (Fraser & Nicholson, 1990, p. 33).

Women comprise more than half of the population. Research approaches to issues of gender, whether conducted by women or men, may vary. Feminist empirical work, as nursing research, is multiparadigmatic (Dzurec, 1989;

Lather, 1991). Westcott (1977) characterizes the feminist scholarship of the 1970s and 1980s as operating largely within the conventional positivist frame, whereas many current feminist researchers view the methodological task as to generate and refine more contextualized, interactive methods in the search for pattern and meaning rather than prediction and control (Lather, 1991).

> When we began theorizing our experience during the second women's movement a mere decade and a half ago, we knew our task would be a difficult though exciting one. But I doubt that in our wildest dreams we ever imagined we would have to reinvent both science and theorizing in order to make sense of women's social experience. (Harding, 1986, p. 251)

One could extrapolate Harding's thought to the words "we [i.e., nursing] would have to reinvent medicine and therapeutics to make sense of the human experience of health care." This is the main point of Jean Watson's 1999 book *Postmodern Nursing and Beyond*. She writes,

> Nursing is presented as a paradigm case for women and the caring-healing dimensions of women's work, work that has been expunged from the traditional western world cosmology, and particularly the modern masculine archetype of traditional science and medicine—the latent and not so latent archetype under which nursing has located itself within this modern era of the 20th century. (p. 6)

Kroker and Cook (1986) state: "Feminism is the quantum physics of postmodernism" (p. 22), and some postulate "postfeminism," that is, issues beyond gender. According to Flax (1990), feminist theories, like other forms of postmodernism, should encourage us to tolerate and interpret ambivalence, ambiguity, and multiplicity as well as expose the roots of our needs for imposing order and structure. She concludes, "If we do our work well, reality will appear even more unstable, complex, and disorderly than it does now. In this sense perhaps Freud was right when he declared that women are the enemies of civilization" (p. 57).

The Convergence of Postmodern Feminism and Nursing: The Time for Reconciliation

None of the approaches discussed in this chapter are axiomatic. This is not a time for a new orthodoxy. Uncertainty and dissonance will persist. Lather (1991) states that her goal is to move research in many different, and occasionally contradictory, directions in the hope that "more interesting and useful ways of knowing will emerge" (p. 69). She supports experimentation, collaboration, and sharing, enterprises supported by feminist approaches. She quotes Polkinghorne (1983):

What is needed most is for practitioners to experiment with new designs and to submit their attempt and results to examination by other participants in the debate. The new historians of science have made it clear that methodological questions are decided in the practice of research by those committed to developing the best possible answers to their questions, not armchair philosophers of research. (p. xi)

As nurses, and knowledgeable consumers of health care, there is very little chance we will become "armchair philosophers of research." There is too much important work to be done.

Nursing theories have "universalizing and generalizing" tendencies that do not address "the diversities of nursing phenomena . . . and thus offer little understanding of people's experiences" (Meleis, quoted in Salas, 2005, p. 19). Salas (2005) notes, "The need to have an organizing framework to order the phenomena of interest for the discipline does not reflect an understanding of the way that nursing is lived in practice" (p. 22). Salas suggests revisiting nursing theory in a "global world." This has relevance for us all as nurses: attention to the marginalized and often exteriorized (Hall, 1982, p. 42). A "path of solidarity" with the exteriorized is postulated as a way of coming to "a deeper understanding and appreciation of the interdependent character of the global community" (Smith, quoted in Salas, 2005, p. 23). Human interdependency demonstrates the need of the weak for the strong, and conversely, at the same time, the strong for the weak. This echoes the important theme of "cyclical continuum" identified by Munhall (2001, p. 5), the idea of "an absolution" to the eternal quantitative-qualitative polarization. Put another way, it suggests "moving to postpositivism and reconciliation" (Stevens, quoted in Munhall, 2001, p. 5).

The global world is the postmodern world. We are there. There is no going back. Take the plunge. The water is fine.

REFERENCES

Agger, B. (1991). Critical social theory, post structuralism, post modernism: Their sociological relevance. *Annual Review of Sociology, 17,* 105–131.

Allen, D. G. (1986). Using philosophical and historical methodologies to understand the concept of health. In P. L. Chinn (Ed.), *Nursing research methodology: Issues and implementation* (pp. 157–168). Rockville, MD: Aspen.

Allen, D., Benner, P., & Diekelmann, N. L. (1986). Three paradigms for nursing research: Methodological implications. In P. L. Chinn (Ed.), *Nursing research methodology: Issues and implementation* (pp. 23–38). Rockville, MD: Aspen.

Baer, E. (1997). Women and the politics of career development: The case of nursing. In A. M. Rafferty, J. Robinson, & G. Elkan (Eds.), *Nursing history and the politics of welfare* (pp. 242–258). London: Routledge.

Bauman, Z. (1992). *Intimations of postmodernity.* London: Routledge.

Bernstein, R. J. (1983). *Beyond objectivism and relativism: Science, hermeneutics and praxis.* Philadelphia: University of Pennsylvania Press.

Browne, A. J. (2000). The potential contributions of critical social theory to nursing science. *Canadian Journal of Nursing Research, 32*(2), 35–55.

Callaway, H. (1981). Women's perspectives: Research as re-vision. In P. Reason & J. Rowan (Eds.), *Human inquiry* (pp. 457–472). New York: Wiley.

Cheek, J. (2000). *Postmodern and poststructural approaches to nursing research.* Thousand Oaks, CA: Sage.

Davidson, J., & Rees-Mogg, W. (1993). *The great reckoning.* New York: Simon & Schuster.

Duchscher, J. E. B. (2000). Bending a habit: Critical social theory as a framework for humanistic nursing education. *Nurse Education Today, 20,* 453–462.

Dzurec, L. (1989). The necessity for and evolution of multiple paradigms for nursing research: A poststructuralist perspective. *Advances in Nursing Science, 11*(4), 69–77.

Flax, J. (1990). Postmodernism and gender relations. In L. Nicholson (Ed.), *Feminism/Postmodernism* (pp. 39–62). New York: Routledge.

Foucault, M. (1980). *Power/knowledge: Selected interviews and other writings, 1972–1977.* Brighton, Harvester: Harvester Press.

Fraser, N., & Nicholson, L. (1990). Social criticism without philosophy: An encounter between feminism and postmodernism. In L. Nicholson (Ed.), *Feminism/Postmodernism* (pp. 19–38). New York. Routledge.

Freire, P. (2003). *Pedagogy of the oppressed.* New York: Continuum. (Original work published 1970).

Habermas, J. (1999). Towards a theory of communicative competence. In E. C. Polifroni and M. Welch (Eds.), *Perspectives on philosophy of science in nursing* (pp. 360–375). Philadephia: Lippincott. (Reprinted from *Inquiry, 13,* 1970).

Hall, S. (1982). The rediscovery of ideology: Return of the repressed in media studies. In M. Gurevitch, T. Bennett, & J. Wollacott (Eds.), *Culture, society and the media* (pp. 30–55). London: Methuen.

Harding, S. (1986). *Sex and scientific inquiry.* London: Routledge.

Hedin, B. H. (1986). Nursing, education, and emancipation: Applying the critical theoretical approach to nursing research. In P. L. Chinn (Ed.), *Nursing research methodology: Issues and implementation* (pp. 133–146). Rockville, MD: Aspen.

Ironside, P. M. (2001). Creating a research base for nursing education: An interpretive review of conventional, critical, feminist, postmodern, and phenomenologic pedagogies. *Advances in Nursing Science, 23,* 72–87.

Jardine, L. (1999). *Ingenius pursuits.* New York: Doubleday.

Johnson, P. (1991). *The birth of the modern.* New York: Harper.

Kendall, J. (1992). Fighting back: Promoting emancipatory nursing actions. *Advances in Nursing Science, 15,* 1–15.

Kroker, A., & Cook, D. (1986). *The postmodern scene: Excremental culture and hyperaesthetics.* New York: St. Martin's Press.

Kunstler, J. (2005). *The long emergency.* New York: Atlantic Monthly Press.

Kuokkanen, L., & Leino-Kilpi, H. (2000). Power and empowerment in nursing: Three theoretical perspectives. *Journal of Advanced Nursing, 31,* 235–241.

Lather, P. (1991). *Getting smart: Feminist research and pedagogy with/in the postmodern.* New York: Routledge.

McCall, E. (1996, April). Horizontal volence in nursing: The continuing silence. *Lamp,* 28–31.

Munhall, P. (2001). Language and nursing research. In P. Munhall, P. (Ed.), *Nursing research: A qualitative perspective* (pp. 3–36). Sudbury, MA: Jones and Bartlett.

Owen-Mills, V. (1995). A synthesis of caring praxis and critical social theory in an emancipatory curriculum. *Journal of Advanced Nursing, 21,* 1191–1195.

Polkinghorne, D. (1983). *Methodology for the human sciences: Systems of inquiry.* Albany: State University of New York Press.

Ritzer, G., & Goodman, D. J. (2004). *Modern sociological theory* (6th ed.). Boston: McGraw-Hill.

Roberts, S. J. (1983). Oppressed group behavior: Implications for nursing. *Advances in Nursing Science, 5,* 21–30.

Salas, A. S. (2005). Toward a North-South dialogue: Revisiting nursing theory (from the South). *Advances in Nursing Science, 20*(23), 17–24.

Skillings, L. N. (1992). Perceptions and feelings of nurses about horizontal violence as an expression of oppressed group behavior. In J. L. Thompson, D. G. Allen, & Rodrigues-Fisher, L. (Eds.), *Critique, resistance, and action: Working papers in the politics of nursing* (p. 79). New York: National League for Nursing Press.

Stevens, P. E. (1984). A critical social reconceptualization of environment in nursing: Implications for methodology. In P. Chinn (Ed.), *Exemplars in criticism: Challenge and controversy. Advances in Nursing Science Series* (pp. 127–139). Gaithersburg, MD: Aspen.

Thompson, J. L. (1987). Critical scholarship: The critique of domination in nursing. *Advances in Nursing Science, 10,* 27–38.

van Manen, M. (1990). *Researching lived experience: Human science for an action sensitive pedagogy.* Albany: State University of New York Press.

Watson, J. (1999). *Postmodern nursing and beyond.* London: Churchill Livingstone.

Weber, M. (2005). The critical social theory of the Frankfurt School and the "social turn" in IR. *Review of International Studies, 31,* 195–209.

Welch, M. (1999). Critical theory and feminist critique. In E.C. Polifroni & M. Welch (Eds.), *Perspectives on philosophy of science in nursing* (pp. 355–359). Philadephia: Lippincott.

Westcott, M. (1977). Conservative method. *Philosophy of Social Sciences, 7,* 67–76.

Wilson-Thomas, L. (1995). Applying critical social theory in nursing education to bridge the gap between theory, research, and practice. *Journal of Advanced Nursing, 21,* 568–575.

Wuest, J. (1994). Professionalism and the evolution of nursing as a discipline: A feminist perspective. *Journal of Professional Nursing, 10,* 357–367.

PART II

Qualitative Methods and Exemplars

Part II of this text invites you to contemplate the potential of qualitative methods with "how to" chapters followed by "here is an example" chapters. You will become aware of the similarities among the qualitative methods as well as variations, which most often depend on the aim of the study.

All the methods in this section are founded on the perspectives described in Part I of this text. You will be introduced to methods in phenomenology, grounded theory, ethnography, case study, historical research, narrative inquiry, and action research. Many methods are most similar to the phenomenological perspective and take into consideration the same concepts described in that chapter (Chapter 6). Although the methods introduced here are the most foundational and commonly used ones, in today's world many other methods are emerging, which are variations of those described in this section.

Each description of a particular method is followed by an exemplar of that method, an actual research study. As mentioned in Chapter 1, the exemplar may not follow the method chapter as a literal example because variations exist. There are different *ways of doing* a specific qualitative research method, and as long as a researcher adheres to the philosophical, and in some cases theoretical, underpinnings of the method, it is acceptable and perhaps characteristic of the respect qualitative researchers have for variations in interpretation.

Studies can vary from the method because a researcher is not aware at the start of a study where the participants may lead the researcher. However, evaluation criteria are available to ensure credibility, trustworthiness, and resonance so we can evaluate our research from the highest standards of research science.

This edition includes new contributing authors for the method chapters and new exemplars. I mention this to encourage you, for further information, to go back and read the method and exemplar chapters in all previous editions, 1987, 1993, and 2001. This can enrich your experience and also introduces you to many of the other leaders in qualitative research development.

I think you will enjoy these chapters and gain appreciation for what qualitative research offers us as human beings, with its intense focus on meaning, understanding, and interpretation of experience. We are always in experience, our patients are always in experience, and so it is incumbent upon us to understand and appreciate their life-worlds, as well as our own, with all the variations and complexities.

To me it is this complicatedness—sometimes called the *messiness* of our human lives—the interconnectedness of phenomena, and the appreciation of intersubjectivity that gives qualitative research the authenticity and existential humanness that has the potential to enrich our lives with the knowledge and insight essential for compassion, care, liberation, and finding meaning in everyday experience.

6

A Phenomenological Method

Patricia L. Munhall

To Think Phenomenologically

The chapters of Part I lay the foundation for our initial foray into the wonderful philosophical world of phenomenology. I hope you are beginning to feel well grounded in the history, language, and epistemology of the qualitative perspective. You will find that what we discuss in this chapter will also apply to the other qualitative methods discussed in this book because most interpretations of qualitative methods are rooted in phenomenological philosophy. However, some qualitative methods also have a theoretical component, such as grounded theory, whereas phenomenology is atheoretical.

Right now, return to Chapter 4 and read the first sentence by Marcia Dombro: "Qualitative research is not a method, it is a philosophical approach that overarches many different ways of collecting and analyzing data" (on page 99). You might be thinking, "But this book is about qualitative methods." Yes, and no! It is entitled *Nursing Research: A Qualitative Perspective*, and that is more appropriate to the underpinning philosophy than is using the word *method* if *method* is a single way of doing something *in a predetermined, step-by-step sequential approach.*

As discussed in Chapter 2, a prerequisite to acceptance as a discipline in the academy or university is to have bona fide research or a "science" for research. To accomplish a respectable status in research, it seems one must use a method and use it correctly for the research to be valid. This we have inherited from the positivistic world of the scientific method as iconic and the necessity of *method*. For qualitative research, it presents a problem. Most problematic is the phenomenological research project. For reasons to be discussed shortly, the words *perspective* and *approach* seem more appropriate. In addition, I suggest in this chapter for you to *think and become* phenomenologic, if you are to embark on phenomenological research, so that this perspective guides your study and your ways of seeing phenomena and understanding experience. This actually is not an unusual direction in that if you were to do scientific laboratory research, you would be encouraged "to think like a scientist." Here is the same helpful suggestion, "to think phenomenologically," and in this chapter it is my aim to help you understand what that means.

WE HAVE METHODS!

So now, because of the language of the academy or university, we have qualitative *methods* for many ways of researching experience, problems, interventions, and acquiring evidence that *do* have steps, rules, checkpoints, and ways of presenting material. But you will find in qualitative research a flexibility that is essential to the inductive approach as discussed. If we start a research project for which not much is known about the subject, often as we explore, we come to "know" something that might make the planned next step of our proposal irrelevant or inappropriate. Whether using phenomenology or another qualitative method, flexibility to change your proposal is essential. This can have dramatic results, as when your beginning study of an experience reveals a factor hidden in the experience that must be studied first for you to understand your first chosen study.

For example, one of my first phenomenological studies was going to be researching the experience of social isolation, when I began to realize that the real phenomenon undergirding this seemed to be the experience of anger. So, then I changed my perspective to seeing when anger appeared, the various faces of anger, and concealed or repressed expressions of this emotion.

However, back to the quote by Marcia Dombro in Chapter 4. This chapter starts out the same way! What if I were to suggest that there really is no phenomenological method for research? If you plan to do a phenomenological study, perhaps you would become dismayed. Now what are you to do? There must be a "way," a "group of steps," a path to follow.

As is mentioned later in this chapter, it is the latter that researchers seek, which is very understandable. We might intuitively know how to get to our destination, but it feels so much safer and secure if we have a map.

So we seek maps that include various roads to get to our destination, always remembering that the map is not the actual territory. Like language, it is a representation. So are research methods. However, before we use the map, we need to know how to interpret it, and also how to drive a car. Too simplistic? Often in the simplest statements are very important, though obvious, truths.

Before we embark on "doing" a phenomenological research study, we must know how to interpret the philosophical underpinnings of phenomenology. We must understand them, and more important, we must know how to "be" phenomenologic in our own being (Sarah Steen Lauterbach in the next chapter discusses her own journey in becoming phenomenologic). This was quite a challenge to me, being brought up in one of the most scientific times in our history. Science was (and still is, to some) an icon, *a single version of truth*. The way the word has come to be used symbolizes a process and product of the material world, seen from an objective stance. As a nursing student, I can remember having the statement "be objective" drilled into my head from the very first day. Today it is easy for me to say, *objectivity is itself a subjective concept*. But at 17 years of age, well, you can just imagine! But objectivity has to be subjective. Who defines it? Who gives a study that kind of status? A subjective opinion. Often those subjective opinions differ. If you have sat through presentations of research, you will recall the many different opinions of various people, which originated from their own perceptions concerning the many different parts of that research project. Granted, the more subjective opinions one can obtain that are similar, the more objective a phenomenon or truth will seem.

However, in my own journey from nursing student to doctoral student, being objective seemed to be the defining characteristic of what was good and scientific. The Heisenberg Principle of Uncertainty withstanding, a problem emerged: often, objectivity is a sterile state, devoid of humanistic characteristics, and it ignores the situated context where the phenomenon is located. When directed to "be objective," what does that actually mean? Don't think about what? Oneself, the other person *in context*, what you would do since you are not the other person? To me it is a most puzzling directive, and I know I cannot be objective in the way the concept of objectivity is presently thought of and that is decontextualized. I want to understand the different reference points, the situated context, and the individual person.

An Overheard Encounter as Exemplar

"Becoming phenomenologic" toward the world is an entirely different view. Here is an example: a student said to a friend, "Why can't you answer me? Must everything be a secret? I was just asking you what you were doing."

For most of us, that kind of dialogue or a variant is not uncommon in communications with a friend or loved one. The scientist hearing the preceding questions might assume *objectively* that the person not answering seems, *objectively* speaking, simply to not want to reveal what he or she is doing. Actually, the questions would not have much interest at all to a scientist! However, for a student who is asking the questions, we have another story. The question could become more complex with an accusation such as: "You are deliberately hiding something from me, you do not like me, you want to be away from me," or more elaborately, "You have been ignoring me for weeks, you don't speak to me, you don't tell me anything, and I am only trying to be reasonable. Why can't you be reasonable as well?" The person asking the question assumes a rational stance to the question, expecting a rational response.

The response might be, "Don't you get it? I don't want to tell you," which is actually pretty rational. But then again it might be more elaborate, with a response, "If you don't stop annoying me, asking me questions, and if I wanted to tell you, I would tell you, and yes everything is a secret if I don't feel like telling you. Who do you think you are, my mother?"

Looking at this potential conflict from a phenomenological perspective, although it is a simple interaction at first glance, it becomes a very significant interaction of which we cannot determine knowledge about anything. Nothing from the questioner, nothing from the responder. Return to this dialogue when you read about intersubjectivity on page 173. Knowing how to think phenomenologically has enormous potential not only to make you a great researcher but a very understanding person. Understanding the dynamics of intersubjectivity can help you avoid many of the conflicts and misunderstandings inherent in human relationships. Thus, becoming phenomenologic is a way of being in the world.

In the preceding interaction, the phenomenological researcher knows there is a situated context and it is embedded in time, space, embodiment, and relationships. We also know that two perceptions are operating here—not an objective truth—two subjectivities, interacting and forming an intersubjective space. Two people are seeing the world through two different social constructions of reality and are even using language differently, though there might be an assumption that they are using the words in similar ways. The two people have two different experiences during this encounter. Perhaps the most important phenomenological realization is that the two different perceptions are going to result in two different interpretations of what seemingly looks like one reality. When doing phenomenological research, thoughts like this should come naturally to you, which is an understanding of communication unlike what might be necessary in doing *quantitative* research, for example.

This is just a brief synopsis of what it might mean to "think" and "be" phenomenologic. Nothing is taken for granted. Everything is held up for questioning. Of course, this would be exhausting if you did this with all communication; however, the more practiced you become with this view of the world, the more automatic this type of thinking becomes for you and actually the better your understanding and communication become. Here is another possible answer to the overheard dialogue: "You know, I had no idea that I was being secretive. I am just preoccupied with something. I would not keep secrets from you. I am going over to the cafeteria." What do you think a phenomenological-type person would think of that answer? It could be a true statement of innocence, but phenomenologically it would never be assumed to be true. By now you probably can think of all the variations that this simple answer might actually be concealing. "Being" phenomenologic is not only hearing language and believing something is being revealed that might be valid, but it is hearing and also contemplating what might be concealed in responses.

RESEARCHING A PHENOMENOLOGIC METHOD

In 1994, in my book *Revisioning Phenomenology: Nursing and Health Science Research* (Munhall, 1994a), I did not articulate a method in a formalized structured manner. I refer you to that work to supplement this chapter, and my aim here is to present a very flexible method that attempts to embrace the possibilities of thinking and being phenomenologic from one's perspective toward living and being. This method has evolved from the work of innumerable doctoral students who used van Manen's method and often utilized work from the "revisioning" book but still raised questions and asked for clarification. In *Revisioning*, I purposely attempted to guide students through the process of inquiry from a phenomenological perspective. I referred the reader to van Manen's approach on the basis of a subjective appraisal that his method was the most consistent with phenomenology as philosophy. Still, I received requests to articulate method because in my teaching I was apparently guiding students with what they perceived as a *method not yet written*. Also, some students, including myself, in contrast to van Manen, did think phenomenologic research could be problem solving and illuminate needed changes in many areas, whether policy or practice. I had begun to respond to Crotty's (1996) emphasis on critique where he states: "The goal of phenomenological inquiry goes beyond identifying, appreciating and explaining current and shared meanings. *It seeks to critique these meanings*" (p. 5; italics added). You will see, then, in this proposed method a "step" not ordinarily found in phenomenological studies, but one that could be added to other phenomenological methods or to any study:

"Write a narrative about the meaning of your study." This answers the "so what" question that has been asked after many research studies have been completed. Here, too, you will find *an emphasis on critiquing the interpretations with implications and recommendations for political, social, cultural, health care, nursing, family, and other social systems, as well as the individual.*

METHODS AND THEMES AND MEANING UNITS

What motivated me to move forward in the previous edition of this text (2001) were some criticisms that were leveled at many of our phenomenological studies. I hoped that, perhaps by integrating those criticisms into the development of this method, our phenomenological research would become more meaningful to practice and policy. I wanted to do this then and now because I do not want phenomenology to be misperceived or have its potential go unrecognized and unrespected, which unfortunately has happened in some instances.

After 20 years of assisting colleagues and students with master's theses and doctoral dissertations, I have become acquainted with common questions and frustrations and with sincere attempts to combine philosophy with method. If we were to accept the proposition that phenomenology as inquiry is aimed at understanding lived experience, as is sometimes written, or that the central purpose of phenomenology is to understand the meaning of being human, then the guiding word, I think, would be *approach*. We would approach the project, the study, and be guided by the emergent material. The experiences themselves would show the way to understanding meaning. However, *approach* does not do well in dissertation proposals or grant applications. The relevant section is simply not labeled "approach" but "method." For now, we must conform and hope the day will come when flexibility in proposal writing will be realized as an essential characteristic of phenomenological study.

"What is the meaning of being human?" is a phenomenal question. I believe the question is asked to come to a phenomenological answer: *understanding* the meaning of being human. For the most part, this question, *the meaning of being,*[1] goes unanswered, and the answer remains a mystery. All the phenomenology in the world is not going to solve the mystery altogether,

---

[1] I acknowledge that many religions have attempted to teach what the meaning of being is, or why we are here. In this text, I take this question out of the religious context while maintaining utmost respect for peoples' religious beliefs.

and I am not sure that we would want all mystery removed. Yet, in many human experiences, the desire for human understanding cannot and should not be ignored. What individuals have done with the foregoing question and its purpose has varied in responses and very different methods, even within the same philosophy of phenomenology. This chapter, though, is not to critique the various ways in which different schools of thought have developed methods to answer this question, but to give examples of how phenomenology has been done using the various humanistic psychological phenomenological methods. Studies following these "psychological" early methods, while well intended and deserving of our gratitude for opening the doors to phenomenologic research, unfortunately have sometimes left us open to a well-founded criticism that these methods reflect a form of reductionism and steplike studies that appear much like those based on logical positivism. Of course, using the same outlines for proposals and criteria for evaluation as those of the scientific method has not helped at all.

Many of these methods came about to gain acceptance within the academy. Many nurse researchers, when reviewing phenomenological research, come away wondering what it all means: lists of themes, lists of essences, structural definitions, categories of abstractions, meaning units, and other reductionistic descriptions of experience. However, these methods eased qualitative research and, in this instance, phenomenology, into the academy with rules to give these methods as much credence and respectability as the icon of the scientific method.

THE UNKNOWN: WHERE BEING REVEALS ITSELF

To be true to the philosophy of phenomenology we must follow *the thing itself* wherever and whenever it appears, while being attentive, conscious, and alert to its appearance or concealment. Know that with appearance there is concealment as well. Explore that and all its possibilities. Liberate yourself from prescribed steps. Methods can place you in a formula where you cannot wander outside, and that critical limitation, while a safeguard in the laboratory, is what will handcuff you and keep you from the spontaneous recognition of the appearance and the crucial exploration of the unforeseen. For years, I have urged my wonderful colleagues to liberate students and let them follow the phenomenological process so that they can be free to journey where "being" reveals itself. My main argument was that where "being" and "understanding" reveal themselves is largely *unknown at the outset* of a phenomenological inquiry. Once again you will see in Sarah Steen Lauterbach's phenomenological work (Chapter 7) that she did indeed wander into places, literally in her city backyard, that she had never known existed! You can see in her first study in the second edition (Munhall & Oiler-Boyd, 1993) a highly structured approach, and in this edition a more phenomenological narrative of her own evolution, which simultaneously produced an evolution of understanding in so many varying aspects of her original "experience" of interest, the understandings she never suspected embedded in the experience of losing a newborn child. The chapter in this edition is not only a phenomenology of her original focus, but also her own journey to ways of discovering over many years the many directions that were not on the map. Sarah states in both pieces that she combined van Manen's method and my approach.

I believe that Sarah had all the freedom she needed to find the unknown, but she was also extremely well grounded in phenomenological philosophy. In Chapter 7, she even speaks to the life-world of temporality that affects her own self-knowledge of phenomenology and indeed influences her study and interpretation. This self-awareness is essential to conducting phenomenological inquiry.

In phenomenological studies that I conduct, I reveal to the reader the situated context of my life experience that brings me to that very instant of interest. I have come to understand in the past 20 years that my own subjectivity, which is often the same as my interpretive belief about phenomenological inquiry as *process* and not as *method*, can be substantiated philosophically. I have, though, also come to understand that nurse researchers and other human science researchers do not have the freedom to go about any inquiry without a *method*.

MORE CONCERNS ABOUT METHOD

In the last edition of this text, I reflected on having a choice to be recalcitrant or, because of my experiential phenomenological understanding of students' experiences, to act on the meaning of their experiences. Will that mean that I am compromising my beliefs? The answer is no. I still believe the phenomenological inquiry is a process of the unknown that gives direction to the study and cannot possibly be known at the outset. How could we possibly come to understand the meaning of being human in experience if we were to follow linear, prescribed steps that create boundaries to exploration?

Each step taken would close that door prematurely; or worse, if it opened another door, we could not go there because it would not be part of the "steps" of the "method." I also believed, at the same time, that such a liberated perspective was not going to be accepted in the academy, unless perhaps (and even this is debatable) one was in a philosophy program. I have also taken note of the phenomenological "methods" and, with the exception of van Manen's, have become sufficiently concerned about the problems inherent in them, such as naming "reactions" to an experience instead of the meaning or even an understanding of the reactions. Most methods, when carried out according to prescribed steps, often start data collection with 6 to 10 "transcribed interviews."

Proceeding in this linear way, one then "extracts" essences or themes and provides a list or, worse, a definition of the lived experience! It is here that we are being critiqued as not understanding phenomenology (Crotty, 1996). I am providing this background as an example of how I have come to use phenomenological understanding to justify presenting a more pliable method. I am troubled by so many studies that present themselves as phenomenological studies, when the researchers have followed a linear method and ironically can come out with, despite the experience under study, often the same list of what I have come to understand as "reactions" to experiences. For example, without naming the experience, studies often have the same essences or themes as findings: fear of the unknown, loneliness, anxiety, anger, depression, helplessness, and isolation.

Listing themes or essences has left us open to the accusation that we are categorizing human experience, much like reductionism, found in quantitative studies. If we recall that the major focus of phenomenological inquiry is understanding meaning of some "thing," some experience, something that is human so that we can better understand the meaning of being human, perhaps the fact that the responses to experiences are often similar may not be surprising. I would venture further and say that we have a fairly good sense of what kind of reactions (themes) people are going to have in a specific experience. However, studies such as Sarah's demonstrate that our preconceived notions of reality can be very wrong.

Where many studies leave off—because, I would suggest, there is no "step" in the method the researcher may be following—is not to inquire into the meaning of these essences/responses for the particular individual. Sarah, however, demonstrates, with her participants, the meaning of isolation in the particular experience. She demonstrates the going back and forth, seeking further explanation, pondering the responses, bringing them to bear on the experience in a unique manner, unique in that experience.

Isolation, for example, has a different meaning in different experiences. The researcher has to be able to narrate for the reader the understanding that enlightens the meaning of isolation in the experience of, for instance, losing a newborn. Reasons are uncovered in the narrative of the participants that surprise us and give new direction to practice and, most important, to an understanding of human beings in experience and over time.

SEARCH FOR SIGNIFICANCE

All this needs to be said because it provides the "situated context" that inspired me to move toward a form of pragmatism and a *search for significance for phenomenological research*. Rochberg-Halthon claims that pragmatism "speaks to the contemporary hunger for significance" (in Crotty, 1996, p. 6). So it was from the perspective of two powerful beliefs of mine: that our phenomenological research *is* significant and that *we can demonstrate* its significance not by numbers, but by stating the implications for change that emerges from the interpretation we glean from our participants on the meaning of various experiences. Results from a phenomenological study can be used for policy development, change in practice, increasing our capacity for care and compassion, and raising our consciousness to what was not known or otherwise erroneous.

On the very practical side of pragmatism, students and researchers are required to present a proposal, which must include a method that is clearly spelled out, that will lead to some kind of findings, and that must also pass the institutional review board. Five years ago I came to a place where I realized that arguing that phenomenology was not a "method" but a process,[2] a way of being toward meaning and experience, was not pragmatic. And so I developed from a very holistic perspective the "suggestions" with which I have guided students and listened to their feedback and now have called a "method."

---

[2] Perhaps you might think I am overemphasizing this, but once into doing phenomenological research, you will understand this readily!

TABLE 6–1   Method for Phenomenological Inquiry Broad Outline

I. Immersion	
II. Coming to the phenomenological aim of the inquiry	
III. Existential inquiry, expressions, and processing*	IV. Phenomenological contextual processing*
V. Analysis of interpretive interaction	
VI. Writing the phenomenological narrative	
VIII. Writing a narrative on the meaning of your study	

*Concurrent processes.

This flexible method is holistic in the sense that students and colleagues participated in a "going back and forth" with me and have been a greater part of this work than I have been. Because of their work, they have demonstrated the method. I have come to understand this experience, mostly from them, and *unbeknownst* to them and me, we were all participants! Table 6–1, which represents the broad outline of this method, and Table 6–2, which presents the method in greater detail, reflect this shared collaboration among former students, colleagues, and me.

PHENOMENOLOGICAL RESEARCH IMMERSION

Immersion is an essential and critical beginning of a phenomenological study. Phenomenological inquiry just cannot be done well or have any meaning if the researcher has not learned the language and come to understand the philosophical underpinnings of phenomenology. This is the place where students often discover that qualitative research can be more difficult than quantitative research is. There may be many reasons for this, but surely one reason, as discussed in Chapter 1, is that students are not prepared for qualitative research in the same way they are prepared for quantitative research, as far as course requirements. Students must master quantitative methods through courses and learn qualitative methods on their own. Thankfully, some changes in this curriculum area are taking place, as was discussed in Chapter 1.

All philosophies are based on assumptions about the world and contain abstractions and concepts to explain, describe, conceptualize, and analyze the nature of being, the universe, truth, meanings, knowledge, ethics, and the many pursuits of philosophy. Criticisms have been directed toward some researchers for simplifying the complexity and text of phenomenology. In fact, this chapter is one of simplification because it is an *introduction*.

It is absolutely critical that, if you use a method, you read, read, read about it. Perhaps you can take a course at your university, or you could request a course or workshop. Online courses are also available. Of course, there is nothing like time and experience to really "get it," and even then there will be people who have really "gotten it" and still do not come to the same interpretation of phenomenology, and that is fine. If we believe all our voices express a polyvocality, then we respect varying interpretations of method. Almost all methods have their own controversies, as mentioned in Judith Wuest's chapter on the grounded theory method (Chapter 8).

TABLE 6–2 Method for Phenomenological Inquiry

I. Immersion	A. Describe and interpret the philosophical assumptions and underpinnings of a particular phenomenological perspective.
	B. Exemplify the meaning of phenomenological concepts.
	C. Elucidate the worldview of phenomenology as an approach to answering questions. (If you know the experience in which you are interested, use it as an example.)
II. Coming to the phenomenological aim of the inquiry	A. Articulate the aim of your study.
	B. Distinguish the experience that is part of your study.
	1. Describe, if circumscribed experience, or delimit context, if broad experience.
	2. Articulate the situated context that is available to you in the moment.
	C. Decenter yourself and come to "unknow."
	1. Reflect on your own beliefs, preconceptions, intuitions, motives, and biases so as to decenter.
	2. Adopt a perspective of "unknowing."
	D. Articulate the aim of the study in the form of a phenomenological question.

	III. Existential inquiry, expressions, and processing*	IV. Phenomenological contextual processing*
III. Existential inquiry, expressions, and processing* IV. Phenomenological contextual processing*	A. Listen to self and others; develop heightened attentiveness to self and others.	A. Analyze emergent situated contexts.
		B. Analyze day-to-day contingencies.
		C. Assess life-worlds.
	B. Reflect on personal experiences and expressions.	
	C. Provide experiential descriptive expressions: "the experiencer."	
	D. Provide experiential descriptive expressions: "others engaged in the experience."	

*Concurrent processes.

TABLE 6–2   Method for Phenomenological Inquiry (CONTINUED)

	E. Provide experiential descriptive expressions: the arts and literature review.
	F. Provide anecdotal descriptive expressions: as experience appears.
	G. Record ongoing reflection in your personal journal.
V. Analysis of interpretive interaction	A. Integrate existential investigation with phenomenological contextual processing.
	B. Describe expressions of meaning (thoughts, emotions, feelings, statements, motives, metaphors, examples, behaviors, appearances and concealments, voiced and nonvoiced language).
	C. Interpret expressions of meaning as appearing from integration.
VI. Writing the phenomenological narrative	A. Choose a style of writing that will communicate an understanding of the meaning of this particular experience.
	B. Write inclusively of all meanings, not just the "general" but the "particular."
	C. Write inclusively of language and expressions of meaning with the interpretive interaction of the situated context.
	D. Interpret with participants the meaning of the interaction of the experience with contextual processing.
	E. Narrate a story that at once gives voice to actual language and simultaneously interprets meaning from expressions used to describe the experience.
VII. Writing a narrative on the meaning of your study	A. Summarize the answer to your phenomenological question with breadth and depth.
	B. Indicate how this understanding obtained from those who have lived the experience calls for self-reflection and/or system reflection.
	C. Interpret meanings of these reflections to small and large systems within specific context.
	D. Critique this interpretation with implications and recommendations for political, social, cultural, health care, family, and other social systems.

In this chapter, I reference material presented in my own text titled *Revisioning Phenomenology: Nursing and Health Science Research* (Munhall, 1994a) and am very open with the reader that reading *that* book does not in any way suffice as the process step of immersion. However, I have been very gratified that readers have thanked me for simplifying what might be more obtuse in other writings on understanding phenomenology. With modesty, I would say that it is a good first book to read. It is conversational and friendly.

Neither does reading van Manen (1990) or Benner (1994) fulfill the requirement for immersion. Look to Chapter 4 to become acquainted with first-generation phenomenologists and continue to research more contemporary ones. For example, to demonstrate how important immersion is to good phenomenological research, the following paragraphs should comprise your knowledge base. As you read them, you might not readily understand the concepts. Because this is not a text on phenomenology, I have compressed some of the most prevalent names and schools to impress upon you what you would read during your immersion process. You need to become familiar with these philosophers, methods, and the different interpretations of phenomenology.

This way, you will have a solid foundation on which to make your own choice of method or focus. This is incredibly important and vital. For some of you, this may seem daunting, but if you find your "home" here, you will *enjoy* the challenge, thoughtfulness, and ideas that reflect the search for meaning and understanding. However, not all philosophers are easy to read. Philosophers trained in the discipline find reading Heidegger exasperating at times. I am aware of the emphasis I have placed on reading the original works of these philosophers, but at the same time I encourage you to read authors who have interpreted the philosophers' works in an understandable format.

In the process of immersion, the following two paragraphs would be easily understood and you would be conversant with the material. For example, as part of your immersion you would read Merleau-Ponty, who is considered more of an existential phenomenologist. His focus is on the importance of perception and the individual's situatedness in the world through experience. Husserl, absolutely essential reading, is thought of as a transcendental phenomenologist for whom consciousness is not empirical but "pure" consciousness.

Hermeneutical phenomenology is most often associated with Heidegger, where the focus is on understanding "being," and you can see that his philosophical influence is prevalent in this chapter. Within Heidegger's phenomenology, one views all phenomenological description as interpretation. As you travel in the immersion process, you will come to ask, "What about analytical phenomenology as contrasted to interpretative? Are they the same?"

The answer to those questions would vary, depending on the phenomenologist. Different answers to the same questions are, in my experience, part of the complexity of phenomenology. Yet, one could continue to categorize these different schools and arrive at one answer to the preceding questions and say that analytical phenomenology has more to do with the semiotic meaning structures of cultural practices, or that gender phenomenology is most concerned with context sensitivity and is truth tentative (M. van Manen, workshop, 1998).

The state of the art of phenomenology reflects the postmodern world that we inhabit in that there are multiple interpretations and multiple realities, as Lynne Dunphy and Joy Longo discussed in Chapter 5. Phenomenology is like a mirror in that it celebrates reflection, where differences and the "particular" are unveiled.

Nursing Research and Phenomenology

My own observations of phenomenological inquiry by nurses include references to one of the French or German phenomenologists, say, the first generation, and then these nurse researchers move to a phenomenologist who has proposed a "method" for inquiry. Among them (for the sake of simplicity, I choose four and refer to them as second-generation phenomenologists) are Georggi, Colaizzi, van Kaam, and van Manen. The first three are from the United States; they became the most influential methodologists for nurse researchers in the 1970s and 1980s. Faced with the requirement of finding a method to conduct a phenomenological study and lacking formal training themselves in this area, nurse researchers understandably chose one of these three phenomenological methods. Many problems seemed to have arisen from this attempt at articulation. Although the researchers became well versed in phenomenological thought by reading the first generation of phenomenologists, the transition to these other methods was often limiting and incongruent with the philosophy.

Historically, this outcome is understandable if we remember the pedestal that "method" was put upon; perhaps more influential and costlier, the closer a method could look like a "scientific method" or "*the* scientific method," the more acceptable it was in the academy. The last phenomenologist mentioned, Max van Manen (1984, 1990), changed this situation dramatically with a human science approach, where his views were often consistent with many of the first-generation phenomenological philosophers. The reason that he is an outstanding phenomenologist for those in the human sciences to follow is that he views phenomenology as a philosophy of being as well as a practice. From this perspective, any methodic location can give a view of experiential understanding by questioning lived experience through reflective writing. Here, and in this way, meaning can be understood and we can become practitioners of the ever-fragile exercise of phenomenological wisdom (van Manen, 1998). Nurse researchers have elaborated on these various methods, including fine works by Paterson & Zderad (1976, 1988), Benner (1994), Parse (1987), Ray (1990), Watson (1985), Newman (1986), and many others. To reiterate, this chapter cannot prepare you entirely to do a phenomenological study. It is an overview, and the whole text is an introduction to many different qualitative methods. In this overview, I would like to place some basic phenomenologic concepts as they appear in *Revisioning*. To really understand these concepts is to dedicate yourself to following up on reading more and more, and then some more.

The Phenomenological *Paradigm*

As an alternative and a historical reaction to the then prevailing hegemony of the positivist perspective, phenomenology construed itself as a philosophy, a perspective, and an approach to practice and research. Philosophically, phenomenology seems to undergird many of the qualitative research approaches (although some argue this point). Because of its importance as a philosophy, some key concepts are presented here. Recognition needs to be given to Husserl, who introduced the idea of phenomenology in response to or in reaction to the context-free generalizations of the positivist approach of the natural sciences. Husserl attempted to restore the "reality" of humans in their "life-worlds," to capture the "meaning" of this, and to revive philosophy with new humanism. Spiegelberg (1976), Cohen (1987), and Reeder (1987) provide excellent discussions of the history of the phenomenological movement. These concepts then, as outlined, reflect an acknowledgment of the inevitability of subjectivity in any exploration or description of reality. This inevitability is not stated with resignation but with the idea that subjectivity expands and enriches the authenticity of perceptions and understandings of phenomenology. It is this perspective that is both essential and desirable.

Key *Concepts of Phenomenology as* Philosophy

As defined by Merleau-Ponty (1962), *consciousness* is sensory awareness of and response to the environment. Consciousness is life: it is not an interior or inner existence, it is existence in the world through the body. The unity of mind and body becomes a means of experiencing, thus eliminating the idea of a subjective and objective world. A person cannot step out of consciousness and be sure of anything. The world is knowable only through the subjectivity of being in the world. Objectivity as a quest for reliability and validity depends on the recognition of this relationship between mind and body, subject and object, and the knowledge that this or any knowing comes about through consciousness.

Embodiment explains that through consciousness we are aware of being-in-the-world, and it is through the body that we gain access to this world. We feel, think, taste, touch, hear, and are conscious through the opportunities the body offers. There is talk sometimes about expanding the mind or expanding waistlines. The expansion is within the body, within consciousness. At any point in time and for each individual, a particular perspective or consciousness exists based on the individual's history, knowledge of the world, and perhaps openness to the world. Human science's focus on the individual and on the meaning events may have for an individual reflects the recognition that experience is individually interpreted.

The *natural attitude* (Schutz & Wagner, 1970) is a mode of consciousness that espouses interpreted experiences. The world as experienced and interpreted by preceding generations is handed down, teaching a great deal about reality in the process. These teachings become assumptions, unquestioned meanings about phenomena, that are a part of a person's "natural attitude" toward the world. To hear or see something contrary to the natural attitude can be disconcerting. This attitude of being in the world is deeply ingrained and usually unquestioned. Understanding the concept of natural attitude can help in understanding, at the individual level, responses to change. Both the perspectival and the physiological alterations associated with a life change are often the result of a *disruption* of the natural attitude.

Experience and *perception* are our original modes of consciousness. Perception, which takes place through the body, is an individual's access to experience in the world. Perception of varying objects depends also on the context in which they are experienced for interpretation and meaning. A person who says the aim of phenomenology is to describe lived experience may be describing his or her own or another's perceptions of that lived experience.

Perception of experience is what matters, not what in reality may appear to be contrary or more "truthful." If a person perceives danger when "in fact" there may be none, in the reality of that person's lived experience, there *is* danger. Perhaps that is why saying "this won't hurt" or "this will only hurt for a little while" is often ineffective in allaying a person's fear. The perception of the lived experience may not even be of pain; the perception may be of a danger far worse than being hurt or feeling pain. Interpretation of the experience from the individual's unique perception of an event is critical. What is important from this worldview, therefore, is not what is happening, but what is perceived as happening. That is the reality to be concerned with — the experience as the individual is perceiving it.

As a philosophy, phenomenology demonstrates these major concepts in the many interpretations that exist concerning its meaning. A phenomenological question here might be asked: "What is it like to try to understand phenomenology?" or, "What makes someone think and talk about phenomenology?" The answers are found in the themes of consciousness, embodiment, the natural attitude, perception, and experience. Again, these two questions would be good grist for the phenomenological perspective as a qualitative approach to research.

Phenomenology as Philosophy: More Key Concepts

The relational view of the person posited by Heidegger (1927/1962) further elaborates on the philosophical theme of phenomenology. Because an individual participates in cultural, social, and historical contexts of the world, to be human is to "be-in-the-world." Language, cultural, and social practices are handed down to individuals who embody the meanings and interpretations of these practices. In Heideggerian phenomenology, the interpretation and self-understanding handed down through language and culture are called the "background" (Allen, Benner, & Diekelmann, 1986). The idea of the background (like the natural attitude) is critical because it provides conditions for human actions and perceptions. It is where the individual is, a history to the present moment, and a view of "what can be." Other Heideggerian ideas include the following:

♦ Meaning is found in the transaction between an individual and a situation so that the individual both constitutes and is constituted by the situation.

♦ Human purposes and concerns "prestructure" the human world so that what is considered significant about an event or object is a function of or embodies that concern (Dreyfus, 1972). The perception of meaning follows from this understanding.

♦ This understanding is predicated on the belief that immediate experience is embodied with organization and meaning, with linguistic, social, and cultural patterning, and with characteristics intrinsic to the experience.

♦ A critical assumption of this phenomenological perspective is its emphasis on language, which imbues and informs experience. Language does not exist apart from thought or perception, for language generates and constrains the human life-world.

Key Concepts of Phenomenology as Research

Max van Manen (1984) offers the following observations about phenomenological research:

+ Phenomenology is the study of the individual's life-world, as experienced rather than as conceptualized, categorized, or theorized. Phenomenology aims for a deeper understanding of the nature or meaning of everyday experiences.

+ Phenomenological research is the study of essences of experience. In phenomenology, the researcher does not ask, "How do nursing students learn to nurse?" but asks instead, "What is the nature of the experience of becoming a nurse?" The aim is to understand the experience. The opportunities for plausible insights bring the investigator in more direct contact with the world.

+ Phenomenological research is the attentive practice of thoughtfulness—a minding, a heeding, a caring attunement, a wondering about the project of living. When the language of a lived experience awakens a person to the meaning of the experience, he or she gains a fuller understanding of what it means to be human.

+ Phenomenological research is a quest for what it means to be human. The more deeply a person understands human experience, the more fully and uniquely he or she becomes human. Such individuals learn to notice and to make sense of the various aspects of human existence. Of course, the more often a person engages in such attentiveness, the more he or she should be able to understand the details as well as the more global dimensions of life. The corollary is that such previously unreflected upon phenomena, the "taken for granted," assume richer meaningfulness.

+ Phenomenology has been called "the science of examples." Phenomenological descriptions are often composed of examples that permit readers "to see" the deeper significance or structure of the lived experience being described.

As emphasized earlier in this book, our colleagues who are preparing to do quantitative studies do so with many methods and statistics courses, and we cannot expect less when we embark on qualitative research. We do ourselves a disservice from the beginning if this formal study of qualitative research is not part of immersion. Reading unfamiliar language leaves the interpretation up to the reader, and it is in this particular activity where caution, in particular in the beginning of learning, needs to be taken. Speaking and hearing others speak of the philosophical ideas, concepts, and assumptions must be part of immersion. This is the area where I have found the most breakdown in phenomenological studies.

I want to again emphasize that the preceding didactic material on phenomenology, concepts, and origins is an abbreviated description, much too little content to really understand the concepts. Unfortunately, some students move directly from reading about a method and how to carry out the method to doing the study. Please don't miss the experience of delving deeper into understanding these concepts. Studying these concepts will eliminate frustration or confusion, and you will be confident in knowing that phenomenology is *more than the study of lived experience.* If you should do a dissertation using phenomenology, you will be comfortable in the knowledge and understanding you have acquired. Am I lecturing? Probably, but it is in your best interest. It is also from my own perspective and experience. For the student who does immersion, all else falls naturally into place. That student has become phenomenologic in being and continues, like Sarah discusses in the next chapter, to continue to become *more so* and *to be in a very good place in this world.*

The Aim of Immersion

The goal of immersion, then, is not unlike the goal of phenomenology: understanding. If you are going to embark on phenomenological inquiry, I urge you to find courses specific to phenomenology. They are becoming more widespread, and you may even find them online. In addition, participating in workshops provides an interaction that enlarges the processes in phenomenological research.* Immersion also requires reading phenomenological studies, which can be a curious sort of immersion. Some of these studies can teach you that some studies are not good ones, such as when you wonder what the point was.

Other studies resonate with you and, after reading such a study, you come to realize that you understand the meaning of being in some experience or another much better than you ever had before, or that you understand a human experience in a way that conflicts with what you once thought, as happens when people read, for example, Sarah's studies; this is good phenomenology. Immersion also means learning what may be called good phenomenology perhaps by reading articles from journals that discuss this

---

*See www.iihu.org for upcoming workshops (Chapter 26)

topic, provide constructive criticism, and remind researchers what must be of importance. The references in the chapters in Part I and this chapter contain important readings, and the Internet sites listed in Chapter 26 are also good sources that can contribute to this process of immersion.

The process of immersion is ongoing. I have found in my own life that the interest in the literature and the pursuit of greater understanding has become a part of who I am as a person. It is as though phenomenology becomes part of who you are, and you become phenomenologically present to and in the world.

Immersion enables you to understand what becoming phenomenologically present to the world means. This is the part that really is a process and cannot be reduced to a method. Over time, one who comes from this perspective will begin to interact differently with others, whether in research or practice. One begins to become less assuming, often abandoning assumptions about another or another's experience, and adopts a stance of "unknowing" (Munhall, 1993, 1994a). In this place, a person can be phenomenologically present to another person. Toward what end? To understand the other. To be open, nonjudgmental, and compassionate.

How can one act toward another in a caring, compassionate way if one has not suspended assumptions or judgments? How can one understand what kind of meaning an experience has for a person unless one suspends one's own preconceptions? In giving of ourselves in nursing and in our personal lives, how do we know what to do, what to say, and when it is better not to say anything if we do not understand the meaning of "something" for the other? This is why immersion is so critical. Becoming phenomenologically oriented requires a new and different way of perceiving reality. Part of immersion is to practice being phenomenological, which is a challenge, but one that is essential to the interviewing step in phenomenological methods. To interview in phenomenological inquiry is to be able to "decenter" and to be fully present to another (this topic is discussed further in this chapter).

If you are philosophically inclined toward understanding, once again I say immersion will be one of the most intellectually stimulating and affectively moving experiences of your educational experience. Without this step, phenomenological inquiry is not possible. Without this step, you will be doing storytelling, journalism, and impressionistic writing. Worse, you will be doing logical positivistic quasi-qualitative research! None of those activities, with the exception of the last one, are negative; but they are not phenomenology.

How to Accomplish the Step of Immersion in an Actual Study

Remember, this method as discussed in this context is for new researchers and for those who might be doing a study for a dissertation or a master's

thesis. Once this step is in process and has become a part of one's ongoing research program, the *step itself does not have to be on every proposal or study*.
However, it has been my experience that I continually enlarge my understanding with new literature as well as by returning to the classical literature.
This step as presented here is for those embarking for the first or second time
who have not done this step before.

Immersion is your research preparation for phenomenology (it is also
preparation for any other method of inquiry; ironically, it is spelled out more
clearly for quantitative studies but is never called immersion). Immersion as
a step, then, is almost pedantic with the aim of achieving a dynamic deep understanding; with practice it can be concretely reported as the first step for
beginning researchers in the following ways. What we are about to do now is
to articulate each step with an explanation of the step as well as the special
considerations inherent in the process of the step of this method as illustrated
in Tables 6–1 and 6–2.

I. Immersion

**A. Describe and interpret the philosophical assumptions and
underpinnings of a particular phenomenological perspective.**
This section should include the evolution of phenomenology, the philosophers, the different schools of phenomenology, and how they differ from one
another. The assurance that section A is done well is that you, your colleagues, and your professor come away from reading this section and agree
that you do have a good understanding of phenomenology. If this is not the
case, more immersion is needed.

B. Exemplify the meaning of phenomenological concepts.
In the process of writing section A, you most likely did not discuss the meaning of the various concepts. In this section, explain what they mean. For instance, give the meaning of the following:

- Situated context
- Intersubjectivity
- Perception
- Decentering
- Unknowing
- Appearance–concealment
- Being-in-the-world
- Consciousness
- Life-worlds: temporality, spatiality, corporeality, relationality
- Contingency

♦ Intentionality
♦ Preconceptions
♦ Shared perceptual fields

These and other phenomenological concepts are described in this chapter as well as in *Revisioning Phenomenology* (Munhall, 1994a) and other references. The assurance that section B is done well is that, with each concept, you demonstrate the meaning of the concept with a real-world example. Again, if colleagues and your professor understand you, you can be assured that you understand the meaning of concepts.

C. Elucidate the worldview of phenomenology as an approach to answering questions. (If you know the experience in which you are interested, use it as an example.)

This process prepares you for phenomenological dialogue/interviews/conversations. After studying decentering as an unknowing process and also understanding intersubjectivity, you practice conversations with others. The best person to practice with is someone who can critique your listening skills. That notwithstanding, after a conversation in which you practice decentered dialogue, write a description of the dialogue with an interpretation. Give this description to the person with whom you conversed to ascertain how and what you heard and whether you overlaid the description or interpretation of the dialogue with your own assumptions or preconceptions. This excellent exercise should be repeated. The assurance that section C is done well is that your description and interpretation of what the "other" was saying is validated by that person. This first step is critical. A lack of immersion is comparable to doing quantitative research without having taken research courses in the scientific method, statistics, and measurement. This step enables you to be the "instrument" for your study. Your role in the study requires high-level skills and learned sophistication in communication.

Existential Interaction.   Remember, in phenomenological inquiry you are going to be in constant interaction in the existential processing of phenomenological material. You will also be in transaction with persons in interviews and conversations and need to develop the consciousness of one who does not know. The researcher is in search of the meaning of a phenomenon, the meaning of being human in experience (phenomenon). Whether the researcher has or has not experienced the phenomenon, he or she needs to come to the phenomenological question as free as possible from assumptions, preconceptions, and forethought about the phenomenon or experience. When you first begin phenomenological inquiry, it is important to be cognizant that you do not and should not have a hypothesis. To this, one may say, "Of course!" However, often we are not aware of some hidden belief we may have and then try to find ways to document that belief. That is why de-centering yourself from your own world of knowledge and hunches is so important.

As you go on with these steps, it is important to understand that, as mentioned, they are not linear. There is a going back and forth, an examining and reexamining, a thought and then a change in thought, and there are many middle-of-the-night ahas!

A major component of phenomenological inquiry is a phenomenon that I call, for lack of a better description, "becoming your study." You become a repository for appearances of the experience or you become an example of the experience, and your attentiveness almost becomes unconscious. You are not actually looking for existential material for your study, but without notice, you will awaken to its presence. Some of us have marveled at the experience "of seeing it everywhere" or of realizing that "it was always there and I did not see it, hear it, understand it." Another way to describe this is to say that the subject of your study, the phenomenon, the experience, takes up residence within you. This will not occur if your inquiry is an academic exercise (although I have heard that, even then, it sometimes happens). The taking up of residence, to me, requires an intense longing to understand meaning—the meaning of something. It becomes a passion, and then the process is so much easier because you have become engaged with the philosophy of phenomenology. Philosophers are thinkers and questioners of a different sort than scientists. One very important distinction is this very lack of linearity.

Heidegger (1927/1962) stated *that language generates and constrains the human life-world* (italics added). As I was writing down a process as a method, I thought it was a wonderful example. I am constrained by language because it is expressed on paper in a linear way—line by line—when this method is, as mentioned, a back-and-forth and circular and sometimes even linear process.

II. Coming to the Phenomenological Aim of the Inquiry

The following four activities will assist you in focusing on the aim of your study. Your aim is to be understandable to others who are taking part in and who are interested in your work.

A. Articulate the aim of your study.

Be very clear about what you want to accomplish in conducting this inquiry. So often, the aim of a study is listed as studying the "lived experience" of some experience, but that is not an aim. It is a means toward an end. You think about what you are attempting to accomplish and for what purpose.

Crotty's (1996) main concern about the way in which North American nurse researchers were conducting phenomenological studies is that phenomenology should offer a philosophical critique. Crotty asks for significance from phenomenological studies—that they go beyond describing and interpreting and suggest possibilities that may enhance or correct some experiences. Others who disagree say that their work is just to describe and interpret and that it is the work of other researchers to point out the problems inherent in the descriptions and to suggest actions leading to change.

My own concern is that, if we do not include critiques or suggestions to alleviate problems, question theoretical incongruencies, or pointedly demonstrate how our understanding illuminates a problem, the critical importance of our studies will go unfulfilled. A critique of the experience may offer infinite possibilities for needed change. At first I was defensive, like many other nurse researchers, in response to Crotty's criticism and leaned toward a purist perspective. But, after much reflection, I came to believe that the addition of critique would certainly have the benefit of increasing the significance of phenomenological work and, in a pragmatic way, provide direction to practice or to theory. Additionally, I was beginning to find it difficult to argue with a suggestion that would ultimately enlarge our purpose and assist individuals in attaining meaning and improve sensitivity, understanding, and change in conditions and approaches that were not enhancing the quality of their lives. In other words, we could use our understanding to improve the quality of life for people.

So, as a researcher, you need to enlarge your aim and be clear about which experience you are going to name, understand, and find the meaning of, as well as critique your findings for larger implications.

You can be assured that this section is complete when you can demonstrate to others the significance of your aim, and they agree that the way you have stated the aim lends itself to phenomenological inquiry.

B. Distinguish the experience that is part of your study.
1. Describe, if circumscribed experience, or delimit context, if broad experience. Describing the experience: here is where researchers seem to go two different ways, and some methodologists may have rules here. From my perspective, either direction is fine. You might choose an actual experience in the form of an activity or procedure or, as in Sarah's study, a life event. Or you might choose an emotion, or feeling state, such as restlessness, comfort, pain, or anxiety. With emotions, or feelings, you must be clear in distinguishing the range of the study. For example: studying pain is an extremely broad experience. Think about what this inquiry is for and for what purpose. Then distinguish in some way the kind of pain or the pain associated with a specific kind of experience that you will focus on.

There is experience within experience, and this is not a problem. Actually, it is part of any experience. No experience occurs in isolation. With this in mind, you might decide to study the meaning of pain experienced in association with a specific condition. If you felt confident and grounded in phenomenology, you could study the meaning of pain to persons who have experienced pain and not actually distinguish a category or condition. That kind of study would be a grand study. All variations of experiences might be associated with pain and, in this type of study, you would distinguish the experience associated with the pain, but it would fall into the background and the meaning of pain would always be in the foreground. One advantage of doing a grand study is that it could become your research program, an area you continuously explore in ongoing studies. Certainly, this type of study requires more time, is a subject for a larger and continuing study, and would find its major understandings narrated in at least one volume.

The assurance that you have distinguished your phenomenon is when your colleagues or professor know that it is "this" that you are studying, not "that" or any other fringe phenomenon along with it. You are able to answer questions, clearly delineating what it is and what it is not that you are searching to find meaning in.

2. Articulate the situated context that is available to you in the moment.   Experience is embedded in life-worlds and various contingencies. In this part of the study, you need to describe the context in which you and the study will be taking place. Life-worlds are described later in this chapter.

C. Decenter yourself and come to "unknow."

1. Reflect on your own beliefs, preconceptions, intuitions, motives, and biases so as to decenter.   It has been said that phenomenology can liberate one from preconceptions. However, ironically, often without their knowing, researchers design their studies or "hear" in a way that substantiates their preconceptions. That is why this decentering process is so critical. The researcher in a phenomenological study is, to use a metaphor, the "research tool" or the "research instrument." To be truly authentic and effective, the researcher is asked to do something that is impossible to do, but to do it to the greatest extent that is possible.

Researchers are asked to clear their vision and thinking from their assumptions, from their prior knowledge, and from their belief systems. In this step, for that to happen, you need to adopt a perspective of "unknowing" in which you listen with "the third ear" free, to the extent possible, of any prejudice or bias. In your journal, record your beliefs, assumptions, preconceptions, what you expect your findings to be, and any other noise that might prevent you from hearing clearly, uninterrupted when you are listening to others by "noise" about the meaning of the experience. This is also an important step in seeing the experience in whatever forms it shows itself. Often, we see something and automatically overlay that sight with our own interpretation. We assumed we knew something about what we were seeing, only to find out that we had misperceived.

Two films come to mind to assist you in this step. The film *As Good as It Gets* is a wonderful portrayal of preconceptions, biases, and prejudices, and *The Tail Wagging the Dog* demonstrates to us that we are on thin ice, believing what we see! Many phenomenological concepts can be understood better by viewing these films from these two different perspectives. It is a wonderful learning experience.

The assurance that you have accomplished decentering is obtained through practice listening/interview/conversation sessions. As in section C of step I, immersion, you can practice decentering with a colleague or friend. Write in your journal what you are decentering from, listen to your friend describe an experience, write a description of what you heard and what meaning your friend ascribed to the experience. Let your friend evaluate how accurately you grasped the essence of what was said.

During this practice, do not use a tape recorder and do not repeat verbatim what was said. Listen to grasp the meaning. Listen to get inside the person's perceptions. This often takes practice with many different people and their experiences. It is quite a revelation to realize how different our perceptions of the same event are and how we take for granted that we both "saw" the same thing. My favorite example of differing perceptions of the same phenomenon are the following two descriptions.

The following passage, written by Jane Smiley (1989), describes the memory of a very young child:

> As I sit on this hard bench I suddenly yearn for one last long look and not only of the phenomenon of little Joe and little Michael, but of the others too; Ellen, four, and Annie, seven months, sharing a peach. . . . As I watch them now as adults the fact that I will never see their toddler selves again is tormenting. (p. 120)

Ann Beattie (1989) writes about the same kind of memory:

> When you are thirty, the child is two. At forty, you realize that the child in the house, the child you live with, is still, when you close your eyes, or the moment he has walked from the room, two years old. When you are sixty and the child is gone, the child will also be two, but then you will be more certain. Wet sheets, wet kisses. A flood of tears. As you remember him the child is always two. (p. 53)

2. Adopt a perspective of "unknowing."   Decentering attempts to achieve the essential state of mind of unknowing as a condition of openness. In contrast, knowing leads to a form of confidence that has inherent in it a state of closure. The "art" of unknowing is discussed as a decentering process from the individual's own organizing principles of the world (Atwood & Stolorow, 1984). Unknowing is not simple but is essential to the understanding of subjectivity and perspectivity.

Unknowing paradoxically is another form of knowing. Knowing that you do not know something, that you do not understand someone who stands before you and who perhaps does not fit into some preexisting paradigm or theory, is critical to the evolution of understanding meaning for others.

To engage in an authentic encounter is to stand in your own socially constructed world and to unearth the other's world, saying: "I do not know you. I do not know your subjective world." A person who engages another human being to form impressions, formulate a perception, and theorize from a place called knowing has confidence in prior knowledge. Such confidence, however, has an inherent state of closure in it. To be authentically present to a person is to situate knowingly in your own life and interact with full unknowingness about the other's life. In this way, unknowing equals openness (Figure 6–1).

Unknowing.   The state of being decentered and unknowing is challenging to achieve. Unknowing is an art and calls for a great amount of introspection. Unknowing is essential to the understanding of intersubjectivity and perspectivity. In other words, it is essential to understand ourselves and each participant in our study as two distinctive beings, one of whom the researcher

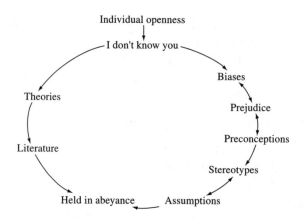

FIGURE 6–1 Unknowing openness.

does not know. Each of us has a unique perspective of our situated context and a unique perspective of who we are as individuals in the world. This is our perspectivity, our worldview, and our reality. When the researcher and the participant meet, two perspectives of a situation need to be recognized. Thus, the process of intersubjectivity begins to create a perceptual space (Figure 6–2).

Intersubjectivity. Intersubjectivity is not difficult to understand, though many writings seem intent on making the concept seem complex. What is complex is practicing it in a wide-awake manner. Intersubjectivity is the verbal and nonverbal interplay between the organized subjective worlds of two people in which one person's subjectivity intersects with another's subjectivity. The subjective world of any person represents the organization of feelings, thoughts, ideas, principles, theories, illusions, distortions, and whatever else helps or hinders that person. The real point here is that people do not know about anyone else's subjective world unless they are told about it. And even then, they cannot be sure. Figure 6–2 illustrates the concepts of intersubjectivity.

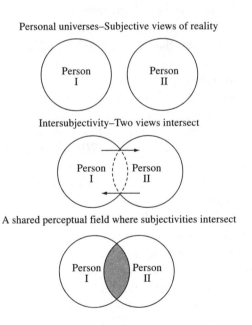

Personal universes–Subjective views of reality

Person I

Person II

Intersubjectivity–Two views intersect

Person I

Person II

A shared perceptual field where subjectivities intersect

Person I

Person II

FIGURE 6–2 Shared perceptual space of intersubjectivity.*

---

*Visually the more interaction, the larger the shared perceptual space.

A film that illustrates how two subjectivities can be extremely different because of the situated context of various life contingencies for individuals is *Whose Life Is It Anyway?* In the perceptual space in which the characters engage in dialogue, there are good examples of how decentering and unknowing by the health care providers in the film would have contributed to an understanding of the patient. The patient is misunderstood, to the point of despair. Watch and listen to a person being heard in a phenomenological manner as the film comes to its conclusion.

D. Articulate the aim of the study in the form of a phenomenological question.

When you know the aim of your study, which is to understand the meaning of an experience, which you have clearly distinguished from other experiences, you are now able to begin to articulate questions. You have decentered yourself so as to be open and receptive to phenomenological material wherever and whenever it appears. These processes of phenomenological inquiry enable you to proceed to the question.

Before Sarah began to articulate questions, she had an overarching interest and aim. Sarah said one day, "I am interested in how the mothers who were mourning for a lost infant and who were part of my first study are doing five years later." Thus, what Sarah wondered was, "Has the passage of time affected the meaning of their experience to them?" The aim of her longitudinal study was to understand the meaning of the experience of losing a child after 5 years has passed (Lauterbach, 2001). In her aim, we can see the question of what it means to be human in such an experience.

This brings us to the critical aims of phenomenology: understanding the meaning of being human (Heidegger, 1927/1962) and, as van Manen (1990) says, becoming more human. We can become more human only through understanding self and others in individual life-worlds, situated contexts, and contingencies and caring about it all.

By internalizing the philosophy of phenomenology, distinguishing the phenomenon, and decentering from our own worldviews, we come now to the process of phenomenological questioning about the meaning of experience for individuals. We can have many questions and will have more as material evolves. However, it is often helpful to have one overarching question. This question can then guide other questions. We must use caution here and not plan more than a few questions. When the existential material "speaks" to us and begs our attention, it will be the material from the study itself that will guide you with questions and provide direction to the study as a whole. The overarching question, *the* question, should reflect the underlying aim, that of understanding the meaning of being human and focusing on the experience that you have chosen to study.

You can articulate the question in different ways, which often has to do with a particular philosopher or school of phenomenology in which you may be most interested. My own experience has led me to find personal meaning in the perspectives of Heidegger, Merleau-Ponty, and van Manen, among other philosophers including the postmodernists. For example, I find Heidegger's curiosity about the question on "being" very compelling. "What does it mean, this idea we call being? What is the nature of being? What is the meaning of being?" To wander down this path, one accepts that "beings" are always in experience. Therefore, we go to the experience in which the human being is to attempt to answer the question of meaning for that human being. The experience may not necessarily be concrete; it may be abstract, such as spirituality or even philosophizing. Beings are always being, even "being" asleep. It is in what beings are being that enables us to find meaning in being! The being is in experience.

The standard answer to the question "what is phenomenology?" evolved from there: it is the study of lived experience. That definition, I believe, has led many astray, as they focus more on the experience than on human meaning in experience. Like "being," "experience" should never be simplified. Merlau-Ponty (1962) believed that experiences are layered with meanings, and he contributes to our understanding by emphasizing how these meanings create the ways in which we perceive experience. This is where the life-worlds, contingency, and the situated context need to be addressed to assist us in understanding the many-layered multiplicity of considerations in any one person's perception of experience.

Articulating the research question calls on us to be very clear about what we are studying. The overall question, from a Heideggerian perspective, would be: "What is the meaning of being human in this experience (entity)?" Many studies begin with the question, "What is it like to be in this experience or to have had this experience?" After many years of reading studies that use the latter question, I have come to believe that if we keep *meaning* in the forefront of our study, we will have a richer study, one in which meaning is usually found in the participants' own words, as they form expressions of meaning. Keep in mind that you will have many questions that can be asked of participants in your study and, "What's it like?" could actually be the first question. Often this will lead to a description of the experience. I think we need to go further. Asking "How were you feeling? thinking?" and other variations can lead to the meaning of the experience, which will then bring into play the life-worlds, the situated context, and contingency.

Now, all this said, usually the academic world demands *the* question be clearly articulated. But too-strict guidelines *might prevent you* from following where the participant wants to go. This needs to be avoided. Use common sense when trying to keep yourself and the participant focused. If the participant wanders from the experience, you must make a decision about the relatedness or, better yet, ask the participant how he or she sees what he or she is saying to be connected. A participant's wandering to areas whose relevance is not obvious to you can be extremely important to the participant. Refocusing participants needs to be done minimally. This wandering is part of the phenomenological study and, as such, has meaning that will be discussed in detail on page 181. Because Sarah's study (Lauterbach, 2001) was not prescribed by dissertation requirements, she was able to let the reader know what she was doing without specifically asking a question, as was heretofore noted. However, how would it be stated if she had to state it in question form? She would simply take her aim and ask the question of it. Her overarching question then might be a version of the following one: What is *the meaning* of having lost a wished-for-baby, with the passage of 5 years? Sarah's aim is to understand the meaning that the passage of time may have had on these women who had this experience.

In one of my own studies, the question that was overarching was: What is the meaning of anger as it is experienced by women who are in therapy? The aim of that study was to begin to understand *the meaning* of anger of women who happened to be in therapy at the time (Munhall, 1994a).

You can see the difference in asking questions and stating aims, which are different from what we have become accustomed to reading. Remember the most frequent definition of phenomenology: the study of lived experience. The "meaning as it is experienced" is a personal preference. I also believe that keeping meaning in the forefront of your study will produce a more phenomenological study. You will not be led astray to structures and categories. Phenomenological researchers do not want to know simply what it is like, but what the meaning of it is. They seek an understanding of the meaning of "things" to individuals. Within the method presented here, that is the ultimate aim and is reflected in the question.

III. Existential Inquiry, Expressions, and Processing

Steps III and IV are two process steps that are conducted simultaneously. Existential inquiry by nature requires our "being-in-the-world" and takes place in the life-worlds of the researcher and the participant. When we engage in dialogue with our participants, in addition to hearing the linguistic expressions they use to describe and interpret their experience, we also need to hear the situated context of their being-in-the-world. This has been called the horizon, or the background, of the experience. Expressions of meaning *cannot be* acontextual. The thoughts, feelings, emotions, and questions are deeply embedded in the context of the participant's life, or life-world. While we are doing the existential inquiry, we are also doing contextual processing. They are separated out for pedantic purposes here and for ease of understanding. This concurrent process can be imagined by overlaying Figure 6–3 with Figure 6–4.

We begin with step III, the existential inquiry, expressions, and processing. Existential inquiry, expressions, and processing constitute the step in which you gather the existential material. This step requires specific processes, such as attentiveness, intuitiveness, constant reflection on decentering, active listening, interviews or conversations clarifying, synthesizing, writing, taking photographs, creating verse, and almost anything that will reflect your participant's and your consciousness and awareness of the experience.

Most phenomenological studies at present use some technique to collapse the material into groupings. This is part of the confounding nature of phenomenological research. Originally, phenomenology was a method used to interpret texts. For example, "What is the meaning of this book?" However, since social and health care scientists started using the method to attempt to learn more about their clients' and patients' experiences, the problem of what to do with all the material has been approached in different ways.

Some methods call for collapsing or condensing the material into themes, essences, meaning units, and (probably the least phenomenological) structural definitions. In many phenomenological studies, we see the prevalence of these approaches in the discussion of themes, essential elements, labeling,

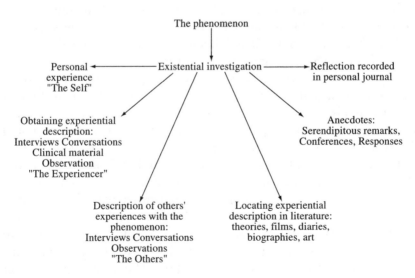

FIGURE 6–3 The phenomenon—existential investigation.

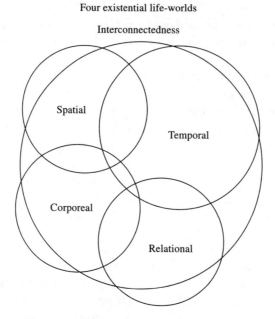

Four existential life-worlds

Interconnectedness

Spatial

Temporal

Corporeal

Relational

FIGURE 6–4 Four existential life-worlds.

clusters, categories—all attempts to provide a description of an experience in a clear, logical listing of some type. Sometimes whichever method the researcher used to organize the material is then placed into a narrative. If there were 10 participants, the researcher searched for similar themes among the 10 with perhaps a note or two about differences, but then wrote the narrative in a way that reflected the mergence of 10 participants.

In a field such as nursing, where we are strongly socialized in a world of signs and symptoms, lists of diagnoses, and other kinds of classifications, we tend to value this "shorthand" for its efficiency in communication. However, a major problem with this approach, especially in a phenomenological study, is that words and signs do not have the same meaning for everyone. Both the health care provider and the patient interpret words differently. These words and signs further lose meaning if they are acontextual. The signs and symptoms manifested by a patient have meaning only when placed in a historical, social, cultural, and individual context. So we have a dilemma. We cannot deliver a study of entire transcribed interviews. What are some alternatives? "Dwelling with the data" used to be a popular phrase, but not so much today. But it is here that I think we need to return. The researcher has either a transcribed interview of one person or notes taken over a series of interview dialogues. Within these texts are expressions of meaning. The expressions convey in words a manifestation of meaning. Throughout the material, the researcher can highlight such expressions. They come as participants express themselves with emotions, thoughts, desires, questions, wishes, hopes, and complaints. It is to this that we need to turn our attention. People do not talk in themes; *we impose themes* on their "language." It seems more authentic to stay close to the participant's language and search through the material for the expressions of meaning.

Dwelling.   I believe it is essential to dwell. There are no shortcuts here. Those who invest the time and make the commitment to authenticity will serve well themselves and their participants. Once again the researcher is called on to be the "instrument." Each individual participant needs our reverence for his or her individuality and way of expressing meaning. You read the text of one participant, highlighting in your head the expressions of meaning, and then you actually do "dwell." *Contemplation* is another word that could be used to describe this part of the study. The researcher needs to be alone to contemplate over a period of time the meaning that this participant was attempting to convey. After a certain amount of time has passed — time not measured in hours — insights, intuitions, and understanding emerge. The researcher begins to write. The researcher returns to the material and uses the language of the participant to illustrate the particular meaning. The researcher also returns to the participant and, depending on the participant's evaluation, will either have successfully captured that individual's meaning or will return after clarification to writing once again. This is a departure from collapsing or categorizing interview materials in that there is no deliberate step of searching for similarities or differences. Each participant stands alone. The ending narrative does not homogenize 10 interviews but tells many different stories of meaning. Of course, the researcher will become aware of similarities and differences and write about them as well, while still holding the individual as the focus for meaning.

  When I review some of my own work, I certainly see how I organized some material into categories, and I suppose for others and myself that there are times when this may be the most efficient way of organizing material. However, there is a chapter (Munhall, 1995) where I narrate Beverly's story, Lynn's story, Lisa's story, Victoria's story, and Carol's story. Each story is different, has different meanings, and challenges different normative commitments and unquestioned myths. Perhaps the experience that I was studying (women's secrets) allowed for the individualistic interpretations, but there is something about the heterogeneity that, for me, has a feeling of "the experiences themselves" and of phenomenology.

So in this part of the study, where the researcher is gathering material that is spoken before it is read, dwelling and contemplation of "the said" needs to take place. This is a thinking through and at the same time a freeing of the mind so that insights spontaneously arise. Every phenomenologist must carry a small notebook in which to write down insights for those spontaneous moments. It is like taking a picture: there is an opportunity, and if you don't capture it, you might lose it. This process will happen to you, I promise you.

This is also the step in which you may, in a proposal, use specific areas to indicate where there will be "human subjects"; in essence this is somewhat analogous to data collection. The difference in phenomenological inquiry is one of perception of the wholeness of the study. Once again, because the process is not linear, you are free to do the various processes of the existential process and phenomenological contemplation in a circular way. In actuality, all the steps should represent a circle. Toward the end of your study, you return to the earlier steps of immersion, coming to the phenomenological aim, and so on. From a language perspective, because phenomenological inquiry has at once a subjective, objective, and intersubjective quality to it, we call the individuals who participate in our study "participants" and we call data "material."

Researcher as Participant and Instrument. Not only is the researcher the most important "instrument," but he or she is a participant as well, as all functions come together to attempt to understand meaning in experience through this existential investigation. In this part of the study, you need to attend to the experience by amassing material and through processes. Again, because this is not a textbook on phenomenology, I cannot possibly do justice to all that needs to be known. Hopefully, you understand the general framework of the inquiry and the processes that are critical to phenomenology. What follows are the process steps of the existential inquiry.

A. Listen to self and others; develop heightened attentiveness to self and others.

Listening and seeing in a phenomenological way need further description. Part of what is required is discussed earlier in the section on the decentering process. Oftentimes in phenomenological studies, as was mentioned, what we have seen consists of 10 or so *transcribed* interviews, with themes extracted, and then perhaps a discussion of those themes. As said in *Revisioning Phenomenology* (1994a), if you feel you need to transcribe interviews in the beginning, you should go ahead and do that. As you progress with this method, taping interviews and writing transcriptions become less necessary because you are able to grasp meaning in what might become a conversation rather than an interview.

When you choose your participants, you do not need to follow the sampling rules of quantitative research. Instead, you need to find individuals who are willing to speak to you about the experience that you are interested in understanding. Another qualification is that the participants want to tell "their stories." Although many other sources assist you in attaining understanding, the language with all its intonation and inflection is the most revealing. Facial expressions and body language are also forms of languaging meaning. Needless to say, then, you want a willing and if possible enthusiastic participant.

Additionally, when you are listening, you must be cognizant that your participants are most likely telling you some things but not all things. As in any self-report, participants may think there is a "correct" way to respond to you. At the outset, this needs to be clarified, and the participants must be reassured that these stories are their own, that you are interested in their own meaning and their own personal experience. The participant is the repository of meaning through narrative. Reminding your participants of their generosity in sharing sometimes painful experiences demonstrates your sincerity. Clarify that there are no "right" answers or better answers and that what you value most is "their" exploring with you, in their own language, the meaning of the experience for them. If a participant asks you, "Is this what you want?" (which is often the case), you need to reassure the participant that it is "what" they want to share with you that you are interested in hearing.

At a dissertation hearing this past year, I heard a student say, "I had to keep bringing her back to the experience." This outcome is frequent; it merits a response and is somewhat like the participant looking for the right answer. Instead, here the researcher apparently had in mind the range of focus that she wanted her participant to stay within. Given that this is not psychotherapy but phenomenology, we do not have the luxury of free association. However, as mentioned earlier, we need to hear what the participant is moving away from and where the participant is going. This in itself can be material from which meaning may be gleaned, and sometimes that meaning is the participant's wish to avoid further discussion. If you ascertain that the participant's comfort level is being disrupted for any reason at all, you need to attend to it and respect the participant's wishes.

Significant Wandering.   However, the participants may be communicating something other than avoidance; the wandering may in the end make significant sense. This is discussed in greater detail later in the section on interpretation, but, for now, note that often there is great meaning in what is concealed. So, we are not only listening to what is said, but what is not said and also to where the participant goes to seek meaning, to another narrative. Moving into a more conversational mode allows the researcher to gently probe as to the meaning of what is said. Saying something like, "Please go on, what are you thinking?" if the participant should fall silent is good for the conversation. Once again, remember how important you are to this process. A good phenomenological researcher has heightened consciousness, focuses intently, and is continuously attentive to self and to the participant. If you, the researcher, find yourself wandering in thought, you must be vigilant and bring your attention back to the dialogue. Make a quick mental note about where you wandered when you might have thought yourself to be distracted. This, too, may have significance in regard to its association.

B. Reflect on personal experiences and expressions.

Phenomenology begins with the personal, the subjective world in which you are present, a part of, and connected to in your own situated context, life-worlds, and different contingencies, which all contribute to you as person. You begin your phenomenological study with self-reflection. Record this self-reflection in a journal. Because this kind of inquiry reflects a coming and going, a back-and-forth between and among parts of the study and the whole, your own personal experiential journey will change you. Your self-reflection includes analyzing your life-world, situated context, and the contingencies, which bring you into relation to this human experience. Why do you, as a person, want to study this experience? How did you become interested in this experience, in meaning, in understanding?

This part of the study is ongoing, and your journal should reflect a deepening of "thinking," a "giving over" to the study, as well as your frustrations, surprises, and questions as your study evolves. Sarah, in the first study (Munhall & Oiler-Boyd, 1993) and in this study shares with us her own experience with what she is studying. She is intricately involved and at once "knows for herself" but puts that in abeyance to see the meaning for others. This often raises the implication of the researcher having had the experience that he or she is studying. By this I mean Sarah had herself "the experience" she was and is studying. Such questions are addressed in *Revisioning Phenomenology*, so in the interest of space I refer you to that book because this component is an important one to think about. The assurance that this personal expression section is being done well is that others who read your study understand in an authentic manner *who you are* in this study, your experiential perspective, and how and why you are engaged in studying the experience.

C. Provide experiential descriptive expressions: The experiencer.

This step pertains to experiences that may have a clinical component. *Clinical* means the experience was in some way related to health care and the nursing domain or the nursing care of individuals living through specific experiences. This is very broad and not limited to individuals who are currently in a clinical setting, but who have had an experience that has a clinical aspect. Examples could be experiences of physical, psychological, or psychosomatic illnesses, diagnoses, and the emotional and physical responses: worry, fear, hope, disorientation, loneliness. Though this step is focused on the experiencer we must always be cognizant that the person is always in interaction with others. This enriches your study and gives additional material for interpretation. Here is a concrete example: In a study related to Sarah's, a doctoral student also studied the same experience with mothers. She also asked the meaning or the experiences of the nurses caring for the mothers and found, as did Sarah, that many nurses did not have an awareness of the grief of the mother. A pragmatic defense seemed to be part of the nurses' and others' reactions to the experience. The belief that the mother had one healthy child for which she should be grateful overrode in almost all descriptions the belief that the mother had a need to mourn. Some "others" were even intolerant of such an idea. Now we find through Sarah's study that this mourning continues and is part of the dailiness of having the surviving twin. The surviving twin is a reminder of the one who died. We have also found out something critical about the attitude of others.

These kinds of studies also remind us of the importance of phenomenology as a critical philosophy and that we need to go beyond interpretation to critique. One can also see that an orthodox data collection of 10 transcribed interviews could not provide the depth and breadth of the existential material. Sarah, I believe, has a real interest in studying the experiential descriptions found in art, literature, music, photography, and other aesthetic works. This interest has increased her focus on that dimension and someday could become a study of its own. One should note how a program of research could be had for those doing phenomenology, and a very meaningful one as the study branches out and continues to shed light on the many facets of an experience. When doing phenomenology, we need to be vigilant of when we find ourselves looking to the rules for research of the scientific method. We do not have the limitations of operational definitions; nor do we have the limitations of linear steps. We are searching for a full-of-meaning-and-detail narrative of experience, which contains whatever adds to meaning. This is a simple and liberating criterion. If something contributes to the meaning of our understanding of an experience, one need not argue whether it belongs or not; of course, it belongs. The material enriches our understanding.

In this step you begin to collect material from individuals who have experienced the phenomenon of interest in your study. *Revisioning Phenomenology* presents structural ways in which you can select themes and essences from transcribed interviews. I refer you to that book for more detail if you believe you need more structure to enable you to elucidate themes. If you feel as though you can listen with "the third ear," asking individuals if they would be willing to share with you their experience in more than one sitting, then you might not need to tape the dialogue, but it is good practice to write immediately afterward as much as you can remember of what was said. Laptops make this a bit easier today.

Some Information about Interviews.   In hermeneutic phenomenological human science, the interview serves very specific purposes: (1) it may be used as a means of exploring and gathering experiential narrative material that can serve as a resource for developing a richer and deeper understanding of a human phenomenon, and (2) it may be used as a vehicle to develop a conversational relation with a partner (interviewee) about the meaning of an experience (van Manen, 1990, p. 66). In our evolution of the past 10 years or so, our phenomenological studies often relied primarily on interviews. Researchers often asked the following questions:

- ♦ What question should I ask?
- ♦ How many people do I need to interview?
- ♦ How do I keep people focused?
- ♦ What do I do with all this material (transcripts)?

As discussed earlier in this chapter, we must be careful in framing our question. The "what is it like" approach is fine, understandable, and concrete. Asking people to tell you about their lived experience of being cared for might prompt different responses from asking people what it is like to feel cared for: the first is asking for examples, and the second is asking for descriptions. There is no need here for either/or; both are fine. Because of individuals' infinite differences, I find interactive dialogue, like conversation, to be very important. Additionally, stories, anecdotes, pictures, and any writing that the individual may be willing to share with you will enrich your study. I find the idea of being in dialogue to be one of a relation between two human beings. In this type of conversation, the unknower is seeking understanding of something from the speaker and not vice versa. It certainly is not a demographic interview, and though often tempting, it does not seek affirmation of your beliefs. Researchers sometimes find themselves saying:

Don't you think . . . ?
Did you find that . . . ?
Do you think it was because they were . . . ?

Such questions may appear harmless, but they have the potential to structure a person's story. They are the kind of questions through which you might be seeking to substantiate some of your own beliefs. The following lead-ins help explicate the person's unfolding of the experience.

- Could you give me an example of that?
- Do you remember how that made you feel (assuming there's a reason for a feeling question)?
- What did that do for you?
- (After a sentence) Go on . . . Could you elaborate more on that?
- (After a period of silence, ask) Can you tell me what you are thinking about?

And never underestimate the "umm . . ." One student, after conducting some of her first interviews, told me that her mouth was sore from smiling. Although you might smile, it is certainly not a requisite and would sometimes be inappropriate. Try to follow the mood of the person you are interviewing. Also be aware of the participant's body, posture, intonation of words, and being. Because the interview has sometimes assumed preeminence in the phenomenological approach, other considerations need to be made:

- If you have never interviewed people before in the form of a dialogic conversation, then you need to practice. Practice with someone who has a background in psychiatric nursing, psychology, or psychoanalysis. In their disciplines, listening is elevated to an art. In phenomenology, listening also becomes an art.
- Listening is an art. Try to hear just what is being said. Try not to be anticipating what comes next. Let there be pauses and silence. Silence is important. An individual says something. You listen. There is a pause. You are both reflecting. The pause will often yield additional reflection. Becoming comfortable with a silence or a *pregnant pause* enables the storyteller to probe deeper within. Let the silence remain until you intuit that a prompt might be helpful.
- Many studies are a result of one-time interviews. As I have suggested elsewhere, two to three interviews with the same person may be more helpful. More "reflected upon" material is usually forthcoming, as is interpretation of what was said in previous interviews. A practitioner or researcher who ends a single interview with, "Is there anything else you might like to add?" is asking the question for that moment. Often, in the week that follows, more reflection occurs and the person desires to tell more about the experience.
- Imagine yourself in the interviewee's place. What might he or she be thinking about? Another reason that I strongly recommend additional interviews is that there is so much to process in the first encounter. You may need to use the first interview to establish trust and rapport, depending on what you are discussing. That effort will ensure the integrity of the material forthcoming.

◆ I believe it is critical to conduct these interviews/conversations where the participant is most comfortable. Sometimes to find participants, you first need to go to where the experience is located; for example, a school, office, clinic, or church.

◆ Be aware of your participant's holistic condition. You do not need to stop an interview because of crying or anger (as long as the interviewer knows whether it is therapeutic). However, you need good judgment. Even though informed consent ensures that the interviewee can stop the interview at any time, sometimes the interviewer needs to recognize that it is time to relax and change direction. Relief time, perhaps a little casual talk, may be comforting. Our intention here is not psychotherapy or nursing intervention. Our role must be clearly known, and we must act accordingly. We need to be cognizant and attuned to our participant's psychological condition. Again, follow-up interviews help protect the psychological comfort of interviewees and demonstrate our genuine interest in them as persons.

Also include in your notes other observations that you or your participant have made. Phenomenology is not only the language of words but also the language of semiotics, the symbols and signs in our environment that "speak" to us and tell us what is going on in this environment. They speak to your participants and are other sources of meaning as participants attempt to make "meaning sense" out of their experience. Your participant will most likely describe his or her own examples or observations, but you as a health care provider can also incorporate your own for comment and feedback. Again, this is an example of the "coming and going," the varying of examples, the varying of perspectives, and the looking upon a reflection with another reflection. This is what makes doing phenomenology so rewarding and worthwhile. The descriptions and interpretations attempt to be as inclusive as is feasible in the study, so as not to present a shallow description but a deeply embroidered tapestry of meaning.

The way you can be assured this step is accomplished is to bring your descriptions and reflections to your participants. If your descriptions and interpretations of the meaning of the experience resonate with the participants, then you can be assured that you did indeed tell the meaning of their story. Now does everyone share the same meaning? Of course not. So, first you go to the person with whom you have had several conversations to see if you captured his or her meaning. At the conclusion of your study, you will have reflected on all the material and will have begun to write a description and interpretation of your study. When that is completed, you once again return to your participants with the material woven into one narrative. Listen to the responses of your participants. Many will read an interpretation and remark that they did not have that experience or share that meaning. This returns us to the reason for separate stories and why it is critical to have in your narrative the similarities and differences found in the meaning of the same experience.

Some studies are written so that it seems that everyone in *a particular study* experienced the phenomenon in a similar manner. That may actually be the case, as with Sarah's mothers. However, other mothers may not have experienced this mourning phenomenon. This we do not know until we widen the scope of the study to include, perhaps, women from different cultures or backgrounds. Or perhaps most mothers do mourn a lost child when there was to be a multiple birth. We do not know and we cannot assume. We cannot generalize, because it is not our intent. However, because of Sarah's studies, our consciousness has been raised to new possibilities and certainly a different way of being with these mothers. However, I need to stress once again that when you write a phenomenological narrative, you must heed the differences in meaning as well as the similarities. Phenomenology is not interested in generalizabilty. It is interested in how various individuals interpret the meaning of experience in their own individual ways.

D. Provide experiential descriptive expressions: "others engaged in the experience."

In this section, your interviews/conversations are with individuals who have lived through an experience in which you are interested but from another perspective. They have not experienced the phenomenon itself but have relationally interacted with the experience. For example, the previously mentioned doctoral student also interviewed the nurses who cared for mothers who had lost one of their twin babies. These individuals become an additional source of material; the material gathered will help vary the examples, provide different perspectives, and actually provide a source for another study or a furthering of one's study.

If you have the desire to broaden the depth of your study, you can talk to those individuals, as in a "going back and forth," to see if you can capture the various meanings from different individuals who may not be "directly" having the experience but who are "directly" involved in the experience. Observing, once again, the language and semiotics of the "others" around the experience at hand is another source of material. The recognition that "others" play a role in phenomenological study comes from the belief that being in experience does not occur in isolation. Imagine yourself painting a picture that is rich in detail and uses different colors and hues. The picture tries to capture, in the expression of individuals, their feelings and thoughts, which is an attempt to let the viewer know the meaning of an experience for those in the picture. Oftentimes, in a museum or elsewhere, individuals gaze at a painting. This is like the phenomenological gaze—searching for something in the picture that will speak to us, to tell us the meaning of this work of art. That is actually what you are doing when you lay out all the pieces of your study, always remembering that it is the pieces, and the individuals themselves, that have provided the meaning in interaction.

In the end, your phenomenological writing will try to make sense of the experience in the many ways in which it has appeared or been concealed; and varying the material will enrich the text and fuse it with meaning. Per-haps the lack of looking beyond interviews with the participants has led to

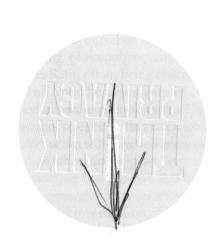

f   n one or two sentences. We
h   henology, and I believe we
s   ology in various ways, using
v   g the freedom to do what
t   thod, we are *guided*. We are
t   ent of some "thing" because
                                                      d is different in intent from
                                                      thod's delimiting steps must
                                                      nt. With phenomenology, if
                                                      ere the experience leads us,
                                                      only some of the meaning, a
                                                      nclude and what to exclude.
                                                      cher have found some mate-
                                                      l to include it, if it helps you

Researcher in Interaction

When nurses do phenomenology, it is not with the same aim, say, as that of a philosopher. We can say very directly that we are conducting a study with the aim of understanding the meaning of experience for our clients. We can acknowledge our values; that is, that *we want to improve the quality of life of those we serve.* So it is different. Nurses are interacting with "beings," and they are "being-in-the-world" in a service profession. Understanding meaning is the best way of designing interventions. I must add, if interventions are called for, better they be designed in consideration of the patient's perspective of the experience than from the caregiver's assumptions. One could argue that it is here where theory development must begin. Before all else, one needs a phenomenological baseline to describe, explain, predict, and control, if that is what is needed in specific circumstances. The argument could be furthered with the observation of how poorly individuals often "comply" with directions or education. If directions, interventions, and education are not derived from understanding what individuals experience and the meaning that they attach to their experiences, we have missed opportunities to be more effective.

Individuals in experience are the ones to inform us of what it is they need, how we could be more helpful, and how we could assist in improving the quality of their health. Only from an understanding of the "other" in experience can we develop theory from "the individuals themselves." Theory needs to be grounded in the authentic experience of what is to be theorized, not from what an authority believes it should be. "Should be" theories usually lead to all sorts of "deficits"; the ideals are not grounded in the everyday lives of individuals.

I would suggest that what is before us and what often cries out for our attention and seeks understanding at the deepest levels is the human experience. I would go even further and say that we have an ethical and moral imperative to use phenomenology to foster the highest and most humanistic standards of care. Wherever, then, you as researcher are able to hear, see, or touch material that has relevance to your study, remember that you are not bounded by rules. Your search is for as much experiential material as is available to you so that your original aim is full of "life." And real life is what nurses are engaged in with others, and our lives are all wonderfully intertwined. We mutually unfold in experience.

E. Provide experiential descriptive expressions: The arts and literature review.

This step embodies the experience that you are studying, in coming into contact with others who have explored it either purposely or tangentially in aesthetic work. The arts are poised to offer us a wealth of understanding if we engage in the search. Leaving yourself open to the experiential appearance, whether by accident or deliberate action, will often capture your imagination in ways that will literally excite you. I say this because I have watched countless students, colleagues, and myself act as though we have found gold when we come upon a film, a novel, biography, paintings, photographs, diaries, or other aesthetic works that announce themselves to us through the experience that we are studying. We are open to appearance. We are also aware of what may be concealed. So we come to these works and keep narratives of them, quotations, verse, a copy of a painting or photograph, lines from films and plays to illustrate the meaning of the experience. We begin to understand more and sometimes stand in awe in regard to where our study has taken us. We stand with the work or we view the film for the third time, we reread the play or the novel, and we search for deeper layers of meaning. This is what we do when we return to an individual for the third time or maybe more. The researcher collects this material or records meaning and understanding gathered from these sources in his or her journal. The process becomes a way of being. You can read how Sarah has found such deep meaning and understanding in aesthetic engagement. However, it is critical to note that she is still engaged in the everydayness of her participants' lives as their own form of art. You can be assured that you have engaged in this process when you have found representations of the experience under study in the form of the various arts. If you find a paucity of material in this realm, begin to write verse, take photographs, or paint to represent what you have heard from your participants or from your own soul and spirit.

Reading the Literature. Regarding experiential material in theoretical literature, you might think of the familiar literature review but, in phenomenology, it is used for a different purpose from a hypothesis. Rather than reading all that is known about an experience in the literature or in theories so as to support a hypothesis, you seek experiential descriptions of the experience or the meaning of the experience that may have been written from different perspectives. The intent is also different in that this step is considered part of your existential investigation, your gathering of material to deepen your understanding of these other perspectives.

Although it has been suggested that you delay this step until after you have had interviews/conversations with your participants so as not to overlay the literature on your "decentered self," literature about the experience may appear when you least expect it. In that case, it is a good idea to read it; just as with other existential descriptions, the content contributes to meaning and understanding.

In phenomenological research, material directs you to areas that you would not have thought of at the beginning of your study. As with all existential material, it shows itself to the researcher to be seen, to be read, to be touched, "as it is" within the life-worlds of the participants. "As it is" for the participants and what is described in the literature at times are very similar and other times very different. What is not in the literature is as important as what is in the literature and in many instances more important. The question of the literature reflecting, contrasting, and/or refuting what you have come to find in your analysis and interpretation is of critical importance to the advancement of understanding and our knowledge base. Often our literature or theories are grounded in the knowledge base of the expert. If that knowledge base is deduced from other literature, from scientific observation of the scientific method mode, and from the perspective of the expert of "knowing," we may find an entirely different account of experience when we "go to the persons themselves." Who can better tell us the nature, the meaning, and the "whatness" of an experience than the person who has had the experience? The question enlarges as previously described when we allow others engaged in different ways with the experience to voice what is going on, what it means, and how they perceive it.

It actually might be preferable to postpone the experiential description in the literature until after you have completed your interviews/dialogues with your participants. It can assist you in staying as close to the participant's narratives as possible, without the influence of a literature review. However, as you progress in sophistication with the processes and the interview/dialogue becomes more conversational, you could introduce to the participant something that you have read and ask what the participant thinks about the material. This once again enriches the study, broadens its scope, and provides another perspective. Whatever happens with this step, it should not appear under "literature review" in a research proposal. If you "must" have a literature review, the review should be of the philosophy of phenomenology and how you are planning to follow its underpinnings and suppositions. Your "literature review" is part of your existential investigation.

More about Decentering.   Here is an important point to clarify. Phenomenological inquiry does have suppositions. The suppositions are clearly articulated in the foundation of the phenomenological approach to being-in-the-world. We do not decenter ourselves from phenomenology; in fact, it guides us through the entire study. What we do decenter from are presuppositions, beliefs, values, knowledge, thoughts, and ideas about the experience that we are studying and attempting to understand without the overlay of prior knowledge. Doing a literature review at the outset only serves the purpose of obtaining additional knowledge from which to separate ourselves. You can be assured that you have accomplished this review when you have gone to the literature on the experience that interests you and have obtained a good description of what is currently in the literature or in theories. This review is another narrative to describe and interpret as it relates to your own findings and understanding of the experience.

F. Provide anecdotal descriptive expressions: As experience appears.
This process step is one that requires a consciousness of the experience or meaning of the experience when you are not necessarily expecting its appearance or concealment. The material appears in a serendipitous manner.

You might be engaged in a conversation with a friend or neighbor who begins to talk about the experience without your prompting. You may hear about this experience at a conference in a formal presentation or in questions that people bring up in various formats. The more commonplace your experience is, the more often this will occur. This type of serendipitous appearance can be a very important source of material because sometimes people, without knowing it, become participants though not formally. They begin to converse with you about how "it is" with them to either be in this experience or to know of someone who is in it and how they are responding to that situation. This is anecdotal and not within the formal frame of your study. You did not expect it; nor did you ask for it. If you wish to pursue this with any one person and engage him or her in the study as a participant, then you must ask his or her permission and follow the same process of informed consent as when you have identified volunteer participants. Informed consent is discussed further in Chapter 21.

Other interesting sources of material for your study are people's responses to the subject. Just their reactions can be fascinating. I recall once discussing with a colleague the study of anger, and she angrily replied to me, "I don't ever get angry," apparently concealing to herself how she does experience anger. Your colleagues can provide feedback on how you are doing with your study and also material from the perspective of their own initial responses to the experience. They may also be potential participants. Again, as you become more familiar with this kind of inquiry, you will find yourself more awake to all experiences and engaging in the world in a different manner. Sometimes it seems to me that "everything" said or seen has potential for a study, that I can collect material and write about "things" that I am not studying at the moment. I feel sometimes as though phenomenology has made me "always" a student of our everyday world. Establishing a phenomenological perspective toward the world at hand stimulates attentiveness to the "everydayness" of life, experiences, and objects, and you begin to see and articulate the taken-for-grantedness of much experience. This attentiveness will further enrich your study with the addition of unforeseen appearances of material reflective within your experience.

You can be assured this process step has been accomplished by evaluating the material that you came upon in a serendipitous way. Serendipitous material comes about because of the aforementioned attentiveness by which a phenomenological study takes up residence within you.

G. Record ongoing reflection in your personal journal.
This process step is ongoing from the *very first day of your study* or from the time you begin thinking about your study. I cannot overemphasize the importance of almost daily entries in your journal. After a conversational inter-

view, the participant's material, your responses, thoughts, associations, what you were feeling, and what you thought the other person was feeling should be written into your journal. This is your phenomenological journal and situates you in the life-world of your study.

What happens to you during this time also should be included. If you don't write as often as possible, you will lose this material; it will naturally be forgotten in the rush of your everyday life. When you embark on description and interpretation, the material in this journal will most likely reflect a greatly enlarged view of the experience and a greatly changed "you," as far as perspective and understanding are concerned. That is why you would never want to lose a record of your own personal growth. Most likely you will see that you have enlarged your perspective in depth and breadth and have become much more sensitive and alert to the "taken for grantedness" of individual people and experiences.

In your phenomenological journal, go beyond description and try to incorporate the meaning of "what is going on" and the meaning of the various experiences that you may be having in the course of this study. All phenomena within this study—the interactions, the responses, the good and the woeful times—will reflect in a back-and-forth way on your study. My journals during studies reflect this back-and-forth, both in tearful entries and in spontaneous "aha" entries. If you are a student doing a phenomenological study for a dissertation, you may have many tearful entries. Stay with it.

Another promise: you will have traveled a journey *to becoming more humanistic and sensitive* than you thought possible. And your world will be enlarged because of it. Your journal will read like a book when you are completed, and I think you will marvel at the richness of your own text as well as your own growth in awareness of meaning and of being human. You will be assured this process step is completed if the preceding sentence rings true!

IV. Phenomenological Contextual Processing

This process step parallels the process step of existential inquiry and processing. In this step you present your thoughts about the material gathered in step III. It is here where you write for the reader, describing the situated contexts of all who take part in the study, where participants are located in the various life-worlds, and the contingencies of those in the study, including the researcher. The experience is not separated from the participant, so that context needs to be articulated as well.

A. Analyze emergent situated contexts.
This concept is actually quite literal. It refers to the situation in which you and others currently are with all the contingencies that exist at the moment and as you progress in the study. Heidegger (1962) uses the term

"thrownness" to express the perspective that the person is always "situated." The person is in context in his or her "being-in-the-world." From what we know thus far, we are without prior consultation, born into a historical time period, a culture, a family with a specific worldview and language. Other parts of the situated context are the experiences that we sometimes choose and other times do not choose. Because of our situated context, some choices are not available to us, and others are not choices but are required within the situated context.

B. Analyze day-to-day contingencies.
Contingencies are most often the reason for our action or inaction, decisions or avoidance of decisions, and voluntary or involuntary change. Whatever the contingencies of one's life, they are within one's situated context and, in actuality, unify with the life-worlds. This unity exerts tremendous influence on the meaning of experience and a person's understanding of that meaning. A person's situated context allows certain actions and simultaneously limits other actions. To truly understand another person, the researcher must engage in hearing and seeing that person by processing the material gathered through the lens of that person's situated context.

C. Assess life-worlds.
The four existential life-worlds are other dimensions from which we need to process phenomenological material to give meaning a perspective that tells us more about it. It is critical to understand that the *life-worlds* shown in Figure 6–4 are a unity and reflect the interconnectedness of all four life-worlds. Contemplating the spatiality, corporeality, temporality, and relationality furthers our understanding of the person in the world. As demonstrated in Sarah's study, a life-world may also "stand out" as something very meaningful to an experience. Both temporality and relationality entered into her understanding of the experience of the mothers.

Spatiality refers to the space in which we are, our environment, which can assume different meanings for different experiences. The phenomenological material needs to be processed once again through the lens of the environment. In regard to my study on women's anger, spatiality was a very important world to discuss in many instances. The home environment for many of these women, especially those living in domestic-violence situations, needed to be part of the interpretation of anger. An experience does not exist alone. It is always embedded and connected.

Corporeality refers to the body that we inhabit and is also referred to as embodiment. Rather than the idea that we have bodies, we think now that *we are our bodies.* Because we often speak as though our bodies and minds are separate, we know that the mind is embodied in this wonderful access to experience, the body. There are times that it is not such a wonderful experience. For this reason, the researcher must contemplate the connectedness of embodiment with experience. Body intelligence is what experiences phenomena. We negotiate experience through the unity of mind and body. Perceptions are what enter the body and therefore become the starting point of meaning. In the example of anger and domestic violence, not only is a woman's physical body shattered or damaged, but her whole perception of self can be shattered and damaged. The woman's embodiment is severely threatened, and readers familiar with the effects of this life-world understand the many different meanings of this experience for a woman. This is how all these ideas are interconnected. *I write "as if this, then this" and need to occasionally focus on the interconnectedness of all these phenomena.* Meaning and experience cannot exist in isolation.

Temporality is the time in which we are living. We are always living through this concept called time. Our embodied bodies occupy a space and that space is located in time. Our participants often bring up the life-world of time, as is illustrated in Sarah's study (Lauterbach, 2001). The passage of time, the temporal life-world, did little to ease the mourning process. Many readers of her study may express surprise, which is a sign of an excellent study. Sarah succeeds here in "liberating" some readers from their preconceptions. The perception of time is another important concept to contemplate when listening to participants and interpreting phenomenological material. The perception of time passing varies, often in incredible ways, with experience and is very meaningful. "Losing track of time" and "the time seemed endless" are phrases that the researcher needs to process with the participant. Actual interventions can be suggested by understanding the meaning of life-worlds in experience. You might recall intensive care unit patients who were diagnosed as being disoriented because they did not know the time and day. They were in rooms without windows, so the orienting dark and light cycles were not present, not to mention that their space lacked clocks that could be seen. This is what might be called "everyday" experience for these patients. I believe the outcome of being in the world in a phenomenological way can lead a nurse to explore the space and time dimensions and arrive at a very practical solution: place large clocks showing time of day and the day of the week where patients can view them. Make sure that they indicate A.M. or P.M. Some would say that it is obvious. Yes, and understanding experience can result in the most obvious solutions. Yet, for years, patients who didn't know the time and day were labeled as "disoriented."

Critical to temporality is history. We not only occupy a place in time, but we are located in a historical period. That period is extremely influential in regard to our behavior, attitudes, beliefs, and where we are located (spatiality). The country and city or town is a critical influence, as is the family.

Relationality refers to the world in which we find ourselves in relation to others. When studying phenomenological material, you need to contemplate the relationships within the experience being studied and as articulated by participants or found in other existential material. The importance of ourselves in relation to others is not just the phenomenologist's interest. This life-world seems to dominate popular culture in all of its manifestations. What is critical to phenomenologists is the recognition that the self is self-interpreting. We now can add "for interpretation" to "to the persons themselves": "to the persons themselves for interpretation"! For example, returning to the subject of women and domestic violence, we as researchers or health care professionals could interpret their situations from all the literature available. There are numerous interpretations, and to adopt the wrong interpretation could be very harmful. To understand a particular woman in this situation, *we must ask her for her interpretation*. Otherwise, we further violate her unique life-world of relationality.

In this process, the researcher begins to contemplate and look for meaning in all the materials gathered in the existential inquiry. Individuals provide meaning in their experiences through the expression of their feelings, thoughts, intentions, reflections, motives, desires, and emotions. These same expressions can be described by using many other existential modes of inquiry. This concurrent contextual processing allows for integration of experience within context. The researcher is beginning to think in a narrative style, there is a wholeness to it, a story with many different expressions of meaning. What is critical is to transcend the natural tendency to generate common emotions, themes, essences, categories, or meaning units. The narratives need to reflect one person's description of the experience with his or her own interpretation of his or her situated context. Where researchers in phenomenology can divert from the philosophy of phenomenology is in the normal inclination to look for similarities, clusters, or themes. This is what has led critics to say that many of our studies are reductionistic. Of course, this reflects the dilemma, discussed earlier, of how to understand individuals. Do we study the parts, in this case, the themes, and then put them back together as a "whole"? We have long rejected the premise that a person is the "sum total of his parts" and have adopted the view that a person is "greater than the sum of his parts." Of all places, then, it is in phenomenology that we need to remember that people *are greater than the sum of their themes*. This is particularly true when we put them in aggregates or categories. This is demonstrated in studies that have as findings for a group of people (an aggregate) a list of themes, which seem to describe the nature of an experience and how it is lived through the perceptions of our sample of individuals reported as a group. This is the principle used in quantitative research and, as challenging as it may be to phenomenology, we need to use our imaginations to report meanings that acknowledge the individual in experience, not a synthesis of meanings. I would venture to say that, in Western culture, that remains the most challenging task of doing phenomenological research.

So, in this step, because it does not have the full richness of depth and breadth until it is combined with the next process step, we need to include in narrative each individual's description and interpretation of the meaning of the experience. The researcher's main task is to choose very carefully from the participant's very long narrative the centrality of meaning that has been communicated and then to integrate the narrative with the life-worlds. One cannot exist without the other, if an authentic meaning is to be the outcome. This is a subjective process in which our own assumptions, prejudices, and predilections can confuse an authentic delineation of what is most significant in one person's story. We cannot do this alone, without our participant's agreement with our much shorter version of the meaning of the experience that was communicated. People do not think or feel in terms of themes and essences, for the most part. That is what researchers have been doing with phenomenological descriptions.

This method varies from the practice of categorization and asks the researcher to search through the material and to begin writing narratives reflective of each participant's experience. The interviews/conversations that you have had with individuals are in verbal form, which by nature is much longer than descriptive summaries in written form. Recall that such narrative summation cannot take place until you have dwelled with the narrative and the memories of the interviews/conversations and have contemplated the meanings that were communicated to you. However, narrative summation takes considerable practice so as not to be writing through your own assumptions and frameworks, and it needs to be returned to the participant as a written narrative with the question, "Does this reflect our conversations (interviews)?"

In the next process step, we will answer the question, "Why did we ever think we could find out the meaning of experience as though there was 'one' meaning?" Although there are common perceptions of experiences, they are quite different from common meanings. These differences depend on each individual's interpretive interaction.

V. Analysis of Interpretive Interaction

A. Integrate existential investigation with phenomenological contextual processing.

This step returns us to step IV, "Phenomenological Contextual Processing." This step needs intensive integration with your existential experiential expressions, or those descriptions will lack authentic meanings. Contextual processing, as described, calls on the researcher and the participant to be historical, political, cultural, and social; in other words, being-in-the-world as it is in a specific time and place. Meaning cannot be found in an acontextual place or in an ahistorical time, if such notions even exist. However, in some descriptions, they have been completely ignored, and meanings gleaned from those studies are without the essentials that create and contribute to meaning.

In this interpretation of the interaction of the situated context in which individuals find themselves while in experience, we can arrive at a meaningful, holistic, simultaneous interpretation of an experience. Each participant in our study brings a personal biography and has already formed an interpretive system from which *they will give voice to their experience*. Each already has his or her own way of interacting with the larger world. Each has different situations in the life-worlds. Particular contingencies will influence his or her description, interpretation, and formulated meaning of experience.

B. Describe expressions of meaning (thoughts, emotions, feelings, statements, motives, metaphors, examples, behaviors, appearances and concealments, voiced and nonvoiced language).

This analysis of the situated context gives the thoughts, feelings, and emotions a horizon, a context, knowledge, and a biography; in other words, a thick web of relational interactional processes that contribute to who the individual "is" among others and that enable the researcher to capture meaning encapsulated in context. In this process of interpretive interactionism, it is critical once again *not to move into thinking in aggregates*, categories, themes, or essences. Because two people were born in the same year or in the same family, town, or society does not mean sameness. We would be guilty of reductionism if we were to think in that manner. In quantitative terms, they are just variables, devoid of meaning. Only in interaction with all the other contingencies of individual life-worlds can we approximate phenomenological meaning. This is so complex that it is always an *approximation* of meaning. I have viewed groups agreeing on a meaning of some "thing," only later to realize how divergent the agreed-upon meaning actually is.

C. Interpret expressions of meaning as appearing from integration.

To reemphasize, it is critical to understand the meaning of being human within context. From these understandings, we can give others the things that will assist them in generating further meaning, the "interventions" that they may need to increase the quality of life or minimize suffering. Such understanding enables us to individualize our approaches to individuals and enlarges our consciousness to a phenomenological way of being with others. *We no longer have only one approach to an experience.* We recognize that meaning for the individual is how we individualize care. Meaning should be at the core of our care, of what we do and plan with others. One might ask, "Then how can we have procedures, policies, treatments, and prescriptive theory?" We can have them, but we need to know why they often fail or meet with "complications," or why we have a high rate of "noncompliance."

There are many reasons why such acontextual, homogeneous approaches do not work. One of them is that large groups of people were reduced to "one" person, whether in a qualitative or quantitative study. The "one" person is a synthesis of many people and, *in actuality, the "one" person does not even exist.* This is critical to keep in the forefront as you do phenomenological inquiry; that is, you are not homogenizing differences. What you are attempting to do is to have your participants and yourself interpret the interactions of their context with the experience at hand and to write a rich description of their experiences. Process steps III & IV combined lead to existential, experiential expressions. Proceeding in this manner, you will have fulfilled many of the philosophical underpinnings of phenomenological inquiry. You will undoubtedly have varied examples, varied interpretations, and varied meanings. In nursing, we espouse phenomenological beliefs and values in our nursing philosophies. We believe individuals are unique organisms in interaction with their environment and then paradoxically attempt to have a nursing care model that fits all. Why this does not work has already been discussed, so let us proceed to the next step and see if it affords us better opportunities to generate knowledge that is more particular than general.

VI. Writing the Phenomenological Narrative

A. Choose a style of writing that will communicate an understanding of the meaning of this particular experience.

In this activity, an analysis of each individual's experiential expressions and interpretive interaction is narrated as one life-world, vivid in description and detail. The narrative is reflective of the complexity of the interconnectedness of all the expressions that were spoken or that "showed themselves" as evidence of the deeper contexualized meaning of experience. There are many different ways to present your findings. For exemplars, I refer you to two books: one by James Hillman (1997), called *Emotion: A Comprehensive Phenomenology of Theories and Their Meanings for Therapy*, and another by Robert Coles (1991), titled *Spiritual Life of Children*. These two books show the variation of presentations, for which there is no formula. Writing is a creative activity, and your subject and content should inspire your own presentation, sparked by your imagination.

The introduction in Hillman's (1997) book is quite good: it presents phenomenology as method and describes how Hillman used the method to write this book on human emotions. It is an example and also provides an interpretation of phenomenology as a method. Coles (1991) states in his introduction that his book is a phenomenological text. It contains one narrative after another about individual children talking about their spiritual life. *Each chapter is one child's story.* Coles finishes with a critique of spiritual life for children and its implications for our society. The book is a good example of presenting narratives for individuals and then doing a critique of the meaning of the study, which is the seventh step of this method. Also, volumes 1 and 2 of *In Women's Experience* (Munhall, 1994b, 1995) contain 21 different phenomenological writings by different authors. As you read them, you will see a wide variation in style and creativity. For further examples, use the many resources discussed in Chapter 26 of this book.

B. Write inclusively of all meanings, not just the "general" but the "particular."

In this method, there is a moving away from the idea of synthesizing experience into one-narrative-fits-all. Surely, there may be similar meanings voiced by individuals, but, when they are contextualized, the interpretations may be different. Perception of experience is always grounded in the historical, political, social, and personal background. One might ask, "Is this not several one-case studies placed together?" There are fundamental differences and they are articulated in phenomenological philosophy, the aim of phenomenology, and the method. The knowledge base of a person conducting phenomenological studies must be sophisticated, and the researcher needs to develop many different practices. The outcome of existential experiential expressions, within a deeply contextual world, produces a narrative that describes and interprets (1) the heterogeneity of responses, which a case study does not do; (2) the heterogeneity of meanings, which case studies do not do; and (3) some similarities, which a case study does not do. However, because this method is phenomenological, we do not want to be reductionistic in "listing" those differences and similarities in the narrative. Once we do that, we have removed the deeply embedded contextual interpretations. In the narrative, similarities and differences will "show" themselves.

C. Write inclusively of language and expressions of meaning with the interpretive interaction of the experience of the situated context.

What we produce in these vivid life-world descriptions of our participants' meanings in experience are the possibilities of being-in-the-world for us to consider when we attempt to understand another individual. In casual conversations, "We are more alike than different" can often be heard. Even if we were to base our theories on such an observation, the differences are probably the most important characteristics to consider when approaching patients, planning patient care, and developing nursing research ideas and projects. The similarities are easy to incorporate, if indeed there are such entities. The differences are what challenge us and make all the difference in meeting the needs of patients. The differences are paramount in our endeavor to understand individuals in their multiple realities, subjective worlds, life-worlds, and individual contingencies.

D. Interpret with participants the meaning of the interaction of the experience with contextual processing (steps III and IV).
This is a process that has been ongoing in your research endeavor and can be referred to as cointerpretation of all the phenomenological material. The best sources the phenomenological researcher has are the participants and the other existential material that he or she has amassed. The researcher goes, as before, back to the participant and asks, "In this narrative am I interpreting the meaning of this experience for you?" This is the "mirror," the capturing of the whole: the participant's experiential descriptive expressions of the meaning of the experience and the participant's situated context. I cannot overemphasize the influence of the situated context on the meaning of an experience for an individual. It contributes to the complexity of understanding experience, but without complexity, a contextual meaning emerges that is essentially meaningless. Every life-world contingency has an influence on the interpretation of meaning of an experience. We do an injustice to individuals by minimalizing their life-worlds in our interpretations of experience or the meaning of being human. From an inclusive interpretation will emerge the material for your own interpretive critique, which can be used for direction for theory, practice, and change. The critique will be enriched if you ask your participant about ways the experience can become more meaningful, tolerable, understood, and how health care professionals can demonstrate understanding of participants' meanings. In Sarah's study, the participants tell her how to understand their experience in ways we might not have thought about because of our own preconceptions.

E. Narrate a story that at once gives voice to actual language and simultaneously interprets meaning from expressions used to describe the experience.
How you capture this complexity in writing about meaning and understanding, I believe, is by narrating the experiences in the language as told to you, in the material that appeared to you, and in the realization of the things that

were concealed from you. The researcher's task is to reflect accurately, as if a mirror, using words in the interpretive analysis of interactions that have given meaning to experience. The integration of all material is essential to the wholeness of experience. The researcher reconstructs from the existential inquiry and contextual analysis a narrative that captures the contingencies and meaning in which individuals have socially constructed for this experience. The researcher narrates findings that were discovered and uncovered in the course of the study. New and unexpected meanings of experience are significant findings and lead to new possibilities of "being."

Discovering.   Discovering the meaning in experience fosters the emergence of authentic encounters with one another. We come to understand the role of perception. We come to question our assumptions. And, often, we take phenomenology as not only a way to do research but also a way of being-in-the-world, in our everyday lives. After becoming phenomenologic, we often develop an entirely new worldview, an entirely new understanding of how to encounter our existence.

VII. Writing a Narrative on the Meaning of Your Study

In this final descriptive and interpretive piece, as nurses, we have a moral and/or ethical imperative to fill. We are ultimately in a profession that has aims and goals to assist others in attaining a better quality of life by enhancing awareness of how life might be lived in a way that has meaning for the individual, in finding meaning in an individual's situated context, and by enabling individuals to understand who they are as persons. Our final research narratives of description and interpretation need to have implications for the profession. What does this meaning have for nursing practice? What does this meaning have for nursing theory? Does the final narrative contain implications that critique current practice? Does the interpretation introduce us to new ways of understanding experience? Does it free us from pre-existing suppositions? In this way, does it liberate us from a way of thinking about an experience or its meaning that is no longer evident as evidenced from our inquiry? I do not believe that we can do phenomenology without answering these questions about its relevance. Relevance must extend beyond listing essences and themes, especially when they are acontextual. We have come a long way in our phenomenological thinking and savvy, and we are more critical of our efforts, which is a sign of confidence and growth in our own understanding. In the final analysis, *if we are studying meaning, the ultimate paradox would be if our study did not have meaning!*

A. Summarize the answer to your phenomenological question with breadth and depth.

For the purposes of this section, you take the narrative from the previous phenomenological writing and condense it into a summary of major interpretations. Here, it is a good idea to once again return to participants and ask them to read the summary. Explain that the summary is not the complete narrative of their experience, that it does not contain that kind of detail, but that it will be used to look for meanings or direction for change in thought or practice.

B. Indicate how this understanding, obtained from those who have lived the experience, calls for self-reflection and/or system reflection.

In the evaluation of your study, ask whether the study itself has meaning. Ask interpretive interaction questions. Make sure your study is embedded in the situated context in which individuals and experiences are located. Be able to articulate clearly the meaning for nursing that your study has explicated and interpreted. Unveiling the meaning of experience contributes to human understanding. We need to remember that this does not lend itself to predictive theory. If we were to entertain the thought that it may lead to descriptive theory, we would have to include many qualifications. The theory would have to be explicit to specific cultures, contexts, and contingencies. Recall that we want to avoid reductionistic formulations; we want to call attention to differences in interpreting realities. Yet, at the same time, usefulness becomes apparent in the realization of similarities. Similarities, as in Sarah's studies, enlightened our understanding and, in many instances, liberated mothers and then nurses from their presuppositions concerning this experience. These mothers can find comfort in the understanding that the meaning of their experience within this group is shared.

C. Interpret meanings of these reflections to small and large systems with specific content.

The outcome of phenomenological description and interpretation can have different purposes, as heretofore mentioned. We cannot lose concentration or the ability to reflect on what we are doing. Even as I write, I reflect and can see another possibility. If you have tolerance for uncertainty, are able to feel a bit unbalanced, and have a philosophical leaning to understand the meaning of experience, phenomenology will enrich your professional life and your personal life as well. It becomes a way of being-in-the-world. Being-in-the-world, from a phenomenological perspective, calls for wide-awakeness and attentiveness. From our phenomenological narrative, we must ask, "Are there implications for change in our situated context?" "Do our narratives contradict prevailing norms, or beliefs, and/or theories?" If we are in agreement that critique should be an intricate part of phenomenology, we must interpret the narratives to find their implications for social, cultural, political, health care, and educational change.

D. Critique this interpretation with implications and recommendations for political, social, cultural, health care, family, and other social systems.

The meaning question asked at the end of a study is, "So what?" We must be prepared to answer this question from a critical perspective. In a previous example, we have considered research about domestic violence. If we ended a phenomenological study with a narrative on the experience of domestic violence as it is experienced by women or men who have been victimized, and then provided an understanding of the meaning of that experience, I believe the study is not yet completed from a moral-ethical perspective. We stand on higher ground if we critique the implications derived from the descriptions and interpretations and state them as direction for change. A call to action is sometimes the most appropriate conclusion of a phenomenological study. All too often, because a critique is not highlighted or narrated, a "very good" study does not fulfill its potential and becomes a narrative without consequence. In a field dedicated to improving the quality of life for members of all societies, we have a mandate to listen, beyond the participant's descriptions and interpretations, to how we can make this a better experience. We do this because in the meaning of our study lies an authentic caring about individuals in experience. We do this kind of research ultimately to shed light on what might otherwise be hidden and then to find ways to act on narratives that include direction and implications for change toward quality experiences characterized by caring.

Coming to an End, for Now

Phenomenology questions our consciousness, how we are in the world, how we experience the world, and how we give meaning to experiences. Meanings and interpretations emerge from our situated context and provide for heterogeneous perspectives on life events. This chapter presents interpretations of how you might do a phenomenological study. It may be flawed in many ways. There are always questions to ask about a claim, and so I must let you know that all claims made herein are tentative. I hope that the method discussed here answers the questions students most frequently ask and clarifies the process of conducting phenomenological inquiry. Research guided by this philosophy seeks to unveil meanings and reveals to us the multiplicity of individual perspectives of our multi-storied world. For example, using the method in this chapter with the prerequisite skills of "unknowing," "decentering," and developing essential listening skills should guide you in the uncovering of what is not yet known. From that place, you provide a critique with suggested changes that foster a better quality of life for our patients and selves, thus fulfilling the purpose of phenomenological research in a human science.

Aren't There a Lot of Steps in This Method?

That is an excellent question. How come there seem to be so many "steps"?

What is presented here is more a multifaceted process that occurs simultaneously and that is impossible to describe without categorizing it into what appear to be linear steps. My intent is to take you step by step through the philosophical process of gathering material, interpreting it, and presenting it with a critique. I have attempted to answer common questions and concerns along the way.

The "steps" can be collapsed and thought of as a process after you have become familiar with phenomenological thinking and being. It will come quite naturally. Take what looks here like a very detailed method and see it as a guide to enable your study to flow from phenomenological philosophy in a systematic way that will satisfy your research "method requirements." Each step leads to a place where you have accumulated "more," in this instance, more understanding, more meaning of a phenomenon, more substance, more significance from a critique. Because I do not believe the journey ends there, you will reach a place that illuminates a focus for the continuation of your next study.

Our Hope for Understanding

As a philosophy, phenomenology is our hope for understanding in this world. If we were to understand the meaning of events and experiences to people, we can approach people in a way that reflects understanding of them specifically, not of theory reflecting aggregates of individuals. Our theories can acknowledge the many ways of being and that one way is not the best or the only way to be-in-the-world. The health care provider cannot be the author of or the authority on much of patient care. Until the meaning of experience for a patient is known, an intervention is acontextual.

"Noncompliance," I believe, results from not understanding the patient and the meaning of a behavior to the patient. Because nurses are often concerned in a caring way about behavior that may be detrimental to a patient, family, or community, they need to understand meaning. At the meaning level, we can offer to patients our understanding, and perhaps this generalization is well grounded: we all wish to be understood.

Phenomenology resists homogenizing responses to experiences, categorizing individuals, and placing them in stages. Unfortunately, individuals are viewed as atypical or, worse, abnormal if they deviate from the "mean" of a statistical equation or the goals of a theory. In contrast, researchers following the path of phenomenology are interested in the "*particular*" of experience, while recognizing that there are similarities. However, they see the meaning of the experience, the context in which the experience occurs, and the contingencies affecting the individual as being integrated and critically influential. With this, there is no attempt at generalizing. The phenomenologist bears witness to individual consciousness and the consciousness of the same event perceived quite differently.

In the end, phenomenological studies raise and expand our consciousness and enable us to understand that at the central core from which all things grow lies meaning. The interpretation of the meaning allows for congruency in communication and in nurse–patient interaction. There is optimism in phenomenology, in its wide-awakeness to experience, in its reverence for differences and the subsequent possibilities, and in its ability to liberate us from our preconceptions and emancipate us from presuppositions that no longer work. Sadler (1969) aptly summarizes:

> Our experience is not less than an existential encounter with a world which has a potentially infinite horizon. This human world is not predetermined, as common sense or physicalist language would indicate; it is a world that is open for discovery and creation of ever-new direction for encounter, and *hence open to the emergence of as yet undiscovered significance.* Because our experience is a creative and thoroughly historical encounter in a lived world, one that is alive with our encounter of it, it is potentially *open to new possibilities* of significant existence. (p. 20)

REFERENCES

Allen, D., Benner, P., & Diekelmann, N. (1986). Three paradigms for nursing research: Methodological implications. In P. Chinn (Ed.), *Nursing research methodology issues and implementation.* Rockville, MD: Aspen.

Atwood, D., & Stolorow, R. (1984). *Structures of subjectivity.* Hillsdale, NJ: Erlbaum.

Beattie, A. (1989). *Picturing Will.* New York: Random House.

Benner, P. (Ed.). (1994). *Interpretive phenomenology: Embodiment, caring, and ethics in health and illness.* Thousand Oaks, CA: Sage.

Cohen, M. (1987). A historical overview of the phenomenological movement. *The Journal of Nursing Scholarship, 19,* 31–34.

Coles, R. (1991). *Spiritual life of children.* Boston, MA: Houghton Mifflin.

Crotty, M. (1996). *Phenomenology and nursing research.* South Melbourne, Australia: Churchill Livingstone.

Dreyfus, H. (1972). *What computers can't do: A critique of artificial reason.* New York: Harper Row.

Heidegger, M. (1962). *Being and time.* San Francisco: Harper & Row. (Original work published 1927).

Hillman, J. (1997). *Emotion: A comprehensive phenomenology of theories and their meanings for therapy.* Evanston, IL: Northwestern University Press.

Lauterbach, S. (2001). Longitudinal phenomenology: An example of "doing" phenomenology over time; phenomenology of maternal mourning: Being-a-mother "In Another World (1992) and Five Years Later (1997)." In P. Munhall (Ed.), *Nursing research: A qualitative perspective* (3rd ed.). Sudbury, MA: Jones and Bartlett.

Merleau-Ponty, M. (1962). *Phenomenology and perception.* (C. Smith, Trans). New York: Humanities Press.

Munhall, P. (1993). Unknowing: Toward another pattern of knowing. *Nursing Outlook, 41,* 125–128.

Munhall, P. (1994a). *Revisioning phenomenology: Nursing and health science research.* Sudbury, MA: Jones and Bartlett.

Munhall, P. (1994b). *In women's experience* (Vol. 1). Sudbury, MA: Jones and Bartlett.

Munhall, P. (1995). *In women's experience* (Vol. 2). Sudbury, MA: Jones and Bartlett.

Munhall, P. (2001). *Nursing research: A qualitative perspective* (3rd ed.). Sudbury, MA: Jones and Bartlett.

Munhall, P., & Oiler-Boyd, C. (Eds.). (1993). *Nursing research: A qualitative perspective* (2nd ed.). Sudbury, MA: Jones and Bartlett.

Newman, M. A. (1986) *Health as expanding consciousness.* St Louis, MO: Mosby.

Parse, R. (1987). *Nursing science: Major paradigms, theories, and critiques.* Philadelphia: Saunders.

Paterson, J., & Zderad, L. (1976). *Humanistic nursing.* New York: Wiley.

Paterson, J., & Zderad, L. (1988 reprinted). *Humanistic nursing.* New York: National League for Nursing.

Ray, M. (1990). Phenomenological method for nursing research. In H. Chaska (Ed.), *The nursing profession: Turning points.* Orlando, FL: Grune & Stratton.

Reeder, F. (1987). The phenomenological movement. *Image: The Journal of Nursing Scholarship, 19,* 150–152.

Sadler, W. A. (1969). *Existence and love: A new approach in existential phenomenology.* New York: Scribner's.

Schutz, A., & Wagner, H. (1970). *On phenomenology and social relations.* Chicago: University of Chicago Press.

Smiley, J. (1989). *Ordinary love and good will.* New York: Random House.

Spiegelberg, H. (1976). *Doing phenomenology.* The Hague, Netherlands: Martinus Nijhoff.

van Manen, M. (1984). *"Doing" phenomenological research and writing.* Alberta, Canada: University of Alberta Press.

van Manen, M. (1990). *Researching the lived experience.* Albany, NY: SUNY Press.

van Manen, M. (1998). Phenomenological Workshop. International Institute for Qualitative Methodology Conference. Edmonton, Canada.

Watson, J. (1985). *Nursing: Human science and human care: A theory of nursing.* Norwalk, CT: Appleton-Century-Crofts.

ADDITIONAL REFERENCES

Allen, D. G. (1995). Hermeneutics: Philosophical traditions and nursing practice research. *Nursing Science Quarterly, 8*(4), 174–182.

Allgood, M. R., & Fawcett, J. (1999). Acceptance of the invitation to dialogue: Examination of an interpretive approach for the science of unitary human beings. *Visions: The Journal of Rogerian Nursing Science, 7,* 5–13.

Anderson, W. (Ed.). (1995). *The truth about truth: De-confusing and re-constructing the postmodern world.* New York: Tarcher/Putnam.

Annells, M. (1999). Phenomenology revisited. Evaluating phenomenology: Usefulness quality and philosophical foundations. *Nurse Researcher, 6*(3), 5–19.

Ashworth, P. D. (1997). The variety of qualitative research (Part 2): Non-positivist approaches. *Nurse Education Today, 17*(3), 219–224.

Asp, M., & Fagerberg, I. (2005). Developing concepts in caring science based on a lifeworld perspective. *International Journal of Qualitative Methods, 4*(2), article 4.

Astedt-Kurki, P. (1994). Phenomenological approach in nursing research: Experiences of health, well-being and nursing are studied from the point of view of clients and nurses. *Hoitotiede, 6,* 2–7.

Atwood, G., & Stolorow, R. (1999). *Faces in a cloud: Intersubjectivity in personality theory.* Northvale, NJ: Jason Aronson.

Baker, C., Norton, S., Young, P., & Ward, S. (1998). An exploration of methodological pluralism in nursing research. *Research in Nursing and Health, 21,* 545–555.

Barnard, A., McCosker, H., & Gerber, R. (1999). Phenomenology: A qualitative research approach for exploring understanding in health care. *Qualitative Health Research, 9*(2), 212–216.

Bishop, A., & Scudder, J. (1990). *The practical, moral and personal sense of nursing: A phenomenological philosophy of practice.* Albany, NY: SUNY Press.

Bruner, J. (1990). *The acts of meaning.* Cambridge, England: Cambridge University Press.

Conroy, S. (2003). A pathway for interpretive phenomenology. *International Journal of Qualitative Methods, 2*(3), article 4.

Corben, V. (1999). Phenomenology revisited. Misusing phenomenology in nursing research: Identifying the issues. *Nurse Researcher, 6*(3), 52–56.

Davis, S. F., & Finlay, L. (1999). Applying phenomenology in research: Problems, principles and practice. *British Journal of Occupational Therapy, 62*(9), 424.

Denzin, N. (1994). The art and politics of interpretation. In N. Denzin & Y. Lincoln (Eds.), *Handbook of qualitative research* (pp. 500–515). Thousand Oaks, CA: Sage.

Ely, M., Vinz, R., Downing, M., & Anzul, M. (2001). *On writing qualitative research: Living by words.* London: Routledge.

Finlay, L. (1999). Applying phenomenology in research: Problems, principles and practice. *British Journal of Occupational Therapy, 62*(7), 299–306.

Forbes, D. A., King, K. M., Kushner, K. E., Letourneau, N. L., Myrick, A. F., & Profetto-McGrath, J. (1999). Warrantable evidence in nursing science. *Journal of Advanced Nursing, 29,* 373–379.

Frankl, V. E. (1984). *Man's search for meaning. An introduction to logotherapy* (4th ed.). Boston, MA: Beacon Press.

Gademer, H. G. (1998). *Truth and method* (2nd ed.). New York: Continuum.

Gearing, R. E. (2004). Bracketing in research: A typology. *Qualitative Health Research, 14*(10), 1429–1452.

Hammond, M., Howarth, J., & Keat, R. (1991). *Understanding phenomenology.* Cambridge, MA: Basil Blackwell.

Irving, J., & Klenke, K. (2004). Telos, Chronos and Hermeneia: The role of metanarrative in leadership effectiveness through the production of meaning. *International Journal of Qualitative Methods, 3*(3), article 3.

Koch, T. (1995). Interpretive approaches in nursing research: The influence of Husserl and Heidegger. *Journal of Advanced Nursing, 21*(5), 827–836.

Koch, T. (1999). Phenomenology revisited. An interpretive research process: Revisiting phenomenological and hermeneutical approaches. *Nurse Researcher, 6*(3), 20–34.

Lauterbach, S. (1993). In another world: A phenomenological perspective and discovery of meaning in mothers' experience with death of a wished for baby: Doing phenomenology. In P. Munhall & C. Oiler-Boyd (Eds.), *Nursing research: A qualtitative perspective* (2nd ed., Chap. 5). Sudbury, MA: Jones and Bartlett.

LeVasseur, J. J. (2003). The problem with bracketing in phenomenology. *Qualitative Health Research, 13,* 408–420.

Laverty, S. (2003). Hermeneutic phenomenology and phenomenology: A comparison of historical and methodological considerations. *International Journal of Qualitative Methods, 2*(3), article 3.

Levin-Rozalis, M. (2004). Searching for the unknowable: A process of detection—abductive research generated by projective techniques. *International Journal of Qualitative Methods, 3*(2), article 1.

Locke, J. (1975). *An essay concerning human understanding.* Oxford, England: Oxford University Press.

Lopez, K., & Willis, D. (2004). Descriptive versus interpretive phenomenology: Their contributions to nursing knowledge. *Qualitative Health Research, 14*(5), 726, 735.

MacLean, L. M., Meyer, M., & Estable, A. (2004). Improving accuracy of transcripts in qualitative research. *Qualitative Health Research, 14*(1), 113–123.

Marques, J., & McCall, C. (2005). The application of interrater reliability as solidification instrument in a phenomenological study. *Qualitative Report, 10*(3), 438–461.

Merleau-Ponty, M. (1999). *The phenomenology of perception.* London: Routledge. (Original work published 1962).

Moerer-Urdahl, T., & Creswell, J. (2004). Using transcendental phenomenology to explore the "ripple effect" in a leadership mentoring program. *International Journal of Qualitative Methods, 3*(2), article 2.

Moran, D. (2000). *Introduction to phenomenology.* London: Routledge.

Moustakas, C. (1994). *Phenomenological research methods.* Thousand Oaks, CA: Sage.

Munhall, P., & Fitzsimons, V. (1995). *The emergence of women into the 21st century*. Sudbury, MA: Jones and Bartlett.

Munhall, P., & Fitzsimons, V. (2000). *The emergence of family into the 21st century*. Sudbury, MA: Jones and Bartlett.

Parse, R. (1990). Parse's research methodology with an illustration of the lived experience of hope. *Nursing Science Quarterly, 3*(1), 9–17.

Paterson, M., & Higgs, J. (2005). Using hermeneutics as a qualitative research approach in professional practice. *Qualitative Report, 10*(2), 339–357.

Picard, C. (1997). Embodied soul: The focus of nursing praxis. *Journal of Holistic Nursing, 15*(10), 41–53.

Pink, D. (2005). *A whole new mind: Moving from the information age to the conceptual age*. New York: Riverhead Books.

Polifroni, C., & King, M. (Eds.). *Perspectives on philosophy of science in nursing: An historical and contemporary anthology*. Philadelphia: Lippincott.

Power, E. (2004). Toward understanding in postmodern interview analysis: Interpreting the contradictory remarks of a research participant. *Qualitative Health Research, 14*(6), 858–865.

Proctor, S. (1998). Linking philosophy and method in the research process: The case of realism. *Nurse Researcher, 5*(4), 73–90.

Ray, M. A. (1994). The richness of phenomenology: Philosophic, theoretic and methodologic concerns. In J. M. Morse (Ed.), *Critical issues in qualitative research methods* (pp. 117–133). Thousand Oaks, CA: Sage.

Rorty, R. (1991). *Essays on Heidegger and others*. New York: Cambridge University Press.

Sandelowski, M. (2002). Reembodying qualitative inquiry. *Qualitative Health Research, 12*(1), 104–115.

Seymour, J., & Clark, D. (1998). Issues in research. Phenomenological approaches to palliative care research. *Palliative Medicine, 12*(2), 127–131.

Smaling, A. (2003). Inductive, analogical and communicative generalization. *International Journal of Qualitative Methods, 2*(1), article 5.

Stubblefield, C., & Murray, R. L. (2002). A phenomenological framework for psychiatric nursing research. *Archives of Psychiatric Nursing, 16*(4), 149–155.

Thorne, S. E., Kirkham, S. R., & Henderson, A. (1999). Ideological implications of paradigm discourse. *Nursing Inquiry, 6*(2), 123–131.

Wolcott, H. F. (2002). Writing up qualitative research . . . better. *Qualitative Health Research, 12*(1), 91–103.

7

Meanings in Mothers' Experience with Infant Death: Three Phenomenological Inquiries: In Another World; Five Years Later; and What Forever Means

Sarah Steen Lauterbach

INTRODUCTION

This chapter discusses my work, which includes the dissertation research (Lauterbach, 1992) entitled "In Another World: A Phenomenological Perspective and Discovery of Meaning in Mothers' Experience of Death of a Wished-for Baby." The 5-year follow-up inquiry, "In Another World: Five Years Later" and the original research were reported in two chapters

Source: Adapted from *Nursing Research* Jan/Feb 1993, Vol. 42, No. 1 © 1993 American Journal of Nursing Company.

(Lauterbach, 1993, 2000) in the second and third editions of this text, respectively. The inquiries have been focused on investigating mothers' experience with death of a baby. In this chapter, a summary of findings from a third inquiry entitled *What Forever Means: Meanings in Elder Mothers' Experience with Infant Death* is described. A fourth inquiry, *Meanings Surrounding Infant Death in the Black Community: In Mothers' Voice* is discussed to animate the research process used in the early development of an inquiry.

The aim of this chapter is to explicate the phenomenological perspective and methodology used in the quest to create human understanding of meanings in mothers' experience with having a baby die. The aim is to discuss the understandings gleaned relating to phenomenology of infant death, human care applications resulting from knowledge, and practice applications in human care resulting from inquiry. The inquiries have used van Manen's (1984, 1990) and Munhall's (1993, 2000) phenomenological perspectives and my own experience with "doing" phenomenology to explicate meanings in mothers' experience.

The reader is referred to the two exemplar chapters in Munhall's text that used van Manen (1984, 1997) and Munhall's (1993, 2000) phenomenological perspectives. In addition, this chapter also uses Munhall's (2000) methodology chapter to narrate the application and outcomes of the phenomenological perspectives and methodologies. Further, I demonstrate the concurrent activities and processes in Munhall's perspective that have been used to integrate the findings in the three completed investigations. Discussion of the fourth inquiry using the methodologies and perspectives of the previous work focuses on the beginning investigation of the phenomenon of infant death in the black community.

The investigations focus on meaning(s) mothers' experience with perinatal loss and the continuing immersion in the phenomenon and inquiry processes have made it possible to integrate findings from three investigations with different populations. Further, a continuing focus has facilitated the development of a retrospective perspective, as well a prospective, longitudinal phenomenological perspective to the investigating mothers' lived experience with infant death.

The longitudinal perspective was developed during the original inquiry, when it became evident in the first interview that one interview would not be sufficient. The first interview served to focus attention on the phenomenon or experience of having a baby die. It was immediately clear that interviews over time would reveal a fuller depth of meaning(s) in mothers' experience. To examine mothers' experience, to fully execute an explication of description and meaning(s) in experience, it was necessary to continue the inquiry over time. The findings of the first and subsequent inquiries have revealed that mothers continue to grieve and mourn the particular infant and loss over time.

The approach used in this research also establishes the importance of methodological consistency in investigations of human phenomena and experience. It is important in investigating and bringing attention to meaning(s) as they have evolved and continue to evolve over time. Participating in research assisted mothers in continuing to develop and explore meaning(s). Over time the researcher becomes a seasoned, knowledgeable observer of the phenomenon and comes to more fully appreciate the nuances, similarities, and differences in mothers' experience. It is now easy to elicit exemplar descriptions and stories from mothers' stories and narrative about their experience.

I used the particular phenomenological methodology to explore other perspectives not originally addressed in Munhall's or van Manen's writings. This chapter shares my understandings gleaned from the process of becoming and being a phenomenological researcher who has been involved in investigating the phenomenon of perinatal loss over time.

SUMMARY OF FINDINGS IN ONE INQUIRY

What Forever Means: Meanings in Elder Mothers' Experience with Infant Death

Begun in 2000, this inquiry used the methodology from my previous research. It received approval for human subjects by the University of Southern Mississippi Institutional Review Board. This inquiry used the perspectives from the two previous inquiries, van Manen's (1984, 1990) work on "doing phenomenology" and Munhall and Oiler-Boyd's (1993) model of existential investigation. This third inquiry has validated findings from the other two inquiries even though it was with a completely different population of mothers.

Nine elder women who were between the ages of 75 and 92 years were involved with interviews, conversations, and shared stories of experience. Serendipitous conversations and comments from five other elder mothers and several narratives shared by other elder women were included in the thematic analysis. Interviews were from 30 minutes to an hour long, depending on the person and the descriptions. One or more interviews and conversations were completed for each participant. When descriptions were detailed and complete, another interview was not scheduled. Interviews with this group of elder mothers were not taped and were much shorter in duration than with the group of younger women. Extensive field notes were kept of the narrative data and written immediately following the contact. In most cases, casual and serendipitous conversations, which contained narratives and stories of mothers' experiences, were written immediately following the contact.

Thematic Groupings of Findings in Elder Mothers' Experience. The thematic groupings from the descriptions, narratives, and stories of elder mothers will be narrated in an integrated text written to articulate elder mothers' *lived experience* with the phenomenon, hoping to create human understanding:

> What forever means . . .
> An ever present, enduring sense of loss, forever . . .
> Grief, lasting much longer than expected, sometimes intense around anniversary or special times . . .
> Phenomenological silence surrounding loss . . . privacy and isolation
> Denial and invalidation of loss — *continuing the silence . . . lack of understanding*
> Temporality of loss meanings experienced and relived again and again
> Embodiment of loss experienced and *relived* again through life review and visits
> Living *with* death and loss in *caring for* other children . . .
> Integration of mourning and death into continuing life, anniversary reminders
> An existential "missing" the baby who died, continues forever . . .

Discussion and Integration of Findings. The following lines are evocative of the overarching theme in elder mothers' lived experience with having a baby die shortly before or after the baby's birth:

> Time past and time present are contained in time future
> And time future in time past. . . (Eliot, 1936, p. 175)

Temporality was the overarching theme, central in narrative data. Mothers' stories from both interviews and serendipitous conversations with elder mothers were quite similar to other inquiries. The experience of having a baby die was an experience in temporality. Elder mothers used the term *forever* to describe this temporal experience. Their descriptions indicated that time, which had passed, was in the present, or in the future, had collapsed into a temporality of meaning where past, present, and future were connected. Temporality was identified as one of the overarching themes in my original doctoral inquiry (Lauterbach, 1992, 1993), and it was a central and overarching dimension for elder women.

The title of the inquiry, "What Forever Means," was described and explicated in elder women's experience. The experience, the silence surrounding grief and mourning over time, is an experience that continues to be felt and remembered in great detail regardless of many years passing. Meanings in younger mothers' experience also continued to develop and unfold over time. One elder mother stated as she described what it was like, "It was forever, until now." "As I get closer to the end, forever is not as long as it used to be." "I used to think I couldn't wait a lifetime . . . but, it's been a lifetime . . . and it seems only like yesterday."

At the time of the death of the baby, several mothers described that they "did not know how to deal with it." One mother stated, "I didn't know if I could stand it . . . you know . . . whether I could ever really deal with it and ever be happy again." Each mother was grateful for the role of mother or wife and that she "had to keep going." Responsibilities required them to function and helped them in "getting on with life." They simply "had to get involved with living."

Several mothers discussed how they learned to "live *with* death" in their experience of caring for other children. One mother cared for her sister's children "as if they were my own." "My sister died, so I raised her children, along with my son. It kept me pretty busy. The niece I raised, I called my granddaughter. Then she lost her daughter, who was 13, in an automobile accident. That was very hard. She has recently had another baby . . . a little girl, who is so beautiful. But, I still really miss my Janie, as if she were my own great granddaughter." Subsequent losses for mothers are often profound experiences.

The integration of mourning and death into continuing life experience is similar to findings in the original inquiry. "You learn to live with it. You don't have a choice." An elder mother stated, "Really, it hasn't been too hard. I've had a full life. But, still I wonder each spring what it would have been like. I still miss her like that."

"It was forever, until now." This mother went on to explain that she had always thought that she would see her baby in heaven. There was an expectation that there would be a reunion with the baby, "when I get up there." "As I got closer to the end, forever is not as long as it used to be. . . . Now, I think I'll have more time [to be with the baby daughter] than ever, because it will be forever together."

Elder mothers also experienced an ever-present, enduring sense of loss, "forever." They described an acute and painful grief lasting much longer than expected. Like the younger mothers in the earlier inquiries, they described that they endured the agony and acute grief, often alone. Four mothers had never even spoken of it to anyone after the acute grief passed. "It was not something you talked about." This mother felt guilty because she felt as if she had neglected her baby daughter in not talking about her. She said, "And you know, sometimes I couldn't help myself. I would just blurt it out. Then I would feel so guilty and bad. I really think I let my baby down. She deserved more from me. I was her mother, for Pete's sake!"

The silence surrounding infant death for elder mothers was quite a surprise to me. Because the deaths occurred many years ago, I assumed that people talked more openly about death, that death was part of life. This preunderstanding was not validated by elder mothers' descriptions and memories. In fact, the silence was very present in the participants' experience of grief and mourning over time. Of the five who had talked about the baby and death, the consensus among mothers was that it really bothered their husbands and families to discuss the baby or its death.

Elder mothers all agreed that they thought about the baby and wondered about the experience and baby a lot, especially at certain times of the year— at holiday times, on birthdays, and at times when they would have celebrated family milestones, such as the anniversary of the pregnancy, anniversary of the death, graduations, weddings, other deaths, and funerals. They shared that they mostly thought about the baby and often wondered what would have happened if the child had lived to maturity. Like younger mothers, infant death prevented a future relationship with the child throughout the child's childhood and with the adult child over the life span. One mother shared that her son would have perhaps been drafted and gone off to the Vietnam War. She felt that at least she knew her son had not suffered there. "Still, it was little comfort," she said.

Elder mothers discussed the experience of "missing" the baby who had died. I called this an existential missing and experience of loss that continues to linger forever, long after the baby died. "I have missed her always." Like the younger mothers in the previous research, elder mothers have excellent recall for child birth and death experiences. Upon reviewing their lives, these memories are recalled in brilliant detail and descriptions.

In the earlier research, with younger mothers, an essential theme in the first inquiry was embodiment, which is experienced as living with the phenomenon felt through one's body. In the 5-year follow-up, embodiment was moved into one of the four overarching themes. In elder mothers, embodiment is one of the thematic groupings. In one woman's words, "I can close my eyes, think about it, and feel it all over again, as if it just occurred."

"I can see my husband, how broken up he was. It was our first baby, and he wanted a son so much. He felt as if he was a failure, that he did not protect me enough. I went into labor as soon as I got in from the field. He never got over it. (silence) And neither did I. But, I know in my mind that I've had a good life. I have no regrets . . . no regrets really, but that." "I wasn't as desperate with the passing of time. But, sometimes it took me by surprise, almost took my breath away." "It's understandable, really. I don't mean I ever really forgot, but it wasn't always on the front of my mind."

"Then sometimes, it would just hit me, that my baby had died, and I felt as bad as I ever did." "I've always wondered why, but I tried to let that thought go. I'm not sure I really wanted to know . . . it might hurt so much." "It has hurt like an acute tummy ache. I couldn't breathe . . . like I had a heavy weight on my chest. It was hard to get my breath. I found that sighing helped. But, no one really knows unless it happens to you. A baby's death really hurts."

THE AIM OF PHENOMENOLOGICAL RESEARCH AND PRACTICE APPLICATIONS

Non ridere, non lugere, neque detestari, sed intelligere.
Not to laugh, not to lament, not to curse, but to understand.

—Spinoza

To become more fully human is the ultimate aim of phenomenology as a philosophy and research perspective. As a human caring science and art, nursing's ultimate goal is to care for persons and human systems experiencing the unfolding life processes by using informed, timely, and appropriate care based on human caring and understanding. Understanding "essences" in experience underpins fully caring for another. Further, "knowing" the person, group, population, or institution is critical in nurse caring. Thus, gaining a fuller depth of understanding of human experience can become actualized in the human care that is an outcome research. It is potentially more humane and reflective of the fuller understanding facilitated by the research.

Nursing phenomenological research perspectives aim to enhance understanding through reflective awareness, describing human experience fully, processing and interpreting experience, and explicating meaning(s) in experience. As meaning is understood, commitment, an intention to care, and informed care become possible. Human understanding comes from conscious, knowing contemplation and commitment. In keeping with the ultimate aim of phenomenology, "to become more fully human," it is my hope that this chapter enables and facilitates you in becoming more thoughtfully human.

Through attending and consciously continuing conversation about sensitive human experience, particularly, nursing has a unique and special role. Caring and inquiry must go hand in hand. Each informs the other.

According to Husserl (1952):

> It [phenomenology] has to place before its own eyes as instances certain pure conscious events, to bring these to complete clearness, and within this zone of clearness, to subject them to analysis and the apprehension of their essence, to follow up the essential connections that can be clearly understood, to grasp what is momentarily perceived in faithful conceptual expressions, of which the meaning is prescribed purely by the object perceived or in some way transparently understood. (p. 174)

Further, phenomenology seeks to explicate personal meanings and to uncover hidden as well as explicit meanings in human experience. Additionally, in the research presented in this chapter, phenomenology has demonstrated its potential to guide the formation of meanings in experience through its investigative processing and research presence in participant mothers' lives as they engage in research activities.

Participation has contributed to mothers' uncovering as well as thorough development of meaning(s) in experience over time. This has been revealed in the continuing research conversations and discussions over several research contacts and in returning to participants from the first inquiry. In each of the three investigations, attending to uncovering and discovering meaning(s) as mothers processed their memories and experience helped them to create new meanings.

With the completion of the first research interview in the doctoral study, I realized that the first interview was just a beginning interview. Three interviews were conducted with participant mothers over the course of 8 months. This strategy has continued in subsequent research.

In the Beginning and Continuing Concurrent Processes: An Immersion in Phenomenology and Human Experience

Phenomenological research involves maintaining a thoughtful, attentive awareness of the phenomenon under investigation. It is an active engagement of the researcher pursuing examples in the existential human world of the phenomenon while at the same time becoming immersed in science as well as human science and creative art and literature. Once begun, an investigation takes on a form and process that is dictated by both what is known and what is unknown about the phenomenon. The researcher begins to "live" the question, or the phenomenological pursuit. In my experience, I began to see examples and references to perinatal loss in the human world where I lived. I began to "see" differently.

Initially, in beginning the focus on mothers' experience with infant death, my personal experience and loss were revisited. Early in the process, there were moments when I thought it did not seem possible to continue. However, when the personal experience and memories were intrusive, with attention, explication, and bracketing I was able to move past the personal experience. I realized, as I had when my loss first occurred, that I had to put the pain and experience aside to continue with responsibilities. Mourning mothers in the inquiry shared that they had bracketed their personal experience to function in roles as wife and mother.

The process of putting aside the early agony and grief had been necessary for me when my loss occurred. To care for my other children, who were at that time 4, 2, and newborn, putting the loss aside to process in private was necessary. Similarly, in beginning the phenomenological research, this "putting aside personal experience" became necessary. Bracketing is particularly important and necessary when the researcher has personal experience and/or knowledge of a phenomenon.

In beginning the research, and in continuing to investigate mothers' experiences with infant death, my primary task was to be capable of conducting research. The process is called "becoming phenomenological" by Munhall (2001) and involves becoming able to "bracket" out personal, knowledge, biases, and experience. Further, it involved being immersed in the literature of phenomenology, of being immersed in the phenomenon of perinatal infant death, and in becoming immersed in methodological activities and existential investigation without interference of personal material.

The experience of becoming phenomenological has continued since the beginning of my investigation of the phenomenon of infant death and in the 24 years since my own loss. As a researcher, one must become accustomed to exploring in-depth descriptions of often painful and sensitive human phenomena and experience. The researcher must suspend judgment and prior knowledge about the experience and phenomena, and must continually try to understand. Munhall calls this adopting a position and stance of "unknowing." With each new description or example of the phenomenon, the researcher must return to the phenomenon, seeking to understand its meaning.

To become a phenomenological researcher, a return to the phenomenology literature for clarification and guidance is necessary. When researching sensitive phenomena, it is imperative that the researcher develop and use personal supportive resources while engaged in research. This is helpful in maintaining the bracketing, so at the same time the researcher can deal with the personal impact of the research on feelings and understandings. My research mentor/sponsor/chair, along with colleagues, were helpful to me and helped me maintain bracketing and perspective.

My family and children were interested in the research and served as wonderful supports. Alexandra, the surviving twin who was 8 years old when my doctoral study began, would set her alarm clock to wake her at 4 A.M. so she could sleep on the bathroom floor with a pillow and blankie while I got ready to travel to New York by train every Friday. Jared would ask, "Are you ready for New York?" Marlow helped her dad make dinner on Friday nights. All posed for pictures for a slide presentation. Marlow, Jared, and Alexandra have written poems about their experience of having a twin sibling die. My mother has participated by editing manuscripts. Each child has participated in cemetery investigations and has become reflective as a result of the family experience and research. Further, as editor, my mother has been helping me clarify, describe, and explicate the meanings and outcomes in clear language. To facilitate human understanding and informed care, it is important that phenomenological research be written and shared in scholarly literature and for the public.

Having a baby die is a family experience. In several of the interviews in the original and follow-up inquiries, children and babies of the participant mother were present. A 2-month-old baby nursed as her mother described two perinatal losses, and the mother stated, "I am really the mother of three little girls." Five years later, this mother of two living children, stated, again, "I am really the mother of six little girls." One mother's 2-year-old daughter crawled under the table around her mother's feet as we talked. In my doctoral research, an unexpected outcome was that the very act of participating served to validate mothers' experience. It also informed mothers about how to guide their families through coping with the loss and mourning. It was particularly helpful to them in addressing, planning, and dealing with anniversary responses surrounding the baby's death.

Back to the Researcher: Becoming Phenomenological, Thinking Phenomenologically, Coming Up with the Phenomenological Questions

Thinking and becoming phenomenological are quite like reframing one's thinking in investigating in depth the qualitative aspects of human experience. The process involves refocusing on the phenomenon with each new description, reflecting on potential meaning(s), and ultimately gaining an enriched, fuller understanding of the phenomenon. It is important to ask these and perhaps other questions:

- "What is/are meaning(s) in this experience or phenomenon?"
- "What is being described here?"
- "What is it like to be a person having this experience?"
- "What is it like for those surrounding the person?"
- "Is this a unique, personal experience, or is it a common, universal experience, and how common?"
- "How is this experience recorded in the human world, in the creative human arts and literature, and in the rituals surrounding the experience?"
- "How is the phenomenon reflected and manifested in human relationships?"
- "What is the evolving meaning(s) that surrounds the phenomenon over time and how does this manifest itself in human experience?"
- "What can be gained in exploring the experience/phenomenon through inquiry?"

Becoming Phenomenological: Using Presence, Becoming the Instrument

In qualitative research and in phenomenological research, the researcher's presence — being fully present with an intention to understand and care — is the ultimate goal. The researcher is the instrument of the perspective or methodology used. It is through the researcher's thinking and processing that meanings in experience are explicated and more fully and deeply explored and understood. The researcher is charged to "see the phenomenon as if seeing for the very first time." This involves explicating researcher bias and prejudice, prior knowledge, and understanding. This material must be bracketed after acknowledgment and placed aside, so that the researcher sees with clear vision. Thus, the researcher must be fully present, with an intention of understanding and caring in explicating the experience and phenomenon.

Becoming Phenomenological: Becoming Therapeutic—The Research vs. Therapeutic Imperatives

In both quantitative and qualitative research, the researcher processes and directs the investigation using a particular methodological perspective. The structure of quantitative research provides the controls through which phenomena are investigated. In qualitative research, the researcher provides the perspective through which phenomena are investigated, but it is much less determined and set. The researcher's knowledge of methodology and the phenomenon being investigated are directive. Qualitative research is more of an approach or perspective than a method. In investigations of human experience, it is much more subject to human direction.

In quantitative research, attention is given to both the research and therapeutic imperatives concerning the research. But the research imperative is key. In qualitative research, there is more of a balancing of the research and therapeutic imperative. In phenomenological research over time, even more attention is given to therapeutic intent. The therapeutic intention is as important as the research intention, and as this occurs, the research and therapeutic imperatives become more balanced.

Outcomes of Phenomenological Research: Practice Applications

The balancing of therapeutic and research imperatives provides a fuller human understanding of the phenomenon under investigation and of the care needed. Human understanding facilitates human care. Understanding has direct care applications: it provides for care that is more fully informed, more sensitive, and timely; and for care that includes more appropriate responses from nurses and others involved with human care work. Herein is the beauty and necessity of doing qualitative research and of the insightful perspectives illuminated by phenomenological research.

Phenomenology transforms care and facilitates the actualization of human potential. It is more assistive in informing providers who are helping others deal with life experience, especially experience and phenomena that involve tremendous human suffering and agony, which often continue for a very long time, a lifetime, and forever after. As elder women approached their own mortality, their life review included a very poignant revisiting of their birth and death experiences. They continued to describe mourning and loss as they prepared for their own death.

Elder mothers' memories, descriptions, and stories were filled with exquisite descriptive details of the experiences from many years ago. Several elder mothers had never spoken to anyone about the experience and the baby's death and were grateful for the opportunity that the research participation provided. One woman wanted me to take her to visit her baby's grave because her son would not do it. Often, family members, if present or alive, worry that talking about the memory or visiting the grave will be too painful. But elder mothers, like younger mothers, welcomed the opportunity.

Several elder mothers had no living relatives or persons who had memory or direct experience of their baby who had died. Several were sole family survivors. In addition, friends of several elder mothers in the research group were all deceased. An elder mother was the only living person who had a memory of her baby. The deaths of those who "knew" are isolating experiences. This mother wanted me to see her baby's grave and wanted to visit it one more time before she died. Because of the family concerns mentioned earlier, we did not go to the grave, regretfully, but such a trip could have been a direct practice application of understanding and of the care needed by this mother. In time, elder mothers can direct their own care and plan experiences that will be helpful.

EXPLICATING THE PHENOMENON: CONTINUING IMMERSION AND DISCOVERY OF PHENOMENOLOGICAL SILENCE SURROUNDING INFANT DEATH AND PERINATAL LOSS

The human experience of infant death is captured by the phrase, "The grief which knows no words." Of death topics, infant death is one of the most sensitive topics and most difficult to discuss. The topic is almost always evocative of powerful human emotions. This is true even for persons closest to the mother. In fact, it may be more difficult for intimate, immediate family and friends. The silence may serve as a protective denial, initially, that makes discussion later more difficult. It contributes to a continuing atmosphere of silence surrounding the death experience.

Mothers in the first investigation described that having a wished-for baby die was an experience of *being-a-mother in another world*. The phenomenologist Heidegger (1927/1962) and his work on being have greatly informed this interpretation. He proposes that in death, the dead abandon the living, but continue to exist in another world. Joseph Campbell's (1988) work on myth proposes that the mythical world is full of connection between life and death. Further, he states that there is support for the thesis that life is supported by an invisible plane, that death is life and life is death.

Using Heidegger's interpretation and an analysis of mothers' descriptions, the title I chose for the first research was "In Another World." It represents the overarching theme identified in descriptions of mothers' experience following the death of a wished-for baby. Five years later, mothers in the original research revalidated the title, saying, in the words of one mother, "It is even truer now than ever before. That's it . . . in a nutshell."

Immersion in Experience: Up Close and Personal

When the qualitative nursing research topic was first identified as the focus for my doctoral dissertation, I, a mother, had experienced the death of a second twin in my last pregnancy 8 years earlier. Even though I was impressed with well-meaning nurses' intentions, the lack of informed care at the time of loss and afterwards was evident. I was impressed with an almost total lack of understanding. In my first contact with a nurse several hours after the twin delivery and emergency, the first question I was asked by the nurse was, "Do you want an early discharge?" This question indicated that the nurse had no idea of what had happened in the almost-perfect midwife delivery of the first twin baby girl, Alexandra, and the tragic delivery of the second twin baby girl, Amy, 32 minutes later with high forceps. Amy was in cardiac arrest, anoxic, and required ventilation. She was seizing and required immediate transport to a neonatal intensive care unit. Uninformed nursing care is less common nowadays but still exists in women's experience. The atmosphere of silence still surrounds the care and experience of mothers and families with infant death.

Explication of Phenomenological Silence: Existential Investigation of the Phenomenon

Ten years after the publication of the first research (Lauterbach, 1993), phenomenological silence was the focus of an article I wrote (Lauterbach, 2003). In the many research presentations since my original doctoral research was completed, I have found that the silence around perinatal loss continues. Further, phenomenological silence also surrounds many other human experiences, especially human experience that involves tremendous human suffering.

In the Pulitzer Prize–winning text *The Denial of Death*, Becker (1973) proposes that man [*sic*] devotes much effort to escape the ultimate burden of life — death. Since the publication of that oft-quoted text and in spite of much media and public attention on death and tragedy, still little public attention is given to infant death. In fact, infant death and pregnancy loss are very common human phenomena. Perinatal death is death of the infant either shortly before or within a month following birth.

Even though changes have been made in nursing protocols surrounding the death of an infant, often a silence still surrounds infant death. In the early 1980s, in response to mothers' and families' wishes, nurses began photographing infants who had died or who were at risk. (Interestingly, when photography was first developed, postmortem photographs were very common because exposure times were longer and a deceased person lay perfectly still.)

In most current birthing and delivery units, babies are photographed right after birth, memorabilia are collected, and memory books are made and given to mothers. From my research, I understand that many years after the experience, mothers' memories are filled with an acute attention to birth and death details, so memorabilia and attention given to mothers' feelings are very important in validating their experiences of grief and mourning. However, mothers' stories continue to reflect that more supportive, informed, and timely attention and understanding are needed in care.

In addition, women describe a continuing development of meaning(s) of loss that unfolds through the years of caring for their families and in attending and acknowledging the memories of the baby who died. Mothers describe the helpfulness of actively planning anniversary and family activities and in guiding their families in coping with loss.

Changes in Mortality Rates

Perinatal and infant mortality rates have diminished from a little over 9.8 per 1,000 at the time of my first research (Lauterbach, 1992) to a little over 5 per 1,000 for whites in northern Florida in 2005. However, for black and non-white mothers, the rate is three or more times the rate for whites in northern Florida. Often, silent phenomena are hidden within biostatistics used as health indicators in populations, which may not be easily viewed by the public or professional eye. The disparities among vulnerable populations increase the likelihood of silence surrounding health care focused on human phenomena such as infant mortality.

It is because of the disparities in white and nonwhite perinatal mortality rates in the rural southeast that my next investigation will explore meaning(s) in mothers' experience with infant death in the black community. I have initiated an exploration of creative literature and an existential investigation of cemetery and memorial art in the black community in the southeastern region of the United States. Of particular interest is the phenomenon depicted in black women's literature. Many excellent resources describe black women's experience with having a baby die.

Having moved back to the farm in northern Florida where I grew up, I have an increased awareness of the silence surrounding the phenomenon of infant death in the rural, Southern community, and particularly in the black community. This heightened awareness reflects a continuing immersion in the human phenomenon under investigation. Over time, this allows me to see what is not readily visible to those without the same personal perspective and experience.

Immersion in the Creative and Memorial Arts and Literature

The creative arts and literature in phenomenological investigations are examples of human lived experience and, as such, are very revealing. As representations of human lived experience with the phenomenon, the mourning and memorial arts can be particularly informative. Creative literature as exists in poetry, short stories, and novels often deals with the experience of infant death. Robert Frost (Untermeyer, 1964) states, "All an artist needs is samples. Without telling all he [sic] suggests all" (p. 31).

For example, Herbert Mason's (1970) verse narrative *Gilgamesh*, discovered during my first existential investigation (Lauterbach, 1992) of creative literature, speaks of a silence surrounding death in general. Additionally, personal experience of the phenomenon for the artist, author, or researcher provides an up close and personal view of the phenomenon that informs. Having experienced as a child the death of his father, Mason's (1997) poem "The Memory of Death" is reflective of his experience:

> It could go on for years and years,
> And has, for centuries
> For being human holds a special grief
> Of privacy within the universe
> That yearns and waits to be retouched
> By someone who can take away
> The memory of Death. (p. 37)

The following quote from *Gilgamesh* (Mason, 1970) is evocative of mothers' lived experience with having a baby die. Mothers also described a much longer period of acute grief than is ordinarily expected with death.

> . . . All that is left to one who grieves
> Is convalescence. . . .
> Few enter without tasting loss
> In which one spends a long time waiting
> For something to move one to proceed. (pp. 53–54)

The following poem titled "Mother's Day" and written by a participant mother (Lauterbach, 1992) describes a mother's lived experience with having her baby die in late pregnancy:

On Sunday I was a mother for a little while.
With one final push the baby was out. . . .
Now I am a mother no longer, left only with a
brief moment, and an emptiness where I had
felt full before. (p. 63)

Robert Frost's poem "Home Burial" (Untermeyer, 1964) describes gender and role differences in the human experience of infant death—among men and women as fathers and mothers.

. . . . God, what a woman! And it's come to this,
A man can't speak of his own child that's dead.

You can't because you don't know how to
speak. If you had any feeling, you that dug
With your own hand—how could you?—his
little grave; . . . (p. 68)

Exploring Mourning and Memorial Art and Photography

Since first exploring poetry and literature, I have continued to pay attention to the examples of the phenomenon as it exists in the real human lived world as well as in literature. Interestingly, from the first decision to focus my doctoral research on the phenomenon, I began to see many human examples of the phenomenon in the world, especially in the mourning art, graves, and cemetery investigation.

At the time of the original research, I passed a cemetery on the way to work for many years without really seeing what was revealed once the research began. There were big differences in how infants and adults were buried and memorialized. Even though postmortem photographs of adults and funeral scenes were common in the mid- to late 1800s, they are very uncommon today. Additionally, there are very few postmortem photographs of infants, and I discovered no funeral scenes that depicted a family surrounding a baby in the casket. However, funeral scenes were very common for adults. The only funeral photographs of infants I found depicted the mother and baby, or the parents with the deceased baby in a casket. This directly speaks to the silence surrounding the phenomenon of infant death in the larger social world.

Immersion in Black Cemetery and Memorial Art

In the decision to investigate infant death in the black community, my cemetery walk-about has revealed many differences in how black and white populations memorialize babies who die. In the first cemetery I visited, my son and I were overcome with a feeling of profound sadness. Only one baby grave was visible in the whole cemetery. It was very revealing that economic contexts surround memorials, cemetery art, and burial rituals and practices. I found this to be true in previous cemetery investigations. In the first cemetery walk-about, in the beginning existential investigation of black cemeteries, I question racial, ethnic, and cultural contexts surrounding infant death.

To address the phenomenon in the black population, the inquiry will focus on black mothers' experience and meanings surrounding infant death. It will also look at the phenomenon and meanings surrounding infant death in the black community. Other contexts of this population, such as cultural, spiritual, and relational, are perhaps involved in the community coping with infant death. An exploration of black women's creative literature has begun. These texts are rich in descriptions of black mothers' experience with infant death and provide narratives and stories of lived experience with infant loss and death of children. Several texts (Naylor, 1980, 1993; Morrison, 1970, 1974, 1987) have been identified and will be included in the existential investigation of black mothers' lived experience with infant death. The immersion in creative art and literature and memorial art will be concurrently explored along with the existential investigation of mothers' experience.

LINGUISTIC TRANSFORMATION: MOTHERS' EXPERIENCE WITH DEATH OF A WISHED-FOR BABY

Introduction to Linguistic Transformation

The following narrative, which van Manen and Munhall refer to as a linguistic transformation, is written as a description of mothers' lived experience with having a baby die. This is the final process in explicating the phenomenology, the meanings surrounding a particular human lived experience. The purpose is to capture in a narrative example the essence of the phenomenon under investigation. I have also written about my own experience in Munhall's (1994) text, *In Women's Experience*. However, the following is a linguistic transformation integrating findings from all of my investigations into the phenomenon of perinatal loss.

The Linguistic Transformation Narrative

"With one final push the baby was out." There was a busyness and silence in the delivery room, which was very unusual for birth. There were no pictures, no congratulations, no putting the baby on the mother's chest, no nursing the newborn baby. There was no cry of the newborn, the usual music of birth. The baby was whisked away without a word except, "fetal demise . . . cord around the neck." There was quiet where there was usually exhilaration and joy. There was an uneasy stillness in the room that was deadening. The whole room was a quiet refuge for this birth. The baby was stillborn. Mary and Joe were holding on to each other, embracing and crying. They were finally relieved that the ordeal of birth and death was over. They had been consumed with agonizing grief and suffering since they first knew something was wrong, and since they finally "found out." It was finally over. Mary kept feeling for the baby in her abdomen. For several days, she would forget at times that she had delivered the baby. She could not take a full deep breath. There was a painful feeling of emptiness in her abdomen that had felt full before.

A couple of weeks earlier, when at a routine prenatal visit at the 36th week, during a check for the fetal heartbeat, it was absent. Mary had worried about the diminished activity of her baby, but had just assumed that it was due to the uterine crowding babies experience in late pregnancy. It was nothing out of the ordinary, she thought. The baby was a big baby, already about 7½ pounds. That was it . . . just a very big baby boy. But, when an ultrasound confirmed the fate, life seemed to stand still . . . as if coming to an end. In the next few days, Mary and Joe both felt as if they would die. Mary experienced the physical ache in her body, her full breasts, and in her empty, heavy arms.

Mary and Joe spent the next few hours after the prenatal visit in agonizing grief, alternating between "Maybe they are wrong," to "Oh, God. . . . Our baby is dead." They alternated between disbelief and reality. They went home, and Joe went back to work. Mary went to bed, completely exhausted. She was unable to sleep, but she lay in a sort of subconscious state. By the time Joe came home, she was in real agony. She found that lying in bed, moaning and crying loudly, and falling down on her knees onto the floor as she walked across the floor, were of some comfort. Joe was a little late coming home from work and the house was dark when he arrived. He came into the dark house with fear and anxiety about Mary. He found her in bed, still in her clothes from the morning doctor's visit.

The decision was to wait until labor began to deliver the baby. At least that way, they could give the baby every opportunity to prove everyone wrong.

And, if true, it would give them the chance to get ready, to prepare for death. By the time the baby was ready to come, Mary was ready. Mary had yelled, fallen down, cried, and fallen into sleep as much and often as she felt the urge. But Joe had continued to try to keep some normality in his schedule, so he went to work each day. He was unable to really cry and thought he had to be strong for his wife. Mary was relieved that she had the privacy she needed, which she continued to need and have in the many months to come.

Mary was still very full and pregnant, though the baby seemed more like a weight. She no longer felt pregnant, just heavy. The baby had dropped, and walking was harder. She caressed her baby son with smooth strokes, often talking to him, comfortingly. With time she realized the worst: her baby boy had not survived the nearly perfect pregnancy.

The family called but did not come over. Mary's sister said, "It is better for something bad to happen now, rather than later. There must have been a genetic defect." Mary could hear her sister's children in the background. Mary's sister invited Mary and Joe over to a 4th of July cookout, with many friends, "to take your minds off of it." Mary and Joe decided to go, but no one even mentioned what they were going through. Still very full and heavy, it was a surreal experience ... pregnant, but no mention. The children splashed in the baby pool and had a great time. The visit made Mary and Joe feel isolated and alone. Joe was able to carry on conversation with the men, who focused on the upcoming football season. Mary and Joe left early and went home.

When they got home, Mary went to bed and Joe watched television while consuming a whole bottle of wine. He fell asleep on the couch with the TV on and awoke at 2:00 A.M. feeling the effects of the alcohol. He got up and got water, and went to bed, trying not to wake Mary. He was unable to sleep and finally got up at 4:30. He was quite lost without work and at that early hour. For the first time, he cried, quietly, but was careful not to wake Mary. He did not know how he could get through the next few weeks. Joe was relieved when it was time for him to get ready for work and Mary was still in bed. He was a little hung over, but he had something to do away from the house.

In the time between learning that the baby did not have a heartbeat and the baby's birth, Mary did the calculations. She figured that she could be delivering another baby, her second, in a little over 40 weeks. She calculated the new delivery date and counted back for the implantation date. They would have to get busy. At the same time she carried her deceased baby in her womb, she began to look to the future. She would be a mother in a year, at least. Joe was less than enthusiastic when she shared her plan. "Let's do one thing at a time," Joe said.

Almost 2 weeks after the ultrasound, Mary was awakened in the middle of the night with the rupture of her membranes. She turned over in bed and felt the warm rush of fluid. She awakened Joe and they silently went to the hospital. The bag packed much earlier had several changes of clothes for Mary and several outfits for her son. She unpacked the extra items and took only one baby outfit and a blanket for the baby. She did not take a change of clothes for herself. Still, there was a flicker of excitement and anticipation of birth . . . and then the harsh reminder . . . the baby was dead.

Upon arrival at the hospital, Mary was quickly moved to a labor room away from the others. The nurses were absent except for taking the necessary vital signs. Joe and Mary were visited infrequently by the nurses. When labor progressed and Mary became very uncomfortable, Joe had to go get help. She was moved to the delivery room. And she thought about anesthesia, but decided against it. She and Joe had practiced and had wanted a natural delivery. The staff was a skeleton staff for this delivery. Labor quickly seemed like real work to Mary. Joe was not sure of what to do. They had used breathing techniques to prepare for delivery, but they seemed to forget about them. It was hard to use the techniques they had learned for delivering a live baby.

The silence in the delivery room was leaden. Finally, it was over. The baby was whisked away. It was a relief for Mary to go back to her room. Joe hugged her and said he would come by right after work. Mary was in her room, had not seen the baby, and had not had a nurse's visit since the delivery. She thought that she must have been given something because she could not even lift her arms. The nurse did not come in for almost 3 hours. The nurse's first question was, "Do you want an early discharge?" Mary was shocked. She had had no postpartum care, had not seen the baby, and was treated as if, because her baby had died, she did not need care. She asked to be helped to the shower so she could get cleaned up. She asked if she had been given something because she was still having difficulty raising her arms. She was informed she had not been given anesthesia.

After helping her to the shower, the nurse left. Finally, after Mary made it back to her bed, still feeling groggy, slow, and like lead, she rang the bell. A nurse arrived and Mary asked to see the baby. "Well, I'm not sure. They may be doing tests. I'll have to check." It was more than an hour before another nurse arrived. She had not been told about the baby's death, and she asked if Mary had nursed the baby. The nurse looked completely shocked when Mary informed her of the outcome. Again, Mary asked to see her baby. The nurse left the room hurriedly. Over half an hour passed before anyone came in. Then it was lunchtime and her tray was brought in. The person said, "What? No baby? Most of our mothers have rooming in." Mary said, rather sharply, "Well, maybe their babies are alive. My baby died." The person apologized and left.

When Joe arrived, Mary had still not gotten to see the baby. She appealed to him to go find out what the problem was. He came back with, "The baby is in the morgue. We have to select a funeral home." By now, Mary was becoming mobilized. She got out of bed and walked rather deliberately, not quietly, to the nurses' station. She asked to see the nurse. The nurse told that if she wanted to see the baby, she would have to go to the morgue. Mary asked why no one had come back to tell her, why she was asked about early discharge, and then not allowed to see the baby. The nurse said that they assumed that because she did not answer the question earlier about early discharge that she did not want it. Mary then stated that she wanted to be discharged, "Now." She went back to her room, quickly packed, and she and Joe stopped at the morgue on the way out.

Mary felt as if for the first time since delivery she had some energy and was feeling propelled into action. Because she was being discharged, she had to ride in a wheelchair accompanied by a nurse. The look at the baby was just that. She was not allowed to hold him, but she did manage to caress him gently as she had done while he was still inside.

When they got home, both Mary and Joe were exhausted. They ate some canned soup and went to bed embracing. They slept soundly, and occasionally, Mary roused with a heavy, groggy feeling like the one she had after the delivery. She also had a physical sensation that she was still pregnant. Her hand moved over her abdomen and discovered the reality of the flattened soft abdomen. How could she forget? She was heartsick, feeling very disappointed when her hand reminded her that her baby had been stillborn. This physical sensation continued for more than a month.

Upon awaking the morning after coming home from the hospital, Joe and Mary cried in each other's arms and finally stumbled out of bed. They made coffee and Joe got ready for work. Mary went back to bed when he left and stayed there until right before he got home. The kitchen was left as it had been in the 2 weeks before the delivery—the sink full of dishes, and the dishwasher filled with clean dishes.

It was many months before this scene changed. Mary spent a lot of time in bed . . . and each weekday Joe went to work. Weekends were most difficult. When Mary's milk came in, she was at a loss in knowing what to do. She developed a breast infection. This required a trip to the doctor. Her postpartum visits were painfully empty without her baby. Just about the time Mary thought she could go out in public to shop, or go to the bank, she would be overwhelmed by the prospect. She went to the mailbox, carefully avoiding the times when schoolchildren were coming home.

Mary declined invitations to go to her sister's house. The children were always audible in the background. Mary's mother was concerned that she "was not getting over it." They had not had a funeral but had cremated the baby. They had not been able to pick the ashes up from the funeral home. Finally, Joe picked them up and put the urn in the garage, not telling Mary, not wanting to disturb her. Mary continued to sneak out of the house and to the post office and bank at times when she did not run the risk of running into someone.

Finally, after 5 or 6 months, Joe and Mary resumed occasional sexual activity. Mary was not using contraception, and Joe did not bring it up. He figured that it could not hurt at that time. Mary kept hoping and looking for signs that she was pregnant. It was around 11 months after the first baby died that Mary missed her period. Immediately, she felt sadness, then euphoria. This roller-coaster emotional experience was over quickly. She was thrilled in a few weeks to find that she was pregnant again. She would be a mother! Joe was more reluctant to be having a baby, but after getting used to the idea a little, he became fully involved and thrilled. Together they went to the first prenatal visits.

After a little more anxiety about the pregnancy outcome, Mary and Joe became very involved with planning and anticipating the arrival of the new baby. Mary's family advised her not to get too committed to the idea. Joe was not so sure about how to proceed, but once the pregnancy was confirmed, it was hard to contain excitement. With each pregnancy milestone, such as the end of the first trimester, the first fetal movement, and when the ultrasound was done, Mary and Joe both revisited the earlier pregnancy and its loss.

Mary was very aware of her body sensations as the pregnancy progressed. As she became more involved with this baby, and as she got closer to delivery, she felt a powerful loss and sadness all over again. "I'm really the mother of two babies," she thought. But, then she returned to the joy and excitement of having a new baby. She and Joe named the baby as soon as they learned that it was another boy. This baby would have Joe's name and Joe's father's and would be called Joe Mack. Mary had always regretted that they had not named the first baby. She always thought about him as "my baby boy."

With the approaching delivery, her family warned her not to get too excited or to get the baby's room ready too soon. Mary simply could not help it. She was involved with the arrival of their second son and becoming more and more excited as time passed and as delivery got closer. She changed some of the baby items and rearranged the baby furniture, but she mostly planned to use the items selected for her first baby. This made her feel a connection . . . her preparation for her first baby was being used for this baby.

Only occasionally did Mary even think that something might go wrong. She already felt as if she had experienced being a mother. In fact, the more attached and involved she became with the new baby, the more she missed and felt connected with the first baby. She was indeed a mother. She had even talked to her first baby after he died. Now, she talked to the new baby and told him quietly about his older brother. She said that when she got very old, they would all be together again. This made the reality of her first baby's death one day, in spite of the loss, seemingly not so bad.

Mary continued to remember and periodically relive the loss of her first baby throughout all three of her subsequent pregnancies. She and Joe ultimately had three living children, two sons, and a daughter. She often spoke to her children of her son who had died shortly before being born. Over the years, she referred to herself as having "three living children." She described that caring for and dealing with her first baby's death had taken almost as much energy as caring for her living children.

Six years after the first baby, when she had three young children, Mary and Joe buried the first baby's ashes in a grave in the family plot in the cemetery. The children visited the baby's grave with her often and asked many questions. The second child said one day, "If he had not died, you would not have me." Mary agreed and noted that this made him very special. Her 6-year-old son, Joe Mack, smiled a big smile.

Over the years, Mary continued to remember the son who died and visited the grave regularly, but especially around the anniversary of the baby's birthday. She also continued to talk to him as if he were listening from the grave. She caressed and hugged the headstone that she and Joe had finally put there. She would quietly tell him about his siblings, how they were doing, and what each was like. She always said how much she had "missed" his living presence, but that he had been there is spirit "with" her and the rest of the family. She also shared that she was so grateful. He was the child who had helped her learn to become a mother, and she had taken care of her living children in the way she had because of him.

When Mary was in her late 80s and Joe had died a few years earlier, she thought comfortingly that she would join her baby and Joe in heaven. Her "baby boy" had died almost 70 years earlier, and her two other sons and daughter, with families of their own, were now grandparents. A granddaughter had experienced two pregnancy losses. The whole family had rallied around the young family and had provided much help and support during the acute grief and in the painful exacerbations at nodal events in the family. They were very involved in actively dealing, discussing, and coping with the family experience of grief. In guiding her own young children and family in dealing with the death of a sibling, Mary and others were able to be active supports to the granddaughter and her husband. They had been guided by Mary and Joe about how to deal with and support a family in times of loss.

Mourning and grief over the loss of a baby are family experiences. As Mary approached her ninth decade, she thought, "It has been a lifetime, but it has gone so quickly." She often found herself thinking about her life lately. It had been a wonderful life, but not without its share of pain. When her baby son had died, she thought she would never live again. It felt as if a part of her died at that time, too. Then she remembered how she and Joe had clung to each other for those first months. He had continued to work. She stayed in bed as much as she wanted. He brought home "take-out" meals, and often they sat in bed eating. In that small way, they had held each other, cried, and gradually had begun to heal.

One day Mary found herself smiling as she began thinking that she and Joe would be with their four children, including her baby boy, and all of the grandchildren again. Having Joe die was not as sad as she had thought it would be because of the idea that he was with their baby son. She was amazed at that . . . the comfort from losing her best friend and husband was that he finally was reunited with their son. The granddaughter's baby was already with Mary's baby son and Joe. It was comforting that one day they would be together, forever.

BRIEF SUMMARY, INSIGHTS, AND INTERPRETATIONS

Mothers who experience death of a baby in late pregnancy or shortly after birth find themselves abandoned by the infant and by the private, intimate and larger social world following the death. The experience is described as an existential experience of being-a-mother in another world. The experience of having a baby die is an experience of temporality in that it is timeless and continues forever.

Grief and loss are felt bodily experiences, which are interpreted as representing the existential experience of embodiment, where loss has physical, bodily manifestations. Mothers' arms ache, they have trouble breathing, and just by closing her eyes the mother often feels pregnant again in the first few months after the death. The active experience of loss and grief continues for a very long time, often years. Over time, the acute exacerbations diminish but can still be very intense during anniversary or other life experience reminders. The experience of grief and mourning over time is an experience of connections and relatedness, which are intimately bound within multiple, recurring, and changing social, relational, and economic contexts of mothers' lives.

Over time, as a result of mothers' thoughtful, reflective attention, there is a development and discovery of new meanings in the experience of having a baby die. The original loss of the particular baby is intimately assimilated and embedded over time into mothers' subsequent lived experience in work and family life. Meanings continue to evolve throughout mothers' lives and are intimately connected to the experience of being a mother to other children.

Ultimately, as mothers anticipate and come closer to their own mortality, they experience a renewed reliving of previously lived birth and death experiences, particularly when a baby had died. There is, at the end of life, a convergence of meanings in the lived experience resulting in mothers' expectation and anticipation of the reunion with the baby. The mother anticipates rejoining the baby, living with and being a mother in another timeless, seamless world where she will be reunited with the child and her whole larger family forever.

CRITIQUE AND CONTINUING QUESTIONS

Note that this research seems to speak to a universal mothering experience of having a baby die, however, findings in each inquiry can speak only for the particular participants and particular babies involved. The three inquiries sought homogeneous samples of participant mothers, where detailed material relating to the human experience was generated through in-depth discussions and interviews. Examples of the phenomenon were sought in the creative arts, literature, and memorial art in cemeteries. However, findings relate only to those participating in the particular inquiry.

I chose to conduct multiple inquiries with smaller sample sizes (fewer participants) to generate full descriptions of experience. This chapter integrates and interprets findings from three separate inquiries, so remember that care must be taken not to overinterpret meanings related to the phenomenon. At the same time, I discovered that the description of mothers' lived experience and the meanings embedded in the experience seem to speak authoritatively to the human experience of the phenomenon under investigation.

In the upcoming fourth inquiry, I expect that findings will be similar, but also different from the results of previous inquiries. This inquiry will begin with conversations with and interviews of black mothers, and it will also look at meanings of infant death in the black community. An ethnographic perspective will be integrated with a phenomenological perspective. This fourth inquiry represents a methodological shift. It will look at black mothers' experience and will use the creative arts, literature, memorial arts, and cemetery art in the existential investigation. Additionally, the inquiry will use phenomenology literature and black literature for interpretive analysis. It will seek to uncover hidden as well as explicit meanings surrounding infant death in the black community in mothers' voices.

Response at the Time of This Writing

As I finish this chapter, the devastation of the Gulf coastal region and New Orleans as a result of Hurricane Katrina is on my mind. For the past week, and especially this weekend after Katrina hit, I have written and have gone back and forth from the television to the computer so that I could see and hear the stories of victims and refugees and the explanations of officials. I have been appalled and find the response to this anticipated disaster to be too late, too little, and often without compassion and understanding. However, as time is passing, there appears to be more understanding of the plight of the thousands of people who were unable to evacuate the city. Much like a phenomenological investigation, the visual images and stories of people suffering, of the poverty and vulnerability of people, facilitate human understanding.

The images and stories are hard to watch and hard to hear. To adequately address what is needed now, following the lack of preparedness and slow response, it is important for us to understand survivors' experience. Hopefully, as understanding is created, care and intentionality will be facilitated. As the people's plight is understood, hopefully change in our nation's preparedness and response is possible.

Similarly, inquiry into mothers' experience with infant death is a silent, hidden phenomenon. It is a difficult topic to discuss, difficult to hear, and it is often difficult for families and friends to "be with" those who have had the experience. Bringing it out of silence into public and private conversations and relationships, hopefully, will facilitate change and support systems to respond in an informed, timely, knowledgeable, caring, and supportive way.

REFERENCES

Becker, E. (1973). *The denial of death.* New York: Basic Books.

Campbell, J. (1988). *The power of myth.* New York: Doubleday Dell.

Eliot, T. (1936). *Collected Poems 1909–1962.* New York: Harcourt, Brace & World.

Heiddeger, M. (1962). *Being and time* (J. Macquarrie & E. Robinson, Trans.). New York: Harper & Row. (Original work published in 1927)

Husserl, E. (1952). *Ideas: General introduction to pure phenomenology* (W. Gibson, Trans.). New York: Macmillan.

Lauterbach, S. S. (1992). *In another world: A phenomenological perspective and discovery of meaning in mothers' experience of death of a wished-for baby.* Doctoral dissertation, Ann Arbor, MI: University Microfilms International.

Lauterbach, S. S. (1993). In another world: A phenomenological perspective and discovery of meaning in mothers' experience of death of a wished-for baby. In P. L. Munhall & C. Oiler-Boyd (Eds.), *Nursing research: A qualitative perspective* (pp. 133–179). New York: National League for Nursing Press.

Lauterbach, S. S. (1994). In another world: "Essences" of mothers' mourning experience. In P. L. Munhall (Ed.), *In women's experience* (pp. 233–293). New York: National League for Nursing Press.

Lauterbach, S. S. (2000). In another world: Five years later. In P. L. Munhall (Ed.), *Nursing research: A qualitative perspective* (pp. 185–208). Sudbury, MA: Jones and Bartlett.

Lauterbach, S. S. (2003). Phenomenological silence surrounding infant death. *International Journal of Human Caring, 7*(23), 38–43.

Mason, H. (1970). *Gilgamesh: A verse narrative.* New York: Houghton Mifflin.

Mason, H. (1997). The memory of death. In J. Y-Mason (Ed.), *The patient's voice: Experiences of illness* (p. 3). Philadelphia: Davis.

Morrison, T. (1970). *The bluest eye.* New York: Penguin Books.

Morrison, T. (1974). *Sula.* New York: Penguin Books.

Morrison, T. (1987). *Beloved.* New York: Penguin Books.

Munhall, P. L. & Oiler-Boyd, C. (1993). *Nursing research: A qualitative perspective* (2nd ed.). New York: National League for Nursing Press.

Munhall, P. L. (2001). *Nursing research: A qualitative perspective* (3rd ed.). Sudbury, MA: Jones and Bartlett Publishers.

Naylor, G. (1980). *The women of Brewster place.* New York: Penguin Books.

Naylor, G. (1993). *Mama day.* New York: Random House.

Untermeyer, L. (1964). *Robert Frost's poems.* New York: Washington Square Press in arrangement with Holt, Rinehart, & Winston. (Original work published in 1930)

van Manen, M. (1984). *Doing phenomenological research and writing.* Alberta, Canada: University of Alberta Press.

van Manen, M. (1990). *Researching lived experience.* London: University of Alberta Press.

van Manen, M. (1997). *Researching lived experience.* Ontario, Canada: Althouse Press.

8

Grounded Theory: The Method

Judith Wuest

GROUNDED THEORY

I became captivated by grounded theory as a graduate student. I was interested in family disruption when children have chronic middle ear disease, and I had been struggling throughout my course work to locate a theory suitable for guiding my thesis research. The most likely match seemed to be stress and coping theory with a specific focus on uncertainty, but I felt uneasy about framing family experience this way. Then, during the qualitative methods course taught by Phyllis Noerager Stern, I encountered grounded theory. Here, *at last*, was an approach that would permit studying the problem from the perspective of the families without force-fitting it into an existing framework. Additionally, the research process felt consistent with my community health background and my way of thinking. Although I began with trepidation a course assignment that required collecting and analyzing three interviews, I became so engaged that my fears vanished. Since then, each grounded theory project has afforded me opportunities to reflect on and reach new understandings of this versatile research approach and its usefulness for generating nursing knowledge.

Barney Glaser and Anselm Strauss in their 1967 text *The Discovery of Grounded Theory* presented grounded theory as a new approach to research developed in their study of dying. Grounded theory is a research approach that results in the development of middle range theory at a substantive or formal level (Glaser, 1978). This explicit goal of theory development makes grounded theory unique among qualitàtive methods. A grounded theory approach demands that the researcher move beyond description of the domain of study toward a theoretical rendering that identifies key explanatory concepts and the relationships among them. The challenge of theoretical analysis and theoretical writing is frequently daunting, especially to novice qualitative researchers. Grounded theory has been embraced by nurses since Glaser and Strauss introduced the method to graduate students at the University of California, San Francisco, in the early 1970s (Stern & Covan, 2001). Grounded theories are useful for directing nursing practice because they are explanatory theories of human behavior within social context. Nonetheless, nurses have found the sociological writing of Glaser and Strauss (Glaser, 1978; Glaser & Strauss, 1967; Strauss, 1987) unfamiliar and have written many articles and books to demystify the method and explicate its contribution to knowledge generation (Beck, 1999; Benoliel, 1996; Chenitz & Swanson, 1986; Hutchinson & Wilson, 2001; Schreiber & Stern, 2001; Stern, 1980; Stern & Pyles, 1986; Wuest, 1995, 1997a, 2000, 2001; Wuest, Berman, Ford-Gilboe, & Merritt-Gray, 2002; Wuest & Merritt-Gray, 2001).

Grounded theory has evolved since its introduction almost 40 years ago. The classic texts (Glaser, 1978; Glaser & Strauss, 1967; Strauss, 1987) continue to provide the best overview. Strauss's approach to grounded theory altered over time, and this shift was captured in his books written with Corbin (Strauss & Corbin, 1990, 1998). Glaser (1992) took exception to Strauss and Corbin's more prescriptive approach to analysis.[1] However, Glaser's more recent writings demonstrate his own evolution (Glaser, 1998, 1999, 2002, 2004). Such shifts in thinking, I believe, are to be expected as any method is used over time within a changing social context. Researchers, therefore, are obligated to disclose their own orientation to the method. In the 1990s, when the differences between the two originators of the method were being disclosed, this was achieved by identifying one's grounded theory approach as Straussian or Glaserian. However, such identification is insufficient in light of the continued evolution of each of those traditions (Glaser, 1998, 1999, 2002, 2004; Strauss & Corbin, 1998).

My own approach to grounded theory is rooted in the earlier writings. Phyllis Noerager Stern, a student of Glaser, supervised my master's research

---

[1]For an excellent comparison of the approaches of Strauss and Corbin (1990) and Glaser (1992), see MacDonald (2001, pp. 138–153).

and, as a mentor and colleague, continues to support my development as a grounded theorist. Marsha Cohen, a student of Strauss, supervised my doctoral work and challenged me to consider critically how my approach fits with the shifting traditions of grounded theory. I have argued elsewhere for the utility of combining feminist theory with grounded theory (Wuest, 1995) and have also wrestled with a more critical participatory approach to the method (Wuest et al., 2002). Thus, my way of doing grounded theory has evolved but remains close to the early work; the text that continues to be most useful to me is *Theoretical Sensitivity* (Glaser, 1978).

In this chapter, my goal is not just to provide an overview of the grounded theory method and its theoretical underpinnings, but also to discuss strategies for handling some of the more common challenges faced by researchers in moving beyond description to theoretical analysis. My intent is not to be prescriptive, because each of us finds our own path to theoretical thinking, but rather to offer some tools that may or may not work for any single researcher. I suggest guidelines to assist novice grounded theorists in evaluating emerging theory. Finally, I will briefly discuss the evolution of grounded theory and its paradigm location.

PHILOSOPHICAL UNDERPINNINGS OF GROUNDED THEORY

Although other researchers have discussed symbolic interactionism as the basic underpinning of grounded theory (Chenitz & Swanson, 1986; Crooks, 2001; Hutchinson & Wilson, 2001; Milliken & Schreiber, 2001), Glaser and Strauss (1967) wrote comparatively little. Strauss (1987) briefly addresses the philosophical traditions that informed the development of grounded theory, noting the influence of pragmatism and the Chicago School of Sociology. He delineates the underlying assumptions: (1) change is a feature of social life that needs to be accounted for through attention to social interaction and social process; and (2) interaction, process, and social change are best understood by grasping the actor's viewpoint. Glaser, in his 1992 writing, explicitly states that an assumption of grounded theory is that people actively shape the worlds they live in through the process of symbolic interaction and that life is characterized by variability, complexity, change, and process. These assertions by the founders of grounded theory suggest that two key underpinnings are symbolic interactionism and pragmatism. More recently, Glaser (1998, 2004) argues that symbolic interactionism is not inherent in grounded theory His critique is not of symbolic interactionism as a philosophical orientation underlying the method, but rather of symbolic interactionism as a dominant theoretical code to guide analysis. I agree that data are not analyzed through the theoretical code of symbolic interactionism. But my understanding of grounded theory suggests that symbolic interactionism and pragmatism inform the underlying assumptions of the method.

Symbolic Interactionism

Blumer (1969) identifies three assumptions of symbolic interactionism: (1) people act toward things and people on the basis of meanings they have for them, (2) meanings stem from interaction with others, and (3) people's meanings are modified through an interpretive process used to make sense of and manage their social worlds. Snow (2001) expands these tenets, reframing the principles of symbolic interactionism as *interactive determination, symbolization, emergence,* and *human agency. Interactive determination* suggests that phenomena exist only in relation to each other and can be understood only by considering interactions and interactional contexts. Because interactions are problematic, they are worthy of observation and analysis. *Symbolization* refers to the process of ascribing meaning to things, people, events, and so on such that they elicit particular feelings and actions. Such meanings become "embedded in and reflective of existing cultural and organizational contexts" (p. 371). Snow asserts that the question then is not how people act in terms of the meanings they ascribe but rather (1) how do meanings become taken for granted or routinized; (2) what contexts, relationships, or structures support such acceptance; and finally (3) are those embedded meanings as a basis for action problematic?

Such questioning leads to *emergence* as a principle (Snow, 2001). By focusing on what is going on in particular social contexts, symbolic interactionism allows for the identification of social, emotional, or cognitive change as it emerges. The final principle of *human agency* refers to the "active, wilful nature of human actors" (p. 373). Social actors make choices or decisions about their actions while taking into account the social or cultural constraints or expectations. Snow argues that the influence of these constraints is often unacknowledged until a disruption makes them visible. At that point, *human agency* drives people toward some sort of corrective action.

Pragmatism

Pragmatism refers to theoretical perspectives that emphasize the practical, giving primacy to usefulness over theoretical knowledge; as such, the goal is transformative (Seigfried, 1998). From a pragmatist perspective, truth cannot be arrived at through deductive reasoning from a priori theory but rather must be developed inductively with constant empirical verification. Truth is modified in light of new discoveries and is relative to time and place. "Pragmatic reflection begins with experience as an interactive process involving individuals and their social and natural environment" (p. 51). Knowledge development is not value free and is historically contextualized. Situated perspectives of the marginalized are seen as more legitimate because they know the limits of the dominant interpretation of reality better than others, but even these perspectives must be reflectively validated. Differences in perspectives are valued and provide a basis for reciprocal problem solving, drawing on existing knowledge and resources, and ongoing revisions of understanding. Under pragmatism the goals of inquiry are judged in terms of their usefulness for making change, and thus values are an inherent part of pragmatism.

Summary

Symbolic interactionism directs grounded theorists to assume that meaning is made and constantly changed through interaction and becomes embedded in social context. Both meaning and social context influence the ways that human agency is enacted. Pragmatism supports seeking revised understandings for the purpose of making useful change through inductive exploration of diverse situated human experience with reflexive confirmation and use of applicable existing knowledge. Thus, pragmatism and symbolic interactionism are the source of foundational assumptions of grounded theory.

GROUNDED THEORY APPROACH

"The goal of grounded theory is to generate a theory that accounts for a pattern of behavior which is relevant and problematic for those involved" (Glaser, 1978, p. 93). Data analysis occurs concurrently with data collection, and the specific research focus or problem emerges as the analysis proceeds. Data analysis involves coding data on a line-by-line basis, asking, "What is this a conceptual indicator of?" and constant comparison of various indicators for similarities and differences. Informal hypotheses and concepts are derived inductively from the data, but then deductively checked out and modified as new data are collected so that evolving concepts fit the collected data. Throughout the analysis process, memos are written to capture emerging ideas about concepts and their relationships.

Sources of data are selected for what they can contribute to the emerging theory and may include formal or informal interviews, field observation, or written data. This process of collecting data to develop the hypotheses and further identify properties and relationships among concepts is called theoretical sampling (Glaser & Strauss, 1967). The emerging theory is further integrated by theoretical coding, a process of examining the data in theoretical rather than descriptive terms. Diagramming relationships among concepts increases the level of abstraction. As data collection and analysis proceed, a core category that explains most of the variation in the behavior pattern is identified (Glaser, 1978). Core categories may be basic social processes if they have at least two stages that "differentiate and account for variation in the problematic pattern of behavior" (Glaser, 1978, p. 97). Once the core variable is identified, extant theory and literature are theoretically sampled for what they can contribute to the developing theory. The final grounded theory report is generally written as a theoretical discussion (Glaser & Strauss, 1967). An important characteristic of grounded theories is their modifiability as new data are generated. Grounded theories may be constantly recast to reflect new variations.

When Is Grounded Theory an Appropriate Approach?

Because a grounded theory captures social process in social context, the grounded theory research approach is most useful when the goal is a framework or theory that explains human behavior in context (Glaser & Strauss, 1967; Glaser, 1978). Thus, human behavior related to health issues, developmental transitions, and situational challenges is well suited to grounded theory research in nursing.

Grounded theory is particularly useful when little is known about the area to be studied, or when what is known is from a theoretical perspective that does not satisfactorily explain what is going on. For example, I carried out a study of women's caring/caregiving using grounded theory because the conceptual understandings of caring (burden and stress [Farran & Keane-Hagerty, 1991; Given & Given, 1991] or fulfillment, satisfaction, and life enhancement [Bevis, 1988; Ray, 1981/1988; Roach, 1992]) that guided this large body of research were conflicting and failed to account for clinical observations of women caring for family members.

The Research Question

Unlike other research methods, the starting point in grounded theory is not a focused research question, but rather exploration of a domain of human behavior. Symbolic interactionism informs the underlying assumption that people in the domain under study share a common social psychological problem, of which they are normally unaware at a conscious level. The researcher will construct both the problem and the way it is processed through inductive and deductive analysis of data.

Thus, rather than a list of research questions or hypotheses, the researcher begins with a statement of purpose, such as "The purpose of this study is to develop a substantive theory of family behavior when a child has chronic middle ear disease (OME)." Because of the constraints of funding agencies and the requirements of graduate programs, researchers may be forced to articulate more specific objectives or research questions. The key challenge here is doing so without making assumptions about what will be most problematic for people in the study domain and without using theory-laden language. The problem that emerges during data collection and analysis may not be what the researcher had anticipated. I had a hunch from my practice that the key problem for families whose children had chronic OME would be related to speech development. The problem that emerged from the data was the family's relationship with the health care system (Wuest & Stern, 1990). Theory-laden language in the statement of purpose or objectives may also derail a study. Had I written my purpose as "to discover how families *cope* with children with chronic OME," I would have situated the study in a well-established body of theoretical knowledge (stress and coping theory). Avoiding language that may link the study to dominant extant theory at the outset is important.

A common way of framing the grounded theory study focus is in terms of finding a *particular* process. This can be problematic because one does not know which process will be discovered. For example, if in my study of women's caring, I had stated that the study goal was "to discover the process of caring/caregiving for family members," readers would have expected an explanatory theory of how women care for family members. Rather, I stated my study focus as the "domain of women's caring." The resultant theory of *precarious ordering* (Wuest, 1997a, 1997b, 2001) did not capture the process of caring, but rather the process of addressing the negative health consequences that stemmed from the problem of competing and changing caring demands. Although this may seem a subtle difference, it is noteworthy. A challenge for novice grounded theorists is distinguishing the situational trajectory of the domain of study from the basic social problem/process. For example, in a study of women having myocardial infarctions (MI), initially the problem might be seen as the MI, and the situational trajectory is *having symptoms, seeking treatment, being treated,* and *recovering.* This sort of trajectory will always be in data, and may be a condition or context, but it is usually *not* the social-psychological problem/ process being sought.

Review of the Literature

The review of the literature is a frequent source of contention in grounded theory studies. According to Glaser (1992), the literature is reviewed after the core variable is generated. The rationale for not conducting an extensive literature review earlier is to avoid beginning the study with preconceived ideas. Stern and Covan (2001) recall that their doctoral dissertation proposals were 10 and 5 pages, respectively, a far cry from the lengthy literature reviews expected today. From my perspective, an initial literature review is necessary in grounded theory research to justify to the thesis committee or research funding agency that a grounded theory study is needed. Additionally, knowledge of what is known in the domain under study enables the researcher to understand how the generated theory is similar to or different from what is known (Morse & Richards, 2002). Through a literature review, the researcher demonstrates a broad grasp of the strengths and limitations of the theoretical and empirical knowledge in the domain under study. If little is known, the literature review is fairly straightforward. On the other hand, if the broad domain has been well studied, a case must be developed for why existing theoretical perspectives are inadequate and why a grounded theory approach is needed. Thus, dominant theories are critiqued for their limitations. Empirical research is reviewed broadly and organized by concepts to highlight the complexity of the domain of study. A detailed critique of individual studies as normally required to provide the groundwork for a theory-testing study is unnecessary. The literature review is completed with a summary in which an argument for the proposed study is made. By summarizing the inadequacies or absence of theoretical frameworks to explain what is going on in the proposed area of study, the researcher builds a case for a grounded theory study. Once the data are collected and the core variable identified, the researcher then theoretically samples the literature relevant to the emerging theory. Most frequently, this involves seeking new bodies of literature previously not explored.

Regardless of how the literature review for the proposal is handled, critique is likely. If a scant literature review is carried out, reviewers may say the researcher has failed to demonstrate knowledge of the field or justification for the research. If a thorough literature review is carried out, reviewers more familiar with the grounded theory approach may argue that such a review violates a basic premise of grounded theory and biases the researcher. Be prepared to defend this assertion. Two foundational elements of grounded theory, *constant comparison* and *theoretical sensitivity,* may inform the counterargument. A key element of the analysis is *constant comparison.* Data are analyzed through coding, that is, breaking the data into bits (phrases, sentences, or paragraphs) that are judged to be indicators of a code, inductively named from the data. Each data bit is compared to each other data bit that is an indicator of the same code for similarities and differences and for what theoretical property of the code it suggests. In this way, a full range of properties of the code is developed, and the name given to the code evolves to fit those properties. One source of data is literature, which is compared in the same way. As long as the principle of *constant comparison* is respected and the codes evolve to fit all data, knowledge from extant theory will not dominate, and the emerging theory will be grounded in the data. Thus, exploration of the literature in advance will not derail the research process, and the phenomenological strategy of *bracketing* is not necessary (Wuest, 2000).

Knowledge of theoretical literature also has relevance for a researcher's *theoretical sensitivity*. "The root of all significant theorizing is the sensitive insights of the observer" (Glaser & Strauss, 1967, p. 251). Theoretical sensitivity refers to an individual's ability to "render theoretically their discovered substantive, grounded categories" (Glaser, 1978, p. 1). Thus, theoretical sensitivity is the researcher's personal capacity to have theoretical insights related to the conceptualization of data and the relationships between concepts based on personal experiences, vicarious experiences, and knowledge of theoretical constructions in many disciplines (Glaser, 1978). Some of this capacity comes from researchers' knowledge of their own disciplinary theories. However, understanding theoretical literature in other fields is also useful for expanding insights regarding what is theoretically possible. Thus, Glaser (1978) advocates reading widely outside the substantive area under study to increase familiarity with theoretical codes. "Theoretical codes are conceptual models of relationships that are discovered to relate the substantive codes to each theoretically" (Glaser, 1992, p. 27). Let me be clear that this does not mean that one takes an extant theoretical framework and uses it to name and organize concepts. Rather, the theoretical codes gleaned from disciplinary knowledge, reading widely, or from using Glaser's (1978) coding families are templates that help the researcher to recognize theoretical properties and relationships among categories. Glaser's coding family, the 6 Cs, commonly sensitizes researchers to the way codes may be related as cause and consequence. Knowledge of feminist theory means that I bring to my analysis a sensitivity to how dominant social structures such as gender, race, and class may be conditions that influence social process (Wuest, 1995; Wuest & Merritt-Gray, 2001). This does not mean that I code for these factors, only that if there are conceptual indicators for them in the data, I am more likely to see them. Thus, when reviewing the literature for the literature review, paying attention not only to the findings but also to the ways that the findings are theoretically organized may strengthen the researcher's understanding of which theoretical relationships are possible.

Theoretical Sampling

Sampling in grounded theory studies is theoretical. Initially, the researcher makes choices about where and how to collect data based on his or her judgment of the best sources of observational, interview, and or document data for the domain of study. Codes are generated inductively from the data, and deductive decisions about where next to collect data are based on what is needed to clarify the properties of and relationships among emerging concepts (Glaser, 1978). Theoretical sampling, therefore, is guided by the demands of theory development. Theoretical sampling takes place by seeking answers to questions or hypotheses that arise during analysis by interviewing new participants who are likely to have relevant experiences, looking for comparisons in data already collected, returning to participants to ask new questions, conducting participant observation, consulting policies or documents, and looking at literature.

Specifying the sample in advance and developing a sampling plan are difficult. Yet, on a practical level, research ethics boards, granting agencies, and institutions expect that the sample will be specified both in terms of population and number, and they are becoming increasingly intolerant toward proposals that refer to emergence as the rationale for not doing so. A strategy for addressing this challenge is to consider broadly the range of people who may offer insight into the domain of study and prepare the proposal inclusively. If the study domain is caregiving for family members with Alzheimer's disease (AD), the researcher might designate the initial sample as English-speaking men and women over 19 years of age who are providing care to a family member with AD. This could be followed with a statement indicating that based on initial theoretical analysis, data may be collected from others such as family members, home support workers, and health care professionals who have knowledge of family caregiving for persons with AD. Including these groups in the initial proposal does not mean that data must be collected from them. Rather, if theoretically necessary to seek data from these sources, the researcher is positioned to do so without gaining additional ethical approval. Prepare consent forms and letters of information in language that will make them applicable to all potential participants. Considering potential sources for theoretical sampling is an informed judgment call, and, unquestionably, analysis may send the researcher in directions previously unimagined.

Nonetheless, some potential sources are obvious, and including them in the proposal may save time later.

Sample Size.   In grounded theory, sample size should not be an issue. Researchers collect data by theoretically sampling until theoretical saturation is achieved; that is, no further theoretical variation in a concept emerges from the data being analyzed (Glaser & Strauss, 1967). The focus of theoretical sampling is discovery, not verification. Saturation is not judged by the number of times similar properties of a concept are identified, but rather by whether a full range of variation in conceptual properties is identified. To some extent, how rapidly saturation occurs depends on how narrowly the study domain is defined. If, in an AD study, the domain studied was constrained to family caregiving when the caregiver is male, lives in a specific community, and is a member of a support group, saturation would most likely be achieved more quickly than if the domain included all family caregivers. Although Glaser (1978) cautions that demographic variables such as age, gender, and location must earn their way into the data and do not necessarily influence variation, some undoubtedly will. Breadth and diversity of study domain are significant when considering time and costs of achieving theoretical saturation.

Still, reviewers, thesis committees, and review boards struggle if no sample size is specified. Morse (1994) suggests that 30 to 50 interviews are needed in a grounded theory study. In my experience, a grounded theory in a narrow domain such as that carried out by masters students usually can be achieved from interviews with 10 to 15 participants. In the case of a broader domain, interviews with about 40 participants are manageable and allow for theoretical saturation. However, much depends on the quality of data collected; these are only estimates to assist with proposal writing. Researchers need to be prepared to be guided by the demands of data for theory building.

Recruitment.   The initial recruitment focuses on ways to access participants who are judged to have good knowledge of the study domain. A specific organization (support group, community agency) or person (physician, clinical nurse specialist, public health nurse) may be approached to give information letters to persons who meet the initial sample criteria. Broader recruitment takes place by putting an advertisement in the newspaper or posters in various community sites. To avoid being deluged by initial volunteers, limit the initial recruitment effort to circulating a small number of letters of information or one newspaper advertisement. When screening participants for inclusion in the study, record demographic characteristics that may influence variation in the study domain as a basis for later theoretical sampling. For example, in the proposed AD study, age, gender, geographic location, ethnicity, help being received, stage of AD, length of time caregiving, and relationship to care recipient might conceivably be salient. This demographic information facilitates later theoretical sampling, if these characteristics emerge as salient.[2]

By limiting initial recruitment, subsequent recruitment can take place purposefully to collect data that are likely to allow hypotheses about properties of, or relationships among, concepts to be confirmed or refined, thus moving analysis toward theoretical saturation. In our study of women leaving abusive partners, we initially recruited women who had been out of the relationship for at least a year (Wuest & Merritt-Gray, 1999). As our understanding of the concept of *leaving* shifted from singular act to multiple acts of breaking free, we sought help from lay and professional helpers to recruit some women who were in the process of leaving to illuminate the variation in the ways and timing of breaking free.

Data Collection

Much has been written about the interview process in grounded theory (Hutchinson & Wilson, 1994; May, 1991; Swanson, 1987; Wuest, 1995). The matrix operation of grounded theory is very difficult if the person collecting the data is unfamiliar with the evolving analysis. Thus, the researcher must be fully engaged in the data collection and analysis process. If a research assistant is employed, I suggest that he or she collect no more than half the data and be involved fully in the analysis. An interview protocol that includes participant tracking forms, processes for screening participants for eligibility, routines for making and confirming interview times and locations, standard interview packages and equipment, and finally a safety protocol for data collectors and participants (Paterson, Gregory, & Thorne, 1999) is important for taking the guesswork out of the data collection process. Familiarity with recording equipment and access to extra tapes, batteries, and an extension cord are advisable if interviews are to be recorded. Glaser (2004) argues against tape-recording interviews, saying that field notes are more useful because they contain only relevant data. Transcripts of tape-recorded interviews often include much data that ultimately are not used because they are not salient to the core variable. However, at the outset the researcher does not know what is relevant, so tape-recording preserves all data until analysis

---

[2]See Wuest (2001) for an explicit depiction of theoretical sampling in a study of women's caring.

results in identification of a basic social problem and core variable. Unless a researcher has solid training in ethnographic traditions of recording field notes during and following interviews, tape-recording may be advisable. Interviews are most fruitful in a setting where the participant feels safe and comfortable, and when there are no interruptions. Although there are diverse opinions on whether fees should be paid to participants, compensating for transportation and/or dependent care is respectful and facilitates recruitment. An information sheet of relevant accessible resources provided at the end of the interview is a useful way to thank participants while providing them with information they may not have.

Grounded theory interviews are semistructured in that the researcher normally has an overview question with some follow-up probes. In our study of caregiving for a family member with AD, we asked participants to tell us what it was like for them to care for their family member (Wuest, Ericson, & Stern, 1994). In general, if the domain of study is important to the participant, the general overview question is a catalyst for participants to share their experience in detail and few additional probes are required from the researcher. If the domain of study seems inconsequential to the participant, the researcher may need to use the prepared follow-up probes more purposefully. In our study of health promotion in single-parent families after leaving, women and children were hesitant in responding to a broad question related to how they attended to their health; specific follow-up probes were essential (Ford-Gilboe, Wuest, & Merritt-Gray, 2005). As data collection and analysis proceed, the interview process shifts in light of the emerging theory. Although I continue to begin with the initial overview question, follow-up probes change; some may prove irrelevant to the developing theory, and new ones are needed to check out theoretical hunches. Analysis sensitizes the researcher to compare what is being said during the interview with what is emerging from the analysis, leading to spontaneous probing or theoretical sampling to obtain further clarification. To confirm, expand, or refine the properties of the emerging concepts or the relationships among them, researchers ask more focused questions as the study progresses. In our leaving an abusive partner study, workplace support emerged as instrumental in fortifying women for leaving, leading us to theoretically sample by probing new participants and old data about how the workplace influenced leaving. For theory development to proceed most effectively, the interviewer builds on data analysis with each subsequent interview.

Novice researchers often struggle with letting participants respond to the overview question in their own ways, often believing at first that they are not getting good data and that they need to focus the interview more. I would caution that we do not know what is salient early on, so give participants latitude. Interviews that are staccato, that is many questions followed by short answers, are less likely to yield rich data. Each of us upon reading our interviews is struck by our obvious errors in interviewing such as interrupting a discussion line, asking a totally unrelated question, or failing to encourage elaboration. Phyllis Stern (personal communication, 1989) asserts that participants are very forgiving, replying politely to our off-base inquiries and then returning to what they really want to talk about. Participants disclose important information after the tape recorder is off, often as the researcher is on the way out the door. Always ask whether this information can be used, and if the answer is affirmative, take a time later to dictate this information, along with any observations, at the end of the tape so that it becomes part of the transcription.

Although transcribing interviews takes a great deal of time for everyone except skilled typists, the benefit is knowing the data very well. If someone else transcribes, more time will be needed to listen to the tape while reading the transcription. Transcriptions need to be accurate and without identifying data, particularly names and locations. I replace names with the relationship of the person named to the participant (DAUGHTER, PHYSICIAN, FRIEND) and location with a more general classification (NEARBY CITY, VILLAGE). Format transcripts such that they are single-spaced with a double space between speakers. Set margins so that text extends only half the page width, leaving room for coding. Finally, number the lines in the interview for easy referencing of conceptual indicators (Int 2: Lines 423–445).

Data Analysis

Analysis in grounded theory is aimed at generating a theoretical, as opposed to a descriptive, account of patterns of behavior in the study domain. Analysis begins through inductive identification of substantive codes to name what is happening in the data, often with more than one code being assigned to a particular data segment (phrase, sentence, paragraph). Eventually, codes are grouped into more abstract categories that reflect the domain of study at a descriptive level. Analysis shifts to a more theoretical level largely through theoretical coding, diagramming, and reduction. Theoretical coding is the process of examining data through the theoretical lens of the coding families (Glaser, 1978). Theoretical properties of categories are identified. Reduction occurs as categories are collapsed into more abstract concepts and linked. The central problem and core variable, which may be a basic social process, are identified. Categories unrelated to the core variable are dropped from the analysis. Additional data are collected through theoretical sampling to further saturate concepts and further clarify the relationships among them. In this process, concepts may be renamed, additionally collapsed, or linked differently. Literature is also theoretically sampled as data to support the emerging theory. Theoretical memos are written to capture the conceptual development throughout this analytic process and become the basis for the final report.

Descriptions, such as this, fail to do justice to the complex and infinitely messy process of grounded theory analysis. The process is far from linear, and the analyst is perpetually moving back and forth from the substantive line-by-line coding, to theoretical consideration, to memoing, and then back to the substantive data. Doing grounded theory is a process of inductively deriving codes, developing hunches about properties and relationships, checking out those hunches deductively in old and new data by theoretical sampling, and developing yet another inductive theoretical hunch.

One aspect of analysis rarely discussed is the need to alternately consider the data at both a macro and micro level. By macro level, I mean considering the larger picture by reading and listening to entire transcripts, asking, "What is going on here with regard to the domain of study?" "What is the problem?" and "What is being done in response to the problem?" This macro-level analysis is important to keep the researcher focused on identifying the core problem and core variable related to the study domain. Data normally include much information that may be background, but not central, to the domain studied. For example, Enman (2004) is studying help-seeking behaviors of caregivers of spouses with AD. Her data contain considerable information about caregiving processes. Hence, she focuses on her domain by asking, "What is the basic problem *related to help seeking?*" Looking at the bigger picture must go hand in hand with the micro-level analysis of line-by-line open coding. Open coding involves focusing on each data bit, asking what it is an indicator of, and assigning a code or label (Glaser, 1978). As codes recur in the data, the researcher compares data bits, asking how they are the same or different and what accounts for the variation. As properties are identified, memos are written separately, tracking theoretical development. Substantive codes are then reviewed for grouping into categories. Throughout the analytical process, the researcher moves back and forth from the micro to the macro level, staying grounded in the data, but thinking about how they are related to the domain of study. In this way, the problem related to the study domain is eventually identified.

Open Coding.   Although open coding seems straightforward, at the beginning it is daunting. Each of us is trying to measure up to an elusive "right way" and thus feels like an impostor. The goal of open coding is to generate as many codes as possible to fit the data. As coding continues, and the researcher compares incidents, some codes recur more than others, others collapse, and categories begin to develop. Often in the initial data, researchers are unable to see indicators of particular codes until later when they emerge in other data. Thus, theoretically sampling data previously coded is important; subsequent discoveries influence how old data are seen. Expect to code and recode data at this substantive level, particularly initial interviews. When selecting words for coding, stay close to the data, choosing words that reflect what is going on. *In vivo* codes, that is, words of the participants that are particularly apt, may sometimes be the best code for what is going on. Avoid words that are theory-laden such as *stress, resilience,* and *denial.* Metaphors and analogies are risky to use for coding because they can begin to drive the analysis, rather like a theoretical framework (Glaser, 1978; Sandelowski, 1998).[3] As open coding continues, codes are constantly compared and gradually grouped together into more abstract categories.

Theoretical Coding.   The process of theoretical coding is challenging and little is written about how to do it. In the following paragraphs, I offer my approach to ensuring that I shift from open to theoretical coding in my analysis. Theoretical coding often begins during open coding with constant comparison when the researcher recognizes that a segment of data is a conceptual indicator of a condition or a consequence of another code. I write memos to track the theoretical development and gradually group the codes into categories. Nonetheless, after approximately 8 to 12 interviews (the number depends on the richness and variation in the data), I find myself swimming in evolving codes and categories. I feel as though I have lost control and need to stop data collection temporarily and focus on analysis.

I list all substantive codes and, through constant comparison, group them into 15 to 20 categories named with a label that best fits the codes combined. Remember, these categorical groupings and their labels are still very provisional, and as data collection and analysis proceed, they will expand and shift to *fit* the data. Some of these categories are processes and have labels that are gerunds (words ending in "ing"); others have labels that are nouns and are more likely to be conditions or context or the problem. I then recode all of the data collected to date in terms of the categories I derived from inductive analysis. The next step is to sort all data by categories. Recoding and sorting can take place in one of several ways: (1) using a computer program focusing on qualitative analysis; (2) coding, cutting up, and sorting hard copies; or (3) cutting and pasting in a word-processing program. I use a qualitative analysis computer program for preparing numbered interview transcripts, coding my data categorically, and generating sorted hard copy output for

---

[3]See Sandelowski (1998) for an excellent discussion of the hazards of metaphor.

each category. However, for all of my initial open coding and categorizing, I work with pencil and printed transcripts.

Once the data are sorted by category, I reflect on the big picture by considering how each category is related to each other, and what each tells me about the basic social problem and how it is being processed. Glaser's (1978) 18 coding families are the basis for theoretical coding and offer diverse lenses for helping researchers see how categories may be related to one another. Having a working knowledge of all of the coding families such as the foundational 6 Cs (cause, consequence, condition, context, covariance, and contingency), process, degree, dimension, strategy, and type enables researchers to consider the relationships among, and the properties of, each category.[4] In short, the coding families act like a template of possible theoretical relationships that assists the analyst to move to a more abstract level, away from descriptive understandings. The researcher may select codes from various families that work to explain theoretically what is going on in the study domain. Diagramming is helpful for visual thinkers to see how concepts relate to one another. This macro-level consideration of categorical relationships helps me to consolidate my hunches related to naming the basic social problem and the core variable, although this remains quite preliminary. Memoing is important to capture theoretical ideas at this point.

My next step is to take one category, preferably a process category that seems important, and examine the data related to it through the lens of theoretical codes. I begin with a large piece of paper, writing the category name in the middle. One at a time, I read each segment of data that has been sorted for this category, asking, "What does this segment tell me about the theoretical properties of this category? Is there anything here about the cause or consequences, the conditions under which it happens, strategies for how it happens, conditions that might influence the degree or frequency or how it happens?" I systematically consider the data through a range of theoretical codes. As I generate theoretical properties from the data, I name and organize them according to whether they are conditions, causes, consequences, strategies, processes, turning points, and so forth, always noting data location (interview and line number). In my study of women's caring, the following data segment had been categorized as "asserting":

Int 2
I knew what I wanted. I felt comfortable with my decisions about breastfeeding and if somebody wanted me to do something that I didn't agree with I would say no. But I was 30 when I had my first child and older and more mature for my other two.

---

[4]See Glaser (1978) Chapter 4 for a full discussion of coding families.

These data indicate that a *cause* of asserting is "someone wanting me to do something I didn't agree with," *conditions* for asserting are knowing what you want (possibly from past experience), being comfortable with your decision, and maturity. A *strategy* for asserting is saying no. As I systematically examine each data segment of a category through the lens of the coding families and record the findings in terms of their theoretical properties and relationships to one another, the page is gradually filled. Each indicator is compared with others, and the various causes, consequences, and so on are grouped conceptually. A range of theoretical properties is recorded. When the theoretical coding of the category is completed, I write an extensive memo that captures this detailed theoretical analysis. I try to pay close attention to Glaser's (1978) dictum to write about the concepts, not about the people. It is good practice for the final report writing and is part of shifting from the descriptive to the theoretical level. I begin by specifying the meaning of the concept: "Asserting is a process of . . . " This conceptual specification is derived from the theoretical analysis as opposed to an *a priori* definition (Glaser, 1978). I discuss the theoretical properties of the concept such as the antecedents, the strategies, the consequences. Of particular importance is identifying the conditions that influence the variation in timing, intensity, or duration of the process. As I finish one category, I move on to theoretical coding and writing memos about the next category. Often, I discover that some categories are actually conditions or consequences of categories I have already theoretically coded. These discoveries help me reduce the number of concepts and integrate the developing theory. When theoretically coding categories that are not processes, the coding families of type, degree, and dimensions may be more helpful. For example, the basic problem for caring women was caring demands. Analysis of the category labeled "demands" focused on the theoretical codes of *types* (competing or changing) and *dimensions* (pervasive, arising daily, simultaneous). Glaser (1978) suggests using typologies (qualitative crosstabulation) to clarify variation according to the presence or absence of dimensions.[5] For example, in the study of women's caring, "caring options" was a condition of the process of "negotiating." By creating a typology or crosstabulation based on the *dimensions* of "suitability" and "availability" of caring options, variation in a caregiver's negotiation with the health care system was explicated: resources are available but not suitable (constantly shopping for other options), resources are available and suitable (satisfied, not negotiating), resources are suitable but not available (taking risks to make suitable options available), resources are neither suit-

---

[5]See Glaser (1978, pp. 65–70) for a discussion of typology construction.

able nor available (no indicators of this in the data, so left blank) (Wuest, 2001). Although unquestionably the construction of typologies is based on an artificial presence/absence of dimensions (some resources may be somewhat suitable), the strategy nonetheless helps the analyst to identify how dimensions make a difference. The analyst may then apply the theoretical code of "degree" to consider further variation when dimensions are somewhat present.

After theoretically coding and memoing for each category, it is important to reflect on the bigger picture again. At this point, the concepts of the emerging theory can be diagrammed, the basic problem named, and the core category provisionally identified. The core category links categories together, explains what is going on, and accounts for variation (Glaser, 1978). Reflection on how well this provisional framework works for explaining the domain of study in terms of the data collected then takes place by a selective theoretical sampling of data to check out whether the relationships hypothesized between concepts hold across cases. I reread transcripts through the lens of my emerging theory, reflecting on data that informed my conceptual construction. When relationships do not hold, I am forced to reconsider my conceptualization, asking which factors account for the variation and how I might increase the level of abstraction to include all data. A second point of reflection is considering which categories are not saturated and which relationships among concepts need confirmation or further development. This reflection continues with conceptual elaboration, that is, systematic deduction from the data of theoretical possibilities in the form of hypotheses that lead to further theoretical sampling and constant comparative analysis (Glaser, 1978).

Theoretical Sampling and Integration.   Based on these reflections, I begin to recruit new participants or seek out other salient data such as documents. Importantly, in these new interviews, the researcher continues to begin with the broad overview question. However, as the researcher attends to the participant, he or she is listening through the lens of the emerging theory, seeking further clarification and expansion of concept properties, conditions that influence variation in process, and relationships among concepts. When new conceptual indicators emerge that are not accounted for by the emerging theory, the researcher again must modify the concept such that it "fits" the data; this normally means increasing the level of abstraction. Data that do not fit the emerging theory contribute to theoretical expansion; they do not disprove the emerging theory (Glaser, 1978). Thus, theory development is a continual process of modification and refinement such that the emerging theory fits the data. Because the researcher is consciously theoretically sampling, he or she is more focused on data salient to theoretical development. Similarly, if returning to participants a second time, the researcher normally has some theoretical purpose. Usually during second interviews, I give the person the opportunity to tell me about what has happened since last we spoke, and then I tell the person about what I am learning, asking further questions. I do this by bringing a diagram of the emerging theory and talking about each concept or process, briefly explaining how the participant's data contributed to its development (Wuest & Merritt-Gray, 2001). Such discussion normally results in additional data that further saturate or refine the concept.

Analysis of data from these continuing interviews is focused to purposefully develop and integrate the theory. Concepts are expanded, sometimes shifted to higher levels of abstraction to account for new data, sometimes collapsed together. Linkages among concepts and conditions that influence variation are more fully saturated. Memos document the ongoing theoretical analysis. Labeling memos according to relevant concepts, including the location of salient data, and keeping them within the conceptual boundaries of the emerging theory provide a useful basis for report writing. Problem, process, and concept names evolve to fit the additional data. Diagrams are revised to reflect the more fully integrated theory. The theory generated at this point may be quite different from the initial framework. Data collection continues until the data being collected are not producing new variation in the emerging theory. Unquestionably, the researcher has some control over this in terms of how broadly he or she theoretically samples.

Once the core process is identified, I begin theoretically sampling the literature well beyond the original literature review. This sampling is guided by the emerging theoretical concepts and extends across disciplines. As I read, I consider the literature as data to expand and densify concepts. I constantly compare for similarities and differences with the emerging substantive theory, and I memo so that I can readily retrieve salient literature for the final report. Sometimes, concepts in extant theory through constant comparison are identified as fitting with the concept specified from the data. In this case, the researcher may decide to adopt the extant theoretical concept through this constant comparative process of emergent fit (Wuest, 2000). However, when this occurs, the researcher acknowledges within the research report that emergent fit has taken place and provides exemplars. In this way, deduction is always in service of induction within the grounded theory process (Glaser, 1978).

At this point, preparation for writing begins. The starting point is to sort previous memos by concepts and to diagram the relationships among the concepts.

Writing the Report

The grounded theory report is a theoretical account of the study domain identifying the basic problem and discussing how the core category addresses the basic problem. Writing theoretically is almost as challenging as theoretical coding. Glaser (1978) urges, "The dictum is to *write conceptually*, by making theoretical statements about relationships between concepts, rather than writing descriptive statements about people" (p. 133). Yet many grounded theory reports are written only at a descriptive level, with cursory naming of concepts or processes, supported by numerous compelling quotes from data. May (1986) cautions that researchers "lapse into pure description and present these data in detail because they are 'too good to throw away'" (p. 148). Pure description can be the result of simply not engaging in the systematic theoretical coding and constant comparison needed to tease out the properties of concepts and the theoretical relationships among them. On the other hand, even after putting extraordinary work into this analysis, some researchers have difficulty carrying their analysis through the writing process such that the end product is written at a theoretical level. This may be related to poorly developed theoretical sensitivity or not having access to a mentor or expert in grounded theory methods.

What are the indicators of a grounded theory report written at a theoretical level? Normally, the findings section of the report will begin with an overview of the theory in which the basic social problem and the basic social process and its core concepts are named and conceptually specified (Glaser, 1978). Conceptual specifications are operational meanings derived from the data, and not from the dictionary, disciplinary usage, or extant theory. They have evolved through constant comparison as the theory is developed. The theoretical linkages among concepts are delineated. Often a diagram is provided to capture the basic social process, particularly movement between stages. This summary of the theoretical scheme provides a map that guides the researcher in the writing of detailed discussion of the theory (May, 1986). When the process identified is somewhat linear, another helpful tool, for both the researcher and the reader, is a chart of the stages in the process. Although many grounded theorists infer rather than specify the problem, I urge researchers to stipulate the problem. Because the theory accounts for what takes place in response to the problem, naming and conceptually specifying the problem helps to keep the researcher focused as the theory is written. Sometimes this is a brief section; other times it is lengthy, leading to a published paper such as our discussion of *intrusion*, the basic problem for health promotion after leaving an abusive partner (Wuest, Ford-Gilboe, Merritt-Gray, & Berman, 2003).

Continue the write-up with a detailed discussion of key theoretical concepts and their properties. At this more detailed level, concepts are conceptually specified, the theoretical properties of the concepts and the conditions that influence their variation are discussed, conceptual indicators are provided from the data, and literature to support the emerging theory is used as data. A limitation of many grounded theories is their failure to explain variation in the substantive concepts or in the basic social process. The theory is written homogeneously, implying that all people move through the basic social process in the same way. Conditions that influence variation may be named but not conceptually specified; nor is the effect of the condition on the timing, duration, intensity, or range of the behavior well developed. Yet a major strength of grounded theory for the discipline of nursing is its capacity to account for variation in behavior. Understanding the conditions that produce variation in the process is often the starting point for nursing intervention or practice change.

In capturing variation, focus beyond how the core variable is affected by the presence/absence of specific conditions and consider how the degree or type of a condition or the interaction among dimensions of a condition makes a difference. Envisioning the variation in this way often moves the theory to a higher level of abstraction. Some conditions influence all stages of the process. The dimensions of these conditions may be described in a separate section. Other conditions are salient only to one subprocess or concept and may be discussed when that subprocess is being explained. But naming and conceptually specifying conditions are not enough. In the detailed discussion of theory, the way that these conditions affect variation in the basic social process or core variable, particularly with regard to degree, duration, and timing, must be delineated and supported with data as conceptual indicators.

Many novice grounded theorists view analysis and writing as separate activities and are shocked to discover how much analysis takes place in the writing process. It is only through writing a coherent storyline about the basic social process or core variable that the inconsistencies in the scope and relationships among concepts emerge, forcing the analyst ever back to the data to confirm and refine through further constant comparison, theoretical sampling, and reduction. Moreover, although one begins writing with an overview of the theory, often the detailed articulation of the properties and relationships among concepts yields further insights that force the researcher to revise the initial overview, moving closer to a clear and parsimonious theory. Some researchers who struggle with getting beyond description find a good starting point is to prepare an outline of key concepts and properties, a procedure similar to preparing overheads for a presentation. Decisions regarding what to include and the words to use in each bullet help the researcher to determine what is core and to reduce the categories to key concepts, thereby increasing the level of abstraction.

One way to avoid writing descriptively is to write the first detailed draft without including conceptual indicators from the data or the literature. Glaser warns, "The *credibility* of the theory should be won by its integration, relevance, and workability, not by illustration used as if it were proof" (1978, p. 134). Writing without data forces the researcher to write about concepts, not cases. Once satisfied with a conceptual discussion of the theory, the researcher can write a second draft, inserting salient data as conceptual indicators. Data or descriptive statements about the data are used only for "illustration and imagery" (Glaser, 1978, p. 134). Data, particularly those collected by talking to people about their experiences, are often beguiling. Hence, researchers are reluctant to abandon rich and detailed narrative in service of theory construction. Consequently, many first drafts, and all too many final papers, of grounded theory studies consist of lengthy direct quotes strung together to tell the "story" of a particular experience. Unlike other qualitative research methods such as narrative analysis, the goal of grounded theory is not to accurately describe an individual's experience. Rather it is to construct a middle range theory that explains how the basic social problem is processed. The researcher takes responsibility for constructing this theory, which reaches far beyond the understanding of any single participant (Pyett, 2004). Although the resulting theory will resonate for the participant, it will not describe the detail of that participant's personal journey. A strength, in fact, of a grounded theory is that the theoretical framework often provides the participant with a new or fuller perspective. Another hazard of being immersed in the data is that researchers may have difficulty using data judiciously. Because the data are so compelling, the researcher may include a lengthy quote in which the conceptual indicator is buried. Select the best indicator of the concept and check that the connection to the concept is readily apparent.

A third writing of the theory focuses on adding in literature. Literature is theoretically sampled and added as supporting data for the theory, or to demonstrate how this conceptualization differs from the current state of knowledge. A challenge in integrating the literature into the write-up, as opposed to dealing with it in a separate discussion chapter, is ensuring that it does not take over. Be succinct and discriminating. Many novice researchers struggle with using literature as data, commonly integrating it "backward." What I mean by this is that they discuss how their findings support the research or theoretical perspectives of others. Rather, the literature should be discussed as data to support the emerging theory. The researcher handles the literature as other data, theoretically sampling, constantly comparing, and integrating what adds to the emerging theory.

Having written and rewritten the grounded theory, adding data exemplars and then literature, the researcher normally has a dense and parsimonious theory. The strength of theory construction is that the outcome can be applied to practice as a lens to interpret people's experience or to direct actions and interventions. Completing the write-up with a section discussing implications helps others to understand the significance of the theory. Often, novice grounded theorists return exclusively to the descriptive data when explaining the implications of their study findings, thus nullifying the power of the explanatory theory. Framing implications of the study in terms of the theoretical process or concepts demonstrates the significance of the framework and offers direction for application. Thus, when writing this final section, consider how this theoretical rendering of the study domain contributes new knowledge to the discipline, and how it might be useful for practice and policy.

BUT IS IT GROUNDED THEORY?

How does a researcher know whether the grounded theory generated is credible? Most qualitative research studies are evaluated in terms of broad criteria for rigor that mirror the post-positivist criteria of validity and reliability. The most broadly referenced are Lincoln and Guba's (1985) guidelines of trustworthiness and authenticity (Whittemore, Chase, & Mandle, 2001). Because these guidelines are broadly applicable to most qualitative methods, the researcher may follow them rigorously and produce a report that is not grounded theory. Glaser's (1978) criteria of *fit* (concepts must evolve to fit the data), *grab* (captures interest because it resonates), *work* (usefulness for explaining, interpreting, and predicting), and *modifiability* (capacity to change in response to new data) are specific to grounded theory. Both Lincoln and Guba's and Glaser's criteria offer more direction for rigor in doing grounded theory than for evaluation of the final product. Over the past decade, I have been increasingly challenged to articulate and justify how I evaluate a qualitative research report that is put forward as grounded theory. Working with graduate students who are learning the method has forced me to begin to consider not just what is wrong with beginning drafts, but also what has to be done to produce a thesis that is defensible as grounded theory. Similarly, review activities for journals, granting agencies, and graduate schools have assisted me in developing clear benchmarks for what constitutes a grounded theory. Those benchmarks have guided the foregoing discussion of how to write the grounded theory report. I am aware that articulating criteria for judging whether a qualitative report is grounded theory may be considered dogmatic given the diversity of grounded theory approaches; however, I believe the following benchmarks will stand regardless of the approach used.

Broadly, my benchmarks for grounded theory are as follows:

- The theory is written at a theoretical level.
- The conditions that account for variation in the basic social process or core variable are delineated and demonstrated in the discussion of the theory.
- Primacy is given to inductively derived concepts/processes in the substantive theory, which are conceptually specified from the data.
- Emergent fit is delineated when concepts/processes are labeled as existing theory-laden concepts already well developed in the literature.
- Data, particularly direct quotes, are used judiciously to demonstrate theoretical properties and variation.
- Existing theory and research are used to support the substantive theory and its uniqueness, as opposed to substantive theory being used to support extant theory.
- The implications of the study are written in terms of the substantive theory, not in terms of the descriptive data.

WHERE DOES GROUNDED THEORY FIT IN THE PARADIGM DEBATE?

Benoliel (1998) in a letter to Pam Brink, editor of *Western Journal of Nursing Research*, observed, "Within nursing . . . the notion of qualitative research has been approached as a way of *doing* more than as a way of *thinking*" (p. 238). She further argued that "the 'hows' of doing research are embedded within basic assumptions about the nature of knowledge and knowing and the paradigms or formats through which the investigator designs and implements specific proposals" (p. 238). These observations resonate with me because in my development as a researcher, I focused initially more on doing than thinking. Yet, I now understand that the way I do grounded theory is influenced greatly by my paradigm orientation. Increasingly, qualitative researchers are expected to be clear about their paradigms or worldviews, that is, assumptions regarding the nature of reality, what can be known, and how it can be known (Guba & Lincoln, 1994). My initial introduction to worldviews was in the first edition of this text (Munhall & Oiler, 1986) where worldviews were presented as received (traditional, mechanistic) and nonreceived (holistic, humanistic) and were, in my mind, aligned with quantitative and qualitative methods, respectively. I classified grounded theory with the nonreceived view. Subsequently, Guba and Lincoln identified four paradigms: positivist, postpositivist, constructivist, and critical. To my surprise, they located grounded theory in the postpositivist paradigm, which is informed by the assumptions that (1) a single reality exists that can only be imperfectly apprehended; (2) objectivity is a regulatory ideal; and (3) findings are confirmed through replication and fit with existing knowledge.

In my judgment, grounded theory is more consistent with the constructivist paradigm. Glaser and Strauss in their early writings (Glaser, 1978; Glaser & Strauss, 1967; Strauss, 1987) discuss how their research approach challenged verification of extant theory, the dominant research approach at that time in sociology. They question the dominant grand theories of their day, suggesting that these theories were not sufficient to explain relevant social issues. In contrast to grand theory, substantive middle range theories, called grounded theories, explain focused areas of sociological inquiry. Grounded theories are generated by first discovering inductively which concepts and hypotheses are relevant to the area being studied. Strauss (1987) asserts that a key assumption of grounded theory is that social phenomena are complex. He observes that a major limitation of much social research is to ignore complexity and study phenomena in isolation, assuming that complexity would be dealt with later. Grounded theory "emphasizes the need for developing many concepts and their linkages in order to capture a great deal of the variation that characterizes central phenomena studied during any research project" (Strauss, 1987, p. 7). Glaser and Strauss (1967) also broke with the dominant research tradition of that time by asserting that the researcher is not "a passive receiver of impression" but rather is actively hypothesizing and checking out hunches to generate theory (p. 39). "Grounded theory is developed in intimate relationship with data, with researchers fully aware of themselves as instruments for developing that grounded theory" (Strauss, 1987, p. 6). How the researcher actively engages in shaping the research process depends in part on the researcher's theoretical sensitivity. This acknowledgment of the researcher as an active participant in the construction of the research outcome was a significant departure from the objectivist position.

A criterion for judging grounded theory is whether it works; that is, interprets what is happening, explains what did happen, and predicts what will happen (Glaser, 1978). Although the notion of prediction is somewhat postpostivist, Glaser recognizes the partial perspective offered by a grounded theory, arguing that grounded theory is modifiable and can be recast as new data are collected and compared. Nonetheless, the language that Glaser and Strauss use in their various writings (Glaser, 1978, 1992; Glaser & Strauss, 1967; Strauss, 1987) is rooted in the positivist tradition of their research training in the mid-20th century. Critics of grounded theory often focus on this language, sometimes ignoring the significant shifts of thinking that align the approach more with what is often called the constructivist paradigm.

Charmaz (2000) wrote extensively about constructivist grounded theory. "Constructivism assumes the relativism of multiple social realities, recognizes the mutual creation of knowledge by the viewer and the viewed, and aims toward interpretive understandings of the subject's meanings" (p. 510). "Causality is suggestive, incomplete, and indeterminate in constructivist grounded theory" (p. 524). She argues that all data are narrative reconstructions of experience, not indicators of an external reality. The constructed theory does not constitute participant reality; rather, it is a theoretical rendering, "one interpretation among multiple interpretations of a shared or individual reality" (p. 523). Charmaz presents her perspective as if it were a total departure from the original position of Glaser and Strauss, failing to give the originators credit for the ways they did challenge dominant positivist thinking. This is particularly evident in the discussion of the epistemology. Charmaz argues that Glaser assumed that "we gather our data unfettered by bias or biography" (p. 592). Yet Glaser and Strauss (1967) were clear that the researcher's theoretical sensitivity influences data collection and analysis and that the researcher is an active participant in generating theory. Thus, Charmaz's strong assertion that the theory is shaped and constructed by the researcher and that coding is an interpretive process is consistent with that of the orginators. Glaser (1978) uses the language of emergence and discovery, but I understand emergence as a process of researcher generation that is consistent with constructivism. Charmaz moves beyond Glaser and Strauss in offering important direction conducting constructivist grounded theory when she calls for exploration of values and establishing relationships with participants so that they may tell their stories their way, preferably through a sustained relationship rather than once only. This direction expands the approach to doing grounded theory and supports the constructivist location.

In recent years, I have debated whether grounded theory could legitimately be located in the critical paradigm (Wuest et al., 2002). Benoliel (1996) notes that although most grounded theory studies result in practical knowledge based on interpretive understanding, "some findings provided an *emancipatory* focus in that they point to interactional and environmental constraints on the freedom and well-being of individuals with health problems . . ." (p. 417). Emancipation and critique are the explicit goals of research in the critical paradigm. The ontology is historical realism; that is, reality has been shaped over time by dominant social, political, cultural, economic, and ethnic factors and ultimately crystallized (Guba & Lincoln, 1994). The investigator and the investigated engage in a dialogic interaction that is value mediated and intended to challenge what has been taken for granted as real. Although Glaser (1978) argues that grounded theory is a starting point for change, change is not normally an explicit goal of the research process. In the development of a program of research focusing on health promotion in single-parent families after leaving an abusive partner (Ford-Gilboe et al., 2005; Wuest et al., 2003), we theoretically sampled data related to policy and services to expand our conceptual understanding of how these social structures influenced the basic social process. Within the critical paradigm, the test of the emerging theory is not just in how it explains what is happening but also in how it opens up alternatives for thought and action about how things could be (Kvale, 1995). We hoped our research would influence policy and services for families and reasoned that change would be more likely to take place as part of the research process if we shared our emerging theory derived from interviews with the families as a starting point for our discussions with policymakers and service providers (Wuest et al., 2002). Our discussions were dialogues that allowed for generation of theory based not only on the perspectives of the family, but also on those of the providers and policymakers.

Similarly, Kushner and Morrow (2003) propose a critical feminist grounded theory methodology, arguing that the conscious use of feminist and critical theory with grounded theory supports "the integration of social structural analysis in the generation of explanations of human interaction in the social world" (p. 41). Clarke (2003) also positions grounded theory in the critical paradigm with her assertion that grounded theory is postmodern. Interactionist grounded theory, according to Clarke, has always had the capacity to reveal perspectives in ways that are congruent with the postmodern situated knowledges. Clarke argues that new methods needed to address the complexity and heterogeneity of a postmodern world "should be epistemologically/ontologically based in the pragmatist soil that has historically nurtured symbolic interactionism and grounded theory" (p. 555). "The methodological implications of the postmodern primarily require taking situatedness, variations, complicatedness, differences of all kinds, and positionality/relationality very seriously in all their complexities, multiplicities, instabilities, and contradictions" (p. 556). Grounded theory, by virtue of producing substantive theory, may be seen as imposing a universal narrative that entrenches a singular viewpoint, rather that encouraging situated knowledge. Grounded theory, especially when conducted from a feminist perspective, allows for the inclusion of difference in the development of explanatory frameworks (Wuest & Merritt-Gray, 2001). Although the core variable or basic social process reflects the commonality of the experience, conditions are identified that influence the variation in the way the theory is enacted. Clarke observes that most methodological approaches in the post-modern center on giving individual voice through narrative and other bio-graphic strategies that neglect social context. In contrast, grounded theory has the capacity to capture complexity within the social context, and thus is an important research approach for the postmodern.

Researchers are using grounded theory across paradigms. Using grounded theory from different worldviews does not violate the intellectual roots of the method. The paradigm in which the grounded theory project is located will influence the relationship between the researcher and the participants and the broad goal of the project (explanation, understanding, or transforma-tion). Thus, sorting out the paradigm location may be helpful for designing the research study.

CONCLUSION

Grounded theory is a versatile research approach useful for generating ex-planatory substantive theory of human behavior in social context. Thus, the research problem must be one that will be illuminated by understanding so-cial psychological process in the study domain. Moreover, grounded theory is only an appropriate method when the researcher intends to go beyond de-scription of the study domain, toward a theoretical rendering. Choosing to use grounded theory is not a decision that should be made without consid-erable forethought. A critical issue is the individual researcher's capacity to think theoretically. Most researchers have a sense of their capacity to handle quantitative research approaches from their education and life experience related to mathematics and basic statistics. Background in qualitative analy-sis is less common. In my experience, most novice researchers handle initial open coding well. However, moving from open coding to theoretical coding and theory construction is much more challenging. Working with experi-enced researchers on an ongoing grounded theory project or engaging in a small pilot project with guidance from an experienced grounded theorist is invaluable in helping researchers determine whether grounded theory is a suitable approach for them. For some, descriptive understanding is much more meaningful and the shift toward conceptualization is painful. Learn-ing that *before* embarking on a grounded theory project is wise.

Doing grounded theory requires persistence, tolerance of uncertainty, ab-stract thinking, ability to make connections, facility with words, and willing-ness to live with an emerging theory always in the back of one's mind. Indeed, often it is when it is in the background that the most useful theo-retical thoughts arise. Grounded theory is also hard work. Open coding, categorizing, theoretical coding, and writing memos all require methodical, diligent effort if the outcome is to be a parsimonious and well-integrated theory. Grounded theories do not magically appear; they are generated from the data, one step at a time. Sometimes the process is slow and tedious, but when theoretical concepts and linkages begin to come together, researchers can experience what Glaser (1978) calls a "drugless high." Researchers find the emerging theory interesting and recognize its usefulness. Work on conceptual specification and theory integration is stimulating and exciting as the theory begins to take shape.

In summary, grounded theory research is all about fit: (1) fit between the research problem and the grounded theory product, (2) fit between researcher capacity and the grounded theory method, and (3) fit between the data and the evolving theoretical construction. The first fit can be determined before getting started. The second can be partially determined in advance through some training experience. The last is up to the researcher once the project is under way.

REFERENCES

Beck, C. T. (1999). Grounded theory research. In J. Fain (Ed.), *Reading, understanding, and applying nursing research* (pp. 205–225). Philadelphia: Davis.

Benoliel, J. Q. (1996). Grounded theory and nursing knowledge. Presented at a symposium sponsored by the College of Nursing, University of Rhode Island, October 1994. *Qualitative Health Research, 6*(3), 406–428.

Benoliel, J. Q. (1998). Letter to the editor. *Western Journal of Nursing Research, 20*(2), 238.

Bevis, E. O. (1988). Caring: A life force. In M. Leininger (Ed.), *Caring: An essential human need* (pp. 49–60). Detroit: Wayne State University Press.

Blumer, H. (1969). *Symbolic interactionism: Perspective and method.* Englewood Cliffs, NJ: Prentice Hall.

Charmaz, K. (2000). Grounded theory: Objectivist and constructivist methods. In N. Denzin & Y. Lincoln (Eds.), *Handbook of qualitative research* (2nd ed.) (pp. 509–535). Thousand Oaks, CA: Sage.

Chenitz, W. C., & Swanson, J. (1986). *From practice to grounded theory: Qualitative research in nursing.* Menlo Park, CA: Addison-Wesley.

Clarke, A. (2003). Situational analyses: Grounded theory mapping after the postmodern turn. *Symbolic Interaction, 26*(4), 553–576.

Crooks, D. (2001). The importance of symbolic interaction in grounded theory research on women's health. *Health Care for Women International, 22*(1–2), 11–27.

Enman, A. (2004). *Help seeking in spousal caregivers of those with Alzheimer disease and related disorders.* Unpublished master of nursing thesis proposal. University of New Brunswick, Fredericton, NB.

Farran, C., & Keane-Hagerty, E. (1991). An interactive model for finding meaning through caregiving. In P. Chinn (Ed.), *Anthology of caring* (pp. 225–238). New York: National League for Nursing Press.

Ford-Gilboe, M., Wuest, J., & Merritt-Gray, M. (2005). Strengthening capacity to limit intrusion: Theorizing family health promotion in the aftermath of woman abuse. *Qualitative Health Research, 15,* 477–501.

Given, B., & Given, C. (1991). Family caregiving for the elderly. *Annual Review of Nursing Research, 9,* 77–99.

Glaser, B. (1978). *Theoretical sensitivity.* Mill Valley, CA: Sociology Press.

Glaser, B. (1992). *Basics of grounded theory analysis.* Mill Valley, CA: Sociology Press.

Glaser, B. (1998). *Doing grounded theory: Issues and discussions.* Mill Valley, CA: Sociology Press.

Glaser, B. (1999). The future of grounded theory. *Qualitative Health Research, 9*(6), 836–845.

Glaser, B. (2002). Conceptualization: On theory and theorizing using grounded theory. *International Journal of Qualitative Methods, 1*(2), Article 3. Retrieved September 11, 2002, from http://www.ualberta.ca/~ijqm/.

Glaser, B. (2004). Remodelling grounded theory. *Forum: Qualitative Social Research, 5*(2), Article 4. Retrieved February 7, 2005, from http://www.qualitative-research.net/fqs-texte/2-04/2-04glaser-e.htm.

Glaser, B., & Strauss, A. (1967). *The discovery of grounded theory.* Chicago: Aldine.

Guba, E., & Lincoln, Y. (1994). Competing paradigms in qualitative research. In N. Denzin & Y. Lincoln (Eds.), *Handbook of qualitative research* (pp. 105–117). Thousand Oaks, CA: Sage.

Hutchinson, S., & Wilson, H. (1994). Research and therapeutic interviews: A post-structuralist perspective. In J. Morse (Ed.), *Critical issues in qualitative research methods* (pp. 300–315). Thousand Oaks, CA: Sage.

Hutchinson, S., & Wilson, H. (2001). Grounded theory: The method. In P. Munhall (Ed.), *Nursing research: A qualitative perspective* (3rd ed.) (pp. 209–244). Sudbury, MA: Jones and Bartlett.

Kushner, K., & Morrow, R. (2003). Grounded theory, feminist theory, critical theory: Toward theoretical triangulation. *Advances in Nursing Science, 26,* 30–43.

Kvale, S. (1995). The social construction of validity. *Qualitative Inquiry, 1,* 19–40.

Lincoln, Y., & Guba, E. (1985). *Naturalistic inquiry.* Thousand Oaks, CA: Sage.

MacDonald, M. (2001). Finding a critical perspective in grounded theory. In R. Schreiber & P. N. Stern (Eds.), *Using grounded theory in nursing* (pp. 113–158). New York: Springer.

May, K. (1991). Interviewing techniques: Concerns and challenges. In J. Morse (Ed.), *Qualitative nursing research* (pp. 180–201). Newbury Park, CA: Sage.

May, K. A. (1986). Writing and evaluating the grounded theory research report. In W. C. Chenitz & J. M. Swanson (Eds.), *From practice to grounded theory: Qualitative research in nursing* (pp. 146–154). Menlo Park, CA: Addison-Wesley.

Milliken, P. J., & Schreiber, R. (2001). Can you "do" grounded theory without symbolic interactionism? In R. Schreiber & P. N. Stern (Eds.), *Using grounded theory in nursing.* (pp. 177–190). New York: Springer.

Morse, J. (1994). Designing funded qualitative research. In N. Denzin & Y. Lincoln (Eds.), *Handbook of qualitative research* (pp. 220–235). Thousand Oaks, CA: Sage.

Morse, J., & Richards, L. (2002). *README FIRST for a user's guide to qualitative methods.* Thousand Oaks, CA: Sage.

Munhall, P., & Oiler, C. (1986). *Nursing research: A qualitative perspective.* Norwalk, CT: Appleton-Century-Crofts.

Paterson, B., Gregory, D., & Thorne, S. (1999). A protocol for research safety. *Qualitative Health Research, 9,* 259–269.

Pyett, P. (2004). Validation of qualitative research in the "real world." *Qualitative Health Research, 13,* 1170–1179.

Ray, M. (1981/1988). A philosophical analysis of caring within nursing. In M. Leininger (Eds.), *Caring: An essential human need* (pp. 25–36). Detroit: Wayne State University Press.

Roach, Sister S. (1992). *The human act of caring.* Ottawa, Ontario: Canadian Hospital Association.

Sandelowski, M. (1998). Writing a good read: Strategies for re-presenting qualitative data. *Research in Nursing & Health, 21,* 375–382.

Schreiber, R., & Stern, P. N. (2001). *Using grounded theory in nursing.* New York: Springer.

Seigfried, C. H. (1998). Pragmatism. In A. Jaggar & I. Young (Eds.), *A companion to feminist philosophy* (pp. 49–57). Malden, MA: Blackwell.

Snow, D. (2001). Expanding and broadening Blumer's conceptualization of symbolic interactionism. *Symbolic Interaction, 24,* 367–377.

Stern, P. (1980). Grounded theory methodology: Its uses and processes. *Image, 12,* 20–23.

Stern, P. N., & Covan, E. (2001). Early grounded theory: Its processes and products. In R. Schreiber & P. N. Stern (Eds.), *Using grounded theory in nursing* (pp. 17–34). New York: Springer.

Stern, P. N., & Pyles, S. (1986). Using grounded theory methodology to study women's culturally based decisions about health. In P. N. Stern (Ed.), *Women, health, and culture* (pp. 1–24). Washington, DC: Hemisphere.

Strauss, A. (1987). *Qualitative analysis for social scientists.* Cambridge: Cambridge University Press.

Strauss, A., & Corbin, J. (1990). *Basics of qualitative research: Grounded theory procedures and techniques.* Newbury Park, CA: Sage.

Strauss, A., & Corbin, J. (1998). *Basics of qualitative research: Techniques and procedures for developing grounded theory.* Thousand Oaks, CA: Sage.

Swanson, J. (1987). The formal qualitative interview for grounded theory. In W. C. Chenitz & J. Swanson (Eds.), *From practice to grounded theory: Qualitative research in nursing* (pp. 66–78). Menlo Park, CA: Addison-Wesley.

Whittemore, R., Chase, S., & Mandle, C. L. (2001). Validity in qualitative research. *Qualitative Health Research, 11,* 522–537.

Wuest, J. (1995). Feminist grounded theory: An exploration of congruency and tensions between two traditions in knowledge discovery. *Qualitative Health Research, 5*(1), 125–137.

Wuest, J. (1997a). Fraying connections of caring women: An exemplar of including difference in the development of explanatory frameworks. *Canadian Journal of Nursing Research, 29*, 99–116.

Wuest, J. (1997b). Illuminating environmental influences on women's caring. *Journal of Advanced Nursing, 26*, 49–58.

Wuest, J. (2000). Negotiating with helping systems: An example of grounded theory evolving through emergent fit. *Qualitative Health Research, 10*, 51–70.

Wuest, J. (2001). Precarious ordering: Toward a formal theory of women's caring. *Health Care for Women International: Special Volume, Using Grounded Theory to Study Women's Health, 22*(1–2), 167–193.

Wuest, J., Berman, H., Ford-Gilboe, M., & Merritt-Gray, M. (2002). Illuminating social determinants of women's health using grounded theory. *Health Care for Women International, 23*(8), 794–808.

Wuest, J., Ericson, P., & Stern, P. N. (1994). Becoming strangers: Changing family relationships in Alzheimer's disease. *Journal of Advanced Nursing, 20*, 437–443.

Wuest, J., Ford-Gilboe, M., Merritt-Gray, M., & Berman, H. (2003). Intrusion: The basic social problem identified in a grounded theory study of family health promotion among children and single mothers after leaving an abusive partner. *Qualitative Health Research, 13*(5), 597–622.

Wuest, J., & Merritt-Gray, M. (1999). Not going back: Sustaining the separation in the process of leaving abusive relationships. *Violence Against Women, 5*, 110–133.

Wuest, J., & Merritt-Gray, M. (2001). Feminist grounded theory revisited. In R. Schreiber & P. Stern (Eds.), *Using grounded theory in nursing* (pp. 159–176). New York: Springer.

Wuest, J., & Stern, P. (1990) The impact of fluctuating relationships with the Canadian health care system on family management of otitis media with effusion. *Journal of Advanced Nursing, 15*, 556–563.

9

Exemplar: Teetering on the Edge: A Continually Emerging Theory of Postpartum Depression

Cheryl Tatano Beck

Mothers suffering from postpartum depression have described themselves as being "afraid to be alive" and feeling like "death warmed up" (Dalton, 1996). Undiagnosed postpartum depression can plunge mothers into the depths of despair and turn their first months of motherhood into blackness. This mood disorder affects, on average, 13% of mothers (O'Hara & Swain, 1996). It has been estimated that up to 50% of all cases of this tragic illness are undetected (Ramsay, 1993). This crippling mood disorder has been described as a thief that steals motherhood (Beck, 1999). In 1993, a grounded theory study of postpartum depression, teetering on the edge, was first developed (Beck, 1993). At the time that study was conducted, there were only two other qualitative studies on the topic that had been published (Beck, 1992; Nicolson, 1990). Neither of these studies used a grounded theory design.

In more than a decade since the original teetering on the edge study was completed, a review of the literature revealed 10 qualitative studies of postpartum depression in women from other cultures. A decision was made to use these studies of this mood disorder in women of different cultures as new data to modify this grounded theory. Postpartum depressed mothers in other cultures were considered as comparison groups because the original teetering on the edge had been developed with a sample of all Caucasian, middle-class women in the United States.

BACKGROUND

One question that has been debated over the years is whether postpartum depression is a Western culture-bound syndrome. Stern and Kruckman (1983, p. 1036) hypothesize "that the negative outcomes of depression and baby blues in the U.S. result from the relative lack of (1) social structuring of postpartum events; (2) social recognition of a role transition for the new mother; and (3) instrumental assistance to the new mother." They list the following six components of postpartum activities, which provide social support for new mothers and help to buffer or prevent postpartum depression (1983, p. 1039):

♦ Structuring of a distinct postpartum time period
♦ Protective measures and rituals reflecting the presumed vulnerability of the new mother
♦ Social seclusion
♦ Mandated rest
♦ Assistance in tasks from relatives and/or midwife
♦ Social recognition through rituals, gifts, and so forth after new social status of the mother

Seel (1986) and Bhugra and Gregorie (1993) are examples of support for Stern and Kruckman's (1983) hypothesis. Seel (1986) purports that rituals and customs surrounding birth and the postpartum period are critical for a woman to feel that her new role is valued by her culture and that a supporting network of family and friends surrounds her. Bhugra and Gregorie (1993) describe four themes within these protective rituals: (1) isolating and secluding the new mother, (2) intensive caring and support of the new mother, (3) behavioral proscriptions on the women such as "doing the month" among the Chinese (Pillsbury, 1978) or dietary restrictions, and (4) suspending of social roles and protecting from previous demands. Seel (1986) refers to these childbirth rituals as "rites de passage" and when incomplete, as in Western society, are associated with an increase in postpartum depression. Seel argues that in the Western society the mother and father are left in limbo. New parents have to fend for themselves as they can. Without these rituals, mothers are stripped of protective layers. This cultural stereotyping is dangerous, however, because of the possibility that postpartum depression in non-Western culture may go unrecognized (Kumar, 1994).

Since the 1990s, findings from transcultural research on postpartum depression have accumulated evidence that the prevalence of this postpartum mood disorder is fairly consistent around the globe. Oates et al. (2004) examine whether postpartum depression was a universal experience with common attributions and how it was described. The research occurred in 11 countries: France, Ireland, Italy, Sweden, United States, Uganda, United Kingdom, Japan, Portugal, Austria, and Switzerland. Three different groups participated in this qualitative study: new mothers, relatives, and health care professionals. "Morbid unhappiness" (postpartum depression) was recognized by women in all 11 countries as a common experience after delivery.

Examples of international rates of diagnosed postpartum depression include 19% in Morocco (Agoub, Moussaoui, & Battas, 2005), 16% in Zimbabwe (Nhiwatiwa, Patel, & Acuda, 1998), 12% in Nepal (Regmi, Sligl, Carter, Grut, & Seear, 2002), 23% in India (Patel, Rodrigues, & DeSouza, 2002), 15% in Italy (Carpiniello, Pariante, Serri, Costa, & Carta, 1997), 28% in Pakistan (Rahman, Iqbal, & Harrington, 2003), 12% in Hong Kong (Lee, Yip, Chiu, Leung, & Chung, 2001), and 17% in Japan (Yamashita, Yoshida, Nakano, & Tashiro, 2000).

The 10 qualitative studies of postpartum depression in women from other cultures focused on Hmong women in the United States (Stewart & Jambunathan, 1996), Canadians (Berggren-Clive, 1998), Middle Eastern women in Australia (Nahas, Hillege, & Amasheh, 1999), Australians (Holopainen, 2002), women in Ireland (Lawler & Sinclair, 2003) and India (Rodrigues, Patel, Jaswal, & deSouza, 2003), black Caribbean women in the United Kingdom (Edge, Baker, & Rogers, 2004), black and ethnic minority women in the United Kingdom (Templeton, Velleman, Persaud, & Milner, 2003), African American women in the United States (Amankwaa, 2003), and Hong Kong Chinese women (Chan, Levy, Chung, & Lee, 2002).

In grounded theory, modification never stops (Glaser, 2001). As new data come in, the substantive theory is modified to accommodate the varying conditions to increase the theory's power and completeness. "All is data" in grounded theory (Glaser, 2001, p. 145). Whatever is happening in the research scene is data, no matter the source. As new literature is discovered, it is compared as simply additional data (Glaser, 1998). Constantly comparing the literature as data yields new properties of the categories. The theory is modified as the data-literature is woven into it.

The scope of a substantive theory can be carefully increased and controlled by making conscious choices of groups for comparison (Glaser & Strauss, 1967). A more general substantive theory, for example, can be achieved by comparison of different groups from different parts of a country or from different countries. It must be remembered, however, that persons are not categorized, but the behavior persons engage in is (Glaser, 1998).

What is searched for are maximum differences among these groups so that comparisons can be made on as many relevant differences and similarities in the data as can be found. Maximizing differences among comparative groups is a powerful method for enhancing the generation of theoretical properties and extending and saturating the theory.

RESEARCH DESIGN

Grounded theory is the systematic generation of theory from data (Glaser, 1998). It is an integrated set of conceptual hypotheses about relationships between concepts. Grounded theory has its roots in latent structure analysis and in conceptual index formation (Glaser, 1998, 2003). It is a theory about the continual resolving of a problem or main concern of the participants in a substantive area. The problem is the main mover of action in a substantive area. Grounded theory accounts for the action, which is the participants' behavior as they continually resolve their problem. The problem is found in the data and must be discovered through the constant comparative method, which entails jointly coding and analyzing the data. Glaser (2001) warns that the problem must be conceptualized and not described. Data can be newly collected or previously compiled qualitative data (Glaser & Strauss, 1967). Every incident is coded for a category and compared with previous incidents in the same category. As coding continues, incidents are compared with properties of the category. One of the rules of the constant comparative method is to stop coding and write up a memo as soon as the researcher thinks of ideas pertaining to the developing substantive theory.

In analyzing data, different conceptual levels emerge. The first level is the data themselves, while the second level is the conceptualization of the data into categories with their properties. The third level occurs with the overall integration into a theory (Glaser, 1998).

There are two types of codes that an analyst generates: substantive and theoretical. Substantive codes conceptualize the categories and their properties that image the empirical substance of the area being studied. Theoretical codes, on the other hand, conceptualize how the substantive codes relate to each other as hypotheses in explaining how the main concern is resolved (Glaser, 2005). The interaction between these two types of codes characterizes grounded theory. Some popular theoretical codes include basic social processes, cutting point, and the 6 Cs (Glaser, 1978). Some newer theoretical coding families include the paired opposite family, scale family, and unit identity family (Glaser, 1998).

The generation of a substantive theory occurs around a core category that accounts for the majority of the variation in the pattern of behavior of the participants in resolving the main core or problem. A core category can be any theoretical code. A popular core category is a basic social process (BSP). A BSP has two or more clear emergent stages. Just as the problem did, a core category emerges from the data and is discovered.

RESEARCH QUESTIONS

♦ What is the specific social psychological problem that women experience during postpartum depression?
♦ What social psychological process do postpartum depressed women use to resolve this fundamental problem?

DATA COLLECTION

In the original grounded theory study (Beck, 1993), data collection took place over an 18-month period. The researcher assisted in facilitating the postpartum depression support group, which met twice a month throughout this time. During the group meetings, the researcher's role was one of nursing consultant to the mothers by answering questions, providing suggestions, and helping to facilitate the group meetings. The number of participants who attended each support group meeting ranged from 1 to 12. Husbands periodically attended the meetings. After each support group meeting, the researcher immediately wrote field notes on the interactions that had occurred during the meeting. Twelve of the mothers who attended the support group were interviewed in depth. The interviews took place in private either in the women's home or in the facility where the support group was held. After obtaining informed consent, the researcher asked mothers to describe their experiences with postpartum depression.

Varied interviewing techniques were used. At the beginning of data collection, interviews consisted of open-ended questions, and the mothers were permitted to talk with no imposed limits. Women told their stories of postpartum depression. As the theory developed, later interviews consisted of specific questions related to the emerging categories. The same emergent interview questions were not asked of all the mothers. As categories became saturated, questions related to those categories were no longer asked in subsequent interviews. Toward the end of data collection, interviews became shorter in length. Interview questions were constantly refined (Table 9–1).

TABLE 9–1   Selected Examples of Interview Questions

Initial Interview Questions

Would you please share with me what it is like to experience postpartum depression?

If you have recovered from your postpartum depression, could you tell me your story from the beginning when your symptoms first appeared and continue through your recovery?

Focused Interview Questions

Once you made the decision to seek professional help, what was your experience with the health care system?

Was there anything or anyone that would trigger your anxiety?

Some mothers have said that when they were suffering from postpartum depression they did not feel real. If you experienced similar feelings, could you please describe them for me?

Theoretical sampling guided data collection and the development of the emerging theory. Data were jointly collected, coded, and analyzed to indicate which data to collect next and where to go to find those data. Theoretical sampling yielded theoretical saturation of categories. Saturation was achieved when comparisons of more incidents resulted in no more properties of the categories (Glaser, 1998, 2001). Throughout data collection, memos were written, for instance, regarding any ideas about codes and their relationships or about direction for theoretical sampling (Table 9–2). At the final stage of the grounded theory process, the piles of memos from the memo bank were sorted into an outline that guided the write-up of the findings.

In this grounded theory modification, the results from the 10 qualitative studies on the experience of postpartum depression in women from different cultures were compared with the findings from the original teetering on the

TABLE 9–2   Example of a Theoretical Sampling Memo

Mothers are repeatedly sharing that they feel so alone because their family and friends don't understand just how devastating the postpartum depression is for them. Mothers are isolating themselves from their husbands/partners, their mothers, sisters, and friends.

Do mothers also distance themselves from their infants? If women are multiparas, do they isolate themselves from their older children? I need to include these questions in my next interviews to explore the properties of the category of isolating oneself.

edge to extend the properties of the categories and to increase the scope of this grounded theory. Described in the following section are the modified results of teetering on the edge.

RESULTS*

Loss of control was the basic social psychological problem in postpartum depression. One mother stated that *"I had absolutely no control and that was the scariest thing because I always had control."* Women lacked control over their emotions, thought processes, and actions. One mother described it as *"I just couldn't get out of the pain. It's like you hurt so bad and you don't want to be that way and yet you lose all control of everything"* (Beck, 1993, p. 44). Hong Kong Chinese women echoed this loss of control (Chan et al., 2002). As one Chinese mother shared, *"I suffered greatly. I could not control my emotion and behavior"* (p. 574). For African American women, *"losing it was associated with the lowest and most difficult point of PPD"* (Amankwaa, 2003, p. 303). African American mothers reported loss of control of their ability to care for their babies, their families, and themselves.

The basic social psychological process of postpartum depression is the process of teetering on the edge, which refers to walking the fine line between sanity and insanity. Women suffering from postpartum depression attempted to cope with the problem of loss of control through a four-stage process (Figure 9–1). The stages that emerged from the data included (1) encountering terror, (2) dying of self, (3) struggling to survive, and (4) regaining control. For each stage, the three levels of coding were identified, compared and contrasted, and collapsed. Figure 9–2 is an example of a portion of the audit trail illustrating the comparing and collapsing of level I and II codes for the construct of dying of self (Beck, 1993).

Encountering Terror

In the initial stage, women were hit suddenly and unexpectedly by the postpartum depression. The syndrome can begin within the first few weeks after delivery or can be delayed until 6 months or more after birth. When postpartum depression hit, mothers felt trapped in a dark tunnel with no foreseeable escape. As one mother poignantly described: *"I was on cloud nine through my whole pregnancy. I was very happy in the hospital. Then it hit me when my baby was 14 days old. One night I had my first severe panic attack. I*

---

*Results are excerpted with permission from the original study: Beck, C. T. (1993). Teetering on the Edge: A substantive theory of postpartum depression. *Nursing Research, 42,* 44–47.

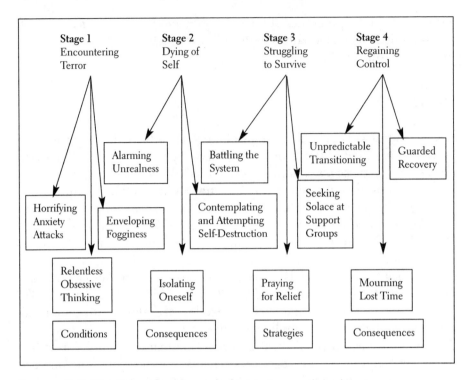

FIGURE 9–1 The four-stage process of teetering on the edge
Source: Reprinted with permission from "Teetering on the Edge: A Substantive Theory of Postpartum Depression," by C. T. Beck, 1993, *Nursing Research, 42,* p. 43.

felt like everything was closing in on me. Something just snapped in me and there was no going back" (Beck, 1993, p. 44).

Mothers described this onslaught as *"going to the gates of hell and back," "your worst possible nightmare," "everything was falling apart piece by piece," "the bottom fell out,"* and *"your whole world turned upside down."* Three conditions of encountering terror can occur during this first stage: horrifying anxiety, relentless obsessive thinking, and enveloping fogginess" (Beck, 1993, p. 44).

Horrifying Anxiety.   When anxiety attacks hit, the mothers felt that they were literally losing their minds. Women repeatedly stated that the anxiety attacks were worse than the depression they felt. Three different mothers described their experiences with anxiety attacks as follows:

> *"When it first hit me at 7 months I had a major anxiety attack. It came out of the blue. I just felt numb all over and I started to hyperventilate.*

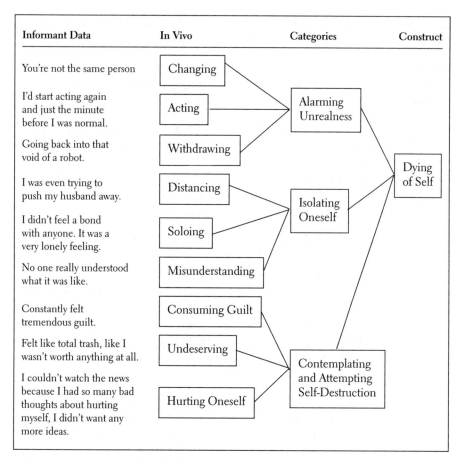

FIGURE 9–2 Partial audit trail for the construct of dying of self

Source: Reprinted with permission from "Teetering on the Edge: A Substantive Theory of Postpartum Depression," by C. T. Beck, 1993, *Nursing Research, 42,* p. 44.

> *I felt this pain in my chest so I started to think, Oh my God, I'm having a heart attack. I'm dying!"*
> "*It was like every nerve in my body was exploding. Like little fireworks were going off all over my body. I felt like I was going crazy.*"
> "*My skin felt like it was literally crawling. I wished I could rip it off and put it on another body. I would try and wipe my skin off.*" (Beck, 1993, p. 45)

Hong Kong Chinese women suffering from postpartum depression were so anxious that something dreadful would happen to their babies that they experienced "phantom crying" (Chan et al., 2002). "Phantom crying was a common experience in which they reported actually hearing their baby cry, but when they went to check, the baby was sound asleep" (p. 575).

Relentless Obsessive Thinking. Throughout their waking hours, the women were bombarded with obsessive thoughts, such as these shared by two mothers:

> *"My thoughts were extremely obsessive. They would never stop. I thought, Oh my God, am I going crazy? What if I have to be admitted to the hospital? And so on. It was just nonstop."*
> *"I was living constantly in these terrible thoughts that I was a horrible person, a horrible mother, and questioning what's wrong with me. I was just obsessed with this all day long."* (Beck, 1993, p. 45)

All this obsessive thinking left the mothers mentally and physically exhausted. At the end of the day, the women could not even look forward to some relief because, as one mother put it, *"I would lay in bed and the thoughts would just go and go and go. I thought I was going to go insane"* (Beck, 1993, p. 45).

Women in India revealed that when a woman thinks too much she becomes weak, drowsy, and loses her appetite. She cannot eat or do anything (Rodrigues et al., 2003). One mother shared that when she feels this way she just wants to end her life.

Enveloping Fogginess. During this initial stage of postpartum depression, the fogginess settled in. Mothers experienced loss of concentration and sometimes of motor skills. This fogginess is clearly illustrated in the following two quotes from mothers:

> *"I could not concentrate to read a book. I had been a very avid reader and could comprehend well. I lost all that in my postpartum depression. I would have to read lines over two and three times. People would talk to me and all I would see was their lips moving."*
> *"Oh, I tried to do something—go out for a run, visit a friend, or take the baby to the mall—but it didn't work. The fogginess would set in."* (Beck, 1993, p. 45)

A Hmong mother with postpartum depression suffered so much from difficulty concentrating she experienced physical symptoms. *"So many problems with concentrating. Sometimes I feel like my breath is short and my head is pounding so big, I feel like I'm going to fade away, so I can't concentrate"* (Stewart & Jambunathan, 1996, p. 325).

An African American mother remembered vividly how she could not even concentrate to wash her face: *"I'd try to get a mental grip. Okay. Go over and pick up the soap, you know, the routine. It is like we have a routine of doing things, and I couldn't really remember what the routine was. It was like, well, wow, I must really be, you know, out of it. I can't even wash my face."* (Amankwaa, 2003, p. 304)

Dying of Self

As a result of the conditions in the initial stage of postpartum depression, the dying of mothers' normal selves occurred during stage 2. This stage consisted of the following three consequences: alarming unrealness, isolating oneself, and contemplating and attempting self-destruction. These three consequences were involuntary responses to the conditions in stage 1.

Alarming Unrealness. In alarming unrealness, mothers' normal selves were no longer present. Neither the women nor their husbands knew who these women were. Husbands asked where their wives had gone. During postpartum depression, women repeatedly said that they did not feel real. They felt like robots just going through the motions of taking care of their babies. They felt void and empty of any caring emotions. Several mothers vividly described this transformation:

> *"One minute I'd be socializing and laughing and talking. All of a sudden I would feel like all those emotions were being physically sucked away from you and you'd go back into that void of a robot, like you'd just start acting."*
> *"It's very scary. You feel as though you are not the same person. You are afraid your children aren't going to have you for a mother."*
> *"The roughest part was between me and my husband. It had gotten to the point where I didn't know him anymore because he didn't know me anymore. He felt like he was living with a Dr. Jekyll and Mr. Hyde."*
> *"My big fear was that I wasn't going to ever be the person I had been before postpartum depression. I was terrified and I'd cry hysterically."* (Beck, 1993, p. 45)

Women in Canada also experienced loss of self (Berggren-Clive, 1998). Postpartum depressed mothers struggled with their identity and asked themselves, "Who am I?" A Canadian mother's quote illustrates this:

> *"You know how water runs over the rock and it eventually smooths them down and then you end up with the Grand Canyon. Well, that was very much what it was like. You can maintain your boundaries for so long, but the water wears you away. It doesn't matter if you are*

*made of rock or steel or you are made of paper, the water wears you
away. I lost completely who I was. Completely."* (p. 112)

Isolating Oneself.   Isolation was another consequence of the second stage
of postpartum depression. Mothers lost all interest in things they had previously enjoyed, their interests and goals, and their families and friends. They
felt alienated and alone because they believed no one understood what they
were going through. They feared that people thought they were bad mothers. Some of the women isolated themselves in their homes because they
were afraid to go anywhere. They repeatedly expressed a lack of interest in
sex. They also experienced a distancing of themselves from their babies: *"I
had these really weird feelings towards my baby. I couldn't be around him. He
gave me anxiety as if he were something bad. I couldn't walk past the door of
his room without becoming anxious"* (Beck, 1993, p. 45).

The isolation that postpartum depressed Middle Eastern women living in
Australia experienced was intensified because of their deep sensation of loneliness (Nahas et al., 1999). The migrant women missed the support from
their families in the Middle East. In Australia, without any close neighbors
from the Middle East, the mothers were left home alone during the day
while their husbands went to work.

Contemplating and Attempting Self-Destruction.   A third consequence
of the first stage of encountering terror was contemplating and attempting
self-destruction. Not only were these mothers pondering death, but some
also attempted self-destruction. Contributing to their thoughts of death was
the guilt they carried as a result of their perceptions of being failures as mothers and their thoughts of harming their babies:

> *I would go into my baby's room and think, put the blanket over his
> head. He's nothing. Then I'd start crying hysterically, I felt like the
> worst person in the world, the worst mother in the world. I felt
> tremendous guilt and just wanted to hurt myself.*

> *I started thinking death thoughts at one point. I didn't plan suicide,
> but I started thinking I'd be better off dead. I had never been that
> low in my whole life when I thought death was the way to go. I just
> wanted to get out of this world. It was like everything was black.*
> (Beck, 1993, pp. 45–46)

Two women not only contemplated self-destruction but also attempted to
carry out these thoughts by overdosing or cutting their wrists.

Canadian women also painfully shared similar thoughts of ending their
lives. As one mother described: *"There were moments when I was opening the*

can, the infalac, and the moment I opened it I wanted to take a knife and cut my wrists" (Berggren-Clive, 1998, p. 112).

Thoughts of harming themselves occurred in Hmong mothers, as the following quotes illustrate: *"Dying is much better . . . but if I die, who will take care of my kids?" "Better off dead than to be alive"* (Stewart & Jambunathan, 1996, p. 327).

Struggling to Survive

In struggling to survive, the third stage of teetering on the edge, women employed the following three strategies: battling the system, praying for relief, and seeking solace in a postpartum depression support group. The consequences in stage 2 became conditions requiring strategies by the women. Consequences of one set of actions can become part of the conditions affecting the next set of actions occurring in a sequence.

Battling the System.   Once the decision had been made to seek professional help, women began a tortuous path to find the appropriate treatment. Disappointment, frustration, humiliation, and anger were experienced by mothers in their initial call to health professionals for help:

> *"I picked up my phone and called my obstetrician. He never even returned the phone call. Three days later I called again and he told me there's nothing he could do for me and not to waste my time coming there just to talk."*
> *"I was very, very disappointed in my obstetrician's response to me. He patted me on the back and was very patronizing and said, 'You're only a mild case. I've had women come in here who were ten times worse.' "*
> (Beck, 1993, p. 46)

Obstetricians gave women the names and numbers of psychiatrists. However, some of these referrals were not successful because not all psychiatrists were knowledgeable about postpartum depression. The search would have to continue until a knowledgeable psychiatrist was found (Beck, 1993).

Use of antidepressants was the treatment of choice by psychiatrists, and Prozac was the drug prescribed most often. Some mothers required shock therapy and psychiatric hospitalization in addition to medications (Beck, 1993).

During their postpartum depression, some mothers found that they began to become hypochondriacs and reported physical symptoms. Some experienced chest pains during anxiety attacks and often went to the emergency room to validate that they were not having a heart attack (Beck, 1993).

Finances hindered some mothers from obtaining the professional help they needed, and health insurance often did not adequately cover the costs of psychiatric care: *"We couldn't afford to see a regular psychiatrist at over $100.00 an hour. We just didn't have that kind of money. So I went to our church for counseling, but they weren't really equipped to help me with my postpartum depression"* (Beck, 1993, p. 46).

Often complicating matters for postpartum depressed mothers living in different cultures than their own was the language barrier. Women from minority ethnic communities (Bangladeshi, Indian, other Asian, and Portugese) living in the United Kingdom often were not diagnosed as suffering from postpartum depression by their general practitioners because of the language barrier (Templeton et al., 2003).

Instead of understanding, Australian women reported patronizing attitudes from physicians toward their symptoms, which increased the mothers' feelings of low self-esteem and guilt (Holopainen, 2002). Postpartum depressed mothers in Ireland expressed negative comments toward health providers, using such words as *"rude, unsupportive, judgmental and constantly questioning my ability to be a good mother"* (Lawler & Sinclair, 2003, p. 39).

Praying for Relief. In addition to battling the system, women turned to prayer as a strategy in their struggle to survive:

> *"The Lord was what really got me through a lot. It was just a lot of prayer and crying to the Lord that helped me get through it."*
> *"I used to go to church and pray for hours. My God, how much more can I endure! You're not a vindictive or hateful God, but why is this happening to me? You have to get me out of this because I cannot take this any longer."* (Beck, 1993, p. 46)

Black Caribbean mothers trying to cope with their postpartum depression drew on spiritual support from black-led churchs. One woman shared, *"The support pulled me through it [postnatal depression]. There's no doubt about it! I was reading my Bible and I do follow the Rastafarian faith"* (Edge et al., 2004, p. 434).

Seeking Solace in a Support Group. Attending a postpartum depression support group was the third strategy women used in their struggle to survive. The support group helped to counter the isolation and loneliness the mothers felt, while introducing them to women who had recovered from postpartum depression. It provided hope that their depression could be overcome and that they would regain control of their lives. Being among other women suffering from postpartum depression helped to confirm the reality of the condition for the mothers. One woman poignantly described the benefits she received from the group: *"My doctor never told me about other women with postpartum depression. I was in the total dark the whole time. It wasn't until I* *started coming to the support groups that I realized, for God's sake, that other women went through this!"* (Beck, 1993, p. 47).

In Australia, mothers also viewed postpartum depression support groups in a positive light, as reflected by this quote: *"Finding people who were going through the same thing, having support I knew someone was there. . . . I never talked about anything, so just talking about it helped me to feel better after"* (Holopainen, 2002, p. 43).

One mother in Australia, however, initially benefited from attending a postpartum depression support group but after a while she became overloaded and could not cope with anyone else's problems. *"I'm sick of going there and everyone just sitting around saying the same thing. I'm fed up with it. . . . I just feel like my head is ready to explode most of the time"* (Holopainen, 2002, p. 43).

In Ireland, meeting other mothers suffering from postpartum depression was cited as one of the turning points in mothers' recovery (Lawler & Sinclair, 2003).

Regaining Control

Regaining control was the fourth and final stage of the substantive theory of teetering on the edge. Regaining control was a slow process consisting of three consequences: unpredictable transitioning, mourning lost time, and guarded recovery.

Unpredictable Transitioning.   The process of recovery from postpartum depression was not sudden. Occasionally, among the bad days, there would be a good one. Gradually, the number of good days experienced would increase until only a few bad days cropped up here and there. These would be unpredictable. This erratic transition to regaining control is illustrated in the following quote:

> *"When I got out of my severest depression, I had more good times than bad times. I had days where I felt like nothing bad ever happened. I mean, I was normal. I really felt such intense love for my baby. I could have a relationship with my husband. Then the next day for no reason at all I'd wake up and just be off."* (Beck, 1993, p. 47)

Mourning Lost Time.   As the mothers progressed in their recovery from postpartum depression, they began to mourn the lost time that they would not be able to recapture with their infants: *"I feel robbed of the first 6 months of my daughter's life. I never really got to hold her as a baby and I feel cheated."*

Another mother repeatedly walked through the baby departments of stores in the mall looking at infants' clothes, mourning her baby's infancy that had been lost because of postpartum depression. Throughout the recovery period, the mothers needed to work through these feelings of being cheated of the opportunity to experience unique periods of their children's lives (Beck, 1993, p. 47).

Women in Ireland also described feeling cheated of the joys of motherhood by their postpartum depression (Lawler & Sinclair, 2003).

Guarded Recovery.   Guarded recovery was the final consequence of the strategies of struggling to survive. This occurred when the mothers felt they had essentially recovered from postpartum depression. Mothers repeatedly noted how at this point in their recovery their husbands would say, *"Thank God, my wife is finally back!"* When mothers felt better, they would talk about how all the symptoms of postpartum depression just eventually faded away: *"When I was sick, I didn't want my baby, I didn't love my husband. I didn't want to work. I hated everything. When I got better, it all melted away"* (Beck, 1993, p. 47).

Postpartum depression, however, left an indelible mark on mothers' lives. Even after regaining control, they repeatedly stated they still feared that at some point in the future they could be stricken with the depression again: *"Postpartum depression makes you very, very vulnerable. You still feel like you're on a fine line between sanity and insanity because when it first happened it came out of nowhere. You're normal and then the next thing you know you're crazy"* (Beck, 1993, p. 47).

Canadian mothers agreed that coming through such a difficult time with postpartum depression left them with many scars. At the same time, however, surviving this ordeal became a source of strength for the women. As one woman expressed, *"I am a different person. Much stronger. I don't know how you could be the same person because so many things happen to make it different. Going through it was really terrible. I have the same family and a better understanding of myself"* (Berggren-Clive, 1998, p. 114).

DISCUSSION

Teetering on the edge emerged from the data as the BSP in this grounded theory of postpartum depression. As Glaser (1996, p. xv) claims, "The practical implications of a BSP gives a transcending picture that helps practitioners access, evaluate and develop desirable goals in a substantive area." The BSP suggests variables that yield interventions and the outcomes from such interventions. For practitioners, the BSP can be used as a guideline or framework for clinical practice to ground their efforts to assist the participants in resolving their main problem or concern. In this case, the BSP of teetering on the edge can become the framework for clinicians working with mothers suffering from postpartum depression. The richness of the four stages of teetering on the edge enables postpartum depressed women to feel understood and to benefit from appropriate interventions tailored to whichever stage of their recovery process they are currently in.

This grounded theory of postpartum depression gives women insightful ways they can gain some degree of control over the situation in which they find themselves. It is a theory of process and addresses the problem postpartum depressed mothers have to contend with in a language understandable to these women. This modified grounded theory now has wider applicability because all properties of its categories have been expanded from data from a number of cultural orientations.

A BSP also helps to organize and transcend the literature in a field (Glaser, 1996). For example, in the health care industry and organizational change literature, teetering on the edge is also operating (Mycek, 1999). When discussing steering health care institutions, Mycek warns that there is a catch to teetering on the edge. "Venture too far and you're in complete and total chaos. Don't go far enough and you become stuck in monotony. The secret lies in operating on the edge" (p. 10). Teetering on the edge is linked to chaos theory. Irons (as cited in Mycek, 1999, p. 11) proposes, "In chaos theory, you have to capitalize on trouble. . . . It's when you walk on the edge of losing control that you make progress." Kaiser (as cited in Mycek, 1999, p. 13) offers, "On the edge, you take responsibility for the creation of your preferred reality."

SUMMARIZING

Teetering on the edge emerged from the substantive area of postpartum depression. It can, however, be used to address problems that are related to loss of control in a variety of substantive areas. Suggestions for future research can focus on elevating teetering on the edge to a formal grounded theory. Its exploratory potential need not be confined to postpartum mood disorders. Loss of control, the main problem this grounded theory helps to resolve, can be found through a range of human conditions, such as binge eating (Johnson, Boutelle, Torgrud, Davig, & Turner, 2000), pathological gambling (Toce-Gerstein, Gerstein, & Volberg, 2003), dementia (Gilmour & Huntington, 2005), nonvocal ventilated patients (Carroll, 2004), emergency patients with unexpected surgery (Pearson & Kiger, 2004), and alcoholism (Bartek, Lindeman, & Hawks, 1999).

Glaser's (1998) four criteria for judging grounded theory include workability, relevance, fit, and modifiability. He calls these criteria product proof.

The proof of a grounded theory is in the outcome. Over the decade since the original teetering on the edge was developed (Beck, 1993), the theory (1) has worked to explain the relevant behavior of women suffering with postpartum depression, (2) has relevance to the depressed mothers and health professionals working in that clinical field, and (3) has fit the substantive area of postpartum mood and anxiety disorders. It is the fourth criterion for judging grounded theory, modifiability, for which this current revision of teetering on the edge has provided evidence. Teetering on the edge was readily modifiable as new data emerged from qualitative studies of cross-cultural experiences of postpartum depression.

REFERENCES

Agoub, M., Moussaoui, D., & Battas, O. (2005). Prevalence of postpartum depression in a Moroccan sample. *Archives of Women's Mental Health, 8*, 37–43.

Amankwaa, L. C. (2003). Postpartum depression among African-American women. *Issues in Mental Health Nursing, 24*, 297–316.

Bartek, J. K., Lindeman, M., & Hawks, J. H. (1999). Clinical validation of characteristics of the alcoholic family. *Nursing Diagnosis, 10*, 158–168.

Beck, C. T. (1992). The lived experience of postpartum depression: A phenomenological study. *Nursing Research, 41*, 166–170.

Beck, C. T. (1993). Teetering on the edge: A substantive theory of postpartum depression. *Nursing Research, 42*, 42–48.

Beck, C. T. (1999). Postpartum depression: Stopping the thief that steals motherhood. *AWHONN Lifelines, 3*, 41–44.

Berggren-Clive, K. (1998). Out of the darkness and into the light: Women's experiences with depression after childbirth. *Canadian Journal of Community Mental Health, 17*, 103–120.

Bhugra, D., & Gregorie, A. (1993). Social factors in the genesis and management of postnatal psychiatric disorders. In D. Bhugra & J. Leff (Eds.), *Principles of social psychiatry*. Oxford: Blackwell.

Carpiniello, B., Pariante, C. M., Serri, F., Costa, G., & Carta, M. G. (1997). Validation of the Edinburgh Postnatal Depression Scale in Italy. *Journal of Psychosomatic Obstetrics and Gynecology, 18*, 280–285.

Carroll, S. M. (2004). Nonvocal ventilated patients' perceptions of being understood. *Western Journal of Nursing Research, 26*, 85–112.

Chan, S. W., Levy, V., Chung, T. K., & Lee, P. (2002). A qualitative study of the experiences of a group of Hong Kong Chinese women diagnosed with postnatal depression. *Journal of Advanced Nursing, 39*, 571–579.

Dalton, K. (1996). *Depression after childbirth*. New York: Oxford University Press.

Edge, D., Baker, D., & Rogers, A. (2004). Perinatal depression among black Caribbean women. *Health and Social Care in the Community, 12*, 430–438.

Gilmour, J. A., & Huntington, A. D. (2005). Finding the balance: Living with memory loss. *International Journal of Nursing Practice, 11,* 118–124.

Glaser, B. G. (1978). *Theoretical sensitivity: Advances in the methodology of grounded theory.* Mill Valley, CA: Sociology Press.

Glaser, B. G. (1996). *Gerund grounded theory: The basic social process dissertation.* Mill Valley, CA: Sociology Press.

Glaser, B. G. (1998). *Doing grounded theory: Issues and discussions.* Mill Valley, CA: Sociology Press.

Glaser, B. G. (2001). *The grounded theory perspective: Conceptualization contrasted with description.* Mill Valley, CA: Sociology Press.

Glaser, B. G. (2003). *The grounded theory perspective II: Description's remodeling of grounded theory methodology.* Mill Valley, CA: Sociology Press.

Glaser, B. G. (2005). *The grounded theory perspective III: Theoretical coding.* Mill Valley, CA: Sociology Press.

Glaser, B. G., & Strauss, A. L. (1967). *The discovery of grounded theory.* New York: Aldine de Gruyter.

Holopainen, D. (2002). The experience of seeking help for postnatal depression. *Australian Journal of Advanced Nursing, 19,* 39–44.

Johnson, W. G., Boutelle, K. N., Torgrud, L., Davig, J. P., & Turner, S. (2000). What is a binge? The influence of amount, duration and loss of control criteria on judgments of binge eating. *International Journal of Eating Disorders, 27,* 471–479.

Kumar, R. (1994). Postnatal mental illness: A transcultural perspective. *Social Psychiatry and Psychiatric Epidemiology, 29,* 250–264.

Lawler, D., & Sinclair, M. (2003). Grieving for my former self: A phenomenological hermeneutical study of women's lived experience of postnatal depression. *Evidence Based Midwifery, 1,* 36–41.

Lee, D., Yip, A., Chiu, H., Leung, T., & Chung, T. (2001). A psychiatric epidemiological study of postpartum Chinese women. *American Journal of Psychiatry, 158,* 220–226.

Mycek, S. (1999). Teetering on the edge of chaos. *Trustee, 52,* 10–13.

Nahas, V. L., Hillege, S., & Amasheh, N. (1999). Postpartum depression: The lived experience of Middle Eastern migrant women in Australia. *Journal of Nurse-Midwifery, 44,* 65–74.

Nhiwatiwa, S., Patel, V., & Acuda, W. (1998). Predicting postnatal mental disorder with a screening questionnaire: A prospective cohort study from Zimbabwe. *Journal of Epidemiology and Community Health, 52,* 262–266.

Nicolson, P. (1990). Understanding postnatal depression: A mother-centered approach. *Journal of Advanced Nursing, 15,* 689–695.

Oates, M. R., Cox, J. L., Neena, S., Asten, P., Glangeud-Freudenthal, N., Figueiredo, B., et al. (2004). Postnatal depression across countries and cultures: A qualitative study. *British Journal of Psychiatry, 184*(suppl 46), 510–516.

O'Hara, M. W., & Swain, A. M. (1996). Rates and risk of postpartum depression: A meta-analysis. *International Review of Psychiatry, 8,* 37–54.

Patel, V., Rodrigues, M., & DeSouza, N. (2002). Gender, poverty and postnatal depression: A study of mothers in Goa, India. *American Journal of Psychiatry, 159,* 43–47.

Pearson, E., & Kiger, A. (2004). How emergency patients cope with their unexpected surgical event: An exploratory study. *Journal of Advanced Perioperative Care, 2,* 11–18.

Pillsbury, B. L. K. (1978). "Doing the month": Confinement and convalescence of Chinese women after childbirth. *Social Science and Medicine, 12,* 11–22.

Rahman, A., Iqbal, Z., & Harrington, R. (2003). Life events, social support and depression in childbirth: Perspective from a rural community in the developing world. *Psychological Medicine, 33,* 1161–1167.

Ramsay, R. (1993). Postnatal depression. *Lancet, 341,* 1358.

Regmi, S., Sligl, W., Carter, D., Grut, W., & Seear, M. (2002). A controlled study of postpartum depression among Nepalese women: Validation of the Edinburgh Postpartum Depression Scale in Kathmandu. *Tropical Medicine and International Health, 7,* 378–382.

Rodrigues, M., Patel, V., Jaswal, S., & deSouza, N. (2003). Listening to mothers: Qualitative studies on motherhood and depression from Goa, India. *Social Science and Medicine, 57,* 1797–1806.

Seel, R. M. (1986). Birth rite. *Health Visitor, 69,* 135–138.

Stern, G., & Kruckman, L. (1983). Multi-disciplinary perspectives on postpartum depression: An anthropological critique. *Social Science and Medicine, 17,* 1027–1041.

Stewart, S., & Jambunathan, J. (1996). Hmong women and postpartum depression. *Health Care for Women International, 17,* 319–330.

Templeton, L., Velleman, R., Persaud, A., & Milner, P. (2003). The experience of postnatal depression in women from Black and minority ethnic communities in Wiltshire, UK. *Ethnicity and Health, 8,* 207–221.

Toce-Gerstein, M., Gerstein, D. R., & Volberg, R. A. (2003). A hierarchy of gambling disorders in the community. *Addiction, 98,* 1661–1672.

Yamashita, H., Yoshida, K., Nakano, H., & Tashiro, N. (2000). Postnatal depression in Japanese women: Detecting the early onset of postnatal depression by closely monitoring the postpartum mood. *Journal of Affective Disorders, 58,* 145–154.

10

Ethnography: The Method

Zane Robinson Wolf

Ethnographic research started with investigators who sought out and experienced worlds different from their own and then tried to understand the meanings of social action within cultures. Thus, the behavior of informants or insiders was translated into social action that was meaningful as represented in ethnographic reports. Understanding the symbols of cultures helped investigators with interpretation. Many researchers distinguished themselves by "going native," by living with, learning and speaking the language of, and participating in the cultures of the people being studied. They valued the life-worlds of the "folk" who lived cultures dramatically different from the anthropologists'. Through their narrative descriptions, researchers revealed the social actions, beliefs, values, and norms of markedly different cultures from their viewpoints as outsiders, keeping the perspectives of informants very much in mind.

Moreover, ethnographers have continued to make explicit the common-sense knowledge of the cultures studied by revealing what the social worlds mean for the persons within the worlds and what they mean as insiders acting within them. Ethnographers portray shared understandings of insiders' worlds. Ethnographers study the processes of sense making that members of cultures use to create the social world and its factual properties (Leiter, 1980). Cultural rules inform, in part, human social behavior (Aamodt, 1982). Ethnographies begin with investigators taking a somewhat naïve position about the culture and its insiders. They are described as exploratory and hypothesis-generating studies.

Ethnographic research originated in the discipline of anthropology, caught the attention of the fields of sociology (Fox, 1959; Goffman, 1961; Liebow, 1993) and education, and appealed to nurse investigators in the 1960s and 1970s (Byerly, 1969; Germain, 2001; Pearsall, 1965; Ragucci, 1972). Later, nurse researchers (Robertson & Boyle, 1984; Thorne, 1991) emphasized the contribution of ethnographic research to nursing and pointed out what might be learned about health and illness phenomena as studied in cultural contexts. The works of ethnographers who produced classics continue to influence researchers (Douglas, 1963, 1966, 1975; Douglass, 1969; Firth, 1936; Malinowski, 1922, 1948; Mauss, 1967; Turner, 1957; Turner, 1967) and have stimulated ethnographers for decades (Spradley, 1970).

The ethnographic approach is a naturalistic, systematic, interpretive approach and relies on observation, interview, and description rather than statistics and experimentation (Ragucci, 1972). Detailed descriptions of phenomena in context and insights gained through interpretation are hallmarks of ethnography. Enthographies rely on two forms of authority, the personal experience of the ethnographer, the research instrument (Atkinson, 1992), and the report, which combines factual writing (Richardson, 1988) and reflects field notes, methodological notes, theoretical notes, and investigator diaries or personal notes.

Culture, according to Sapir (1924), embraces

> in a single term those general attitudes, views of life, and specific manifestations of civilization that give a particular people its distinctive place in the world. Emphasis is put not so much on what is done and believed by a people as on how what is done and believed functions in the whole life of that people, on what significance it has for them. (pp. 311–312)

Culture is also defined as the total way of life of a group and the learned behavior that is socially constructed and transmitted. Some questions of interest to ethnographers include what knowledge people use to interpret experience and mold their behavior within the context of their culturally constituted environment, what the nature of culture is, how culture emerges, how it is transmitted, and what the functions of culture are. Individuals in a culture hold common values and ideas acquired through learning from other members of the group. Ethnographies describe the unique and distinctive processes of culture. Cultural phenomena, beliefs, values, rules, and norms are ethnographic emphases.

Ethnography refers to a description of a culture or subculture. The term *ethnography* includes an account of the people of the culture and involves writing that depicts the culture. Ethnographic studies differ from other forms of qualitative research by their focus on the cultural perspective. By generating cultural descriptions, ethnographic investigations examine what the world is like for people who have learned to see, hear, speak, think, and act in ways that are different from dominant cultures or not yet described. Ethnographers do not attempt to alter the lives of the natives, folk, insiders, or informants.

Concepts of structure, function, and symbol orient ethnographic studies (Fetterman, 1989). Structure indicates the social structure of the group, such as how various positions and job descriptions function on a patient unit. Function points to the social relationships and interactions among the members of the group. Symbol, as condensed meaning, operates like a "cognitive reflex" and evokes "powerful feelings and thoughts" (Fetterman, 1989, p. 36).

Often, investigators acquire skill in the research techniques of ethnography during apprenticeships. Nonetheless, in spite of learning the rules under the guidance of a seasoned fieldworker, the ethnographic process is personalistic because no ethnographer works just like another. Also, one of the challenges for nurse ethnographers is the fact that nurses are also clinicians who study individuals in the circumstances of health and illness (Brody, 1981; Field, 1989). Research, not therapy, is the intent of ethnography. Nurse ethnographers always defer to the therapeutic imperative, however, when the welfare of patients is at stake, and data collection is suspended temporarily.

PURPOSES AND RESEARCH QUESTIONS

The process of identifying the purposes of ethnographic studies is a complex one. Investigators often have a general idea of a topic that interests them and gradually realize that an ethnographic study might be the best strategy to discover the meanings and understandings of a cultural group or subgroup of society and a topic about which little is understood. A review of the literature might take researchers outside of their discipline as they recognize how few studies have been conducted on the topic by nurse investigators. Eventually, they focus the purpose(s) and research questions because it is not possible to study the topic to complete understanding of cultural groups. Two examples from nursing ethnographies follow:

> Purpose: A descriptive analysis of the nature of nursing rituals was the focus of the ethnographic study. Questions: (1) What actions, words, and objects make up nursing rituals? (2) What are the types of nursing rituals demonstrated by professional nurses caring for adult patients on a unit? (3) What explicit or manifest meanings do these rituals

have to nurses, patients and their families, and to other hospital personnel, such as physicians, licensed practical nurses, and nursing assistants? (4) What implicit or latent meanings are identified by the nurses, patients, and other hospital personnel, and by the investigator? (5) How are patients, physicians, licensed practical nurses, aides, and orderlies involved in theses nursing rituals? (6) How are nursing rituals embedded within the context of the routines, procedures, and reports of the nursing unit? (Wolf, 1986, pp. 2–3)

The main question to be answered was: How do elders survive in the midst of "drug warfare" in an inner-city community known for its dangerous streets and public spaces? (Kaufman, 1995, p. 231)

Although problem definition and the purpose of studies are common expectations for investigations, ethnographers often discuss the evolving nature of the purpose as participant observation gears up. Emergent decisions characterize ethnographies and are ongoing as investigators reflect on what has already been learned. However, the members of institutional review boards, acting as guardians protecting human subjects from harm, demand specificity from proposals, such as the amount of time to be spent in the field; the expected number, gender, and race of informants; and how much time individual informants will be observed and interviewed. Although this is challenging, ethnographers must create a plan for data collection that best addresses how they intend to achieve the purpose of the study. They are called upon to notify institutional review boards of changes in data collection plans and sampling frames as issues emerge that warrant additional attention.

ETHNOGRAPHIC METHODS

Ethnographic methods are distinctive because of use of self as an observer, on-site fieldwork, prolonged engagement in the fieldwork, interviews ranging from informal (unstructured) to formal (structured), event analysis, and document and artifact analysis. Fieldwork is considered a rite of passage for the "genuine" anthropologist, sociologist fieldworker, or ethnographer (Ward & Werner, 1984). Data collection is qualitative and inductive. The ethnographer creates a raw record during data collection that is written as text. The thick description (observing, recording, and analyzing a culture so that signs are interpreted to gain meaning and understanding within the culture) (Geertz, 1973) produced by investigators takes a naturalistic stance in which the detailed patterns of cultural and social relationships are disclosed and placed in context. Interpretation is based on the meanings that actions and events have for members of the culture. Ethnographers' work with key informants leads to interpretations that cannot be separated from time, place, events, and actions of people. The culture to be studied through ethnography might be a society, community, subculture, organization, group, or phenomena such as beliefs, rituals, events, routines, interactions, or any other aspect of human existence.

Participant Observation

Participant observation is defined as the method by which investigators join the insiders of a culture so that human relationships, events, patterns, and sociocultural contexts in which people live and work can be studied (Jorgensen, 1989). Investigators participate in the daily life of the members of the group. Participant observation, achieved through the experience of investigators' fieldwork, is a chief source of data. Ethnographers use themselves as participant observers as they gather data during fieldwork by observing and interviewing. Through this involvement, they achieve on-site, temporary membership in the culture. Everyday life is studied and accessed through observations that are open-ended, flexible, opportunistic, factual, and situated in settings. The physical and social environment of the informants being studied provides the context. Total immersion in the culture, accomplished by living with the natives or insiders, is preferable for participant observers.

Some ethnographers use a team participant observation approach, whereas others conduct studies alone. Participant observation is useful for the study of alien, foreign, or exotic cultures; topics about which little is known; or everyday circumstances about which knowledge is assumed, but not necessarily examined. During participant observation, researchers learn the use of insider language and later seek clarification and understanding during interviews. Patience and open-mindedness are required characteristics of ethnographers.

Participant observers are strangers to the communities to be studied and gradually and temporarily become members of the group (Stocking, 1983). They have been called "marginal natives" (Freilich, 1970). In contrast, Shokeid (1988) disputes this idea and prefers the term "professional stranger," one who develops closeness, detachment, indifference, and participation with informants. Developing face-to-face relationships is essential, and acceptance by the insiders, especially the gatekeepers, who may or may not be key informants, is crucial. Building trust and establishing relationships early in the first stages of the research are important aims. The quality of relationships is important as is the position and status of informants and investigators.

Participant observation is performed as a data collection strategy and helps ethnographers reduce the problem of reactivity. Fieldworkers are able to formulate interview questions using the native language. Participant observation enables investigators to answer research problems that are not easily answered by other methods. It takes time and requires ethnographers to learn the roles of informants, understand their language, learn the functions and structures of the culture through explicit and implicit interpretation, build knowledge about the topic through increasingly focused participant observation, maintain curiosity and a naïve approach, and build the writing and analytic skills demanded by descriptive and analytic field notes and the ultimate product of the study, the ethnography.

Participant observation demands that investigators remain ethical by overt, that is, with the knowledge of insiders', involvement. Covert investigations have been conducted; however, human subjects' considerations have ideally eliminated them. Overt participant observation demands observations to be direct, on-site, and to return over an extended period of time. According to Spradley (1980), culture, the knowledge that people learn as members of a group, cannot be observed directly. However, the ethnographer directly observes the group of insiders. Cultural knowledge is gained through tacit and explicit understandings developed over the introductory, focused observation, and coding stages (Keith, 1986) of projects. Inferences are developed by investigators. Observation is open-ended, and the surprises of fieldwork demand that investigators are flexible and opportunistic, following the inquiry where it leads. They define sources of data and identify informants as the investigation progresses.

Junker (1960) describes participant observation roles of fieldworkers: participant as observer, observer as participant, complete participant, and complete observer. The complete participant may gradually become participant as observer. Another complete participant may never leave the role, however, and will remain completely ethnocentric and never become a social scientist. The complete observer may have a better chance of becoming a social scientist, emphasizes observation more than participation, and eventually moves to observer as participant. Although Junker's notions of the role seem somewhat artificial, they do describe the dynamic nature of individual participant observers as they enter the field. Initially, fieldworkers observe more often. They gain the trust of informants, ask permission to observe, and gradually move among the various roles, depending on the situations and people at the center of attention. Thus, the idea of participant observer presents like a continuum of roles, where the movement from pure observer to pure participant depends on the social scene, how comfortable the ethnographer is at the moment, and which aspect of the culture calls for more study. Before the ideal participant observer role is achieved, investigators often find themselves explaining the purpose of the study repeatedly to potential informants. Furthermore, relationships with informants, once established, must be carefully maintained as everyday life is studied as unobtrusively as possible (Jorgensen, 1989). However, the more ethnographers participate, the less likely they are to observe, limiting access by restricting the time available for recording and analyzing events, actors, and everyday life.

In contrast to Junker (1960), Adler and Adler (1987) describe varying roles of membership involvement, peripheral membership, active membership, and complete membership. Peripheral membership is the most marginal, yet these ethnographers interact often and closely with informants through direct, firsthand experience. They do not assume functional roles within the group of informants. Active membership goes further, with the researchers becoming more engaged with the central activities of the group. They become co-participants in the research. Complete membership requires ethnographers to achieve equal status with informants. They are completely immersed in the field; some become the phenomenon, while others are more opportunistic (Adler & Adler, 1987). Similar to the point made about Junker's (1960) notions of participant observation, the nature of fieldwork demands movement among the various role classifications, with ethnographers ideally not frozen in one.

Participant observers are outsiders who gradually gain insider knowledge of the culture. Often they transform to insider status and perform various roles over the course of the study. For example, in a study that took place on a nursing unit, one investigator (Wolf, 1986) transported laboratory slips, helped with patient care when a member of the nursing staff needed assistance caring for patients, and listened to the complaints of the staff about working conditions. Others assumed the "socially acceptable incompetent" (Lofland & Lofland, 1984, p. 38) position in which a nurse made beds, fetched and carried, and made tea (Hopkins, 2002) and provided comfort and emotional support (Varcoe, 2001). Such roles must fit within the scope of the investigators' expertise (Jorgensen, 1989) and are limited by the chief purpose that brought them to the field, the study. The "socially acceptable incompetent" position helps ethnographers to assume the role of the ones to be taught. It may be necessary to refuse to perform some duties, either because of human subjects' considerations consistent with restrictions of institutional review boards, awareness that the activity might blur fieldworkers' role with informants, or conflicts about threatened patient safety.

Fieldwork

Fieldwork is a disciplined mode of inquiry that engages the ethnographer firsthand in data collection over extended periods of time. It combines art and science so that the accomplished ethnographer produces a narrative that offers insight and understanding of human social life to a "discerning audience" (Wolcott, 1995, p. 251). Ethnographic fieldwork has a bias toward cultural interpretation, involves the study of people in social interaction, and aims to understand the culture from the native point of view (Spradley, 1980; Wolcott, 1995). Fieldwork informs ethnographers about the cultures of groups. Doing fieldwork demands that observations are recorded in a systematic manner. It requires that ethnographers make a commitment to the individuals being studied; intimate, long-term acquaintances result. Fieldwork by participant observation is a hallmark of ethnography (Stocking, 1983).

During fieldwork, ethnographers attempt to carry out the purpose of the study, although some of the subsequent questions asked, interviews conducted, and observations scheduled are emergent. Participant observation begins with performing broad descriptive observations, analyzing data, making focused observations, and conducting increasingly more focused interviews. Through fieldwork, ethnographers gain primary data from informants in context, moving among various situations, crises, and events.

The 12-month standard of ethnographic fieldwork has been accepted for many decades. However, this guideline is tempered by a judgment of the adequacy of the knowledge accumulated during uninterrupted or interrupted field encounters (Wolcott, 1995). Instead of specifying the length of time, some refer to the length of engagement as long-term immersion in the field.

Although the ethnographer's role of the "pure" participant observer is an ideal and must be visible to insiders, researchers benefit most when people carry out everyday activities so that fieldwork is conducted unobtrusively. Informants become so accustomed to the presence of investigators that investigators seem part of the typical surroundings of the settings for the study. This takes time. Ethnographers try to conduct the study without having an impact on the lives of informants. Also of note is the fact that in spite of well-developed plans for data collection, fieldwork for all first-time ethnographers is learned by doing.

Because ethnographers are strangers to informants, it takes time for ethnographers to establish themselves in the culture of the group. Courtesy and patience are required during participant observation. Ethnographers have to show up, day after day, so that people begin to learn their commitment to the study (Wolcott, 1995). They share stories and food and often develop rapport or friendships.

Fieldwork requires ethnographers to collect data using a variety of sources: structured and unstructured direct observations of events, including interaction analysis and situations; observation and recording of the characteristics of the physical environment through drawings, maps, photography, and videotapes; audiotapes; social network analysis; unstructured, semistructured, and structured interviews with informants; document analysis; and artifact analysis.

Fieldwork taxes the energy of investigators and is intellectually challenging, particularly as data collection and analysis progress. The work that is accomplished between field notes and the readable prose generated at the completion of studies is significant (Agar, 1986). It is also stimulating and exciting as ethnographers illuminate taken-for-granted worlds and sensitize readers to commonsense knowledge.

Fieldwork also demands making explicit what is intuitively understood about what is going on in contexts. When rapport is established with members of the group, ethnographers learn to act with them. Next, they pull back to plan additional observations, write field notes, analyze data, think critically, and return for more interviews and observations. Cultural knowledge is gained on a daily basis during fieldwork; ethnographers return repeatedly to the field.

Access to the Cultural Group and Informants

Ethnographers rely on gatekeepers to help them gain access to potential informants. For example, prominent administrators of a hospital or school and community leaders are approached to review proposals. They act as valuable consultants to the investigation and often give advice that benefits studies. They might sponsor the proposal during review by institutional review boards. Gatekeepers provide names of potential primary informants (DeSantis, 1990), and investigators use leaders' names to establish credibility within the group.

It may be very difficult to select and gain access to settings. Many ethnographers rely on personal acquaintances to review the potential fit of settings with the topic of the investigation (Jorgensen, 1989). In one ethnographic study, a physician colleague suggested the hospital where he was employed as an ideal setting. Subsequent meetings with nurse administrators led the nurse investigator to realize the group's lack of commitment to nursing research and the proposed ethnography. Although political pressure could have been brought to bear on the nurse administrators, the investigator soon realized the futility of such efforts despite her disappointment. Later, a nurse administrator who was eager to support research within his hospital provided access and continued support for currently proposed and future investigations. Initial acceptance into the field by gatekeepers and later by informants is critical to the success of investigations.

Within the same study (Wolf, 1986), the investigator realized that some aspects of the nursing unit were more closed to fieldwork than were others. Whereas most of the nursing staff of the night shift welcomed her, two licensed practical nurses were suspicious of her motives and seemed to fear negative reports to supervisors. The investigator conducted fieldwork for a few nights and decided to rely on the permanent night nurse's talents as a key informant. Much of the data collection was visible to all staff, conducted front stage. Some participant observation episodes were private and backstage, such as witnessing nurses bathing patients and performing postmortem care.

Informants, actors, or insiders are members of the cultural group. They are knowledgeable about topics and understand how things work in the culture. Informants must be willing to share knowledge with ethnographers by providing detailed explanations from insiders' points of view and providing the time and opportunity to be interviewed and observed. Key and other informants are crucial to the task of the ethnographer. Informants are chosen to share information about the research topic and the cultural group. Key informants are chosen after time is spent in the field during preliminary data collection. Each informant may or may not be able to explain subtleties of the culture. Different individuals serve different functions. Some are key, some are primary, and some are secondary. Ethnographers are informant-centered, and as such actively participate in the research process. Because interviews and participant observation are key data sources, the ethnographer must work to develop trust relationships and collaborate with informants (Kleinman, 1988). It is through trust that informants allow ethnographers entrée to insiders' knowledge. Investigators often learn during fieldwork that informants ascribe their own interpretations to the nature of the research and form their own versions of the method. Many informants welcome investigators; however, at times a few do not. These few may remain suspicious over the course of data collection, seeing the study as an "I spy" opportunity for researchers that might situate informants at risk in the community or at work.

As the investigator conducts interviews and performs the work of participant observation, close relationships often develop. On the one hand, the intimate, meaningful, and trusting relationships among informants and fieldworkers are a privilege that investigators cherish for a lifetime. On the other hand, analysis forces ethnographers to stand back periodically and detach as coding and interpretation progress. It is wise to develop rapport with informants rather than friendships (Glesne, 1989). The time investigators are in the field enables them to develop relationships distinguished by confidence and trust. Rapport serves the interests of ethnographers in that they can acquire data easily while reducing the distance between informants and themselves, quieting informants' anxiety about being observed and described, and building trust. In contrast, friendships may hinder access to cultural knowledge because informants may overidentify with investigators. Some informants may be so preferred that data gathering is limited, or informants act in atypical ways or to impress researchers (Glesne, 1989). The distance between informants and fieldworkers arises chiefly because of theoretical reflections and analysis. However, understanding the life-worlds of informants is achieved by entering into the subjectivity of their experiences during fieldwork (Adler & Adler, 1987). Intimate familiarity with the culture is a goal (Lofland, 1976).

The nature of relationships and the insider knowledge gained are protected by the ethical codes of investigators. It is not likely that the anonymity of informants is totally protected because the data collection period is prolonged and other study informants have also shared in the situations and events of the field research. However, to protect confidentiality, researchers use pseudonyms, limit access to data and records, secure records, and may eliminate or change small facts when writing the results of the study at informants' request or to protect disclosure of informants' identities that may place them at risk. Informants might become distrustful of members of their community if all possible protections are not used. Also, the uses of the study results may not be under the control of investigators (DeSantis, 1990). Nonetheless, ethnographers do their best to adhere to the strategies that protect human subjects and sites. Members of institutional review boards might have limited knowledge of ethnographic research so that prior to approval and entry into fieldwork, investigations may need to establish the legitimacy of the design (Reid, 1991).

One of the chief strategies that ethnographers use to protect informants is providing direct access to the narrative results prior to publication or public presentation. This is referred to as "member check" by Lincoln and Guba (1985). Informants might request that the investigator suppress or change findings, might refuse to permit the study to be published, or might restrict data collection (Hammersley & Atkinson, 1983).

Investigators develop ongoing relationships with key or primary informants. Because of the close relationships that investigators develop with informants, it is necessary for ethnographers to maintain distance by being visible as researchers, by adhering to the focus of the study and the evolving nature of data collection, and by respecting the confidentiality of the people studied.

The number of informants varies according to the topic. A study of a nursing unit includes a more limited number of potential informants, who may all be included in observations and interviews, than does one of a community or large group. Preliminary participant observation helps investigators to focus and restrict the number of informants. Some use purposive sampling to include the fullest range of informants, events, and situations being studied. This approach helps to obtain a more manageable number of interviews and observations.

Field Notes

Ethnographers try to gain an inclusive and extensive picture of the group under study. How people act and the descriptions of activities are main sources of cultural knowledge and are gained through interpretation. Although it is not possible to gain understanding of the whole culture or group, ethnographers work toward understanding a holistic outlook of the purpose of the study. The main data source of ethnographic records is written field notes. "Field notes make 'the field' manageable and memorable" (Atkinson, 1992, p. 18). Field notes involve writing, in which observations and interviews are constructed and reconstructed, and reading the notes (Atkinson, 1992) when interpretation is performed. Field notes identify the dates, days, times, settings and the names, status, and activities of informants being observed. They often combine native language and observer language. Ethnographers record in the language they use in everyday situations (Spradley, 1980). Accurate records of what informants say are documented through verbatim transcriptions of audiotaped and videotaped interviews. When unstructured interviews are conducted, investigators paraphrase in field notes what informants say as soon as possible.

Field notes are written with a great amount of detail. Concrete language is used to reveal the physical and social details of each observational episode. Because initial field notes often are condensed and preferably recorded on the spot, ethnographers return to expand them as soon as possible. Computers have facilitated this process.

During fieldwork, ethnographers develop habits of recording observations through narrative records. Care is paid to identifying the informants as actors, identifying the location, date, and time of the episodes observed, as well as retaining duplicate copies of field notes and storing them in separate, safe locations. Field notes enable the published results to adhere to the "thick description" standard espoused by Geertz (1973). Field notes help investigators describe and analyze cultures; the data recorded are rooted in the realities of the episodes, situations, informants in action, and events witnessed by ethnographers. As they observe and record field notes, ethnographers think and reflect on social events, the use of space and artifacts, and informant conduct. Field notes begin with extensive detailed description with little evaluation or summary; they note language events, situations, leadership roles (formal and informal), and informants of importance. Next, they become more focused; tentative hypotheses may be stated about themes and patterns in observations. Ethnographers conduct more focused interviews, perform final coding, and often return to the field for more focused observations and field notes that are again coded to understand patterns in question. The finished product with the best "thick description" reveals the abstract and general patterns and traits of social life in cultures. Readers get a sense of the emotions, thoughts, and perceptions of informants.

It is wise for ethnographers to remind themselves to remain nonjudgmental about individuals and cultural practices (Fetterman, 1989). Keeping personal notes separate from field notes might assist ethnographers to guard against biases and help prevent them from imposing their own culture on the one being studied.

During fieldwork, ethnographers make decisions about how to include and exclude events and informants, staying true to the research topic. Informants and their actions are observed along with the manner in which they interact with each other. Participant observation assists ethnographers in making choices about who to interview and which situations to witness. Interviews follow next in which informants, as members of the group or culture, are asked to explain what they see and how they perceive what is going on, and to share their interpretations of events, rules, and roles. Systematic field notes, recorded by the ethnographer day after day, reflect what is learned through the perspectives of investigators. No matter whether the field notes record the events and actors during typical or atypical days, the ideal notes are characterized by "thick description." Such a narrative conveys the cultural scene, with details that other readers would appreciate almost as if they were witnesses. It is important that ethnographers pay attention to describing the language of informants and the language researchers select to depict each observation.

Field notes accumulate over time. Well-written field notes reveal the interplay of informants in natural contexts. The individuals, events, and situations change rapidly; crises occur. This results in ethnographers shifting attention to capture interaction. Field notes record the documentation of unexpected events. Precise control of factors is irrelevant. By capturing the stage or context, the actors, the behaviors involved in interaction, and the meaning and significance of the symbolic parts, field notes and, later, analysis, help investigators gain understanding of the culture.

The physical depiction of the site is described in field notes, including photographs, drawings, and the use of space and time. Time during 24-hour, weekly, and monthly cycles frames events and behavior. The amount of field notes and other documents collected demands that investigators develop organized systems of data retrieval. Computer files, backup files, and scanned documents are stored in logical, indexed formats. They need to be organized initially and sequentially to facilitate data analysis. These files are arranged in an easily accessible manner and are augmented by other documents, photographs, maps, and available materials that expand the material on which data analysis depends.

Some investigators print field notes and organize them chronologically in loose-leaf binders. Backup printouts of field notes should be stored in a separate location. Backup file copies are stored on floppy disks and compact discs or external hard drives. Additional files that include demographic profiles of informants, institutional review board permission letter(s), signed consent forms, and a record of informant names with corresponding pseudonyms are also stored. Two indexes corresponding with field notes can be kept: first, an index of the analysis or coding, and second, an index of maps, drawings, photographs, and so forth. Videotapes and audiotapes should be accurately labeled and stored in easily accessible containers. Verbatim transcriptions of videotaped and audiotaped interviews are either combined with field notes or filed in another chronologically organized, loose-leaf binder. "Field records must . . . be properly organized and preserved if their future research potential is to be realized" (Ruwell, 1985, p. 1).

Other Types of Records and Notes

Field notes are maintained separately from other ethnographic notes. Field journals are often kept by investigators. They serve as a calendar of events for the ethnography in combination with scheduled appointments with informants and gatekeepers. Field journals provide running, chronological records of fieldwork.

Ethnographers often record personal notes, in which reflections, feelings, hunches, and speculations are documented (Wilson, 1989). "The personal experiences, anxieties, and fears are marginalized" (Richardson, 1988,

p. 203) and sometimes have appeared in the memoirs of classic ethnographers. As personal reflections, they are introspective and also include mistakes, ideas, confusions, and epiphanies. It is preferable that personal notes are written as soon as possible. Paper records predominate because they are often recorded on-site and are expanded later using computers to reflect ethnographers' insights. However, investigators might lose laptops to theft. Short notes work best in the field and can later be expanded and converted to electronic form as investigators reflect on what happened during a day's field observations.

Methodological notes help to describe how the study was conducted and to formulate additional plans for data collection as the study progresses. They remind ethnographers of the next steps in data collection. Methodological notes include analyses of cultural meanings, interpretations, and insights into the culture studied. Most of the tasks in the remaining steps involve detailed analysis and can be recorded in this category of field notes (Spradley, 1979, p. 76). Methodological notes assist ethnographers in writing final reports because they describe the methods used in studies.

Development of theoretical notes begins by coding field notes and interviews as codes or themes are identified and labeled. Investigators look for patterns and relationships among the facts of the data sources and may record interpretations and inferences in notes separate from the coding recorded directly on field notes. Theoretical notes could double as an index of codes that takes investigators back to specific pages in which thematic structures (themes, codes, categories, patterns, etc.) and indicators (chunks of data from field notes) are located.

Context

Because meaning changes with context, ethnographers are careful to place observations into larger perspectives (Fetterman, 1989; Leiter, 1980). By contextualizing data, a greater understanding is achieved by researchers and readers of the study. First, the physical context of the group being studied is detailed. This includes drawings, videotapes, or photographs for documentation. Multiple physical settings may be described, for example, meeting rooms, break rooms, patient rooms, classrooms, and dining rooms. These settings may also be placed in the larger context and physical description of a patient unit, school of nursing, or assisted living facility and community senior setting. Second, the social context requires attention and detailed description. For example, how the informants work together over the course of a 24-hour day, administer medications, manage patients' symptoms, care for patients with chest pain, and respond to a nursing professor during class or clinical assignments reveal the nature of the cultures being studied. Interactions and relationships are detailed as much as possible through field notes covering conversations. The elements of the context are constantly shifting, as does the meaning of the episodes and events being described (Leiter, 1980).

Interviews

Ethnographers depend on interviews to gain understanding of informants' worlds during participant observation opportunities. They are motivated by respect for insiders throughout the course of the study. Cultural understanding and interpretation are chief on the agenda for all types of ethnographic interviews. What people say leads investigators to cultural understanding. Ethnographers, working alone or with a team of investigators, carefully record the date, time, location, and names of informants in field journals as well as on verbatim transcriptions of tape-recorded or video-recorded interviews.

Interview questions vary (Spradley, 1979), from grand tour questions that help to position subsequent questions, to contrast questions that inquire about, for example, what happens if events go as planned or do not go as planned, what was good or bad about a crisis, or how to classify the benefits or detriments of a mistake. Grand tour questions often present informants with "Tell me about . . . " leads. For example, an investigator might ask, "Tell me about what typically happens during your shift." More specific questions such as "What was going on then?" "What do you do when you administer medications?" and "What are the steps that you take when you determine that a patient has chest pain?" help to uncover cultural meanings. Questions are also described as open-ended and closed-ended.

Prior to scheduling formal ethnographic interviews, researchers take part in friendly conversations that help build rapport with insiders. Informal conversational interviews are open-ended and flexible (Patton, 1990). When the conversation shifts to a structured interview, the purpose of the conversation is explicit to informants and has been planned by interviewers (Spradley, 1979). Ethnographers remind insiders of the purpose of each interview and often tape-record the session. Permission to record interviews is always asked whether consent is accomplished on a consent form, verbally, or electronically. If informants deviate from the purpose, ethnographers courteously bring them back to focus. Frequently, ethnographers interview key informants, or key actors (Fetterman, 1989), repeatedly over the course of data collection. By this time, ethnographers have realized who among the informants is best able to speak expertly about the cultural scene and to provide native explanations. On the other hand, ethnographers must avoid overreliance on one or two key informants. Not only could this lead to insufficient or inaccurate understanding, but it could isolate investigators from those informants who view the key informants jealously or adversarially.

Semistructured interviews are less formal than are structured ones. Investigators might start with a vague idea in mind, question informants, and follow the conversation to greater understanding as questions gradually become more focused. Probing questions or prompts are often used to augment interviews.

Investigators meet with informants during participant observation occasions. They have already greeted each other casually and may be exploring various aspects of informants' concerns. At this time, ethnographers conduct unstructured interviews as topics present themselves suddenly and seem relevant to one of the various directions of the study. Interviewers follow leads, explore issues, and examine various points of view. Ethnographers allow their imagination and ingenuity to help them test hypotheses during the course of the dialogue (Becker & Geer, 1957). Different tactics and types of questions are used to help to gain explanations and descriptions of social interaction. However, it is important to consider how the presence of other informants influences the dialogue with a single informant (Weiss, 1994). Private interviews preserve informant confidentiality.

Event Analysis

Geertz (1973) suggests that ethnographies produce momentary examples of behavior. Nonetheless, during the process of participant observation, transient events take place that divert ethnographers to more focused observations. Event sampling and analysis evolve according to crises, chance occurrences, and planned observations. For example, in a study of nursing rituals (Wolf, 1986) in which postmortem care was considered an event that might evoke nursing rituals, the investigator realized that the recurrent context of postmortem care was events in which do not resuscitate decisions were made. She decided that when these decisions took place, she had to study such events along with postmortem care events. Additionally, cardiopulmonary resuscitation events or codes were also witnessed and provided context. Describing events involves a description of the setting, artifacts, documents, actors or informants, and conversations.

Document Analysis

Documents are records collected by ethnographers that represent a broad range of cultural phenomena, such as technological, historical, demographic, and economic phenomena (Stocking, 1983). As sources of data or facts about a culture, they instruct ethnographers about what is going on and who is doing it. Documents include texts, such as journals, diaries, biographies, and histories; files; maps; charts; and other records that lead to a fuller understanding of the culture.

Artifact Analysis

The way insiders use artifacts informs ethnographers about the culture. The use of objects in the contexts of physical settings and social interaction serves as another source of data. How the objects are used often assists investigators in comprehending tacit knowledge.

Emic/Etic Distinction

Emic perspectives, or those from the insiders' sense of the world around them, are valued in ethnographic studies more than etic perspectives, or those perspectives of the investigators. Emic understandings rely on understanding the culture, language, and situations of the insiders through the way members of the culture see their world. Emic is shortened from the word *phonemic* and is borrowed from linguists who used it to study native classificatory systems. Etic, from *phonetic*, originates in analyses produced by the investigators (Leininger, 1987). The etic dimension originates in the intent of investigators to understand tacit knowledge, which is beneath the surface and hidden. It originates in outsiders' interpretation of experiences of the culture. Etic dimensions include interpretation of meaning, theoretical explanations, and understanding of symbols.

Types of Ethnographies

Spradley (1980) places types of ethnographies on a continuum, from microethnography to macroethnography. His classification refers to the size and complexity of the social units studied. Cultures vary in complexity, for example, complex society, multiple communities, single community, multiple social institutions, single social institution, multiple social situations, and a single social situation. Omery (1988) concurs with Spradley, noting that macroethnography is the study of complex societies and is broad in reach. Microethnography is limited to a subunit of a single institution, such as a nursing unit. Spradley further explains the distinct focus of studies, citing Hymes (1978). Comprehensive ethnography describes a total way of life. Topic-oriented ethnography restricts the study to one or more aspects of life. Hypothesis-oriented ethnography is characterized by studies in process by which ethnographers engage in testing hunches about the way cultural practices might influence human development. Another classification for types of ethnographic studies is descriptive or conventional ethnography and critical ethnography, in which power and hidden agendas are studied.

Ethnography may be holistic in which a society is described as a whole. This type is compared to focused ethnography, where the focus is on specific problems or situations within a larger social scene. Another example, cognitive ethnography, seeks to determine what things mean to participants and how those meanings are created. Often, students are assigned miniethnographies; these studies are small scale (Leininger, 1985) and can be conducted in a shortened time period, such as 6 weeks, with data collection on a single cultural practice taking place one day a week. Students are directed to the Human Relations Area Files (eHRAF), the detailed classification scheme and multicultural database.

eHRAF is unique because each culture or ethnic group contains a variety of source documents (books, articles, and dissertations) that have been indexed and organized according to HRAF's comprehensive culture and subject classification systems: the *Outline of World Cultures* and the *Outline of Cultural Materials*. These retrieval systems extend search capability well beyond keyword searching, thus allowing for precise culture and subject retrieval, even in a foreign language. *The Development and Applications of the HRAF Collections* can provide investigators with an extended overview of these resources. (http://www.yale.edu/hraf/collections.htm).

Maxiethnographies are "comprehensive studies of general and particular features of a designated culture" (Leininger, 1985, p. 35). Comparative ethnographies are those whereby two societies are studied so that cross-cultural comparisons can be made. Other types of ethnographies have emerged as disciplinary boundaries have blurred; examples are autoethnography and reflexive ethnography (Ellis & Bochner, 1996).

ANALYSIS

Many ethnographers record field notes using a great amount of detail. Field note construction has been facilitated by computers, scanners, digital cameras, audiotapes, and videotapes. This contrasts markedly with the methods of early ethnographers whose notes were not always easily accessible, organized, or followed by other readers, for example, by peer reviewers who are asked to follow audit trails when assessing the rigor of studies.

The gold standard for field notes and completed studies is best expressed by Geertz (1973). "Thick description" refers to the characteristic of a study that is written artistically, like a story; the finished ethnography is so complex and descriptive that readers are able to see the social action in context. The thick description of field notes helps ethnographers recollect experiences in the field and provides sufficient data for analysis. The quality of field notes, transcribed interviews, document analysis, and other data sources strongly influences the quality of the study. The narrative of the finished ethnography must remain faithful to informants' perspectives in context. Additionally, Ward and Werner (1984) suggest a deeper analysis of data when discussing thick description: "Thick description is that description in which the ethnographer has made a full and conscious attempt to resolve (rather than adjudicate) the discrepancies among inconsistent data" (p. 233).

Data analysis is time and energy intensive as well as complex (Robertson & Boyle, 1984). The aim of data collection for ethnographic studies is to portray the culture as informed by the knowledge of the best informants. Analysis requires that ethnographers remain familiar with all of the data throughout the course of studies. It begins almost immediately as field notes are recorded and ends when researchers are satisfied with their interpretations and the written report. They make choices throughout the process and pay attention to the details and the larger contexts. Intuition also is important. As thematic analysis continues, themes are sorted and related to other themes. Critical thinking ability and skills in synthesis are important (Fetterman, 1989) as are persistence, writing, and rewriting.

To reflect informants' perspectives when writing drafts of final reports, ethnographers select indicators or extracts from field notes, such as examples, comments, phrases, or detailed descriptions to match the purpose of the investigation. This provides evidence of the skillful analytic techniques of investigators, because they make sense of cultures and beliefs, values, norms, structures, functions, and symbols. Commonsense knowledge and ethnographic descriptions produce impressionistic and at the same time detailed accounts for readers that "reveal, rather than hide" their "context-dependent character" (Leiter, 1980, p. 91). From the start of fieldwork, data collection and analysis have interacted in the thoughts and records produced by ethnographers. The analytic cycle, described by Jorgensen (1989), involves data analysis in which research materials are broken up into units (themes, etc.); are sorted and searched for categories, patterns, or wholes; and are reconstructed in a meaningful and comprehensible way. The theories that emerge begin with thematic analysis and end as explanations appearing in the final record of ethnographies. Different disciplinary traditions use a variety of terms to describe units of analysis.

> A society's culture consists of whatever one has to know or believe
> in order to operate in a manner acceptable to its members. . . . It is

> the form of things that people have in mind, their models for per-
> ceiving, relating and otherwise interpreting them. . . . Ethno-
> graphic description . . . requires methods of processing observed
> phenomena such that we can inductively construct a theory of how
> our informants have organized the same phenomena. It is the the-
> ory, not the phenomena alone, which ethnographic description
> aims to present. (Goodenough, 1964, p. 36)

Ethnographers are active participants in both data collection and data analysis (Aamodt, 1982). Data analysis begins with the first field notes and continues throughout the time necessary for completion of ethnographic studies. Not only do ethnographers rely on themes or codes induced during content analysis, but they also rely on memory (Mulkay, 1985). According to Mulkay, ethnographic writing involves a reconstruction and produces a secondary text alongside the original text, a narrative that is superior to the original. Social worlds are reconstructed that depict tacit knowledge discovered by ethnographers and revealed as written into existence. The collective memory of the group (Halbwach, 1980) is disclosed, and a likeness of the original cultural model, the culture being studied, is produced.

Data analysis procedures for ethnographies involve content analysis of text. Cultural data, as recorded in field notes, are drawn from abstractions of behavior about what people do and what they say they do (Aamodt, 1982). Investigators keep the research purpose and questions in mind so that they adhere to the original focus of ethnographic proposals. At this juncture, they are familiar with field notes and return to them again and again. They read and review the text and begin the analysis. Each time analysis is performed, investigators read textual material to get a feeling for and make sense of the data. Coding assists researchers in identifying key words, themes, patterns, essences, conceptual models, indexes, concepts, social processes, and descriptive theories. Coding is accomplished by reading texts line by line and then identifying codes (category labels) (Miles & Huberman, 1984) or themes (thematic structures) in margins of the field notes or other material. Next, significant statements (words, phrases, sentences, paragraphs) are extracted that correspond with the listed structures (themes).

Thematic or categorical analysis is accomplished through the process of coding. Coding is a process of classifying and interpreting data and reveals deep and surface structures. This suggests that meaning and symbols (deep structure, latent, hidden, symbolic, high inference, implicit) are identified as are explicit (surface structure, manifest, overt, explicit, descriptive, low inference) results. Whether major or minor themes (codes, categories), patterns (explanatory or inferential codes or meta-codes, also referred to as clusters or major themes), and clusters (grouped and conceptualized objects with similar patterns or characteristics, using comparison) (Miles & Huberman, 1984) are identified, nevertheless they serve to produce the narrative of reports along with theoretical formulations. Data analysis is typically etic, with consistent attention to emic dimensions, reflective of informants' cultural knowledge.

Software programs are used to facilitate the data analysis process. Qualitative software, such as Ethnograph and Non-numerical Unstructured Data Indexing Searching and Theorizing (QSR N4), has been developed to assist in data management and analysis. Additionally, some ethnographers use Microsoft Word to create and manage all aspects of the study and produce the audit trail, from field notes to thematic analysis to the final product.

Broad structures (categories, patterns, clusters) most likely exist in the thoughts of investigators as they begin data analysis early in fieldwork and continue throughout the study. The structures fit the research purposes and questions identified at the inception of the ethnography. Inference produces the themes and patterns that are labeled when analyzing textual accounts. Ethnographic inference helps ethnographers achieve coherence, in that different pieces of knowledge (from field notes, transcribed interviews, etc.) are linked, and then connect the knowledge to explanations of the culture being studied (Agar, 1986). Perhaps situations, informants, objects, actions, and goals are connected through the inferences of ethnographers, and greater clarity and understanding are gained regarding aspects of the culture. A simple way to achieve inference and reveal part of the process might be for ethnographers to create a table as a three-column organizer that helps them sort, compare, contrast, and synthesize indicators into themes and patterns. For example, the columns are labeled "Indicators," "Themes," and "Interpretive statements." In a table such as this, the indicators are selected from field notes and other data sources. They are considered to be facts or chunks of data when used in ethnographies as either a low-level inference (surface structure, descriptive, explicit) or a high-level inference (deep structure, symbolic, latent) to support an explanation. Symbolic meaning might be realized as investigators label and explain deep structures.

Inference and interpretation require investigators to make choices as they select data during analysis and disregard other material. The analytic processes of conducting ethnographic studies focus on generating themes (codes, categories), which are the structural features of the cognitive map of a society, and discovering relationships between these categories, such as describing how the structural features relate to one another (Aamodt, 1982).

Fetterman (1989) explores the idea of crystallization as thought processes, much like "aha" moments, take ethnographers to insights and conclusions during the course of data analysis. Whether a mundane or extraordinary event, crystallization is the coming together of themes into a pattern or category or a clear understanding of beliefs, values, or norms of a social group. Crystallization is a result of reflection, interpretation, and conscientious work. As studies are written, often the writing and revision process brings additional crystallizations as thoughts converge in meaning. Ethnographers might then return to field notes and other sources of raw data to locate confirmation of such insights with similar field note examples.

It is worthwhile for ethnographers to create a table of contents for all textual material generated during ethnographic studies in which field notes and other materials that show evidence of content analysis are organized into broad or main categories. The table of contents is further subdivided within those main categories into lists of themes with page numbers that correspond to the exact locations of those themes with significant words, phrases, and paragraphs, throughout the raw records (field notes, transcribed interviews, etc.).

INTERPRETATION

All ethnographers interpret. Interpretation helps ethnographers create and uphold the factual character of the social and cultural world as represented in the ethnographic report. They use interpretation to translate the behavior of informants into meanings. Interpretation is framed by data analysis, the study's purpose and questions, the answers or report, the explanations (interpretations) produced, the data sources that are the evidence provided to accomplish the purpose and interpretation, and the organization of these elements (purpose/questions, data, interpretation) into an argument. Informants' words and actions are important for interpretation. Ideally, throughout the study, ethnographers have been immersing themselves in the data sources (Roper & Shapira, 2000). They are familiar with emerging themes, patterns, clusters, and explanations, and are sensitive to emerging meanings. Behavior is explained through socially constructed structures, functions, and processes of meaning.

Ethnographies are subjective as well as systematic, rigorous studies. The creativity of investigators as they analyze and interpret data is balanced with written explanations, supported by evidence and applied ethnographic methods (Whittemore, Chase, & Mandle, 2001).

Wolcott (1994) distinguishes ethnographic description from analysis and interpretation and proposes that they are the "three primary ingredients of qualitative research" (p. 49). He also notes that a balance must be achieved among all three with no particular combination or percentages of one to the others considered the best. He suggests that ethnographers might link interpretations to theory but cautions that such links might not be the best solution.

FINDINGS OF ETHNOGRAPHIC STUDIES

Ethnographic texts are written as stories that emerge from the data. Data have primacy; the theoretical framework is not predetermined by the data but derives from them. Ideally, ethnographic reports are artistically presented and accessible to more readers than the members of the discipline. As narratives, they include straight and analytical description. Hypotheses about behavior, interpretive theories, concepts, constructs, associated theoretical definitions, taxonomies, and typologies might also emerge as findings.

When ethnographers begin to write the ethnography, they already have codes, categories, and patterns created when developing the rationales supporting their interpretations. Pieces of information are presented as objective reality through the raw data of field notes, recorded observations of subjects' words and behavioral actions, and verbatim transcriptions of audiotaped or videotaped interviews. The pieces of information are empirical indicators of codes, themes, categories, patterns, and so forth.

Straight description is characterized by ethnographic details in which a situation might be revealed, including actors, their roles and behaviors, the artifacts used, conversations, and outcomes that were previously recorded in field notes and copied into the final product. As the writing of the report progresses, the text is then recontextualized to build understanding of the pattern of social and cultural action. There is a back-and-forth switch between the explicit/descriptive and the latent/symbolic.

Analytic description, also considered interpretive description, refers to the decontextualized narrative in which analysis and interpretation are exposed. The beliefs, norms, values, social structure, function, and symbols are revealed by the results of ethnographers' thoughts and creative insights.

Interpretive theories originate in themes or concepts and are built inductively from the raw material of field notes, transcribed interviews, analysis of documents, and the like. The interpretive theory of ethnography could be considered a descriptive formulation that is disciplined (Jorgensen, 1989).

The explanations that are provided in ethnographic reports could be functional, associative, or causal. The explanations about a group's way of life provide a beginning and are never finished or absolute because cultures continue to develop and change.

Themes are repetitive, recurrent topics that emerge during analysis. Themes "cluster" or form patterns. Patterns are natural configurations of observations (van Manen, 1990). Concepts are abstract ideas generalized from the particulars revealed in the factual material of field notes, transcribed interviews, and the like. They may be equated with themes. Constructs are concepts constructed by the mental synthesis of ethnographers. Both concepts and constructs require theoretical definitions in which they are defined circularly, that is, a synonym or substitute for one or several words replaces the concept or construct name. For example, following are circular definitions: *ritual* is patterned, symbolic action that refers to the beliefs, values, and goals of a social group; *nursing ritual* is patterned symbolic action that refers to the beliefs, values, and goals of a group of nurses (or nurses in general); *therapeutic nursing rituals* are symbolic actions that improve the condition of patients; and *occupational nursing rituals* (rites of socialization) are symbolic actions that facilitate the transition of professional neophytes into their professional role.

Hypotheses are conjectural statements about the relationships between two or more concepts. Ethnographic studies produce hypotheses inductively as data collection and analysis proceed. An example is this: the greater the nurse identification of a patient as temporary family, the greater the nurse's difficulty in performing postmortem care. Taxonomies are orderly classifications grouped according to presumed natural relationships; they are used to organize and interpret findings. Taxonomies include domains within the classificatory scheme. The domains are labeled (Powers, 2001). Taxon is the name given to a taxonomic group in a formal system of nomenclature. For example, the taxonomy for a code called in the event of cardiopulmonary arrest includes full code, no code, slow code, and almost no code (Wolf, 1986). Typologies are classification schemes and are useful in forming hypotheses and discovering themes.

RIGOR, OR SCIENTIFIC ADEQUACY, OF ETHNOGRAPHIES

It is important that ethnographers establish the rigor or scientific adequacy of saturation ethnographic accounts. The methodological literature, although sparse initially (Ward & Werner, 1984), has been elaborated over recent decades (Reid, 1991; Shokeid, 1988). Many ethnographers have followed the methods of Lincoln and Guba (1985).

To document the rigor of studies, investigators attempt to establish their trustworthiness (Lincoln & Guba, 1985). For the credibility criterion to be achieved, they engage in reading and reflecting on the material of studies, including field notes, transcribed interviews, documents, diaries, appointment records, and so forth. At the end of studies, they might attempt to achieve theoretical triangulation by matching published theories or concepts to the interpretive theories discovered in the study. They might request that a trusted, qualitative investigator review transcripts, field notes, essential themes, indexes, documents, and the ethnography. To achieve member check, investigators mail the results of the study to informants, meet with informants, or in other ways share drafts of studies and invite informants' assessment of the accuracy of the description and solicit their insights. Ethnographers look for transferability in nonstakeholder persons, those who were not informants but who share knowledge of the culture and can read and comment on the study.

To establish dependability, audit trails are made available for review by peer reviewers and other interested investigators. Data trails include field notes, documents, photographs, maps, drawings, personal notes, transcribed interviews (raw data), coding schemes, themes and indicators, and the text of the finished ethnography (data reduction and analysis products). Ideally, the results are confirmed through the manuscript as well as through implications and recommendations of the study. In contrast to Lincoln and Guba (1985), Whittemore, Chase, and Mandle (2001) reconceptualize validity in qualitative research, organizing crtieria according to primary criteria, secondary criteria, and techniques.

REFLEXIVITY

Reflexivity is defined as the process by which researchers recognize that they are an integral part of the research and vice versa (Cutcliffe, 2003; Pellatt, 2003). Similar to other qualitative research, ethnographic studies achieve reflexivity when investigators are aware of themselves in relation to the informants, the data, and their own roles in the study (Lipson, 1989). Reflexivity recognizes the circularity of the relationship of investigators to the data; how and when different aspects of the interpretation emerge in the reports and in prior and various forms; how open investigators were to inducing breakdowns in their understanding of the data; and how their confidence in interpretations was challenged and tested over the course of study. They are aware of their role in the interpretation of the material and are sensitive to the meanings and patterns. The relationships and communication among researchers and informants, the influence of each in the knowledge produced in the study, as well as their reflections on the actions and observations in the field, are important. Reflexivity may be achieved when readers judge the validity of the researcher's work (Kahn, 1993).

Cutcliffe (2003) discusses different strategies used to establish reflexivity and ways to establish credibility of the study. He proposes that tacit knowledge/knowing is important for qualitative research and that it is difficult to explain investigators' flashes of insight. Cutcliffe encourages investigators to bring "creative, intellectual, and analytical processes to bear on any qualitative analysis" (p. 147) and to "let the magic happen" (p. 147). Allen (2004) discusses the dilemmas posed by the dual practitioner–researcher identity. However, the ethical codes of investigators help nurse ethnographers to always act on behalf of the welfare of patients when conducting studies. For example, if patient safety is threatened or if practitioners are behaving illegally, investigators must act, such as filing reports with administrators. While this might threaten the trust earned from informants, it is the best course.

CONCLUSION

Cultures are displayed in the writing of ethnographic studies. The process of doing ethnography is systematic and subjective and involves stating the purpose(s) and problem; collecting data through a variety of sources, chief of which is fieldwork, participant observation, and interviewing; and describing, analyzing, and interpreting the data. The best ethnographies display an interpretive understanding of social and cultural action in context. They are interesting to read and illuminate the worlds of informants. Table 10–1 includes a selection of ethnographic studies conducted by nurses.

TABLE 10–1 Examples and Methods of Ethnographic Studies by Nurses

Citation	Type	Purpose	Participant Observation/ Field Notes	Interview	Document Analysis	Artifact Analysis	Time in Field	Findings
Allan, H. (2001). A 'good enough' nurse: Supporting patients in a fertility unit. *Nursing Inquiry, 8*, 51–60.	Focused critical	To describe two activities central to the nursing role in a fertility unit: caring and noncaring	X	Semistructured	—	—	2 years	Taxonomy; definition; narrative description; analytic description
Brathwaite, A. C., & Williams, C. C. (2004). Childbirth experiences of professional Chinese Canadian women. *JOGNN, 33*(6), 748–755.	Focused	To provide detailed information about how Chinese culture influences the childbirth experience and how health care providers can support cultural expression and positive outcomes for these women, their children, and their families	X	Structured; semistructured	—	—	—	Narrative description; analytic description
Cleary, M. (2003). The challenges of mental health care reform for contemporary mental health nursing practice: Relationships, power and control. *International Journal of Mental Health Nursing, 12*, 139–147.	Focused	The way mental health nurses interpret their practice in an acute inpatient psychiatric unit in light of the current challenges, demands, and influence brought about by service reforms	X	Focused; discussion groups	—	—	5 months	Narrative description; analytic description

Connelly, L. M., Keele, B. S., Kleinbeck, S. V., Schneider, J. K., & Cobb, A. K. (1993). A place to be yourself: Empowerment from the client's perspective. *Image: Journal of Nursing Scholarship, 25*(4), 297–304.	Focused	To describe the effects of chronically mentally ill consumer involvement in a client-run community support services drop-in center	X	Semistructured	—	—	5 weeks	Process domains; definition; model; narrative description; analytic description
Costello, J. (2002). Do not resuscitate orders and older patients: Findings from an ethnographic study of hospital wards for older people. *Journal of Advanced Nursing, 39*(5), 491–499.	Focused	To explore the way in which terminal care was provided to older patients; in the context of a larger study with the purpose: To explore the way in which DNR orders were a socially constructed part of the practices of both nurses and doctors	X	Semistructured; unstructured	Medical notes (charts); nursing notes; field diary	—	9 months	Major themes; narrative description; analytic description
Cricco-Lizza, R. (2005). The milk of human kindness: Environmental and human interactions in a WIC clinic that influence infant-feeding decisions of black women. *Qualitative Health Research, 15*(4), 525–538.	Focused	To explore WIC's influence on the infant-feeding decisions of inner-city black women enrolled in a New York metropolitan area WIC clinic	X	Structured; semistructured	—	—	18 months	Patterns; themes; narrative description; analytic description

continues

TABLE 10–1 continued

Citation	Type	Purpose	Participant Observation/ Field Notes	Interview	Document Analysis	Artifact Analysis	Time in Field	Findings
Gates, M. F., Lackey, N. R., & Brown, G. (2001). Caring demands and delay in seeking care in African American women newly diagnosed with breast cancer: An ethnographic, photographic study. ONF, 28(2), 529–537.	Focused	To describe the caring experiences in terms of the behaviors and demands of African American women newly diagnosed with breast cancer and to consider the influence of that caring on the women's decisions to delay prompt diagnosis and maintain continuing treatment	X	Semistructured	Journal; photographer	—	—	Themes; narrative description; analytic description
Germain, C. P. (1979). The cancer unit: An ethnography. Wakefield, MA: Nursing Resources.	Holistic	Description of a community hospital adult oncology unit as a subculture	X	Structured; unstructured	—	—	12 months	Narrative description; constructs
Hall, J. M. (1994). Lesbians recovering from alcohol problems: An ethnographic study of health care experiences. Nursing Research, 43(4), 238–244.	Focused	To describe lesbians' experiences in alcohol recovery and identify barriers to help-seeking and recovery from their perspective	X	Semistructured	—	—	—	Themes; narrative description; analytic description

Hopkins, C. (2002). "But what about the really ill, poorly people?" (An ethnographic study into what it means to nurses on medical admissions units to have people who have harmed themselves as their patients). *Journal of Psychiatric and Mental Health Nursing, 9,* 147–154.	Focused	To gain an understanding of what it means to nurses on medical admissions units to have people who have harmed themselves as their patients	X	Semistructured	Reflective fieldwork journal	—	1 month	Themes; narrative description; analytic description
Kauffman, K. S. (1995). Center as haven: Findings of an urban ethnography. *Nursing Research, 44*(4), 231–236.	Focused	To describe how elders survive in the midst of "drug warfare" in an inner-city community known for its dangerous streets and public spaces	X	Formal; casual conversations	—	—	3 years	Pattern; narrative description; analytic description
Lipson, J. G. (2001). We are the canaries: Self-care in multiple chemical sensitivity sufferers. *Qualitative Health Research, 11,* 103–116.	Focused	To describe the daily life experiences and ways of coping, of multiple chemical sensitivity (MCS) sufferers', coping subcultures, current social/cultural/political issues associated with this condition, dealing with negative reactions from health providers and others who do not believe in	X	Semistructured; chat rooms	Newsletters, news articles, TV programs	—	2 years	Categories; themes; narrative description; analytic description

continues

TABLE 10–1 continued

Citation	Type	Purpose	Participant Observation/ Field Notes	Interview	Document Analysis	Artifact Analysis	Time in Field	Findings
Miller, M. P. (1991). Factors promoting wellness in the aged person: An ethnographic study. *Advances in Nursing Science, 13*(4), 38–51.	Focused	this illness, and self-care and medical treatment of MCS To ascertain the factors contributing to well elderly persons' wellness state	X	Semistructured	—	—	—	Brief narrative; constructs
Neufeld, A., Harrison, M. J., Stewart, M. J., Hughes, K. D., & Spitzer, D. (2002). Immigrant women: Making connections to community resources for support in family caregiving. *Qualitative Health Research, 12*(6), 751–768.	Focused critical theory	To understand how Chinese and South Asian immigrant women caring for an ill or disabled family member gain access to support from community resources and identify the barriers to support that they experienced, including those arising from their social and material circumstances	X	Semistructured; focus group	—	—	—	Narrative description; constructs

Powers, B. A. (2001). Ethnographic analysis of everyday ethics in the care of nursing home residents with dementia. *Nursing Research, 50*(6), 332–339.	Focused critical	To critically examine ethical issues of daily living and to construct a descriptive data-based taxonomy	X	Structured; semistructured	Newsletters; activity calendars; daily care worksheets; in-service education calendars and teaching tools; annual reports; documents of ethics committee	—	2 years	Concept; taxonomy (4 domains); narrative description; analytic description
Varcoe, C. (2001). Abuse obscured: An ethnographic account of emergency nursing in relation to violence against women. *Canadian Journal of Nursing Research, 32*(4), 95–115.	Focused critical	To examine the relationship between the social context of practice and the ways in which nurses recognize and respond to the plight of women who have been abused	X	Semistructured; unstructured	—	—	2 years	Patterns; narrative description; analytic description

continues

TABLE 10–1   continued

Citation	Type	Purpose	Participant Observation/ Field Notes	Interview	Document Analysis	Artifact Analysis	Time in Field	Findings
Wolf, Z. R. (1986). *Nursing rituals in an adult acute care hospital: An ethnography.* Ann Arbor, MI: University of Pennsylvania School of Nursing, University Microfilms.	Focused	What actions, words, and objects make up nursing rituals? What are types of nursing rituals as demonstrated by nurses caring for adult patients on a hospital unit? What explicit or manifest meanings and implicit or latent meanings do these rituals have for nurses, patients, physicians, and other hospital personnel? How are nurses, patients, families, physicians, and other hospital personnel involved in these rituals? How do nursing rituals emerge in the context of the routines, procedures, and reports of the nursing unit?	X	Semistructured; unstructured	Patient charts; nursing unit minutes; kardexes	Unit furniture; nursing care equipment; primary board	12 months	Patterns; narrative description; analytic description; taxonomy; definitions

Source: Adapted from "The Health of Teenagers: A Focused Ethnographic Study," by J. K. Magilvy et al., 1987, *Public Health Nursing* 4(1), 35–42.

REFERENCES

Aamodt, A. M. (1982). Examining ethnography for nurse researchers. *Western Journal of Nursing Research, 4*(2), 207–221.

Adler, P. A., & Adler, P. (1987). *Membership roles in field research.* Newbury Park, CA: Sage.

Agar, M. H. (1986). *Speaking of ethnography.* Beverly Hills, CA: Sage.

Allen, D. (2004). Ethnomethodological insights into insider-outsider relationships in nursing ethnographies of healthcare settings. *Nursing Inquiry, 11*(1), 14–24.

Atkinson, P. (1992). *Understanding ethnographic texts.* Newbury Park, CA: Sage.

Becker, H. S., & Geer, B. (1957). Participant observation and interviewing: A comparison. *Human Organization, 16*(3), 28–32.

Brody, E. B. (1981). The clinician as ethnographer: A psychoanalytic perspective on the epistemology of fieldwork. *Culture, Medicine and Psychiatry, 5*(3), 273–301.

Byerly, E. L. (1969). The nurse researcher as a participant-observer in a nursing setting. *Nursing Researcher, 18*(3), 230–235.

Cutcliffe, J. R. (2003). Reconsidering reflexivity. *Qualitative Health Research, 13*(1), 136–148.

DeSantis, L. (1990). Fieldwork with undocumented aliens and other populations at risk. *Western Journal of Nursing Research, 12*(3), 359–372.

Douglas, M. (1963). *The Lele of the Kasai.* London: Oxford University Press.

Douglas, M. (1966). *Purity and danger.* London: Routledge and Kegan Paul.

Douglas, M. (1975). *Implicit meanings: Essays in anthropology.* London: Routledge and Kegan Paul.

Douglass, W. A. (1969). *Death in Murelaga: Funerary ritual in a Spanish Basque village.* Seattle: University of Washington Press.

Ellis, C., & Bochner, A. P. (Eds.). (1996). *Composing ethnography: Alternative forms of qualitative writing.* Walnut Creek, CA: Altamira Press.

Fetterman, D. (1989). *Ethnography: Step by step.* Newbury Park, CA: Sage.

Field, P. (1989). Doing fieldwork in your own culture. In J. M. Morse (Ed.), *Qualitative nursing research* (pp. 91–104). Newbury Park: CA: Sage.

Firth, R. (1936). *We, the Tikopia.* London: Allen and Unwin.

Fox, R. C. (1959). *Experiment perilous.* Philadelphia: University of Pennsylvania Press.

Freilich, M. (Ed.). (1970). *Marginal natives: Anthropologists at work.* New York: Harper & Row.

Geertz, C. (1973). *The interpretation of cultures.* New York: Basic Books.

Germain, C. P. (2001). Ethnography: The method. In P. L. Munhall (Ed.), *Nursing research: A qualitative perspective* (3rd ed.) (pp. 277–306). Sudbury, MA: Jones and Bartlett, National League for Nursing.

Glesne, C. (1989). Rapport and friendship in ethnographic research. *Qualitative Studies in Education, 2*(1), 45–54.

Goffman, E. (1961). *Asylums: Essays on the social situation of mental patients and other inmates.* Garden City, NY: Anchor Books.

Goodenough, W. (1964). Cultural anthropology and linguistics. In D. Hymes (Ed.), *Language and culture and society: A reader in linguistics and anthropology.* New York: Harper & Row.

Halbwach, M. (1980). *The collective memory.* New York: Harper Colophon Books.

Hammersley, M., & Atkinson, P. (1983). *Ethnography: Principles in practice.* New York: Tavistock.

Hammersley, M., & Atkinson, P. (1995). *Ethnography: Principles in practice.* London: Routledge.

Hopkins, C. (2002). "But what about the really ill, poorly people?" (An ethnographic study into what it means to nurses on medical admissions units to have people who have harmed themselves as their patients.) *Journal of Psychiatric and Mental Health Nursing, 9,* 147–154.

Human Relations Area File. eHRAF. Retrieved July 7, 2005, from http://www.yale.edu/hraf/collections.htm.

Hymes, D. H. (1978). *What is ethnography?* (Sociolinguistic Working Paper 45). Austin: TX: Southwest Educational Development Laboratory.

Jorgensen, D. L. (1989). *Participant observation: A methodology for human studies.* Newbury Park, CA: Sage.

Junker, B. H. (1960). *Field work: An introduction to the social sciences.* Chicago: University of Chicago Press.

Kahn, D. L. (1993). Ways of discussing validity in qualitative nursing research. *Western Journal of Nursing Research, 15*(1), 122–126.

Kaufman, K. S. (1995). Center as haven: Findings of an urban ethnography. *Nursing Research, 44*(4), 231–236.

Keith, J. (1986). Participant observation. In C. L. Fry & J. Keith (Eds.), *New methods for old age research* (pp. 1–20). South Hadley, MA: Bergin & Garvey.

Kleinman, A. (1988). A method for the care of the chronically ill. In A. Kleinman (Ed.), *The illness narratives: Suffering, healing, and the human condition* (pp. 227–251). New York: Basic Books.

Leininger, M. (1987). Importance and uses of ethnomethods: Ethnography and ethnonursing research. *Recent Advances in Nursing, 17,* 12–36.

Leininger, M. M. (Ed.). (1985). *Qualitative research methods in nursing.* Orlando, FL: Grune & Stratton.

Leiter, K. (1980). *A primer on ethnomethodology.* New York: Oxford University Press.

Liebow, E. (1993). *Tell them who I am: The lives of homeless women.* New York: Penguin Books.

Lincoln, Y., & Guba, E. (1985). *Naturalistic inquiry.* Beverly Hills, CA: Sage.

Lipson, J. G. (1989). The use of self in ethnographic research. In. J. M. Morse (Ed.), *Qualitative nursing research* (pp. 61–75). Rockville, MD: Aspen.

Lofland, J. (1976). *Doing social life.* New York: Wiley.

Lofland, J., & Lofland, L. (1984). *Analyzing social settings: A guide to qualitative observation and analysis* (2nd ed.). Belmont, CA: Wadsworth.

Malinowski, B. (1922). *Argonauts of the Western Pacific.* London: Routledge and Kegan Paul.

Malinowski, B. (1948). *Magic, science and religion*. Prospect Heights, IL: Waveland Press.

Mauss, M. (1967). The gift: Forms and functions of exchange in archaic societies. New York: W. W. Norton.

Miles, M. B., & Huberman, A. M. (1984). *Qualitative data analysis*. Beverly Hills, CA: Sage.

Mulkay, M. J. (1985). *The word and the world: Explorations in the form of sociological analysis*. London: Allen and Unwin.

Omery, A. (1988). Ethnography. In B. Sarter (Ed.), *Paths to knowledge: Innovative research methods for nursing* (pp. 17–31). New York: National League for Nursing.

Patton, M. Q. (1990). Qualitative evaluation and research methods (2nd ed.). Newbury Park, CA: Sage.

Pearsall, M. (1965). Participant observation as role and method in behavioral research. *Nursing Research, 14*(1), 37–42.

Pellatt, G. (2003). Ethnography and reflexivity: Emotions and feelings in fieldwork. *Nurse Researcher, 10*(3), 28–37.

Powers, B. A. (2001). Ethnographic analysis of everyday ethics in the care of nursing home residents with dementia. *Nursing Research, 50*(6), 332–339.

Ragucci, A. T. (1972). The ethnographic approach and nursing research. *Nursing Research, 21*(6), 485–490.

Reid, B. (1991). Developing and documenting a qualitative methodology. *Journal of Advanced Nursing, 16*, 544–551.

Richardson, L. (1988). The collective story: Postmodernism and the writing of sociology. *Sociological Focus, 21*(3), 199–208.

Robertson, M. H., & Boyle, J. S. (1984). Ethnography: Contributions to nursing research. *Journal of Advanced Nursing, 9*, 43–49.

Roper, J. M., & Shapira, J. (2000). *Ethnography in nursing research*. Thousand Oaks, CA: Sage.

Ruwell, M. E. (1985). Introduction. In M. A. Kenworthy, E. M. King, M. E. Ruwell, & T. Van Houten (Eds.), *Preserving field records* (pp. 1–6). Philadelphia: University Museum, University of Pennsylvania.

Sapir, E. (1924). Culture, genuine and spurious. In D. G. Mandelbaum (Ed.), *Selected writings of Edward Sapir in language, culture, and personality* (pp. 308–311). Berkeley, CA: University of California Press.

Shokeid, M. (1988). Anthropologists and their informants: Marginality reconsidered. *European Journal of Sociology, 29*(1), 31–47.

Spradley, J. P. (1970). *You owe yourself a drunk: An ethnography of urban nomads*. Boston: Little, Brown.

Spradley, J. P. (1979). *The ethnographic interview*. New York: Holt, Rinehart & Winston.

Spradley, J. P. (1980). *Participant observation*. New York: Holt, Rinehart & Winston.

Stocking, G. W. (1983). *Observers observed*. Madison: University of Wisconsin Press.

Thorne, S. E. (1991). Methodological orthodoxy in qualitative nursing research: Analysis of the issues. *Qualitative Health Research, 1*(2), 178–199.

Turner, V. (1967). *The forest of symbols: Aspects of Ndembu ritual*. Ithaca, NY: Cornell University Press.

Turner, W. (1957). *Schism and continuity in an African society.* Manchester: Manchester University Press.

van Manen, M. (1990). *Researching lived experience.* Albany: State University of New York Press.

Varcoe, C. (2001). Abuse obscured: An ethnographic account of emergency nursing in relation to violence against women. *Canadian Journal of Nursing Research, 32*(4), 95–115.

Ward, J. J., & Werner, O. (1984). Difference and dissonance in ethnographic data. *Communication and Cognition, 17*(2/3), 219–243.

Weiss, R. S. (1994). *Learning form strangers: The art and method of qualitative interview studies.* New York: The Free Press.

Whittemore, R., Chase, S. K., & Mandle, C. L. (2001). Validity in qualitative research. *Qualitative Health Research, 11*(4), 522–537.

Wilson, H. S. (1989). *Research in nursing* (2nd ed.). Redwood City, CA: Addison-Wesley Publishing Company Health Sciences.

Wolcott, H. F. (1994). *Transforming qualitative data: Description, analysis, and interpretation.* Thousand Oaks, CA: Sage.

Wolcott, H. F. (1995). *The art of fieldwork.* Walnut Creek, CA: Altamira Press.

Wolf, Z. R. (1986). *Nursing rituals in an adult acute care hospital: An ethnography.* Ann Arbor, MI: University of Pennsylvania School of Nursing, University Microfilms.

11

Exemplar: The Milk of Human Kindness: WIC Influence on the Infant Feeding Decisions of Black Non-Hispanic Women

Roberta Cricco-Lizza

Infant feeding decisions have important public health implications. Health care professionals have formally acclaimed the advantages of breastfeeding for maternal child health (American Academy of Pediatrics, 2005; American College of Nurse-Midwives, 1992; American College of Obstetricians and Gynecologists, 2000; American Dietetic Association, 1997; American Public Health Association, 1982). The Healthy People 2010 initiative calls for an elimination of racial disparities in health and has set a goal of having 75% of mothers breastfeed after birth, 50% at 6 months, and 25% at 1 year (U.S. Department of Health and Human Services, 2000). Current breastfeeding rates do not meet these goals and reflect disparities related to race, ethnicity, and income.

Source: Adapted from Cricco-Lizza, R. (2005) The milk of human kindness. *Qualitative Health Research*, 15(4), 525–538.

The Special Supplemental Nutrition Program for Women, Infants, and Children (WIC) is charged with improving the nutritional health of vulnerable mothers and children (U.S. Department of Agriculture, 1995). This program supplies supplemental foods, infant formula, health care referrals, and nutrition education for lower income women and children. For reasons that are not clearly understood, the lowest breastfeeding rates in the United States are found among women who are enrolled in WIC (Ryan, Wenjun, & Acosta, 2002). The breastfeeding rates for mothers enrolled in WIC are 58.8% for initiation, 22.1% for 6 months duration, and 12.8% for 12 months duration (Ross Products Division of Abbott Laboratories, 2003). These low breastfeeding rates are particularly disturbing because approximately 50% of all infants in the United States receive WIC benefits (Fox, McManus, & Schmidt, 2003).

WIC serves a diverse population. In 2000, 37% of all WIC enrollees were White, 35% were Hispanic, and 22% were Black non-Hispanic (Fox et al., 2003). Li and Grummer-Strawn (2002), using data from the Third National Health and Nutrition Examination Survey (1988–1994), stratified breastfeeding rates by race, ethnicity, and sociodemographic characteristics and determined that lower income, Black, non-Hispanic women had the lowest rates.

Does enrollment in WIC influence infant feeding decisions? Schwartz, Popkin, Tognetti, and Zohoori (1995) report that WIC enrollment during pregnancy, in conjunction with breastfeeding advice, significantly increases breastfeeding initiation. Few studies have specifically focused on WIC influence on the infant feeding decisions of Black non-Hispanic women. Beal, Kuhlthau, and Perrin (2003) found that being African American was associated with less likelihood of breastfeeding advice and greater likelihood of bottle-feeding advice from WIC nutritionists.

Since 1972, WIC has supplied formula for infants enrolled in its program. In 1989, the Child Nutrition and WIC Reauthorization Act designated funding for breastfeeding promotion and support (U.S. Department of Agriculture, n.d.). Do these WIC activities influence infant feeding decisions of Black non-Hispanic women? In an ethnographic study in St. Croix, Virgin Islands, Corbett (1999) indicates that WIC's provision of free formula might adversely influence breastfeeding duration. Other studies suggest that breastfeeding promotional activities might offset this influence. Counseling and motivational videotapes increased breastfeeding duration in African-American WIC participants who initiated breastfeeding in a WIC clinic in Baltimore, Maryland (Gross et al., 1998). Breastfeeding education programs with additional incentives also increased exclusive breastfeeding among urban, primarily African-American WIC participants in western New York (Finch & Daniel, 2002). Additional studies are needed to investigate the influence of WIC.

In this research, I explore WIC's influence on the infant feeding decisions of inner-city, Black non-Hispanic women enrolled in a New York metropolitan-area WIC clinic. The women's beliefs and experiences with WIC are described over the course of pregnancy and the postpartum period. This report is part of a larger ethnographic study on the infant feeding beliefs and experiences of these same women (Cricco-Lizza, 2002). The findings of this larger investigation demonstrate that formula feeding was the norm for these mothers. The women also described a preponderance of loss and daily stress in their everyday lives and reported experiences with financial hardship, housing, racism, and fears for safety. Infant feeding beliefs of these mothers reflected responses to their life experiences. The study participants also reported that nurses and physicians provided limited education and support for infant feeding during their pregnancy and postpartum care. It is within those contexts that the present report should be considered.

RESEARCH METHOD

I used an ethnographic approach to explore WIC's influence on the infant feeding decisions of Black non-Hispanic women. Eight months of preliminary fieldwork at a local affiliated WIC clinic facilitated my entry into the field. During this time, I obtained staff input about the clinic and their perceptions about the concerns of the women served. I obtained approval for observations and interviews from the WIC agency and the human subjects committees with a requirement for written consents for tape-recorded interviews.

Participant Observation

I conducted observations over an 18-month period with participants of a New York metropolitan-area WIC clinic. This clinic served a primarily Black and Hispanic population, but the research was centered on the Black non-Hispanic women. Maxwell (1996) states that participant observation can reveal tacit understanding and perspectives that participants might be reluctant or unable to share in direct interviews. I observed WIC clinic operations with a particular focus on 130 mothers' interactions with 15 Black, Hispanic, and White WIC employees (6 nutritionists, 6 clerks, 1 lactation consultant, and 2 breastfeeding peer counselors).

Participant observation can vary along a continuum from pure observation to active participation in the daily activities of study members (Gold, 1958). In this investigation, I dressed informally and sat with the WIC participants in the waiting room and the group nutrition education classes. For the most part, I listened and observed but also engaged in reciprocal activities such as holding doors and assisting with child care. When I initiated discussions with the women, I introduced myself as a nurse studying infant feeding, and the participants seemed receptive in response.

Observation sessions in the WIC clinic were about 2 hours long and took place two or three times per week at varying times and on various days during the study period. The data obtained from these observations were documented immediately after these encounters.

Interviews

From this group of mothers, I purposefully selected 11 key informants who were African American or Caribbean American, primiparous, English speaking, and willing to be followed through pregnancy and postpartum. These women reported a variety of infant feeding beliefs and experiences as they made their transition into motherhood. They signed written consents and agreed to two or three in-depth formal, audiotaped interviews over time. During these interviews, each key informant discussed infant feeding in light of her childhood experiences, pregnancy, childbirth, hospitalization, recovery, and return to work or school. The women were specifically queried about the influence of WIC on their infant feeding decisions. These informants were told that pseudonyms would be used throughout the research process.

With the key informants' continuing permission, these formal interviews were extended by informal interviews during face-to-face meetings and telephone calls. I met the key informants in the WIC clinic, homes, hospitals, malls, and fast-food restaurants to see how infant feeding fit into the context of their everyday lives. I also called them frequently on the phone to hear about the ongoing factors that influenced their infant feeding decisions over pregnancy and the first year postpartum. There were 147 telephone calls to the key informants over the course of the study. During these calls, I made no recommendations about specific feeding methods, but I did refer women for help as requested.

The formal interviews were audiotaped and transcribed verbatim. I reviewed the transcripts and tapes line by line for accuracy. The informal interview field notes from the meetings and telephone calls were consistently typed immediately after each session.

Data Management, Analysis, and Verification

By the end of the study, I had 63 detailed observations of 319 people (130 mothers, 116 children, 20 grandmothers, 17 fathers, 11 friends, and 25 other relatives). There were 11 to 32 data points for each key informant. Each data point signified a formal tape-recorded interview or an informal interview through a telephone call or face-to-face meeting. All of these sources of data about the key informants, along with WIC clinic observational data of all of the study's general participants, and analytic memos were entered into the computer software program QSR NUD*IST. This program facilitated management and analysis of the data. I developed codes inductively from the data and collected them at nodes on an index tree in this program. I examined these nodes and restructured them during analysis, checking for recurring patterns and themes.

I verified the findings through prolonged engagement with the participants over the 18-month study, triangulation of interviewing and observation techniques, and member checks (Creswell, 1998). These verification procedures were a good fit with the ethnographic method and enabled me to check findings from WIC clinic observations with the key informants for further elucidation. I was also able to take specific data obtained from the key informants and look among the general WIC participants for verification. In addition, I confirmed findings with WIC employees, the local Maternal Child Consortium, and representatives of eight subgrantee agencies of the Healthy Mothers/Healthy Babies program. I shared raw data and NUD*IST analyses with a peer group of doctoral students for verbal and written critiques.

FINDINGS

The 130 mothers observed in the WIC clinic varied in age and parity. Most of these women reported formula feeding to the clerk during intake procedures in the waiting room. Bottle feeding was common in the waiting room, and only one time during the course of the study was a Black non-Hispanic WIC participant observed breastfeeding in the WIC clinic. More detailed, prospective data were obtained about WIC influence on the infant feeding decisions of the 11 key informants. Ten of these key informants were born locally, and 1 was born in the Caribbean. Their ages ranged from 18 to 34 years with a mean of 22.9 years. They had 10 to 15 years of education with a mean of 12.5 years. Ten of 11 of the key informants were single. In the postpartum period, 6 of these key informants formula fed, and 5 initiated breastfeeding. One of the breastfeeders weaned at 6 weeks, 2 at 3 to 4 months, and 2 others had breastfeeding durations of 1 year.

The context of infant feeding decisions in WIC is detailed in the following sections. In particular, I describe the environmental and human interactions in WIC, the women's beliefs about WIC, and the influence that these beliefs and interactive experiences had on infant feeding decisions over pregnancy and the postpartum period.

The WIC Clinic Environment

As noted previously (Cricco-Lizza, 2004), the women in this study experienced a preponderance of loss and stress in their everyday lives. These problems did not go away when they went to WIC. A trip to the WIC clinic often required much effort for the women. Some were barely a few days postpartum, whereas others made the trip with babies and toddlers in hand. Some walked to the clinic; others arranged for rides or took buses. Because many of these women returned to work in the early postpartum period, mothers also reported that they had to take time off from their jobs to come to WIC. It was also not uncommon to see fragile babies attached to apnea monitors and hear mothers' accounts about prematurity and neonatal intensive care unit (NICU) experiences.

The WIC clinic that served as the main research site was located in a storefront on a busy, main street in the heart of a downtown, inner-city area. From the street perspective, one could not help but notice the colorful displays in the large glass windows at the entrance to the WIC clinic. These artfully arranged displays of juice, milk, cereal, bread, and vegetables were changed frequently to reflect holidays and seasons.

Through the front door of the WIC clinic, one entered a bright, open space that served as the waiting room. The reception desk was directly ahead on the right side of the front of the room and was staffed by two clerks. The WIC waiting room was decorated festively for every holiday, and one could always count on seeing life-size homemade ghosts, Christmas carolers, hand-cut valentines, or other seasonal decorations. The staff expended extra effort to make the clinic look warm and cheerful. One of the nutritionists said that she wanted to make the clinic more "inviting" for the women and children, and I did frequently observe children pointing to the decorations.

The waiting room had 24 seats, which were arranged in groups of 4 to 6 that faced each other. This physical structure facilitated social interactions among people waiting to be seen. During my observations, women chatted together and often helped in the care of each other's babies. If a mother was struggling with a crying baby or restless toddler, WIC employees or other mothers would freely offer assistance with child care and/or words of support. For example, one teen mother looked overwhelmed while she cared for her newborn and tried to keep her 22-month-old child from running around the room, climbing on tables, and pulling on the cord of the public telephone. Two mothers listened to her talk about her difficult labor, how tired she was, and how hard it was to get to the WIC clinic that morning. They told her that it was normal for the toddler to act out when a new baby was born and reassured her that things would settle down with time. They took turns helping her care for the children while this teen mom talked about her concerns. She seemed calmer after these interactions in the WIC waiting room.

The WIC clinic environment was also welcoming for children. Children frequently gathered around a small wooden toddler's table or played with a bead board attached to the wall. On one occasion, a middle-aged mother gathered some restless children to play school. She let them take turns being the teacher and taught them the colors on the bead board.

Human Interactions in WIC

The WIC clinic has stringent governmental guidelines to determine eligibility for WIC enrollment. The WIC clerks checked proof of residence, income, identity, and height, weight, and blood work information from referring professionals. Typically, a woman would present this information to the clerk and then see a nutritionist for evaluation and counseling. Pregnant women also saw a lactation consultant or peer counselor for breastfeeding promotion. On designated food voucher distribution days, the women attended a nutrition education program in the classroom.

I witnessed these procedures repeatedly over the study period. Quite often, the WIC enrollee would be missing part of the eligibility documentation for presentation to the receptionist. In some instances, the woman would become angry and other times tearful. The clerks at the front desk consistently remained calm and pleasant during these times. One particular clerk had a special knack for dealing with the women. She was kind and empathetic in varied difficult situations and invariably found the right words to soothe even the most stressed women. She altered the procedures as much as she could and demonstrated respect and caring for the women. She would leave her desk to help women who were struggling to get around after cesarean sections. Frequently, she would hold and soothe their babies as these mothers completed the WIC paperwork. She distracted overtired toddlers and gently encouraged exhausted mothers. In one situation, she successfully appeased an angry father, and he was soon laughing with her about all of the things that had gone wrong during his day. The people who came to this WIC clinic responded quite positively to her and visibly relaxed after talking with her. I also overheard positive comments about her from women in the waiting room. She apparently knew many women from the community, and I witnessed several people walk in off the street just to say hello to her. In one situation, she had kind words to say to a woman who came in to tell her that

like the main thing. So WIC is one of the best programs that they came up with.

Imani expressed similar beliefs about WIC:

> It helps provide you with things that you need, to help the baby grow. And you know everybody don't always have money, and it's helpful like that you know that you can go to the store and get like food and stuff. You would be amazed like how many kids don't eat.

WIC Influence on Infant Feeding Decisions

WIC's Influence on Prenatal Infant Feeding Decisions.   During prenatal interviews, I asked the key informants if WIC was a source of influence on their infant feeding decisions. Ella responded like many when she said, "No, nobody but me." Imani told me that the decision for infant feeding was "not really up to them." Nevertheless, further interviews and observations suggested that WIC did influence the women on several fronts and sometimes in contradictory ways. Cherise said, "When you're applying to WIC, you know the [formula] milk is free, so why wouldn't you take it?" Most of the key informants claimed that their friends and relatives bottle-fed. These women came to the clinic with the expectation that they would get free formula from WIC. On arrival at the clinic, the women were immediately exposed to posters displaying images of breastfeeding women. A large poster prominently displayed directly behind the receptionist's desk featured a Black woman breastfeeding a baby. This poster was entitled "Breastfeeding for you." Phrases underneath the title included: "Feel better about yourself, feel closer to baby, enjoyable, rewarding, no messy bottles, no one will notice, burn off more calories, more WIC benefits for you." On the left wall of the waiting room was a huge banner with the words "Loving Support Makes Breastfeeding Work." The walls of the entire clinic were covered with multi-ethnic posters about breastfeeding, the food pyramid, recommended immunization schedules, and healthy nutrition.

I specifically asked the key informants what messages they received from the posters. Most of the women identified that the posters in the WIC clinic encouraged healthy eating. Many of them also identified the emphasis on breastfeeding. Aja said that the posters were "usually about breastfeeding." Brenda also said, "I be's seeing a lot of breastfeeding" in the posters. Dena said that she saw posters about "breastfeeding, yeah, they want you to breastfeed . . . cause they feel that's very important." Gloria told me that the posters encouraged her to breastfeed. She said, "It's just something that's so natural and so sweet about it." Helena, Karen, and Imani also said that they noticed the posters. Imani specifically said, "I'm always reading something or looking at something, always learning something."

The key informants said that the nutritionists encouraged breastfeeding during individual counseling sessions. Julie claimed that she was told, "Breastfeeding is the best way." Helena was full of pride as she talked about the positive feedback that she received during her session. She told me that the nutritionist said, "I had an excellent diet and I would be an excellent candidate for breastfeeding."

The lactation counselors contacted pregnant enrollees during the prenatal period to offer individual and group educational sessions about the health benefits of breastfeeding. I attended several of these sessions and noticed mixed reactions from the participants. Some of the women were engaged in the discussion, others were quiet, and some looked annoyed. One particular mother interrupted the session to complain that WIC did not offer the brand of formula that she preferred.

During the prenatal interviews, I asked the key informants to tell me about these breastfeeding promotion sessions. Many of the key informants told me that the first time they had heard about the health advantages of breastfeeding was at the WIC clinic. Their responses to this new information varied. Brenda said, "It ain't gonna change my mind." Some of the key informants were initially suspicious about this information. Cherise and Aja, in particular, voiced concern that WIC might be promoting breastfeeding as a way to save money on formula. Cherise also told me that she felt a little "intimidated" by the breastfeeding promotion because she fully intended to feed formula to her baby. She remained committed to this course of action until after her baby was born. In her early days postpartum, I was surprised when she told me that she was breastfeeding. She said:

> You know, some of the facts that they give you about breastfeeding, to me, they were, I found them important. And especially like when they said, well, you know as far as, they can't get shots for two months. And if the breastmilk builds up the immune system a little stronger and I have a winter baby, the weather's going to be crazy, the chances of cold and flu are so much higher. That's what made me really think, well, if I, I'm gonna breastfeed, if I can make her a little healthier and chances of getting sick a little lower, I'm gonna take it.

Other key informants were intrigued by the health advantages or the bonding benefits that were described in breastfeeding promotion sessions. After attending these sessions, Febe said, "I started thinking about it a lot." She claimed that WIC "makes me want to try it [breastfeeding]." She claimed, "I think the milk from your breast has a lot more things than formula milk can provide. So I think it's important." Gloria and Helena specifically mentioned that they wished to avoid digestive problems or ear infections in their babies. Helena said that the WIC peer counselor told her that her own breastfed baby was very healthy and never had any ear infections as an infant. Helena then said, "I lost part of my hearing in this ear about a year ago and that's due to having grown up with a lot of ear infections from when I was little. If breastfeeding will take the odds of that happening down on my kid, it's worth it to me."

Helena claimed that the peer counselor was "really nice" and influenced her to decide to breastfeed. She said, "After talking to her, I said I don't care what they [friends] say about my breasts being small."

WIC's Influence on Postpartum Infant Feeding Decisions.   The women who formula-fed returned to WIC very early after delivery. They enrolled their babies in the WIC program and received vouchers to obtain formula. This process was familiar to them and followed patterns used by their families and friends. Some of the key informants told me that their babies experienced difficulties tolerating the formula. Karen said, "I'm having problems with her formula." She said that when she switched from the hospital brand to WIC's brand of formula, "It gave her diarrhea and an upset stomach, so I had to take her to the doctor . . . so now her milk has to be changed."

WIC waiting room observations supported this experience. A few women mentioned to me that babies have digestive problems with certain formulas. It was accepted as normal that formulas would be changed a few times before the right one was found. Cherise told me that in the beginning, the mother has to work on "getting the right formula with the right bottle." The WIC clinic employees worked with the mothers to make these changes.

The five key informants who initiated breastfeeding reported a variety of experiences in the postpartum period. All of them were unfamiliar with breastfeeding techniques, and most of them reported minimal breastfeeding assistance during their hospitalizations. Two of them had babies in the NICU. These breastfeeding key informants independently, creatively, and resiliently faced feeding challenges in their own individual ways. Cherise and Gloria called the hospital hotline for breastfeeding advice, whereas Febe received some breastfeeding recommendations from her pediatrician during an early infant checkup. Their families and friends recommended formula when feeding questions arose.

The key informants did not independently contact WIC for breastfeeding support and guidance. I asked Cherise whom she would call if she had any feeding questions or problems, and she said that she would call the hospital hotline. I asked if she would call WIC, and she said that she did not need any formula, so she was planning on waiting before she went back to WIC. It was noteworthy that she immediately associated WIC with formula rather than breastfeeding assistance. At a later interview, I assessed her perception of breastfeeding support from WIC. I asked her if the nutritionist made any recommendations about how she should feed the baby when she did return to WIC for a routine appointment. Cherise said, "Breastfeeding, as much as possible to try to stick to it, stick to the breastfeeding."

Most of the key informants who initiated breastfeeding did not contact WIC when they encountered problems. Aja, Cherise, and Febe never met with the lactation consultant in the postpartum period. Aja did not get in touch with WIC when her baby was in the NICU for the first 2 weeks of life. She only pumped her breasts when she was visiting the baby at the hospital. When her breast milk supply decreased after a few weeks, she weaned. Cherise and Febe breastfed without major problems on discharge from the hospital. They both faced difficulties combining work and breastfeeding at 3 to 4 months postpartum and weaned at that time.

Gloria told me that she called the hospital hotline for assistance when she had initial questions about breastfeeding. She said that she also had some early difficulties with yeast infections and pain in her breasts. She said that while she was at WIC for a prescheduled appointment, she stopped to see the lactation consultant. She told me that the lactation consultant gave her some recommendations that helped her to overcome her problems. She was very satisfied with this assistance and consulted her again a few months later when she had questions about her milk supply. She continued to breastfeed for one year.

Helena had major problems initiating breastfeeding after her daughter was discharged from the NICU. She had purchased a lower-priced pump that damaged her nipples, and she had a very difficult time with engorgement. She had no experience with breastfeeding and did not know what to do to start. Helena said that her mother told her that she should just "get a pill to dry up those things." Helena was frightened by her daughter's serious neurological problems and was also recovering from an infection after delivery. She was crying when she called me on discharge. I listened to her concerns and referred her to WIC for hands-on assessment and treatment. When I talked with Helena afterward, she said that the lactation consultant was helpful when she called her and told her to come down to WIC right away. She said that the lactation consultant immediately took her in the back room, closed the curtain, showed her what was wrong, and helped her fix it. Helena said that the lactation consultant got her baby latched on and then talked with her for 40 minutes. Helena told me that she felt so much better after that. She said her breasts were softer and the pain went away. Helena said

> That made *all* the difference. When I finally got her latched on, she showed me this pillow that I could lay her on and sit her on my waist. And I went and I got the pillow . . . brought that home and got her to latch on. My breasts didn't hurt any more from that day on.

Many months later, Helena still talked about how kindly she was treated that day at WIC. She credited WIC with her successful initiation of breast-feeding, and she continued to breastfeed for a year.

DISCUSSION

This study contributed valuable information about the environmental and human interactions that influenced the infant feeding decisions of Black, non-Hispanic women enrolled in WIC. Formula feeding was the norm for the women in this study. They heard positive messages about WIC from family and friends, and most of the key informants initially came to this WIC clinic expecting free formula for their babies. For many of the women, their first encounter with breastfeeding promotion was at this WIC clinic. This study documented their responses to this breastfeeding promotion and captured the changes in beliefs and experiences that occurred over time.

Besides offering basic breastfeeding information, WIC provided environmental support through its window displays, breastfeeding posters, and banners. These physical props were sensually appealing and featured culturally sensitive role models. They also used messages that have been deemed to be relevant to this population (Bryant, Coreil, D'Angelo, Bailey, & Lazarov, 1992; Corbett, 2000; Underwood et al., 1997). In addition, the physical layout of the waiting room encouraged interaction among the WIC participants. The women received support and encouragement from both strangers and known friends in the waiting room. This was particularly important for women who reported high levels of stress and loss in their everyday lives (Cricco-Lizza, 2002).

The "milk of human kindness" (Thackeray, 1993, p. 352) was freely dispensed at this WIC clinic. The study findings suggest that designated health care professionals are not the only ones who influence health care behaviors. The clerks that served as the frontline receptionists set a tone of caring and concern for the women that used this clinic. WIC's influence on these women began at the door with the kindness of the clerks and extended through the encouragement of the nutritionists and lactation counselors. The WIC providers were attuned to the needs of the women and children and demonstrated caring and respect throughout WIC procedures. They listened to the women's concerns, and they personalized education to meet individual needs. Interpersonal skills including understanding patients' individual experience, expressing caring, communicating clearly, sharing power, and honesty and respect have been linked to patients' experiences of trust with their physicians (Thom & Campbell, 1997). Raisler (2000) reports that breastfeeding women enrolled in WIC valued personal and caring breastfeeding peer counselors. The women in this study were consistent in their positive evaluation of WIC as a trusted source of aid. Within the context of these trusting relationships, the women seemed to be more open to hearing the breastfeeding promotion by WIC employees. In their concept analysis of trust, Lynn-McHale and Deatrick (2000) found that an outcome of a trusting relationship between family and health care provider was support of health care provider treatment recommendations. This study demonstrated that breastfeeding information might not initially be received well by WIC participants who have bottle-feeding as their norm. However, when WIC employees listened to the concerns of women, treated them with caring and respect, and tailored messages according to their needs, infant feeding beliefs changed for about half of the key informants. The longitudinal nature of this study allowed for the capture of changes in WIC influence over pregnancy and postpartum. These findings concretely reflect that caring human and environmental interactions might hold strong potential to decrease health care disparities.

WIC was a trusted source of assistance for the participants; however, there was also evidence of missed opportunities. The women did not regard some of the videotapes positively. This finding is different from that reported by Gross et al. (1998) and could be related to differences in cultural sensitivity of videotapes. The women in this study paid greater attention to the nutritionist-led educational sessions. The human link was more effective, and the women responded to the personal give and take of these pragmatic, nutrition-oriented discussions. In a similar fashion, the breastfeeding women told me that the lactation counselors were supportive and kind to them during their encounters. Nevertheless, not all of the women who chose breastfeeding had postpartum visits to the lactation counselors. The women seemed unaware that they could receive breastfeeding assistance or advice about returning to work. For the most part, they did not actively seek assistance but independently dealt with problems on their own. The mothers did not report that either WIC or other agencies or providers contacted them in the postpartum period to offer outreach and support.

One of the striking findings in this study is that although bottle-feeding was the norm among this sample of women, almost one-half of the key informants initiated breastfeeding. It is a testament to the strength of this group that these women persisted to find their own styles to fit their everyday life demands despite so many barriers. Nevertheless, it behooves professionals to structure services to facilitate rather than impede women's efforts to initiate and continue breastfeeding.

CONCLUSION AND IMPLICATIONS

The findings of this study suggest that human and environmental interactions might be important for health behavior changes. In this investigation, caring, respectful interactions with health care workers led to trusting relationships in which new health behaviors were initiated. These particular study findings indicate that WIC can play an important role in decreasing health disparities in breastfeeding for Black non-Hispanic women. This investigation points out the need for more support postpartum. The participants also highlighted the need for practical assistance with return-to-work feeding issues. WIC should consider active outreach during the postpartum period and increased collaboration with local hospitals and providers to create a web of support after childbirth. Education should also be targeted to family members, significant others, and employers to extend this support into the community.

Different WIC clinics might vary in the influence they exert on infant feeding decisions. Additional ethnographic studies are needed with other WIC agencies and populations.

REFERENCES

American Academy of Pediatrics. (2005). Breastfeeding and the use of human milk. *Pediatrics, 115,* 496–506.

American College of Nurse-Midwives. (1992). *Clinical practices statement on breastfeeding.* Washington, DC: Author.

American College of Obstetricians and Gynecologists. (2000). *Breastfeeding: Maternal and infant aspects.* (ACOG Educational Bulletin no. 258). Washington, DC: Author.

American Dietetic Association. (1997). *Position of the American Dietetic Association: Promotion of breastfeeding.* Washington, DC: Author.

American Public Health Association. (1982). *Breastfeeding.* (APHA Public Policy Statements no. 7403 and no. 8226). Washington, DC: Author.

Beal, A. C., Kuhlthau, K., & Perrin, J. M. (2003). Breastfeeding advice given to African American and White women by physicians and WIC counselors. *Public Health Reports, 118,* 368–376.

Bryant, C. A., Coreil, J., D'Angelo, S. L., Bailey, D. F., & Lazarov, M. (1992). A strategy for promoting breastfeeding among economically disadvantaged women and adolescents. *NAACOG's Clinical Issues, 3,* 723–730.

Corbett, K. S. (1999). Infant feeding styles of West Indian women. *Journal of Transcultural Nursing, 10*(1), 22–30.

Corbett, K. S. (2000). Explaining infant feeding style of low-income women. *Journal of Pediatric Nursing, 15,* 73–81.

Creswell, J. W. (1998). *Qualitative inquiry and research design: Choosing among five traditions.* Thousand Oaks, CA: Sage.

Cricco-Lizza, R. (2002). Thirst for the milk of human kindness; an ethnography of infant feeding decisions of Black women enrolled in WIC. *Dissertations Abstracts International* (UMI No. AAT 3031299).

Cricco-Lizza, R. (2004). Infant feeding beliefs and experiences of Black women enrolled in a New York metropolitan area WIC clinic. *Qualitative Health Research, 14,* 1197–1210.

Finch, C., & Daniel, E. L. (2002). Breastfeeding education with incentives increases exclusive breastfeeding among urban WIC participants. *Journal of the American Dietetic Association, 102,* 981–984.

Fox, H. B., McManus, M. A., & Schmidt, H. J. (2003, August 14). WIC reauthorization: Opportunities for improving the nutritional status of women, infants, and children. *National Health Policy Forum,* 1–36. Retrieved August 12, 2005, from http://www.nhpf.org/pdfs_bp/BP%5FWIC2%5F8%2D03%2Epdf.

Gold, R. (1958). Roles in sociological field operations. *Social Forces, 36,* 217–223.

Gross, S. M., Caulfield, L. E., Bentley, M. E., Bronner, Y., Kessler, L., Jensen, J., et al. (1998). Counseling and videotapes increase duration of breastfeeding in African-American WIC participants who initiate breastfeeding. *Journal of the American Dietetic Association, 98*(2), 143–148.

Li, R., & Grummer-Strawn, L. (2002). Racial and ethnic disparities in breastfeeding among United States infants: Third National Health and Nutrition Examination Survey, 1988–1994. *Birth, 29,* 251–257.

Lynn-McHale, D. J., & Deatrick, J. A. (2000). Trust between family and health care provider. *Journal of Family Nursing, 6*(3), 210–230.

Maxwell, J. A. (1996). *Qualitative research design: An interactive approach.* Thousand Oaks, CA: Sage.

Raisler, J. (2000). Against the odds: Breastfeeding experiences of low income mothers. *Journal of Midwifery and Health, 45*(3), 253–263.

Ross Products Division of Abbott Laboratories. (2003). *Breastfeeding trends—2002.* Columbus, OH: Author.

Ryan, A. S., Wenjun, Z., & Acosta, A. (2002). Breastfeeding continues to increase into the millennium. *Pediatrics, 110,* 1103–1109.

Schwartz, J. B., Popkin, B. M., Tognetti, J., & Zohoori, N. (1995). Does WIC participation improve breastfeeding practices? *American Journal of Public Health, 85,* 729–731.

Thackeray, W. (1993). *Vanity fair.* Kent, Great Britain: Mackays of Chatham.

Thom, D. H., & Campbell, B. (1997). Patient-physician trust: An exploratory study. *Journal of Family Practice, 44*(2), 169–176.

Underwood, S., Pridham, K., Brown, L., Clark, T., Frazier, W., Limbo, R., et al. (1997). Infant feeding practices of African-American low-income women in a central city community. *Journal of Community Health Nursing, 14,* 189–205.

U.S. Department of Agriculture, Food and Consumer Service. (1995). *Study of WIC participant and program characteristics 1994 final report.* Washington, DC: U.S. Department of Agriculture, Office of Analysis and Evaluation.

U.S. Department of Agriculture, Food and Nutrition Service. (n.d.). Legislative history of breastfeeding promotion requirements in WIC. Retrieved August 12, 2005, from http://www.fns.usda.gov/wic/breastfeeding/bflegishistory.htm.

U.S. Department of Health and Human Services. (2000). *Healthy people 2010: Conference edition—Volumes I and II.* Washington, DC: Author.

12

Case Study: The Method

Patricia Becker Hentz

According to Yin (2003), case study methods are well suited when the researcher's aim is to retain the holistic and meaningful characteristics of real-life events. Reasons for choosing case study method include the desire to understand complex social phenomena with the belief that the research approach needs to explore the contextual conditions related to the phenomena. Before delving into case study method, it is important to point out that there are no hard and fast rules on how to do case study research. It has been used by many disciplines for a range of purposes. What can be agreed upon when it comes to case study research is that there is no standardization (McKee, 2004). Case study research can be simple or complex; it can focus on a single individual, a group of individuals, organizations, processes, neighborhoods, institutions, and events. It is used extensively in social science research, including psychology, sociology, political science, anthropology, history, and economics. It is also used in practice-oriented fields such as urban planning, public administration, public policy, management science, social work, nursing, medicine, and education. In reviewing the literature on case study method, it is evident that the focus of the case studies varies greatly. What is also evident is that there is marked divergence regarding how case study research has been defined and conceptualized. In addition, the processes of data collection and analysis also vary because they are reflective of the research question and aims of the study. Finally, case studies may be small or large and may be qualitative or quantitative.

This chapter presents an overview of case study method with emphasis on how it can be used as a qualitative approach. The usefulness of the method is discussed with an attempt to focus on the common features as presented in the research literature. One key aspect of case study research is the emphasis on identifying the "object of study within its social context." This is discussed in more depth within the chapter.

The concept, case study, is applied in a variety of ways with a range of definitions. Therefore, as a starting point, it is critical to clarify what case study method is, and what it is not. Case study, in its broadest definition within the social sciences, has been divided into four categories; however, only the fourth category depicts the research method. One definition of case study refers to a teaching case. Teaching case studies do not need to accurately depict a person, event, or process. The aim is to enhance learning. The second category is case histories. Case histories are used for a purpose of record keeping. Casework, the third category, is used to describe the management of health care for a patient or population. Case research or case study research, the fourth category, is for the purpose of "investigating activities or complex processes that are not easily separated from the social context within which they occur" (Cutler, 2004, p. 367).

Case study is defined by Gerring (2004, p. 341) as an intensive study of a *single unit* (a relatively bounded phenomenon) with an aim to generalize across a larger class of similar phenomena. The *single unit* is the phenomenon under investigation, also referred to as the object of study. What is essential in case study research is that the unit or phenomenon be clearly defined. Another critical feature of case study research, as discussed by Yin (2003), is that case study inquiry investigates a phenomenon within its real-life context, when the boundaries between phenomenon and context are not clearly evident. At first glance, these two definitions may seem somewhat contradictory in regards to how boundary is applied. In actuality, both agree that the unit or phenomenon needs to be clearly defined. To a large extent the research literature describing case study research has been in agreement that the unit or phenomenon needs be linked to life or social context. What is also characteristic of case study research is that the boundary between the phenomenon of study and the social context is quite blurred. It is common in case study research that the researcher has little or no control over the context within which the phenomenon exists. This last condition is one of the major justifications for choosing case study method. In essence, understanding the social context is vital for one to have a comprehensive understanding of the phenomenon. Cutler (2004) makes the point that if clarity of boundary is vague or porous, the situation is not a case. Again, it is important to note that the boundary to which he is referring is the boundary of the single unit or phenomenon, not the boundary between the phenomenon and the social context. An example illustrating the blurring of social context and phenomenon can be seen in Columbia Tristar Films' 2003 movie *Monster*. The movie depicts the life story of the first female serial killer. Clearly, the phenomenon or object of study is the female serial killer. What is also evident, as her life story unfolds, is that the troubling aspects of her life and the sequence of events leading to her becoming a serial killer are seamlessly interconnected.

CHARACTERISTICS OF QUALITATIVE CASE STUDY RESEARCH

Stake (1995) discusses the following characteristics of qualitative case study research, which are helpful when considering case study as a methodology:

- ♦ *It is holistic.* Focus is on a comprehensive understanding of the phenomenon with rich contextual detail. The sum of the whole is greater than its parts.
- ♦ *It is empirical.* The researcher maintains a naturalistic orientation for data collection.
- ♦ *It is interpretive.* The research acknowledges the importance of researcher–subject interaction. The researcher needs to be aware of preunderstandings and biases.
- ♦ *It is empathic.* Qualitative case study research as human science maintains the value and respect for persons.

Case study research offers flexibility in choosing data gathering processes with the aim of understanding the phenomenon embedded within its contextual background. Anderson et al. (2005) describe case study as a way of exploring a phenomenon as an integrated whole drawing upon complexity theory as a way of elaborating on the nature of case study research. Additionally, Yin (2003) describes case study research as a "comprehensive research strategy" rather than a particular methodology for data collection. As such, researchers can employ a variety of data collection methods (Cutler, 2004). This flexibility might also be a drawback of case study research, making it difficult to operationalize. The question this raises is, "If the method is so flexible, how does one go about case study research?" Considering the fact that case study method draws upon various methodologies, the researcher embarking on this approach needs to be well grounded in a range of qualitative methods. In addition, one needs to remember that it is the level of the question that directs the data collection strategies, data analysis, and how the study will be presented. It is beyond the scope of this chapter to present the range of possible approaches; however, some highlights from phenomenology, grounded theory, and ethnography are discussed. It is recommended that the reader refer to these chapters within the text for more detailed information.

Understanding the lived experience is an aim in phenomenological studies. As such, researchers choosing case study research aimed at understanding individuals' life experiences would benefit from reading sources on phenomenology. It should be noted that phenomenological narratives should not be equated as case study research even though there may be many similarities. Case study research places greater attention on the contextual aspects related to an experience. Researchers may also draw upon grounded theory in regards to sampling and data analysis strategies and as a means of generating cases for theory development. In addition, theoretical sampling may be employed as a means of creating comparative cases. Ethnographic approaches, such as observation strategies, are often incorporated into case studies and are worth exploring.

DETERMINING THE RESEARCH AIMS: INTRINSIC, INSTRUMENTAL, AND MULTIPLE CASE STUDY

Before embarking on any research study, the question of what one hopes to learn from the research needs to be explored. Case study research has been conceptualized in a variety of different ways. Stake (2005) presents one approach for categorizing case studies that involves three types; intrinsic interest, instrumental interest, and multiple case study. The first, intrinsic interest, refers to a case study aimed at understanding a particular case of interest. The research aim is not to generalize to other cases, although it may. An example would be Liebow's (1967) *Tally's Corner*, a study that focused on a single group of men living in a poor, inner-city neighborhood (Yin, 2003). The results of this research have in fact been generalized, providing insights into a subculture that existed within many U.S. cities. The second, instrumental case studies, endorses the aim of providing insight and advancing understandings that can be generalized. Goffman's (1961) classic study of mental institutions describes a culture "underlife" that has provided insights that have been instrumental in understanding similar institutions. Third, an example of multiple case study involves a number of cases to investigate a phenomenon, population, or general condition. The study *The Family Encounters the Depression* (Angell, 1936/1965) depicts the experiences of university students whose families had suffered a loss of income during the Depression.

FIVE TYPES OF SINGLE-CASE STUDY DESIGNS

Yin (2003) highlights five different single-case designs:

- *Critical case in testing a well-formulated theory.* In these case studies, "the theory has specified a clear set of propositions as well as the circumstances within which the propositions are believed to be true. To confirm, challenge or extend the theory, a single case can then be used to determine whether a theory's propositions are correct or whether some alternative set of explanations might be more relevant" (Yin, 2003, p. 40).
- *Extreme or unique cases.* Examples of these cases may be seen in clinical psychology where a specific disorder is so rare that a single case is worth examining. It could also involve the description and analysis of a unique organization or community.
- *Representative or typical cases.* These cases represent a common experience or pattern.
- *Revelatory cases.* These cases involve situations where the researcher explores and analyzes a phenomenon previously inaccessible. An example is Goffman's (1961) study of mental institutions.
- *Longitudinal cases.* In longitudinal case studies, the same single case is viewed at different points in time.

MULTIPLE-CASE DESIGN

The unit or phenomenon of study can involve a small or large N. Several cases may be involved that are representative of a phenomenon. When several cases are utilized to represent a phenomenon, the researcher needs to take care not to blur the boundaries of the unit or phenomenon. If the phenomenon is too broad, too loosely defined, and/or the social context too varied, the study may resemble an exploratory study but not an exploratory case study.

CASE STUDY DESIGNS: DESCRIPTIVE, EXPLORATORY, EXPLANATORY

The research design is the logic that links the data and the research findings to the initial research question. Because case study research focuses on a unit of study or phenomenon rather than a research methodology, it can be used at any level of knowledge development, including for exploratory, descriptive, or explanatory purposes. Case study research is also used to describe processes, generate theory, and test theory. Therefore, the data collection approaches and data analysis strategies need to be tailored to the research aims. Given the divergent nature of case study method, researchers need to familiarize themselves with the data collection and analysis approaches appropriate for the type of case study research. Thus, in descriptive studies that focus on individuals' experiences, a review of interviewing approaches and phenomenology may prove invaluable. For multiple-case studies that are comparative in nature, a review of grounded theory research, including theoretical sampling, and constant comparative approaches to data analysis would be useful.

TYPES OF DATA FOR CASE STUDY RESEARCH

As expected, the data one collects reflect the research question as well as what one hopes to understand from conducting the research. Yin (2003) presents six common types of research evidence: documents, archival

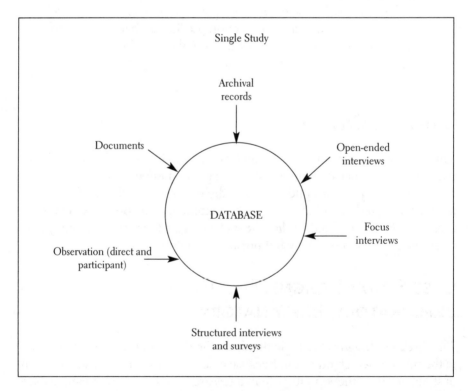

Figure 12–1 Convergence of evidence (triangulation). Adapted from Yin (2003). *Case Study Research* (3rd ed.) Thousand Oaks, CA: Sage.

records, interviews, direct observation, participant observation, and physical artifacts. The choice of combination of data collection options is dependent upon the research question and how the data collection strategy can uncover the complexity of the phenomenon. The use of multiple approaches, termed triangulation of data, aids in providing different perspectives, which adds depth to the case study. (See Figure 12–1, Convergence of Evidence.)

COMPONENTS OF CASE STUDY RESEARCH

The components of qualitative case study research are similar to other qualitative methods. What is complex about case study method is its flexibility. With the focus on the object of study and the social context, case study research borrows from a variety of qualitative research methods in regards to data collection approaches and strategies for data analysis. Thus, researchers who choose to adopt a case study approach need to be familiar with a range of qualitative approaches. The following sections highlight examples of the major components of case study research.

Identifying the "Object of Study": Defining the Boundaries

The first step is to identify topic of interest and whether case study method is appropriate. As stated earlier, the boundaries regarding the single unit or object of study need to be identified clearly. The social context should also be evident. The following represent exemplars of case studies with the "object of study" highlighted.

> *Single-case example: "The Jack-Roller"*: Shaw (1930) presents comprehensive data on one individual, a juvenile delinquent who is the object of study. The case study is presented as a life history, written by him, with material about him from several other sources. The boundaries of this case are clear: a single juvenile delinquent. Consistent with case study method, the social context is a critical component of the study.
>
> *Mutiple-case study: "Street Corner Society"*: Whyte (1943/1955) focuses in detail on two gangs and their local social context, a street corner. The object of study is "street corner gangs." The research is exploratory in nature using participant observation as the primary data collection approach.
>
> *Case study with the emphasis on social process: "Boys in White"*: Boys in White (Becker, Greer, Hughes, & Strauss, 1961) focuses on a process

within a social context. The researchers' major interest was in the effect of medical school on students. Here the process is the object of study. Participant observation was utilized in this study. The researchers focused on different points of time in medical school rather than on the study of individuals in medical school (Platt, 1992).

Explanatory case study: Teaching effectiveness: In the late 1950s and 1960s, a group of educators wanted to understand why the changes they had made in educational approaches did not improve test results (Yin, 2003). Case by case, they explored the complexity of the teaching process in practice, widening the lens from classroom activity to the organizational, cultural, economic, and policy contexts in which learning and teaching occur. The object of study involved the education approaches within the social context.

Evident in each of these examples are clear boundaries identifying the object of study. The second characteristic of these case studies is the focus on the interface between the object of study and the social context.

What Is the Research Question?

Case study research can be descriptive, exploratory, and explanatory. Descriptive case studies describe the phenomenon, as shown in the previously mentioned case study involving the life of a juvenile delinquent. Exploratory studies such as the *Street Corner Society* (Whyte, 1943/1955) are employed when little is known about a phenomenon. An explanatory case study seeks to answer the question why, as in the preceding example examining the effectiveness of educational approaches. For more information on types of research questions, refer to other chapters within this text that highlight different qualitative approaches.

What Are the Purpose and Aims of the Research?

The purpose and aims of the study are derived directly from the research question. What is distinct about case study is its desire to understand complex social phenomena and retain the holistic and meaningful characteristics of real-life events (Yin, 2003).

What Types of Data Are Needed to Answer the Research Question?

Case study research uses a variety of data collection strategies, depending on the aims of the research. Refer to Figure 12–1 cited earlier for examples of data. In addition, refer to other qualitative methods such as phenomenology, ethnography, and grounded theory for data collection approaches.

What Sampling Strategies Are Needed?

It is probably fairly clear by now: there are no simple answers to this question. Sampling may be a single case based on the uniqueness of the case or may be purposive sampling based on the representative nature of the case. Sampling follows the question and aims of the study. As stated earlier, case studies can involve one subject, a group, an event, or a process. Multiple-case studies can be used to look at similar cases. Comparative case studies may be similar to those used in grounded theory studies and may benefit from sampling approaches such as theoretical sampling. Again, referring to different approaches for sampling is advised.

DATA MANAGEMENT, ANALYSIS, AND WRITING UP THE RESULTS

Data analysis requires attending to the different types of data and creating databases. Because of the diversity of case study research, each study can incorporate a range of approaches. See chapters in this text on ethnography, grounded theory, and phenomenology for more information. Writing up the results also reflects the types of data used as well as the type of case study. A general recommendation is to develop a rich narrative that attends to the social context and answers the research question.

CONCLUSION

This chapter offers an overview of key aspects of case study method. Case study method might best be viewed as a broad-spectrum method. It can range from descriptive to explanatory, from single case to multiple case, and can employ a variety of data collection and data analysis approaches. Although significant differences in opinion regarding the definition of case study and its scope exist, most concur that its aim is to understand complex social phenomena in a manner that is holistic and humane.

REFERENCES

Anderson, R. A., Crabtree, B. F., Steele, D.J., & McDaniel, R. R. (2005). Case study research: The view from complexity science. *Qualitative Health Reseach*, 15(5), 669–685.

Angell, R. C. (1965). *The family encounters the Depression.* Gloucester, MA: Peter Smith. (Original work published 1936)

Becker, H. S., Greer, B., Hughes, E.C., & Strauss, A. L. (1961). *Boys in white: Student culture in medical school.* Chicago: University of Chicago Press.

Columbia Tristar Films. (2003). *Monster.* Sony Pictures. Directed by Patty Jenkins, written by Patty Jenkins.

Cutler, A. (2004). Methodical failure: The use of case study method by public relations research. *Public Relations Review, 30,* 365–375.

Gerring, J. (2004). What is a case study and what is it good for? *American Political Science Review,* 98(2), 341–354.

Goffman, E. (1961). *Asylums: Essays on the social situation of mental patients and other inmates.* Garden City, NY: Anchor Books.

Liebow, E. (1967). *Tally's corner.* Boston: Little, Brown.

McKee, A. (2004). Getting to know case study research: A brief introduction. *Work Bases Learning in Primary Care, 2,* 6–8.

Platt, J. (1992). Cases of cases . . . of cases. In C. C. Ragin & H. S. Becker (Eds.), *What is a case?* New York: Cambridge University Press.

Shaw, C. (1930). *The jack-roller.* Chicago: University of Chicago Press.

Stake, R. E. (1995). *The art of case study research.* Thousand Oaks, CA: Sage.

Stake, R. E. (2005). Qualitative case studies. In N. K. Denzin & Y. S. Lincoln (Eds.), *Handbook of qualitative research.* Thousand Oaks, CA: Sage.

Whyte, W. F. (1955). *Street corner society: The social structure of an Italian slum.* Chicago: University of Chicago Press. (Original work published 1943)

Yin, R. K. (2003). *Case study research* (3rd ed.). Thousand Oaks, CA: Sage.

13

A Case Study Exemplar: Health Outcomes of People with Serious Mental Illnesses

Terry A. Badger

Case studies are one strategy for mental health systems researchers to examine health care systems to improve behavioral health care. Although case studies can be conducted with individuals, groups, institutions, and organizations (Sechrist, Steward, Sickle, & Sidani, 1996; Yin, 2003b), mental health nurses have primarily used case study research methods to study outcomes of individuals. This method has been used less frequently to evaluate public mental health systems. The conclusions from such case studies can be used to inform policy and to provide recommendations for changes in the behavioral health system. The purposes of this case study were to describe health outcomes (functioning; quality of life (QOL); service use, need, and satisfaction) of clients with serious mental illnesses who used regional public mental health services in a southwestern state, and to describe what the public mental health system did well or needed to change to better satisfy clients' needs. The system selected for this case study served a five-county area, providing public mental health services to approximately 16,500 clients annually. The case study method was selected for this research because it allowed for an investigation of the phenomenon within its real-life context (Yin, 2003b), that is, the current public mental health system. This case study was first published in *Perspectives of Psychiatric Care* in 2003.

As shown in Figure 13–1, a case study can use multiple sources of data (Yin, 1994). Each data source adds to the case study evidence and to our understanding of the phenomenon of interest. In this study, there were three primary sources of data: (1) the quantitative data from the questionnaires used in the larger study; (2) the qualitative responses of the clients to the questions about the system; and (3) the providers' responses. The quantitative results from the larger experimental study are reported elsewhere (Badger, Gelenberg, & Berren, 2004). In the larger multimethod study, 58 participants were assigned to either an intervention or control group, with the intervention participants receiving an in-depth evaluation and a consultative intervention with their community service providers, plus their usual care. The control group received only usual care. Client outcomes (functioning, quality of life, service use and need, costs, and satisfaction) were examined

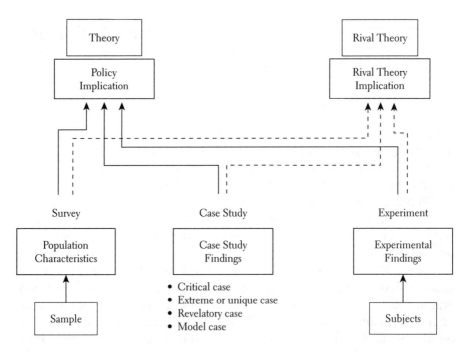

Key:
Solid Line - Data from survey, case study, or experiment support hypotheses/theory.
Dotted Line - Data from survey, case study, or experiment do not support rival hypotheses/theory.

Figure 13–1 Case Study Methodology
Source: Used with permission from Badger T, et al. (2003). *Health outcomes for people with serious mental illness: A case study.* Malden, MA: Blackwell Publishers.

over time. Data were collected at baseline upon enrollment in the study, 6 to 8 weeks after the consultative intervention, and 9 months post baseline. A second source of data resulted from participants, who were encouraged to elaborate about their lives, the mental health services currently used and needed, and their satisfaction with services beyond the fixed responses on the questionnaires. These client perspectives are often absent in evaluations, yet provide important information about how well the system meets or does not meet treatment needs. Finally, community service providers added their perspectives about what the system did well or needed to change to better meet client needs.

Methods

This case study used a multiple-case study design (Mariano, 2001) with a group of cases that were representative or typical of participants who used the regional behavioral health system. In this chapter, the qualitative findings are reported. The 15 participants (cases) were carefully selected from the 58 participants (cases) who participated in the larger experimental study. These participants had also completed all three interviews. Data from the community service providers (case managers and psychiatrists) were analyzed from discussions with these providers. The responses from both participants and providers provided validation of each other's perceptions of the system and ensured a richer description of the system.

Data Analysis

A model case study analysis strategy was used (Yin, 2003a, 2003b). Model cases are those considered representative or typical. When using this strategy, the researcher must have a sufficient understanding of the population served to select typical or model cases; thus, all members of the research team had extensive psychiatric–mental health experience with clients with serious mental illnesses who use public mental health systems.

Data were analyzed using four steps:

1. Two members of the research team developed case histories for each participant from the client's responses to verify each other's data interpretation. The six questions (Table 13–1) used to frame the case histories are stated in the first person because it was important to describe the clients and their systems of care from the unique perspectives of the clients.

TABLE 13–1   Questions Used to Frame the Case Study Analysis

Who am I?

What is my life like on a daily basis?

What services do I receive?

What services do I need?

What do I think the system does well?

What do I think needs to change so that I get better care?

2. These data were counted and collapsed into categories. These categories described client characteristics, quality of life and functioning, service use and need, and what the system did well or needed to change to give better patient care (consumer satisfaction).

3. All five members of the research team verified the data used to develop these categories.

4. To ensure accuracy, the primary researcher (Badger) conducted a secondary review of all case histories; any differences in interpretation were noted and discussed with the research team until consensus was achieved.

A complete audit trail of the data analysis process was used. The process involved noting all data sources and recording interpretations through detailed notes. Methods to ensure the trustworthiness of the data and the quality of the research were used throughout the study (Lincoln & Guba, 1985; Yin, 2003b).

Measures

Four measures were used. The Structured Clinical Interview for Diagnosis and Global Assessment of Functioning (First, Spitzer, Gibbon, & Williams, 1997) provided a diagnosis and global assessment of functioning. Interrater reliability was ≥90%. The Brief Quality of Life Index (Lehman, 1995; Lehman, Kerna, DeForge, & Dixon, 1995; Lehman & Postrado, 1995) measured QOL. Participants rate their satisfaction on health, safety, finances, social relations, family relations, daily activities, hobbies, and general life satisfaction. Participants determine frequency of social contacts, family contacts, and daily activities, and evaluate their financial adequacy.

The OARS Multidimensional Functional Assessment Questionnaire (Badger, 1998; Fillenbaum, 1988) measured service use and need. Participants were asked about their use of and need for 24 generic services: medical help (mental health services, psychotropic medications, nursing care, medical/psychiatric services, supportive services and prostheses, physical therapy), transportation, financial (financial assistance, food, groceries, housing), home help (personal care services, continuous supervision, checking, homemaker-household, meal preparation), administrative, legal and protective, social/recreational, other (employment, remedial training, sheltered employment, educational services, relocation and placement), and assessment and referral.

The Consumer Satisfaction Survey-Adult Services measured consumer satisfaction (Berren, 1998). Participants were asked how long they had received services through the mental health system, how much they participated in aspects of their treatment, and how satisfied they were with their case managers/therapists and psychiatrists. Case managers/therapists and psychiatrists were the only staff category included on this survey because they provided the majority of direct services in this system. All questionnaires had satisfactory reliability and validity.

RESULTS

Participant Characteristics

The typical participant was white, middle aged (38–48 years), and single. About half were women. The majority had a high school education. None was employed by the third interview, but had previous employment as janitors, maids, or in some other type of unskilled labor. Some had previously participated in vocational rehabilitation. Most stated they could only work for a few hours at a time and could not work the 4 to 6 consecutive hours that many part-time jobs required. Typical responses were, "When I do get a job, it only lasts for a month or two," or "I'd like to work, but it's too stressful. I just can't." All participants lived in their own apartments, grouped together with supervisory staff on site. A representative comment was, "I live in my own apartment. I really like that I can do whatever I want to do." The majority (80%) had children who were not living with them, with women more likely than men to report having children.

The major diagnoses were of the schizophrenia spectrum of disorders or bipolar disorder, and all participants were prescribed medications to treat their illnesses. Most participants (93%) reported an onset of illness in their late teens or early 20s. Responses included, "I heard voices in high school and quit," or "I had a nervous breakdown at 19." Many (80%) reported a history of illegal drug use, particularly in their early 20s. A typical participant described his drug use this way: "I have used rush, speed, marijuana, crack, or just about anything I can get." About one-third reported a family history of mental illness, most commonly bipolar disorder, and a childhood history of physical, sexual, or emotional abuse. About half had past suicide attempts, but none during the course of the study. All had at least one episode of court-ordered treatment.

Participants reported between 1 and 50 hospitalizations, but none in the year prior to study enrollment. Most reported no hospitalizations in the last 5 years. Most attributed their fewer hospitalizations to decreased symptoms. A typical comment was, "I have been in and out of the hospital in the past, but it's been about 5 years since my last admission. I've tried suicide but not recently. I now take a combination of drugs and they seem to work well." In sum, the participants in this study were typical of people with serious mental illness who use public behavioral health systems (Lehman et al., 1995; Noble, Douglas, & Newman, 2001).

Quality of Life

Participants rated their QOL as mixed or mostly satisfied on the QOL instrument, yet it was their qualitative responses that provided insights into specific problem areas for intervention and system change. The majority of responses focused on general health and social functioning. Many reported unhealthy lifestyles such as smoking, overeating, and lack of exercise. As one participant stated, "I know I should quit smoking. I'd really like to get this extra weight off me that's come in the last 2 years." Although most participants who realized their lifestyles were unhealthy had insurance, few used preventive health practices or participated in any health programs. The majority reported no routine health care even if prompted by mental health staff because "I just don't think about it." A typical woman stated: "I haven't had a Pap or mammogram in years." Participants clearly needed assistance to arrange for routine health care. Further, health education programs, including those addressing the weight gain that often accompanies taking certain psychotropic medications (Hester & Thrower, 2005; Newcomer, 2005), were noticeably absent.

All participants discussed at length their social functioning in four areas: limitations in usual social roles (e.g., parent and worker), integration, contact, and intimacy and sexual functioning. These four areas are consistent with those reported in previous research (Covington & Cola, 2000; McDonald & Badger, 2002; Patrick & Erickson, 1993).

The Limitations in Usual Social Roles.   The limitations noted in usual roles were for the roles we all typically enact—employee, parent, and home-maker. In contrast to the myth that clients did not want to work, participants wanted to work but were incapable of performing on the job even on a part-time basis. Other participants could not continue working because the money received would interfere with their benefits. One woman who worked as a maid quit when she found her benefits would be discontinued. This woman had been ill since her early 20s and, given her potential for relapse, decided that she needed her health benefits more than the work. Most participants wanted to see their children, but agreed they were incapable of parenting on a full-time basis. A typical comment was, "I haven't seen my children in a long time. I wish I could. They are better off with. . . ."

All participants lived in subsidized apartments and received assistance with their roles as homemakers. A typical comment about the advantages to the residential programs was, "Staff checks my apartment and makes sure it's cleaned up. If not, I get some help with it. I like having staff around. They take us on outings sometimes or to the grocery store." Nearly all participants interviewed experienced severe role limitations as employees, parents, and homemakers.

Integration in the Community.   The second area of social functioning focused on community activities, social/recreational or leisure activities, membership in organizations, and community safety. Most participants were not involved in community activities except for church, although a few used the public library. Lack of transportation and money were reasons participants were not more actively involved in the community. However, a few of the participants stated their lack of involvement was because of the symptoms of their illnesses (e.g., increased paranoia, panic attacks, and poor physical health).

All participants discussed how essential leisure activities or social/recreational activities were to maintaining their QOL. A typical comment was, "You must stay active to fight the boredom. You must stay active, that's how you stay out of the hospital." Although participants generally recognized the need to manage their time wisely, many were unsuccessful in managing their time because of poor activity choices or the need for assistance to participate in activities. For example, one participant stated he was "tired of hanging around and doing nothing." Another noted, "Mostly we just sit around every day . . . smoking cigs, watching TV . . . until staff says do something, but what?" Table 13–2 outlines a typical daily schedule.

A particularly significant finding was the general dissatisfaction with the types of recreational or daily activities available to participants. One participant stated, "I go to the recreation place they have for us, but I am getting tired of ceramics. And we really don't do much there." Another commented, "I have a hard time sitting still, so there is no point in having 'watch TV' on my treatment plan." Along with inappropriate activities that often reflected standardized rather than individualized treatment plans, participants also stated that lacking money and transportation were major deterrents to

TABLE 13–2   Typical Daily Schedule Reported by Participants

7 AM	Wake up and ADLs, breakfast
8 AM	Medication management, talk to staff, "hang out"
9 AM to 12 PM	Day program: arts/crafts, ceramics, talk with other clients
12 noon	Lunch
1 PM	Housekeeping
2 PM	Sit around and talk with other clients, call mother
3 PM	Nap
4 PM	Watch TV
5 PM	Listen to radio, talk with other clients
6 PM	Dinner, wash dishes
7 PM	Medication management, community meeting
8–10 PM	Watch TV
10 PM	Bedtime

Source: Used with permission from Badger T, et al. (2003). *Health outcomes for people with serious mental illness: A case study.* Malden, MA: Blackwell Publishers.

participation in outside activities. It was difficult to go to the movies with friends when one had no money or means of convenient transportation. Public transportation was limited, especially in the evenings.

About half the participants reported less dissatisfaction with their daily activities by the third interview. One commented, "I'm doing more reading. I like that." This increased satisfaction may be caused in part to the participants initiating some changes that the research nurses recommended. The nurses discussed the importance of improving diet, increasing exercise, managing medication, increasing daily activities (e.g., getting a library card to enable the participant to obtain novels). They further recommended appropriate community activities (e.g., YMCA, parks and recreation programs) and/or lifestyle changes (e.g., walking with a friend).

The majority of comments about organizational membership focused on being members of "the mental illness community." Comments primarily focused on participants' relationships with their case managers and psychiatrists in the community. Most expressed dissatisfaction with these relationships, especially with the case managers/therapists. As one participant stated, "I want the case manager to go the distance. Why don't they go the distance with me? One quit on me and she didn't even call. It really hurt me." The final theme related to integration was community safety. Many participants voiced concerns about their community safety. Typical comments were, "I feel unsafe in this apartment complex," or "I want to move to a better place." The case managers voiced similar concerns about some of the neighborhoods where the subsidized apartments were located.

Contact.   The third area was family and friend contact. The majority (80%) reported family contact, with about half seeing family members daily. Others reported weekly or monthly contact. One participant commented that "I see my mom once a week." Another stated he talked with his parents two to four times a month. A few reported no family contact, but reported that "my friends who live here are my family." By the third interview, the majority of participants reported almost daily contacts with friends. Most participants reported contact with behavioral health staff as very important sources of their contacts with others. Typical comments were, "Staff help me if there's a crisis," and "Staff plan outings for us sometimes." In general, most participants were not isolated and had contacts with others.

Intimacy and Sexual Functioning.   The final social functioning area was intimacy and sexual functioning. Participants discussed the desire for closeness and a relationship. Typical comments included, "I want a girlfriend," "someone to talk to and do things together," or "someone to help me out." Several participants expressed the desire for marriage or a more intimate type of relationship than friendship. As one participant stated, "I [would] like to find a compatible partner, long-term relationship. Someone to have sex with." The large number of comments related to this theme was unexpected, but suggests areas for treatment. As one participant commented, "I would like a girlfriend, but I feel nervous around women, about what to do." Other participants voiced similar concerns about their lack of skill and knowledge about intimate relationships and the lack of discussions by health care providers about this area of their lives. As one participant stated, "I would like to attend some therapy group [to learn how] to make a friend and find a girlfriend." In sum, the typical participant believed that his or her life was generally satisfactory. The two areas of greatest dissatisfaction were general health and social function.

Service Use and Need

Participants reported using case management services, psychiatrist services, pharmacy assistance, Social Security, disability, subsidized rent or residential programs, food stamps, state Medicaid, and some recreational activities and vocational rehabilitation. When asked about what services they needed, the top three needs were for increased case management services, social/recreational activities, and vocational rehabilitation. Typical responses were, "I need staff support to get my GED, voc rehab training, psychotherapy, a car, and more time with my case manager," or "I need more time with my case manager . . . planned activities, a diet plan, and an exercise group." Another participant stated, "I'd like a day program, socialization, budget skills, employment, recreation, and to continue my independent living. I'd like to maintain my sobriety, AA meetings would be nice. I'd like more time with my case manager and more frequent appointments with my psychiatrist for counseling." Other unmet needs included physical exams and dental and eye exams. For example, "I need to see a dentist to get my teeth cleaned and an eye doctor for glasses." These services were not covered by insurance, or the co-pay was too high to enable participants to obtain these services.

All participants believed their medications were essential for health, and they requested classes to improve their ability to manage medications and maintain independent living. Typical comments included, "I need to stay on my meds because I get very ill without them. How I function and my freedom is really important to me," or "I like my medicine. It helps me think clearly without feeling tired. If I don't take it, I end up in the hospital." By the third interview many of the patients had been switched to atypical antipsychotic medications that improved control of their symptoms. These findings are validated by qualitative comments such as: "Clozaril helps me with stress and makes me feel better on a daily basis." In general, participants believed the newer medications were more effective in controlling many of their symptoms and in improving their quality of life and abilities to function than were their previous typical antipsychotics. In sum, participants clearly identified needs for services not currently available. Most needs were neither surprising nor new.

Consumer Satisfaction

Overall, the participants were mostly satisfied with their care. When asked, "What do I think the system does well?" they identified the staff's commitment to providing good care. Participants acknowledged they had been switched to newer medications (atypical antipsychotics) that were much more effective and that the staff tried to provide greater support for their daily lives. For example, one participant stated, "The case manager and nurse are wonderful people who help me and know how to explain things to me. I really like it when the case manager speaks Spanish [client's primary language] to me."

Staff turnover and case manager/therapist services dominated the discussions about how the system needed to change to better meet the needs of clients. Most participants had two to three case managers over the course of the study. A typical participant stated, "I see a case manager about every 2 weeks. I've had three this year and I don't remember the last one's name."

Participants also voiced concerns about the psychiatrists, but not as strongly. Most participants were seeing a psychiatrist every 3 months, but there was also psychiatrist turnover. Many reported they felt like they "had to start over every time the doctor changes." One participant called his psychiatrist "Dr. Nobody" because he didn't feel he had any relationship with him. It is not surprising there were fewer comments about the psychiatrists because most participants viewed the case manager/therapist relationship as the one with more frequent interaction and, therefore, judged that the case manager should provide more services.

It was not surprising that the psychiatrists and case managers also voiced dissatisfaction over their inability to provide adequate services and their lack of time. As one provider stated, "Sometimes I just give up because the case-load is so impossible. I don't really get to know my clients. There is absolutely no time to adequately coordinate care." This comment was heard repeatedly from various case managers and psychiatrists. In sum, the fact that dissatisfaction with the case managers/therapists was the number one service complaint from participants provides a clear target for system improvement.

Discussion

The goals for this project were to describe outcomes (functioning; QOL; service use, need, and satisfaction) of clients with serious mental illnesses who used regional public mental health services, and to describe what the public mental health system did well or needed to change to better satisfy clients' needs. The use of both qualitative and quantitative methods strengthens the confidence in these findings because the two different, but complementary, methods validated the results. However, the qualitative data from the case study method provided more in-depth insights, that is, the how and why, for specific problem areas.

Two major themes influenced the quality of the clients' daily lives. First, the general health of the participants was poor. Many participants were obese, lacked physical fitness, had poor nutrition, or smoked. Most structured programs or activities did not address such health issues. The poor health of these clients with serious mental illnesses will become of greater concern for providers as this population grows older and their chronic illnesses increase (Casey, 2002; Dixon, Postrado, Delahanty, Fischer, & Lehman, 1999; Harris & Barraclough, 1998). The lack of preventive health care, the frequent delays in seeking health care, and the unhealthy lifestyles of the participants will ultimately increase costs to the health care system.

A second area that influences participants' QOL was social functioning. Social functioning, along with the newer and more costly atypical antipsychotic medications, is critical to clients' QOL and to prevent relapse and rehospitalization (Bengstsson-Tops & Hansson, 1999; Eklund & Backstrom, 2005; Lehman, 1995). In this study, as in previous literature (Aquila & Korn, 2002), participants found that the newer atypical antipsychotic medications were better in controlling their symptoms and were critical to maintaining their independence in the community. As the newer, albeit more expensive, antipsychotic medications successfully clear thinking and improve abilities, these more functional patients will have different rehabilitation needs (Badger et al., 2004). Individualized treatment plans will be needed to increase daily activities with pastimes that are sufficiently stimulating, interesting, or challenging. Additional educational programs and activities will also be needed to improve employability and functioning in all areas, including sexual functioning. Ultimately, clients who receive more individualized care that addresses their unique needs may require less overall care with fewer hospitalizations, costing the system less over time.

Along with social functioning needs, staff issues dominated the discussions. Participants complained about frequent turnover in staff. Case manager turnover was about 75%, according to participant and provider responses. Turnover is costly not only in recruiting and training new staff, but also in the time it takes for new staff to become acquainted with clients. Inexperienced staff often must make patient care decisions based on limited knowledge, which may result in poor quality care. This finding also suggests that a major initiative is required to recruit and retain qualified case managers/therapists. Efforts were needed to decrease turnover by decreasing caseloads and providing increased supervision and increased salaries. Given that case managers/therapists are regarded as critical to maintaining those with serious mental illnesses in the community while reducing costs, a study examining qualifications, salary, optimal caseloads, or other factors that may influence case managers is needed. Further, the roles of nurses in this system must be addressed. During the course of the study, the system hired nurses in primarily one of two roles—as an inpatient staff nurse or infrequently as a nurse practitioner. Although the inpatient nursing role was recognized and defined in the inpatient setting, nursing roles (e.g., nurse case manager, community mental health nurse) that provide direct care in the community were less well recognized or defined.

During the course of this study, one of us coined the phrase "the cost of chaos." Overextended systems with overworked staff have insufficient time and little emotional energy to provide the neediest and ill clients with quality care. This system issue has a major impact on continuity of care and satisfaction with care. Investment in staff selection, training, and retention is a good economic investment.

POLICY AND PRACTICE IMPLICATIONS

One criterion for evaluating a case study is that a case study should make a significant contribution to the understanding of the phenomenon and provide evidence from multiple perspectives to support the conclusions and recommendations (Mariano, 2001; Yin, 2003a, 2003b). This case study did in fact make such a contribution. These case study findings were used by the regional behavioral health system, in part, to support needed system changes in the years following the release of the final study report (Badger & Gelenberg, 2001). Most notable were the changes made to address the staff turnover rate and case manager dissatisfaction. The number of case managers was increased, the salary structure for the case managers was improved, a greater emphasis was placed on training and supervision of case managers, and individual case manager caseloads were reduced. Ultimately, these changes reduced staff turnover by about half and improved quality of care and client satisfaction. An additional contribution of this study was that the case study method, given the richness of the data generated, was incorporated within the system to systematically evaluate aspects of the behavioral health system. Also, an increased number of advanced practice mental health nurse practitioner (APRNs) was hired by community service providers to provide more direct client services in the community.

Although mental health nurses are still underutilized in the system, there is greater recognition that nurses have both the community mental health and case management skills to provide cost-effective, quality direct patient care in the community. Nurses must continue to convince mental health systems they have the essential knowledge and skills to provide cost-effective quality care (see Talley [2002] for discussion of essentials for graduate psychiatric nursing). Psychiatric–mental health APRNs can facilitate group therapy that addresses intimacy and sexuality issues, can use cognitive behavioral therapy techniques to teach job skills or social behaviors, and can assist clients to practice those behaviors in the community. We continue to have a dearth of convincing outcome data, however, to document the effectiveness of the various nursing roles in mental health systems. As more APRNs have increased responsibility for direct patient care, future research must evaluate client outcomes to document the effectiveness of nursing care.

Second, because of nurses' abilities to address physical and mental health care, we must take a proactive leadership role in addressing the comorbid health conditions common among people with serious mental illnesses. The APRN who specializes in adult and/or women's health can use the community health nursing model to plan health programs at the residential sites and perform physical and gynecological exams. Health teaching would follow naturally. A cadre of health professionals (e.g., nutritionist, dentist, exercise specialist) could be incorporated into a multidisciplinary practice. Nurses must decrease the sedentary activities inherent in the treatment plans and aggressively address poor health habits. As the newer medications help clear thinking and improve functioning, mental health nurses can develop and implement programs to improve employability, increase daily activities that are sufficiently stimulating and challenging, and address intimacy and sexual functioning. APRNs have the requisite knowledge and skills to provide quality, cost-effective care using an individualized holistic approach to care.

CONCLUSION

Case studies are an extremely effective way for nurses to evaluate the health care systems where they work, and if done well, case studies can have a tremendous positive influence on the health care system. Results and conclusions of case studies can be used to inform policy and suggest changes to the health care system. My research team, using this method, was able to determine QOL, system strengths, and areas for improvement in one regional behavioral health system, directly influencing the quality of patient care. The public mental health system is always changing because of societal and political issues, reimbursement issues, and new treatment methods; thus, mental health providers must continually evaluate their systems, including the perspectives of the patient/clients/consumers they serve, if providers wish to improve care and better satisfy patients' needs.

ACKNOWLEDGMENTS

Funding for this study was provided by Community Partnership of Southern Arizona, Tucson, Arizona, and St. Luke's Health Initiative, Phoenix, Arizona. The author thanks the clients, staff, and health care providers of Community Partnership of Southern Arizona and members of the research team, Cheryl McNiece, Elizabeth Bonham, Jennifer Jacobsen, and Alan Gelenberg. Portions of this paper were presented at the International Society of Psychiatric Mental Health Nurses 3rd Annual Conference, Phoenix, Arizona, April 2001, and were published in *Perspectives of Psychiatric Care*. Permission to use was granted by Blackwell Publishing.

REFERENCES

Aquila, R., & Korn, M. L. (2002). *Promoting reintegration chronic schizophrenia*. Retrieved April 10, 2002, from http://www.medscape.com/Medscape/psychiatry/Clinical Mgmt/CM.v06/public/index-CM.v06.html.

Badger, T. A. (1998). Depression, physical health impairment and service use among older adults. *Public Health Nursing, 15,* 136–145.

Badger, T. A., & Gelenberg, A. (2001). *Mid-cost and high-cost utilizers study: Final report.* Unpublished report.

Badger, T. A., Gelenberg, A., & Berren, M. (2004). Consultative intervention to improve outcomes of high utilizers in a public mental health system. *Perspectives of Psychiatric Care, 40,* 53–69.

Bengstsson-Tops, A., & Hansson, L. (1999). Clinical and social needs of schizophrenic outpatients living in the community: The relationship between needs and subjective quality of life. *Social Psychiatry and Psychiatric Epidemiology, 34,* 513–521.

Berren, M. (1998). *Community partnership of Southern Arizona consumer satisfaction survey—Adult version.* Unpublished instrument.

Casey, D. E. (2002). Atypical antipsychotics: Enhancing healthy outcomes. *Archives of Psychiatric Nursing, 15*(3, suppl 1), S12–S19.

Covington, L., & Cola, P. A. (2000). Clozapine vs haloperidol: Antipsychotic effects on sexual function in schizophrenia. *Sexuality and Disability, 18,* 41–48.

Dixon, L., Postrado, L., Delahanty, J., Fischer, P. J., & Lehman, A. (1999). The assessment of medical comorbidity in schizophrenics with poor physical and mental health. *Journal of Nervous and Mental Disorders, 187,* 496–502.

Ecklund, M., & Backstrom, M. (2005). A model of subjective quality of life for outpatients with schizophrenia and other psychoses. *Quality of Life Research, 14,* 1157–1168.

Fillenbaum, G. (1988). *Multidimensional functional assessment of older adults: The Duke older Americans resources and services procedures.* Hillsdale, NJ: Erlbaum.

First, M. B., Spitzer, R. L., Gibbon, M., & Williams, J. B. W. (1997). *Structured clinical interview for DSM-IV Axis I disorders—Patient edition* (SCID-I/P, Version 2.0, 4/97 Version). New York: Biometrics Research Department.

Harris, E. C., & Barraclough, B. (1998). Excess mortality of mental disorder. *British Journal of Psychiatry, 173,* 11–53.

Hester, E. K., & Thrower, M. R. (2005). Current options in the management of olanzapine-associated weight gain. *Annals of Pharmacotherapy, 39*(2), 302–310.

Lehman, A. (1995). *Evaluating quality of life for persons with severe mental illness.* Baltimore, MD: Center for Mental Health Services Research.

Lehman, A., Kerna, E., DeForge, B., & Dixon, L. (1995). Effects of homelessness on the quality of life of persons with severe mental illness. *Psychiatric Services, 46,* 922–926.

Lehman, A., & Postrado, L. (1995). Quality of life and clinical predictors of rehospitalization of persons with severe mental illness. *Psychiatric Services, 46,* 1161–1165.

Lincoln, Y. S., & Guba, E. S. (1985). *Naturalistic inquiry.* Beverly Hills, CA: Sage.

Mariano, C. (2001). Case study: The method. In P. L. Munhall (Ed.), *Nursing research: A qualitative perspective* (3rd ed.) (pp. 359–384). Sudbury, MA: Jones and Bartlett.

McDonald, J., & Badger, T. A. (2002). Social function of persons with schizophrenia. *Journal of Psychosocial Nursing and Mental Health Services, 40*(6), 42–50.

Newcomer, J. W. (2005). Second-generation (atypical) antipsychotics and metabolic effects: A comprehensive literature review. *CNS Drugs, 19*(suppl 1), 1–93.

Noble, L. M., Douglas, B. C., & Newman, S. P. (2001). What do patients expect of psychiatric services? A systematic and critical review of empirical studies. *Social Science and Medicine, 52,* 985–998.

Patrick, D. L., & Erickson, P. (1993). *Health status and health policy.* New York: Oxford University Press.

Sechrist, L., Steward, M., Sickle, T., & Sidani, S. (1996). *Effective and persuasive case studies.* Tucson, AZ: Evaluation Center.

Talley, S. (2002). Improving outcomes: Clinical and educational challenges for psychiatric nurses. *Archives of Psychiatric Nursing, 16*(3, suppl 1), S20–S26.

Yin, R. K. (1994). *Case study research: Design and methods* (2nd ed.). Thousand Oaks, CA: Sage.

Yin, R. K. (2003a). *Applications of case study research* (2nd ed.). Thousand Oaks, CA: Sage.

Yin, R. K. (2003b). *Case study research: Design and methods* (3rd ed.). Thousand Oaks, CA: Sage.

14

Historical Research: The Method

M. Louise Fitzpatrick

The purpose of this chapter is to introduce nurse scholars to the field of historical research in nursing. Specifically, the recent developments in historical inquiry as a scholarly pursuit, the objectives of historical research, and, most importantly, the methods, approaches, and procedures associated with historical investigation, analysis, and interpretation will be explored. Historical inquiry, by its very nature, implies a degree of subjectivity in the interpretation and narration of past events. However, the rigor of the research process, corroboration of facts, and comprehensive examination of available data serve to provide the objective evidence on which analysis and interpretative historical exposition rely. The balanced combination of objectivity and subjectivity in the process of the research distinguishes history from the chronicling of events at one extreme and unsupported anecdotal narrative at the other. Like all scholarly investigations, historical research requires careful attention to method and procedure and adequate training of investigators in both the method and the contextual background of the subjects that they select for study.

HISTORICAL INQUIRY IN NURSING

Historical inquiry in nursing, as a legitimate scholarly pursuit, received increased attention and interest in the past three decades. The renaissance of

375

interest in the profession's heritage reflects the concern of a mature profession with its antecedents, not only as a means of informing itself, but to gain a backdrop for current and future directions. It also reflects a renewed concern with the role and contributions of nurses as part of important but more contemporary world events, such as World War II, and society's increased attention to historic events of the twentieth century at the time of the new millennium. History serves a pragmatic purpose as well as a contextual one. It connects us with a heritage and confers on us an identity, personally and professionally. Simultaneous with this heightened interest in nursing's roots has come an expansion of opportunities for doctoral study in nursing. Logically, some individuals found historical research an exciting and productive path to take as part of their doctoral studies and, ultimately, their preferred research agendas.

Understandably, there was resistance to this movement in some sectors. In some universities, there were no nurse historians prepared to guide students. In others, history departments were reluctant to guide students who had not had previous education and experience in historical research methods. In a majority of situations, there was documentation by nurse faculty who, understanding the need for greater research productivity in the field, emphasized the need for clinical research over all else and did not place a value on history or on scholarly attempts to interpret the profession's past.

Scholtfeldt (1975), in her classic article titled "Research in Nursing and Research Training for Nurses," encouraged history and the preparation of historiographers for nursing and commented on the dearth of prepared historiographers (p. 181). She contended that reasons might be the extent to which nursing history is presented to neophytes in ways that capture and nurture their interests and the unavailability of educational opportunities designed to prepare nurses for historical inquiry.

Persistence, administrative support in certain universities, and maintenance of a high standard of performance and rigor in the preparation of nurse historians provided catalysts for the renaissance in the 1970s. Finally, a revised opinion has developed of history's value and worth as a scholarly research endeavor among nurses prepared for such investigations.

From a small cadre of individuals, a growing community of nurse historiographers has emerged. Funding for historical research in the field is possible to obtain, and centers for nursing history and research have developed in selected universities where doctoral study in nursing history is encouraged. Additionally, organizations such as the American Association for the History of Nursing have evolved, thereby providing a network for colleagues in the field and a focus for programs, research conferences, and related activities concerning historical research in nursing. Increasingly, there are international conferences and opportunities for nurse historians to share the results of their research.

THE OBJECTIVES OF HISTORICAL RESEARCH

History, like philosophy, concerns itself with the thought side of human existence. As such, it has worth in and of itself. There is usually a tendency to justify historical research in professional fields such as nursing from the standpoint of its helping to inform future decisions and to avoid repeating past mistakes. Such arguments have only slight merit because they serve a reductionist belief that historical facts can be distilled with a formula. History, although its goal is the establishment of fact that leads us to truth, cannot be reduced to statistical proof. The historian views events as unique. Therefore, it is impossible to ensure that any set of variables, acting in concert, will arithmetically result in some outcome. In human affairs, there are always intervening variables that make it impossible to control or precisely predict destiny. In addition, as Tholfsen (1977) posited, there is danger in demythologizing everything, and an understanding of the limits imposed by the past is what makes liberation and revolution possible (p. 247).

Commager (1966) contended that the scientific historian studies the past because it is part of the evolutionary process and that this process is the key to solving problems (p. 10). Allen Nevins believed that history is to be enjoyed, not endured, and attempted to popularize the results of scholarly research without corrupting it (Billington, 1975, p. xxi). In a practice discipline, the sharing of the results of historical inquiry in ways that are interesting and useful to a majority of the profession's members is probably an important consideration. Narration, presentation, and connection of solid historical interpretation with current trends, issues, and areas of professional interest are the keys to the utilization of such research findings by the contemporary professional and to the education of students about their corporate heritage.

If one of the reasons for pursuing historical research is to build up the body of knowledge in nursing, it is also essential that ways be found to make findings useful to other historians and to the public. The relation of nursing's contributions and activities to the history of women, women's work, and women's studies needs to be strengthened. A related area is the public's perception and image of nursing. History, effectively used, can serve as the collective memory of nursing's accomplishments, not just its struggles; therefore, it can be a principal socializing agent for new members of the profession.

Increasingly, the products of historical research can be viewed in action-oriented dimensions. They can provide prototypes for the development of leaders, they can inform strategic plans of an organizational and political nature, and they can contribute to the development of clinical practice. The outcomes of the historical research process can provide useful analysis of the recent past, as well as an evaluation of events and circumstances that have been well-tempered by time. Without compromising the quality of scholarship, the products of historical research for public consumption can effectively shape the public's perception of nursing, by better informing others about the profession and its contributions.

Synthesizing the past and present through useful insights contributes to the work of those who are architects of the profession's future and brings historical research in nursing into an active and useful mode while continuing to expand the knowledge and understanding of the profession's genesis and evolution for more esoteric reasons. Although the value of historical inquiry needs no justification as a scholarly pursuit when it is applied within professional disciplines, those within the disciplines of both history and the professional fields may still require reassurances concerning the preparation and ability of the investigator, the rigor of the research method, and the utilization of findings. For these reasons, among others, maintaining high quality in the research process and in the narrative exposition is extremely important.

Increasingly, nurse scholar–historians, like other career-minded researchers, are embarking on a line or program of related research activity that they pursue throughout their careers. This effort has the net result of increasing their expertise, making a more sustained contribution to the field, and contributing in-depth substantive data to historical knowledge in the profession.

The development and evolution of nursing as an organized profession, a scholarly practice discipline, and a system of education provide a rich source of potential areas for study. Nursing's relation to world events also provides endless opportunities for study and research. Although valuable and credible historical surveys that highlighted major benchmarks in the profession's development were written as texts from the 1920s to contemporary times, more in-depth scholarly investigations and historical analyses about specific events, institutions, individuals, and changes in clinical practice have emerged in the past 30 years. During this more recent period of scholarship, foundational work has given way to more conceptual areas of study such as feminist themes and their relation to nursing's development.

THE NATURE OF HISTORICAL INQUIRY

Various schools of thought have influenced the field of historiography, just as they have affected all disciplines and professions. The extent to which investigators subscribe to or are influenced by their philosophical approaches to history has critical effects on the research activity and influences the products of the studies. Historical inquiry, like all research, has the discovery of truth as its objective. It is systematic in its method, and objective evidence is determined and judged by using tools of validity and reliability (commonly referred to as methods of internal and external criteria) in historical research.

Today, the schools of thought that traditionally influenced historians are rarely in evidence in their extremes. Rather, an eclectic use of approaches from several schools is generally operational among contemporary scholars. One example of a school of thought that has had both negative and positive influences on the course of historical research was the Positivist, or Neopositivist, school. In this reductionist approach, the historical method attempts to parallel empirical methods in the natural sciences. There is an attempt to reduce history to universal laws. Discovery, verification, and categorization of data are used to provide objective evidence that in and of themselves serve as the interpretation of past events. There is an effort to quantify, to show cause–effect relations, and to force interpretation of data through preexisting formulas, models, and generalizations. This school of thought concerns itself with conditions as predictors of outcomes, rather than attempting to discern what specific conditions caused the known outcome. This school of thought employs the use of hypotheses liberally.

The use of constructs and frameworks has a place in historical explanation, but there should not be an attempt to force the development of universal axioms to explain a unique phenomenon—the historical event. It is possible, however, to use some survey methods and statistical analyses commonly employed in the social sciences to enhance the presentation of objective evidence. This has been successfully accomplished in nursing by Kalisch (1981), in particular. These measures in and of themselves do not lend themselves to good historical interpretation but can support it.

Another school of thought that has had influence on contemporary history and interpretation is the Idealist school, which places procedure, intuition, and experience as ingredients for interpretation. This line of thinking posits that all events have an inside and outside view and that the historiographer must get inside the event and rethink the thought of the originator in the context of his or her time, place, and situation, to make adequate historical interpretations.

Today, historiography is influenced by elements of both schools. From the Positivist school have come attention to rigor in method, use of hypotheses, and instruments of statistical investigation and historical explanation. From the Idealist school have come an emphasis on making interpretations within an appropriate temporal and social context and the importance of viewing events as unique and diverse. From the Positivist school, we acknowledge the possibility of describing patterns that seem to exhibit themselves over time; this possibility is shared by the Idealists, who ascribe what is exhibited to unique and interrelated circumstances. Interconnectedness, or the relation of the parts to the whole, is necessary if coherent and meaningful historical explanation is to result from the research. Although the use of hypotheses is not common among inexperienced investigators, hypotheses can be used effectively in historical inquiry. The danger in their use is a tendency for the investigator to be attracted to a hypothesis and to therefore collect only data that will assist in upholding it while inadvertently ignoring other data. This potential bias in data collection can influence the analysis and interpretation of a historical study and is therefore discouraged for novice investigators.

The use of theoretical frameworks, models, or approaches in the conduct of historical studies and their interpretation requires familiarity with the framework and sophistication in the analysis and interpretation of history. The more common or popular frameworks and approaches used by historians include:

1. **Great person:** This approach focuses attention on individuals and their personal power within a social context. It is particularly useful when the objective of the research is a biographical study or there is a desire to emphasize the people who make changes, rather than the changes themselves.
2. **Deterministic:** This approach minimizes the importance and power of individuals in shaping history and relies primarily on predetermined moral/ethical or religious codes for making judgments and explaining historical phenomena.
3. **Sociological:** This approach emphasizes the primacy of social forces and their influence on people and groups as determinants of historical events. With such a framework, historical phenomena are explained through the use of social trends and cultural events as instruments for the interpretation of specific occurrences.
4. **Political/economic:** This approach may employ the use of an ideology as a framework for the interpretation of historical events and is frequently used in combination with the "great person" approach. The use of Marxism or other ideologies as a framework for explaining historical events is one example of this approach.
5. **Psychological:** This approach requires a solid grasp of psychology as well as facility in the historical method of research. It attempts to explain the thinking, motivations, and behaviors of individuals in a historical sense, using psychological theories as instruments for

analysis and explanation. Erikson's biography *Young Man Luther* (1962) is an example of such an approach. Both historians and psychologists have frequently raised valid concerns about the adequacy of either group when it takes on such complex interpretation.

THE PROCESS OF HISTORICAL RESEARCH

The initial stages of development in a historical study are critical to the process and the successful production of the product. Selection of a topic should be considered carefully and in light of its value as a contribution to the field. Frequently, seminal work in an area can provide the foundation for a logical extension and expansion of research on a specific topic. The degree of preparation of the investigator in the historical research method, as well as the investigator's knowledge, history of the period under study, and background in nursing history, can considerably influence the ease of application of the research process and the confidence that can be placed on the result of the investigation. Frequently, the exposition of true interpretative history, in contrast with the development of chronicle, turns on these variables.

When a topic has been selected for study, the framing of the title becomes critical: the title takes on the same significance as the research question in other kinds of studies. Each word in the title is critical to communicating the thesis of the study and the relative emphasis that will be given to specific dimensions named in the title. Frequently, a time period will be specified, and words in the title will become devices to delimit the topic and determine the study's scope.

Early in the process, a thorough investigation and location of sources should ensue. It is possible that the most fascinating topics will become impossible research challenges unless, at the outset, the investigator can ensure the existence of sufficient data to study and research. Location of potential sources such as archives, libraries, and personal collections of individuals can be of great value in determining one's ability to execute the research and to further justify the study. In many instances, embarking on a historical study is like becoming a detective who leaves no stone unturned. Written sources and individuals can be of significant assistance in locating data and ensuring its adequacy for the investigation. Location of sources logically leads to an initial inventory of items that become helpful in shaping the process of the study and collecting data later.

The importance of taking sufficient time to craft the study design systematically, to consider the appropriateness of using or not using hypotheses or specific constructs, and to develop a plan and system that facilitate data collection and analysis cannot be minimized. Although data collection in such research tends to be time consuming, additional time spent in preliminary steps will ensure more ease of analysis, interpretation, and exposition when the study develops beyond the data-collection phase. Developing topical and chronological classification systems can be extremely helpful for filing collected data in ways that make it possible to retrieve them and to read notes in a variety of configurations preliminary to analysis and interpretation.

SOURCES OF EVIDENCE

Contemporary scholars generally agree that a variety of relevant sources, both primary and secondary, are valuable in providing data for historical investigations. Primary sources, either written or in the form of individual verbal responses, provide a firsthand account of an event by one who was present. Examples of primary sources include official documentary material, such as verbatim minutes and proceedings, and interviews with individuals who were present at an event. Although recollection can be faulty and some documents may reflect the subjectivity of the recorder, in general, these primary sources are considered to provide strength to the discovery of truth and establishment of fact.

Secondary sources also can provide rich data. These data are accounts of events at least once removed. They are not hearsay; they are data that can be accepted with confidence despite the fact that they are interpretative reports of events. Some of these sources may include articles written about an event, notes taken at a meeting or summaries of meetings, or narrative descriptions of events by individuals who were not present at the occurrence. Reliability of sources is not related to a particular category. Frequently, a secondary source may be more reliable than a primary one, such as an interview, which may be colored by egocentrism, hyperbole, and selective memory. Guiding and important principles in selecting and collecting available data are: (1) take measures to ensure balance when sources disagree, and (2) include sufficient amounts of available data to establish reliability.

The data-collection stage, the longest stage of the historical research process, can be tedious and isolating. To guide data collection, it is helpful to develop a research outline that raises pertinent questions under each topic or time period. This outline serves to guide the investigator and maps the area of exploration that needs to be addressed through the process of data collection. The outline, though usually broad, should help to focus the investigator and sharpen the parameters of the study in relation to the thesis contained in the title. Ideally, it leads to the articulation of specific questions to be asked of the data. The advent of the electronic age and changes in patterns of communication constitute a formidable challenge to historians. Although the presentation of materials is more sophisticated, human communications are frequently conducted through the use of the computer, and the identification and presentation of existing data become more difficult. The effect of the computer age on the retrieval of historical data as well as the presentation of contemporary documents has both positive and negative aspects.

ESTABLISHING FACT FROM OBJECTIVE EVIDENCE

Two important elements in the research process are measures of validity and reliability that form the basis for establishing fact. In historical inquiry, validity takes on the form of external criticism of the data. Questions may be raised about authenticity, origin, and originality of documents. Techniques to verify the authenticity of an author's handwriting, and the composition of paper at various time periods, also may be expressed in more elaborate studies. Reliability is the primary means by which fact is established. The strength of the data leading to conclusions that result in the determination of fact depends on tests of reliability. When absolute fact cannot be established, probability and possibility become alternatives. Corroboration of data becomes the critical element in the process. In contrast with validity, reliability is related to the internal criticism of data. Therefore, a correct understanding of language, which itself evolves and changes over the decades, is important. Because parlance changes over time, accurate interpretation of the meaning of words in their particular social and temporal milieu becomes essential. Related to this type of interpretation is the adequacy of understanding the customs of a time period, which may be reflected through the language. Placing both words and events within an appropriate context is a basic ingredient for good analogies and interpretation.

Although there is resistance today to the use of formulas for the determination of historical fact, the following guidelines may be helpful to the investigator when setting out the requirements for establishing fact. Two independent primary sources that corroborate one another establish fact, as does one primary source corroborated by an independent secondary source that contains no substantial contrary evidences. When this guideline cannot be followed, probability can be the goal. This goal requires data from one primary source with no substantial contradictory evidence or data from two or more primary sources that disagree only in some minor aspects. If neither fact nor probability can be established or if corroboration is from only secondary sources, possibility can be established by using data from a primary source that cannot be critically evaluated. In short, reliability in historical research is an attempt to establish truth. Validity and reliability become critical elements in the conduct of the research and in the critique of the quality of a completed study. Historical evidence and proof are cited in references and footnotes. Frequently, multiple references are used to reflect the process of corroboration. Content footnotes that further explain information in the text also are useful devices for the historiographer.

Interviews, whether they are primary or secondary source materials, are usually best conducted after data collection from documents has taken place. This sequence provides an opportunity for further clarification and corroboration of written material. Frequently, anecdotal material provided in interviews helps to connect disparate pieces of already collected data and assists the historiographer in interpreting the evolution and pattern of events.

When all known data have been reviewed and collected, the investigator usually becomes aware of a repetition that emerges in further data collection and is able to complete the process, confident that essential information has been gathered.

DEVELOPMENT OF THE INTERPRETATIVE REPORT

The next phase of the study, sometimes taking weeks, comprises careful review, reading, and analysis of the collected data. Simultaneous with this process is the construction of a highly specific writing outline. The more detailed the outline, the easier it becomes to engage in the interpretative and narrative phase of the investigation. A good writing outline helps to form the gestalt. The particular and unique are viewed in relation to the whole without losing their integrity. In addition, careful reading of the data provides an understanding of the interconnectedness of events and moves the process from analysis to synthesis and, finally, to interpretation. Perhaps synthesis is the most difficult of the processes, development of the narrative the most creative, and giving meaning to facts through interpretation the most critical. Historical explanation expressed through the use of a unifying construct or framework or narration based on the predetermined topical or chronological outline emerges through expository writing. At this point, subjectivity plays an essential part in bringing the research process to its logical conclusion. Subjectivity in the interpretation of objective evidence is central to the historical research process and distinguishes history from chronicle; researcher bias in the collection and selection of data must be carefully avoided. In the search for truth, objective evidence and facts provide the foundation for understanding the past; but interpretation by the individual investigator provides the perspectives and views that fill out our understanding of the past and raise new questions for study.

SUMMARY

The use of the historical research process in nursing is a valuable approach to expanding nursing's understanding of itself, as well as for interpreting the field and its contributions to others. It provides a scholarly means of connecting the field to the whole of human experience. Its liberating and liberalizing quality assists the profession to further define its identity through an understanding of its heritage and to provide direction for its future. As a research method, it links nurse scholars with their colleagues in the humanities. As a scholarly pursuit within the professional field, historical inquiry, properly executed, has become essential to the refinement of nursing's understanding of itself.

REFERENCES

Billington, R. (Ed.). (1975). *Allan Nevins on history.* New York: Scribner's.

Commager, H. S. (1966). *The study of history.* Columbus, OH: Merrill.

Erikson, E. (1962). *Young man Luther: A study in psychoanalysis and history.* New York: Norton.

Kalisch, P. (1981). Communicating clinical nursing issues through the newspaper. *Nursing Research, 30*(3), 132–138.

Scholtfeldt, R. (1975). Research in nursing and research training for nurses: Retrospect and prospect. *Nursing Research, 24*(3), 177–183.

Tholfsen, T. (1977). The ambitious virtues of the study of history. *Teachers College Record, 79*(2), 245–257.

ADDITIONAL REFERENCES

Fealy, G. M. (1999). Historical research: A legitimate methodology for nursing research. *Nursing Review (Ireland), 17*(1/2), 24–29.

Hewitt, L. C. (1997). Historical research in nursing: Standards for research and evaluation. *Journal of the New York State Nurses Association, 28*(3), 16–19.

Lusk, B. (1997). Historical methodology for nursing research. *Image: Journal of Nursing Scholarship, 29,* 355–359.

Rafael, A. R. F. (1999). From rhetoric to reality: The changing face of public health nursing in southern Ontario. *Public Health Nursing, 16,* 50–59.

Russel, R. L. (1998). Historiography: A methodology for nurse researchers [Guest editorial]. *Australian Journal of Advanced Nursing, 16,* 5–6.

Szabunia, M., & Buhler, W. K. (1998). Nursing history: Repositories and the Web—historical methodology for nursing research. *Image: Journal of Nursing Scholarship, 30*(2), 109–110.

Turner, C., & Lawler, J. (1999). Mouth care practices in nursing and research-based education: An historical analysis of instructional nursing texts. *International History of Nursing Journal, 4*(3), 29–35.

15

Exemplar: "Called to a Mission of Charity": The Sisters of St. Joseph in the Civil War

Barbra Mann Wall

> Make your meditation in the morning after your prayers and be not
> troubled if you can say no other prayers of the community, not
> even if you are deprived of mass on Sundays.
> —Mother St. John Fournier, n.d., possibly April 19, 1862

Anticipating the difficulties of fulfilling Catholic religious routines, Mother St. John Fournier, superior of the Sisters of St. Joseph of Philadelphia, wrote these words to her sister–nurses at Fortress Monroe in 1862 as they were about to board hospital ships during the Peninsula Campaign of the American Civil War. Her letter is an example of the sisters' flexibility and readiness to accommodate themselves to "times and circumstances," an inherent part

Source: From © Wall, B. M. (1998). "Called to a mission of charity": The Sisters of St. Joseph in the Civil War. *Nursing History Review,* 6, 85–113. Used by permission of Springer Publishing Company, Inc., New York 10036.

of their spirituality since their founding in France in the seventeenth century (Byrne, 1986, p. 249). The Sisters of St. Joseph's spirituality provided a consistent identity for them to serve diverse groups of people, including soldiers from the North and South, Catholic and non-Catholic, during the Civil War. More importantly, as these women lived out their religious roles, they contributed significantly to advances not only in nursing practice but also to the social acceptance of American Catholicism.

This history of nuns' work in the Civil War illustrates the gendered story of what was to become the nursing profession. It also illuminates the interplay between religious and secular influences on nursing and the place of that interplay in American social history.

METHODOLOGY

Historical methodology is used to construct and interpret the wartime nursing experiences of one congregation of sisters; the manner in which they coped with the exigencies of war; and the ways in which religion, gender, class, and ethnicity shaped their experiences. The most significant primary sources were the Sisters of St. Joseph's letters, journals, and records, which are housed in the Archives of the Carondelet, Wheeling, Philadelphia, and Brentwood (New York) congregations. The quality and completeness of these records vary. The archives contain data on individual nuns, including dates of their entrance to the community, place of birth, family background, records of deaths, and lists of sisters' work assignments. One important source is a chronicle of events in 1864, thought to be authored by Mother de Chantal Keating, superior of the Wheeling congregation during the Civil War. Some religious communities kept annals, but many of the reports are fragmentary. Compounding confusion regarding sources on Catholic sisters is that they often did not sign their names to their writings, reflecting their attempts to avoid calling attention to themselves. Such was the case with the Wheeling annals. For information on the military hospital in Wheeling, Army monthly reports and muster rolls located in the National Archives were used. The Philadelphia congregation has more primary sources on the Civil War than the Wheeling group. In 1859, Sister Assisium McEvoy entered the Philadelphia community, and she served as its first archivist. She continually documented congregational events and in 1870 recorded the Philadelphia sisters' nursing activities in the Civil War, although she did not accompany the sister–nurses. Secondary sources included written histories of women's religious congregations, histories of medicine and nursing, women's histories, Civil War books, and sources on ethnicity and religion.

CARING FOR STRANGERS

. . . Notwithstanding the tragic nature of the Civil War, this human event provided an ideal proving ground for medical and nursing practitioners. Throughout the four-year conflict, more casualties resulted from disease and infection than the battlefield. Most women of the Civil War era provided nursing care in the home as part of their domestic duties, but it was limited to family members or friends. They were unaccustomed to attending to strangers outside the home. There were a few "professed" nurses who did in fact care for nonfamily members to provide incomes for themselves (Reverby, 1987, p. 16). In contrast to most women of the day, however, Catholic sisters had extensive experience in nursing people outside the home environment. When they joined a religious congregation, they knowingly accepted the inherent role of caretaker to persons beyond their own circle of family and friends. During epidemics, when others fled the cities, nuns remained to care for the sick and dying. In response to massive waves of immigration, they opened approximately 25 Catholic hospitals between 1823 and 1860. While no formal training programs existed, sisters learned by experience in their hospitals and by visiting the sick at home (Maher, 1989; Rosenberg, 1987; Stepsis & Liptak, 1989).

. . . In the four decades prior to the Civil War, there was a great increase in the number of Catholics in America as a result of the mass immigration of the German and Irish. . . . Anti-Catholic nativist sentiments rose in direct proportion to their growing numbers. There was widespread belief that Catholics were a threat to democratic institutions. In Philadelphia, for example, anti-Catholic and nativist hysteria spawned riots that resulted in 20 deaths, more than 100 injuries, and the burning of two churches in 1844 (Billington, 1938; Feldberg, 1975; Franchot, 1994). Nor were Catholic sisterhoods spared vitriolic contempt. Anti-convent discourse vacillated between views of celibacy as a prison to shocking tales of unrestrained sexuality. Some critics considered the idea of autonomous women avoiding their procreative duties as dangerous to the natural, patriarchal order (Kennelly, 1989; Mannard, 1986). These threatening perceptions of Catholic women persisted in spite of the fact that nuns' work of teaching, nursing, and caring for orphans actually conformed to traditional domestic ideologies of the times. Catholic leaders counterattacked such nativism by attempting to demonstrate the church's compatibility with American democracy. Because of the prevailing anti-Catholicism and nativism, Catholics formed strong attachments to their own institutions. To serve the needs of their own people and to preserve the Catholic identity, bishops and pastors founded schools, orphanages, and hospitals, and they recruited Catholic sisters to administer these institutions (Dolan, 1992).

In 1836, the first six Sisters of Saint Joseph arrived in St. Louis from France to administer schools as well as homes for orphans whose parents had died in epidemics that periodically had swept cities (Byrne, 1986; Mother St. John Fournier, 1873, printed in Logue, 1950). In 1847, Mother St. John Fournier and three other Sisters of St. Joseph from St. Louis came to Philadelphia to take over a boys' orphan asylum. By 1849, they expanded their ministry to include hospital work when they assumed the administration of Philadelphia's predominately Irish Catholic St. Joseph's Hospital. From 1847 to 1857, the Sisters of St. Joseph expanded to other cities as well: they had established foundations in St. Paul, Toronto, Wheeling, Buffalo, Hamilton, Brooklyn, and Albany (Byrne, 1986).

Like all Catholic women religious, the Sisters of St. Joseph took vows of poverty, chastity, and obedience. Through their vow of poverty, they experienced the deprivations of the immigrants they served. They were obedient to their ecclesiastical superiors, either bishops or priests, and to the superiors of their own congregations. And throughout most of Catholicism's history, chastity was a defining behavior for anyone in search of religious sanctity (McNamara, 1996; Wittberg, 1994). . . . Vows gave nuns a public dimension. They were able to go into the community and demonstrate a compassion devoid of sexual connotations, and they could care for strangers in ways other women could not. Furthermore, vows freed sisters from marriage and family responsibilities.

. . . Class and ethnic backgrounds of the Sisters of St. Joseph helped integrate them into local communities as they ministered to a variety of ethnic groups. Religious communities typically recruited women from the common people they served. The original Sisters of St. Joseph who came to the United States were French, including Mother St. John Fournier, but the majority in the 1850s were American-born, primarily born to immigrants. Thus membership also consisted of a large number of Irish women, a smaller group of Germans, and other nationalities. In the period before the Civil War, the Sisters of St. Joseph mostly were from rural or poor laboring classes, although some belonged to the middle class, and they could easily identify with the needs of persons whom they served (Byrne, 1986; Gleason, 1992).

"Unwilling to Trust Any But . . . [Philadelphia's] Sisters of St. Joseph"

At the beginning of the Civil War, the medical departments of both the Union and Confederacy entered the conflict unprepared. . . . Hospitals were often wooden buildings with dirty walls and filth-soaked floors. Sanitation was almost nonexistent, and lack of ventilation and basic cleanliness contributed to a high rate of illness. . . . It was in this setting that 14 sisters from the Philadelphia community of the Sisters of St. Joseph entered. They served in Union army hospitals in Pennsylvania and on hospital ships in Virginia in 1862. Ten others from the congregation in Wheeling, West Virginia, opened their own hospital to the military in 1864 (Roster, n.d.).

On January 9, 1862, Dr. Henry Hollingsworth Smith appealed to Mother St. John Fournier, requesting that her sisters serve as nurses at Pennsylvania's Camp Curtin. Letters between Mother St. John, the superior of the Sisters of St. Joseph at Philadelphia, and Dr. Smith, Surgeon General of the Pennsylvania Volunteers, during 1862 provide opportunities to explore not only the sisters' nursing experiences but gender and religious issues that influenced them. Smith had served on the staff of St. Joseph's Hospital in Philadelphia with the Sisters of St. Joseph and was aware of their reputation as nurses. On January 22, Smith, who often wrote in the third person, communicated with Mother St. John: "Whilst beset by applicants, every female nurse has been refused, Dr. Smith being unwilling to trust any but his old friends the Sisters of St. Joseph" (Smith, H. H., to Mother St. John Fournier, 1862). Smith's preference for Catholic sister–nurses may have been a reflection of the images physicians held of other women nurses at that time.

Nursing had yet to shed its stigma as a job for untrained hospital workers. . . . In military hospitals, male nurses were the norm, and many male army officers and physicians resisted the introduction of women in military nursing. They viewed unskilled female volunteers as useless annoyances and perceived women's delicate natures to be unsuitable for nursing (Brodman & Carrick, 1990). Authority became a point of contention between some of the secular women and male Army officers and doctors, many of whom the women saw as incompetent. Conversely, army officers and doctors saw the women as insubordinate and "quarrelsome, meddlesome busybodies" (Adams, 1952, p. 182; Wormeley, 1863). Some doctors preferred sister–nurses who were accustomed to hierarchical authority and who were more obedient and less likely to question physicians' orders. Sisters also were used to hard work and discipline and were reliable (Brinton, 1914).

On January 23, after obtaining consent from Mother St. John and Bishop James F. Wood of Philadelphia, three sisters arrived at Camp Curtin Hospital, a temporary and roughly constructed frame building. These women were under the direction of Mother Monica Pue, former superior of St. Joseph's Hospital in Philadelphia. One day after their arrival, three more sisters reported to Church Hospital in Harrisburg under the charge of Sister Mary John Kieran. The building was a converted Methodist church, and there the sisters nursed sick soldiers as they disembarked from trains. The initial task of the nurses was to thoroughly clean the hospitals since no sanitary regulations had been observed (Assisium, 1870).

. . . Most of these women were either Irish born or first- or second-generation Irish immigrants from working-class families, and they were accustomed to a tremendous amount of physical work. In 1834, for example, a traveler to Ireland saw "women carrying sacks of potatoes, weighing about 250 pounds. . . ." And after a long day's work, domestic chores of cooking and spinning wool awaited women at night (quoted in Fitzpatrick, 1987, p. 166). Thus, when Surgeon-General Smith wrote to Mother St. John on February 2, 1862, after visiting the Harrisburg hospitals, he praised the sisters' discipline and hard work. The nuns had "no complaints after one week's trial of the inconveniences and exposure attendant on military life. Already each hospital shows the blessings attendant on their presence: everything is now neat, orderly and comfortable" (Smith, H. H., to Mother St. John Fournier, 1862).

. . . At the end of March 1862, the soldiers at Camp Curtin went to the battlefront, and the Sisters of St. Joseph left Camp Curtin on March 27 and Church Hospital the following week (Assisium, 1870). At this time, the war was a year old, and the carnage was escalating. By the first week in April, the Army of the Potomac massed around Fortress Monroe in Virginia. This became the major point from which General George McClellan planned to attack the Confederate capital of Richmond in what was to be known as the Peninsula Campaign. Secretary of War Stanton planned for medical assistance with the New York and Pennsylvania medical authorities, but he did not prepare for transports, nor did he engage nurses. This became the task of the United States Sanitary Commission (Maxwell, 1956; McPherson, 1988).

The War Department approved a project by the Sanitary Commission to equip, supply, and manage hospital steamers. The Commission was a voluntary organization whose mission was to provide Northern troops with supplies and medical care (U.S. Sanitary Commission, 1863). During the Peninsula Campaign, the hospital ships brought the wounded and sick from southern battlefields to northern cities that had better medical facilities. Frederick Law Olmsted provided overall direction of these floating hospitals, and he stressed that the Commission should bring order and discipline to the care of the soldiers. Olmsted wrote, "Whoever comes here on our business, comes not to do such work as he thinks himself fit for, but such as he will be assigned to, and under such authority as will be assigned him. He or she must come as distinctly under an obligation of duty in this respect as if he or she were paid, and must be expected to be treated with the same discipline"

(Olmsted, 1862, quoted in Censer, 1986, p. 341). Catholic sisters did not have to be taught the importance of working as a team, nor did they need additional instruction on discipline. As vowed women religious, their observance of obedience, discipline, and selflessness made them ideal recruits as nurses on the Commission's hospital ships.

The Sanitary Commission employed physicians, stewards, medical students, and male and female nurses. Among the females were Protestant women nurses of the middle and upper classes, such as Georgeanna Muir Woolsey, Eliza Newton Woolsey Howland, and Katharine Prescott Wormeley. As supervisors of nurses, they administered medications and food to the wounded soldiers, and they saw their organizing skills as their greatest asset. African-American women and white working-class women also worked on the ships, performing tasks of cooking, washing, and other physical labors in the care of the sick and wounded. These assignments reflected common class distinctions, yet they were not as severe or as rigidly applied as in the Confederate states (Giesberg, 1995; Ross, 1992; Woolsey, 1870; Wormeley, 1863). The Sanitary Commission did not discriminate against women on the basis of religious denomination, and Catholic sisters also nursed.

The Sisters of St. Joseph worked with Surgeon-General Smith from Pennsylvania, who took charge of two hospital ships. . . . Eventually nine sister–nurses, predominantly Irish-born, went aboard hospital steamers to attend the wounded and sick soldiers (Assisium, 1870). The Confederates evacuated Yorktown, Virginia, on May 4, 1862, after they held off McClellan's advance one month. To allow the retreat, on May 5 a Confederate army fought a delaying action near Williamsburg, where they suffered 1,700 casualties to the Union's 2,200. Three Sisters of St. Joseph accompanied Surgeon-General Smith down the James River on the *Commodore* to bring up the wounded from the battlefield. The transport team members loaded injured soldiers onto the hospital vessel throughout the night. Many Confederate soldiers were taken prisoner, and the sisters attended them indiscriminately as they also treated non-Catholic patients (Assisium, 1870; Foote, 1986; McPherson, 1988).

On June 9, 1862, Smith wrote to Mother St. John informing her that the federal government was taking charge of all the state hospitals, and he would not have to trouble her again for nurses. The Sisters of St. Joseph of Philadelphia completed their active duty in June of 1862 (Smith, H. H., to Mother St. John Fournier, 1862). Amid all the suffering, the nuns not only performed housekeeping duties but also administered medications such as stimulants and coffee, acted as dieticians and cooks, fed patients, and cared for spiritual needs of injured or dying soldiers.

"We Are Regularly Engaged as Nurses"

As the Sisters of St. Joseph of Philadelphia withdrew from their Civil War service, those from Wheeling, Vest Virginia, began theirs. . . . The Sisters of St. Joseph began their work there in 1853 when six nuns came to administer Wheeling Hospital at the request of Bishop Richard Whelan. In 1856, the hospital moved to a newly completed institution on Main Street . . . that housed approximately 50 to 60 patients. . . . By 1864, the sisterhood included 10 nuns, primarily of Irish and Irish-American backgrounds (Keating, Mother de Chantal, 1864–1865).

"Annals" written in 1864, probably by Mother de Chantal Keating, the Irish-born and educated superior of the Wheeling congregation, gives an account of the sisters' activities during that crucial year. While some entries contain only the bare outline of the most important happenings in the community, others lend insight into nursing practice at that time. During the early years of the Civil War, the sisters visited prisoners of war in the Athenaeum, or city jail, in Wheeling, supplying them with food and reading material; and on March 4, 1864, they took charge of all the sick military patients there. On that day, Mother de Chantal made arrangements for 47 patients to be transferred to the hospital, and soon it was filled to capacity (Keating, Mother de Chantal, 1864–1865). . . .

One month later, on April 13, 1864, the army rented the south wing of Wheeling Hospital for $600 a year and placed a military surgeon, Dr. John Kirker, in charge. On April 23, the writer of the "Annals" reported that four soldiers had died, "a small number considering that there were so many cases of serious illness among them." On May 6, the annalist wrote that "things are not in proper working order as yet and will be better bye and bye [sic]" (Keating, Mother de Chantal, 1864–1865). On July 26, 1864, a military captain came to the hospital and ordered Dr. Kirker to take charge of the entire hospital for government use. The Shenandoah Valley had again become a scene of conflict, and 200 ill and injured soldiers unexpectedly arrived in Wheeling on the 26th by ambulances and trains from Harper's Ferry, West Virginia, and Cumberland, Maryland (Arrival of sick and wounded soldiers, 1864; Keating, Mother de Chantal, 1864–1865). . . .

By the first of August, despite the sudden arrival of so many patients, order and discipline prevailed in the hospital. On that day, the annalist wrote: "We are regularly engaged as Nurses," and the duties of that calling "are sufficiently laborious." Mother de Chantal accompanied Dr. Kirker on his morning rounds and took his orders for the patients. She added that "the wounded are attended to as soon as Mass is over; they have no beds to lie on and are uncomfortable" (Keating, Mother de Chantal, 1864–1865).

. . . Military records indicate that the hospital kept from 150 to 200 patients during the autumn and winter months. The hospital also received military and private patients and Confederate prisoners of war. Available primary documents describe a variety of patient diseases but do not specify patients' country of birth. Kirker wrote, however, that because the hospital was near the scene of active military operations, it constantly received patients from the battlefront and from other hospitals. "We have patients transferred to us from all parts of the country," he added (Monthly report of sick and wounded in the U.S.A. Post Hospital, Wheeling, WV, 1864; Muster roll, 1864; Kirker, J., to Brigadier General Barnes, 1864).

Several weeks later, on September 17, 1864, the annalist added: "We are busy still. Sr. Vincent has taken charge of the Prescription Book and we are kept at active duty much of the time" (Keating, Mother de Chantal, 1864–1865). . . . While little evidence survives to explain the details of the sisters' day-to-day nursing care, the picture that emerges is that they gave supportive care through the provision of nutritional diets and hygienic care, provided structure to situations where disorder formerly prevailed, administered nonspecific drug therapy, and worked with doctors to carry out their orders for care.

As an Irish nun and an immigrant to America after the Irish Famine, Mother de Chantal strongly emphasized economic security, which reflected her cultural heritage. With a solid sense of self, Irish women particularly "flexed their muscle and acted" on issues which they considered important (Diner, 1983, p. 152; Hoy, 1995). For example, on February 8, 1865, Mother de Chantal personally appealed to authorities at the War Department in Washington, D.C., when the army was delinquent in paying rent to the sisters for use of their hospital. She presented her accounts and certificates and would not leave until she obtained the money due the sisters. After a two-week wait, a quartermaster informed her that her application had been granted and all arrears would be paid (Keating, Mother de Chantal, 1864–1865). At the end of the war, the government withdrew its control of Wheeling Hospital, and the sisters once again resumed their pre-war duties as nurses and administrators of the hospital.

"YOU ARE THIS DAY CALLED TO A MISSION OF CHARITY"

As they nursed in hospitals and on hospital ships, the Sisters of St. Joseph had to relate to diverse ethnic groups. A variety of records provides a sample of the heterogeneous mixture of soldiers in the Union army. While the overwhelming majority of the men were native born, Irish and Germans were the most numerous foreign-born soldiers, followed by the English, Canadians, Scandinavians, and other groups. There were some predominantly Irish and German regiments, but the sisters' records do not indicate that they cared exclusively for these groups during the war. Examination of previous occupations of white Union soldiers reveals that the majority were skilled and unskilled laborers followed by farmers, with members from the professional or white-collar classes the most markedly underrepresented (Gould, 1869; Lonn, 1951; McPherson, 1988; Wiley, 1951). Equally important, then, is that the sisters came from working-class backgrounds similar to those whom they nursed during the war. Sisters were not strangers to hardship and poverty, which could help them recognize the soldiers' needs.

Religious meaning permeated the sisters' nursing. . . . As they were about to go on board the floating hospital ships in Virginia, Mother St. John Fournier wrote them from Philadelphia: "You are this day called to a mission of charity in a more particular manner than you have hitherto been. . . . I recommend you to be faithful to your trust . . ." (Fournier, Mother St. John, to Sisters of St. Joseph, n.d., possibly April 19, 1862). Yet for all their work, the Sisters of St. Joseph still had to minister within the sphere of rampant anti-Catholicism. . . . For example, Dorothea Dix, the superintendent of the Union Army female nurses, held resolutely anti-Catholic and anti-immigrant attitudes and refused appointments to Catholic sisters (Dix, 1856, in Snyder, 1995). In addition, Dix's nurses were not from the working class as were many of the Catholic sisters. Despite Dix's attitudes, government officials and medical and military officers sought nurses from Catholic communities, and sister–nurses were not under Dix's jurisdiction.

Some Protestant women nurses criticized sisters as lacking warmth and likened them to machines. Jane Stuart Woolsey, a nurse for the Union army, reflected this view when she stated: "The Roman Catholic system had features which commended it to medical officers of a certain cast of mind. The order and discipline were almost always good. The neatness, etc., were sometimes illusory." She continued, "taking the good, leaving the bad, and adapting the result to the uses of the country and the spirit of the time, we might have had an order of Protestant women better than the Romish 'sisterhoods,' by so much as heart and intelligence are better than machinery" (Woolsey, 1870). True to their Catholic identities, the sisters relied heavily on personal and religious discipline. Yet while Woolsey and some other women considered nuns robotic, Katharine Prescott Wormeley defended the need for discipline on hospital ships: "No one must come here who cannot put away all feeling," she stated. "Do all you can, and be a machine,—that's the way to act; the only way" (Wormeley, 1889, p. 102).

Some historians have attributed the criticism to envy over nuns' prestige, organization, and willingness to adapt to harsh circumstances. By joining convents, religious life brought status to Catholic working-class women, and their enhanced status possibly bothered upper-middle-class women who had to share their authority. To counter their feelings of threat and envy, many upper- and middle-class women nurses sought to reaffirm their perceived superiority in matters of upbringing and social status, asserting that their refinement and life experiences in managing households rendered them eminently more qualified than sister–nurses to care for the patients.

Catholic sisters' religious mission in life was to serve others. By contrast, elite women of the U.S. Sanitary Commission were not swayed as much by religious sentiments and built their nursing identities upon the more secular foundations of professional competence and order. In so doing, they claimed organization and efficiency as peculiar to their own class and background (Ginzberg, 1990; Ross, 1992). They had to acknowledge the discipline and order of the sister–nurses, yet they perceived those qualities as being externally imposed by the Catholic church. Hence, they saw the nuns as unthinking machines and convinced themselves that their own discipline reflected true internal strength derived from superior refinement and education.

Others with whom sisters worked expressed positive attitudes toward the nuns. . . . A hospital surgeon who worked with the sisters at Fortress Monroe in Virginia was relieved when the sisters did not ask for "the thousand and one attentions" he had been asked to give secular women (Assisium, 1870). . . . Dr. John Kirker expressed his satisfaction with the Sisters of St. Joseph at Wheeling: "I am much pleased with their services. . . . As they have had much experience in nursing, and caring for the sick, in my opinion their places could not be filled by enlisted men" (Kirker to Blaney, 1864). Soldiers attested to the active role Catholic women religious played in the Civil War and to the changes in their public images. . . . When the Sisters of St. Joseph first went to Camp Curtin, they met hostility from Protestant male nurses. The sisters overcame initial prejudice, however, and eventually won the respect of the infirmed soldiers and hospital staff, who showed their respect through numerous military salutes to the nuns (Assisium, 1870). . . .

Ecclesiastical authorities reflected the changed image of Catholics after the war. The pastoral letter of the American Bishops' Second Plenary Council of Baltimore in 1866 did not specifically praise the sisters' wartime nursing, but the bishops expressed gratitude to the nuns, "whose devotedness and spirit of self-sacrifice have, more perhaps than any other cause, contributed to effect a favorable change in the minds of thousands estranged from our faith" (Pastoral letter, 1866, in Guilday, 1923, pp. 222–223). . . .

As Catholic sisters increasingly came into contact with greater numbers of Catholics and non-Catholics through their nursing in the Civil War, they helped dispel religious prejudice. . . . While nuns played pivotal roles in preserving the faith of immigrants in antebellum America, sisters' nursing of diverse groups of people during the Civil War helped break down the walls of separation that isolated Catholics from the rest of society. By changing public perceptions and opening new social and professional pathways, Catholic sisters' collective influence as agents of social change was both real and substantial.

REFERENCES

Adams, G. W. (1952). *Doctors in blue: The medical history of the Union Army in the Civil War*. New York: Henry Schuman.

Arrival of sick and wounded soldiers. (1864, July 27). *Wheeling Daily Intelligencer*. Ohio County Public Library, Wheeling, WV.

Assisium, Sister. (1870). Copy, The Sisters of St. Joseph at Camp Curtin, Harrisburg, and other places during the war. *Archives of the Sisters of St. Joseph*. Mount St. Joseph Convent, Chestnut Hill, Philadelphia, PA.

Billington, R. A. (1938). *The Protestant crusade 1800–1860: A study of the origins of American nativism*. New York: Macmillan.

Brinton, J. (1914). *Personal memoirs of John H. Brinton: Major and surgeon U.S.V. 1861–1865*. New York: Neale.

Brodman, E., & Carrick, E. B. (1990). American military medicine in the mid-nineteenth century: The experience of Alexander H. Hoff, M.D. *Bulletin of the History of Medicine, 64*, 63–78.

Byrne, P. (1986). Sisters of St. Joseph: The Americanization of a French tradition. *U.S. Catholic Historian, 5*, 241–272.

Censer, J. T. (Ed.). (1986). Olmsted, F. L., to John Foster Jenkins (1862, May 20). In *The papers of Frederick Law Olmsted*. Vol. IV: *Defending the Union: The Civil War and the U.S. Sanitary Commission, 1861–1863*. Baltimore, MD: Johns Hopkins University Press.

Diner, H. R. (1983). *Erin's daughters in America: Irish immigrant women in the nineteenth century*. Baltimore, MD: Johns Hopkins University Press.

Dolan, J. P. (1992). *The American Catholic experience: A history from colonial times to the present*. Notre Dame, IN: University of Notre Dame Press.

Feldberg, M. (1975). *The Philadelphia riots of 1844: A study of ethnic conflict*. Westport, CT: Greenwood Press.

Fitzpatrick, D. (1987). *The modernisation of the Irish female. Rural Ireland 1600–1900: Modernisation and change*. Cork, Ireland: Cork University Press.

Foote, S. (1986). *The Civil War, a narrative: Fort Sumter to Perryville*. New York: Vintage Books.

Fournier, Mother St. John, to Sisters of St. Joseph. (n.d., possibly April 19, 1862). *Archives of the Sisters of St. Joseph.* Mount St. Joseph Convent, Chestnut Hill, Philadelphia, PA.

Franchot, J. (1994). *Roads to Rome: The antebellum Protestant encounter with Catholicism.* Berkeley: University of California Press.

Giesberg, J. A. (1995). In service to the fifth wheel: Katharine Prescott Wormeley and her experiences in the United States Sanitary Commission. *Nursing History Review 3,* 49.

Ginzberg, L. D. (1990). *Women and the work of benevolence: Morality, politics, and class in the nineteenth-century United States.* New Haven, CT: Yale University Press.

Gleason, P. (1992). *Speaking of diversity.* Baltimore, MD: Johns Hopkins University Press.

Gould, B. A. (1869). *Investigations in the military and anthropological statistics of American soldiers.* New York: Hurd and Houghton, for the U.S. Sanitary Commission.

Guilday, P. (Ed.). (1923). Pastoral letter of 1866 (of the Second Plenary Council of Baltimore). In *The national pastorals of the American hierarchy (1792–1919).* Washington, DC: National Catholic Welfare Council.

Hoy, S. (1995). The journey out: The recruitment and emigration of Irish religious women to the United States, 1812–1914. *Journal of Women's History, 6,* 64–98.

Keating, Mother de Chantal. (1864–1865). Annals. *Archives of the Sisters of St. Joseph.* Mount St. Joseph Convent, Wheeling, WV.

Kennelly, K. (1989). *American Catholic women: A historical exploration.* New York: Macmillan.

Kirker, J., to Surgeon Blaney [Medical Director, Department of West Virginia]. (1864, August 14). National Archives SGO L.R. RG 112, Box 51.

Kirker, J., to Brigadier General Barnes. (1864, November 4). National Archives SGO L.R. RG 112, Box 51.

Logue, M. K., Sr. (1950). Fournier, Mother St. John, to the Superior General of the Sisters of St. Joseph in Lyons (1873). In *Sisters of St. Joseph of Philadelphia: A century of growth and development 1847–1947.* Westminster, MD: Newman Press.

Lonn, E. (1951). *Foreigners in the Union Army and Navy.* Baton Rouge: Louisiana State University Press.

Maher, M. D., Sr. (1989). *To bind up the wounds: Catholic sister nurses in the U.S. Civil War.* New York: Greenwood Press.

Mannard, J. G. (1986). Maternity . . . of the spirit: Nuns and domesticity in Antebellum America. *U.S. Catholic Historian, 5,* 305–324.

Maxwell, W. Q. (1956). *Lincoln's fifth wheel: The political history of the United States Sanitary Commission.* New York: Longmans, Green.

McNamara, J. A. K. (1996). *Sisters in arms: Catholic nuns through two millennia.* Cambridge, MA: Harvard University Press.

McPherson, J. M. (1988). *Battle cry of freedom: The Civil War era.* New York: Oxford University Press.

Monthly report of sick and wounded in the U.S.A. Post Hospital, Wheeling, WV. (1864, September; 1864, December; and 1865, January). Wheeling Hospital Archives.

Muster Roll of the Hospital Department at Wheeling, WV. (1864, August 31). National Archives RG 94, Box 107.

Reverby, S. M. (1987). *Ordered to care: The dilemma of American nursing, 1850–1945*. Cambridge, England: Cambridge University Press.

Rosenberg, C. (1987). *The care of strangers: The rise of America's hospital system*. New York: Basic Books.

Ross, K. (1992). Arranging a doll's house: Refined women as Union nurses. In C. Clinton & N. Silber (Eds.), *Divided houses: Gender and the Civil War*. New York: Oxford University Press.

Roster. (n.d., approximately 1860s). *Archives of the Sisters of St. Joseph*. Mount St. Joseph Convent, Chestnut Hill, Philadelphia, PA; and Wheeling, WV.

Smith, H. H., to Mother St. John Fournier. (1862, January 22, February 2, February 18, April 14, April 21, May 16, June 9). *Archives of the Sisters of St. Joseph*. Mount St. Joseph Convent, Chestnut Hill, Philadelphia, PA.

Snyder, C. M. (Ed.). (1995). Dix to Millard Fillmore (October 22, 1856). In *The lady and the President: The letters of Dorothea Dix and Millard Fillmore*. Lexington: University of Kentucky Press.

Stepsis, U., & Liptak, D. (Eds.). (1989). *Pioneer healers: The history of women religious in American health care*. New York: Crossroad.

U.S. Sanitary Commission. (1863). *Hospital transports*. Boston, MA: Ticknor and Fields.

Wiley, B. I. (1951). *The life of Billy Yank: The common soldier of the Union*. Indianapolis: Bobbs-Merrill.

Wittberg, P. (1994). *The rise and fall of Catholic religious orders: A social movement perspective*. New York: State University of New York Press.

Woolsey, J. S. (1870). *Hospital days*. New York: Van Nostrand.

Wormeley, K. P. (1863). *The United States Sanitary Commission: A sketch of its purposes and its work*. Boston, MA: Little, Brown.

Wormeley, K. P. (1889). *The other side of the war with the Army of the Potomac*. Boston, MA: Ticknor and Company.

16

Narrative Inquiry: The Method

Maureen Duffy

Narrative inquiry is a form of qualitative research that uses the collection of stories as its source of data. These stories are the storied experiences of people's lives as told by themselves about themselves or as told by others about them. In other words, the collected stories may be autobiographical, biographical, or a combination of both. Stories are the primary way that people make sense of their experience and through some form of oral or written conversation reveal and share that experience with others. Riessman (1993), in describing narrative research, states that "the purpose is to see how respondents in interviews impose order on the flow of experience to make sense of events and actions in their lives" (p. 2). The meanings that people give to their experience and that shape their lives are collected and organized into story form. Narrative research is a systematic form of inquiry that aims to gather these stories and re-present or re-story them to readers and stakeholders. In this chapter, *story* and *narrative* will be used interchangeably.

However, narrative research does not simply explore the meanings that individuals give to experience or examine the ways in which people tell the tales of their lives. Narrative research is typically more complex than that. Narrative research explores how language reflects the social worlds of people and, in so doing, constitutes their very identities. In other words, narrative inquiry functions at the interface of personal and social identity and of the very social world, which is constitutive of such identities. Narratives reveal, sometimes consciously and often unconsciously, the meanings, conventions, dominant beliefs and values of the time and place in which a person lives and develops an identity.

The question of whether narratives collected in research are "true" or not has come up in discussions of narrative research (Phillips, 1997; Schafer, 1992; Spence, 1987). Spence and Schafer, coming from a clinical psychotherapeutic perspective, maintain that factual or verifiable "truth" is much less important than the stories people build up about their experiences, lives, and why they live the way they do. Spence and Schafer maintain that it is the coherence and congruence of a person's life story that determines how the person will live or perform his or her life story, not whether the story reflects actual events that are often impossible to verify anyway. Phillips, coming from an educational perspective, is more concerned about the "truth" of stories, given that educational policy decisions may be made based on good stories that do not necessarily reflect actual events. Educational policy has real effects on children and families that Phillips worries could be based more on the persuasiveness of a good story rather than on the persuasiveness of actual events. The issue of "truth" in narrative research is unresolved and will probably remain so, given that the whole basis of truth involves differing epistemologies and paradigms that are incommensurable. In this chapter, my bias on the question of truth is toward narrative or storied truth rather than empirical truth.

In keeping with the bias toward meaning and storied truth in this chapter, the following questions reflect important underlying issues of narrative standpoint and philosophy. They deal largely with authorial voice, that is, the cultural discourse or worldview that influences the shaping of personhood and creation of personal identity. At any given time and place, there are many discourses circulating within a culture, but one or two tend to predominate and more powerfully affect the ways in which people come to understand themselves and perform the identities they take on in their lives:

♦ Can there be a life without a story?
♦ Who is the authorial voice of that life/story?
♦ Is the authorial voice the person who is telling his or her own story, or has the authorial voice been taken over or colonized by another or others who have usurped authorship of someone else's life? (Often, such colonization is "below the radar" of the person telling his or her life story because that person has internalized and performed versions of life dictated by the dominant social discourse of the time and place without much awareness of doing so.)
♦ Does the authorial voice change over the course of a lifetime and during critical life transitions?

♦ In what ways do multiple authorial voices help enrich the creation of a unique story or identity?

♦ In what ways do multiple authorial voices steal agency and identity from the story of a life?

♦ Are there many voices authoring the story of a person's life at any given time?

♦ Who decides and according to what criteria is the dominant version of a person's life told?

♦ How do people become aware of alternative stories and meanings that might equally or even more satisfactorily describe their lives?

♦ To what extent is the person aware of the influence of the social world on his or her constructions of a personal identity?

♦ How would persons' stories of themselves change if and as they became aware of the connection between their individual life story and the dominant stories about life that circulate in their culture?

From these questions, it should be clear that narrative research is not a passive activity in which the researcher collects frozen memories of life events. Rather, the narrative researcher is a coparticipant in the exploration of how a life story came to be understood by someone in the way that it has. Through that very process of mutual exploration, the narrative researcher is often an agent of change, encouraging people to critically look at how their own life story and identity are so intimately connected to the wider beliefs and values of their families and cultures. Such reflective examination of one's own life and identity, in collaboration with a skilled narrative researcher, frequently results in a changed understanding of one's past, present, and future. In this sense, narrative research can be seen as a radical intrusion into the ecology of a person's life, and therefore the narrative researcher must seriously attend to the ethics of narrative research practice.

QUESTIONS AS SOURCES OF BOTH DATA AND ANALYSIS

Although the preceding questions are central questions for the narrative researcher interested in how individual identities reflect dominant social realities and themes, the questions can also be used to analyze the narrative in terms of how it reflects the relationship between individual and social identity. Narrative researchers interested in attending to the kinds of questions listed are generally situated in the social constructionist paradigm. Within the social constructionist paradigm, researchers are most interested in how meanings are coordinated among participants in local communities and how knowledge generated within local communities can be understood and validated only within them and not outside of them in a larger, more universal way (Schwandt, 1998). Hence, how people come to understand themselves as gendered, sexualized, sociopoliticized, racialized, ethnicized, privileged, or marginalized persons reveals itself through the study of narratives within the social constructionist perspective.

Clearly, narrative research is interested in sense making, meaning making, constructions, and reconstructions of identity and not in an abstracted factual account of "the truth" of a life story. Coherence of a narrative account, congruence between a person's point of view and how the person makes sense of things, and how well a story is put together are more important and more interesting to the narrative researcher than the positivist illusion of "truth" is.

CAN THERE BE A LIFE WITHOUT A STORY?

Bruner (2004) says, "We seem to have no other way of describing 'lived time' save in the form of a narrative" (p. 692). He takes a decidedly constructionist point of view when he says that the heart of his argument is that "eventually the culturally shaped cognitive and linguistic processes that guide the self-telling of life narratives achieve the power to structure perceptual experience, to organize memory, to segment and purpose-build the very 'events' of a life. In the end we *become* the autobiographical narratives by which we 'tell about our lives'" (p. 694). Narrative research, therefore, does not take life stories at face value, but rather explores how the meanings about life stories were built up, amended, deconstructed, and reconstructed again or, in some cases, over and over again.

The case of Terri Schiavo in the spring of 2005 is illustrative of the power of the authorial voice to make critical life and death decisions for another, and, in so doing, to move and shape social dialogue and social meanings. Terri Schiavo had been in what some physicians and her husband called a "persistent vegetative state" for 15 years. They held that her life was basically meaningless because she was for all intents and purposes "dead" and no longer able to process information or in any way to live meaningfully. Her parents and others strenuously disagreed and held that Terri Schiavo was a person in the full sense of the word and that it was possible she was able to process some information and respond to some stimuli, thereby being "alive" and worthy of being kept alive by retaining her feeding tube (Somers, 2005).

The United States and much of the Western world were fascinated by this case and, in the end, maintained a worldwide death watch while also weighing in on the critical issues involved in her case; namely, who had the right to speak for Terri and when, why, and how should a person's life be declared over? Terri's husband and the courts were given the power of authorship over Terri's physical life. In terms of the story of the meaning of Terri's life, her parents, family, friends, and a world of others, as well as her husband and the courts, continue to tell about and author Terri's experiences, values, desires, wishes, and the implications of her life. Although she is dead, her story is very much alive and goes on being deconstructed and reconstructed again. As the end time of Terri's life approached, multiple, competing identities of Terri were constructed and circulated by the many authors of her life.

THE STRUCTURE OF NARRATIVE

By necessity, narrative researchers are interested in the structure of a narrative and its structural elements. In a general sense, a narrative is a story that is told according to a time line or chronology. The story has protagonists or central characters and other characters playing major or minor roles. It has a plot line with critical events that unfold and have consequences and implications for the characters. The story has a theme and tone, which provide hints of the meanings generated by the storyteller(s) and characters. The story often can be classified into a genre; for example, a romance, a tragedy, a tragic comedy, or a story of heroism, among so many other possibilities. And finally, a story includes the act of making sense out of the characters, the actions, and the events that have occurred within the plot. Who tells or narrates the story, of course, is of critical importance. In other words, who has agency in the story must be identified.

Labov (1972) pays particular attention to the form and structure of narrative, and it is not uncommon for some narrative researchers to use a structural analysis of a narrative during the analysis and interpretation phase of the research project. Labov and Waletsky (1967) and Labov (1972) identify the major elements in the structure of a narrative as the following:

The abstract, which introduces and summarizes the story

The orientation, which provides details of character, time, place, and events

The complication, which details critical events in the story

The evaluation, which describes the implications and meaning of the actions and events

The result, which gives the outcome (if only a partial one) of the story

The coda, which links the story in the past back to the present of the storyteller's life

Even though Labov's work can be used to wall off the individual from the broader culture by focusing only on the individual's actions and meanings in the story, a narrative researcher interested in how individual meaning is linked to cultural meaning can also find Labov's structural elements useful by analyzing each element in terms of how it both reveals and contributes to the development of a personal identity that is social rather than private.

In a different vein, Burke (1969) describes the elements of a narrative as consisting of act, scene, agent, agency, and purpose. In this schema, Burke is interested in what the act was, what the background or context for the act was, who did the act, how the actor did the act, and what the purpose for doing the act was. The focus of Burke's structural elements in narratives is clearly that of the power and meaning of agency and motive.

STEPS IN THE NARRATIVE RESEARCH PROCESS

Formulating the Research Question or Focus

The heart and soul of all qualitative research is the development of a research question or focus that lends itself to a qualitative method. In narrative research, common research questions focus on the life story or life history of an individual or a group, as told by individuals. Such narrative research can consist of autobiography, biography, oral history, life history, autoethnography, narrative case studies, and other methods that require collecting the stories of people as the main data sources.

Clinical psychotherapy (Freedman & Combs, 1996; Schafer, 1992; Spence, 1987; White & Epston, 1990) has also demonstrated a strong narrative turn and has focused on helping people to free themselves from constraining life stories and to adopt more satisfying and liberating ones. In the process of focusing on the narrative as a reflection of the manufacture of a person's identity rather than as an essential inborn identity or personality, clinical psychotherapy has made important contributions to narrative research, especially in the area of question construction about the creation and performance of an identity story.

Some representative narrative research questions might include the following:

How did you get the idea that unless you were rail thin you were not acceptable?

Where do you think this idea came from and how do you think you got
  caught up in it?
Are there any ideas or notions that are interesting to you yet challenge the
  idea of needing to be rail thin to be acceptable?
And where did these competing ideas come from?

These are clinical research-based narrative questions that seek to explore the development of an identity, in this case a spoiled identity (White & Epston, 1990).

These are more sociological-based narrative research questions linking the experience of an individual to that of a larger cultural diaspora:

What has the experience of being a first-generation Irishwoman in the
  United States with no extended family been like for you?
Who or what did your family fall back on during hard times or during
  times of crisis?

Responses to the following questions would result in a collection of memories or oral histories from people associated with the revolutionary grandfather and would also include use of archival materials to create a biographical story of a captured and tortured founder of the Irish Free State:

In speaking to members of your extended family and collecting their stories
  and recollections, as well as reviewing historical and archival material,
  what have you come to learn about your grandfather who fought in the
  Irish Revolution during the founding of the Irish Free State?
What do you know about his imprisonment in England and his systematic
  torture by the British by being dragged out in front of a firing squad on
  multiple occasions without actually being executed?

A follow-up identity and relationship-building question with an ancestor the granddaughter never met that requires reflection and imagination might be this: *How do you think that your grandfather, whom you never knew personally but knew of in so many important ways through others, would view your contributions to carrying forward the commitments and values to which he was so dedicated? What would he see in how you live your life that would make him swell with pride and delight?*

This question would generate oral and life histories collected in story form about one of the darkest periods of our time, powerfully connecting personal stories with political events: *What are the recollections and experiences of survivors of the Holocaust?*

Back to clinical research: *How do you recall your early experiences with your parents or primary caregivers?* This is a question that could be examined narratively for congruence and coherence rather than for historical truth.

The focus on coherence and congruence would set the research question apart from traditional psychological or psychoanalytic research questions that seek historical or actual rather than narrative truth (Schafer, 1992; Spence, 1987). The narrative researcher would generally hold that narrative truth is more important than factual or historical truth because such "factual truth" is always situated or contextualized, not least by the plasticity of memory. In fact, the widely used Adult Attachment Inventory (George, Kaplan, & Main, 1996), developed to assess adult attachment styles, uses a narrative interview format and analyzes the interview and assesses attachment style based not on the degree of trauma a person experienced as a child, but rather on the coherence, congruence, and completeness of the person's narrative account about the trauma experience. In other words, in the Adult Attachment Inventory, attachment style is assessed based on the degree of a person's ability to tell a coherent, complete story about his or her early life without significant gaps of time or memory.

The following question could result in a sociological or symbolic interactionist narrative study: *How do you manage your newly appointed job as associate dean when you have just earned your doctoral degree and will be evaluating faculty at full professor rank?* Such a study might inquire about roles and presentation of self in everyday life similarly to the kinds of questions that fascinated Erving Goffman (1959, 1963, 1974), the classic and utterly original sociologist. Goffman (1963) would have been interested in how a person without appropriate credentials manages that fact on the job site and would have viewed such a set of circumstances as stigmatizing, and therefore, as an instance of spoiled identity.

These examples of narrative research questions illustrate some features of formulating a narrative research question to which the narrative researcher must pay attention. No single story will ever capture a life, or even a part of a life. Therefore, the narrative researcher must limit the scope of the research question and focus on the aspects of the person's life or identity building that are most important or most interesting to the researcher.

The researcher must also clearly identify who is the narrator of the story. The narrator could be the person who experienced the set of events or it could be a witness to the experiences. First-person accounts and witness accounts are both powerful forms of storytelling. For example, an aging mother would provide a witness account of the story of her daughter's struggle with infertility and the callousness and insensitivity of her daughter's husband to her daughter's experience and emotional torment. Witness interviews and stories can also be called collateral interviews and stories. The daughter herself would provide a first-person account of the experience of infertility and her husband's reactions to her.

In biographical and historical narratives, the narrative researcher may collect multiple witness accounts and/or examine the written and oral texts in archival and documentary materials that provide a wealth of witness information. In reflecting on the silence, disguised as love, that prevented her from sharing her own fears with her dying mother, and in wondering how to share her fears about her own cancer experience with her daughter, Kathy Weingarten (2000) invokes the power of witnessing: "We are all always witnesses. People speak, we hear, whether we choose to or not. Events explode in front of us, whether we want to see or not. We can turn on television, see people in moments of extremity, and know their fate before they do" (p. 392).

I would like to suggest that the narrator of a story, even when the narrator is the first person or the person who experienced the events, does not always represent the authorial voice. The authorial voice, especially in examining scripts of identity, is more likely to be the dominant discourse of the culture as represented by key figures in the person's life and by critical cultural signifiers such as the media and advertising. For example, Weingarten (2000), in recounting her mother's impending death, describes the dominant discourse, or we could say, the authorial voice, as the belief that silence and secrecy were the appropriate moral responses to the plight of a middle-aged woman with terminal cancer. It is important, therefore, for the narrative researcher to examine the source(s) of the authorial voices in a person's life and not to confuse those with who is assuming the role of narrator. Authorial voice does not mean the voice of authority in the strictest sense, but rather the voice of the dominant values, beliefs, and attitudes of the culture that are internalized by the person who is providing an account of experience. For a fuller discussion of dominant discourse and its internalization by persons, see the works of Michel Foucault (1970, 1973, 1976, 1978).

Summary.   **Key Steps in Formulating the Research Question or Focus.**

- ♦ Limit the scope of the research question.
- ♦ Identify who is the narrator of the story.
    - ♦ Is the account a first-person account?
    - ♦ Is the account a witness account?
    - ♦ Does the account include both first-person and witness stories?
- ♦ Understand the distinction between the narrator and the authorial voice.

Data Collection Procedures

The primary vehicle for data collection in narrative research is the interview. The interview could consist of a personal face-to-face interview with the person or persons who is (are) the participant(s) or subject(s) of the research project and could also include witness or collateral interviews with people who know or knew the subjects of the narrative study. Documentary, historical, and archival materials are also important sources of data collection in narrative research. These sources help add to the developing narrative and to confirm or triangulate the accuracy or validity and richness of the information already collected.

Kvale (1996) provides excellent guidelines that could easily be used as standards for assessing a narrative interview. He emphasizes that the purpose of the interview is to gather information about the life-world or everyday experience of the interviewee and that the researcher has the task of seeking and interpreting the meaning of these everyday experiences. Kvale also reminds researchers that global statements from the interviewee are usually not useful and that the researcher has the task of eliciting detailed, specific descriptions of everyday events and their meanings from the interviewee.

Another quality Kvale (1996) outlines as important for the narrative interview is that the researcher have a flexible interview focus, neither too constraining nor too open and unfocused. He also reminds researchers that it is important to develop a willingness to accept ambiguity as a part of the reality of life and therefore to avoid forcing clarity or specificity from an interviewee who is ambivalent or ambiguous about a life situation. Kvale regards the knowledge generated in an interview as an interpersonal act and conversation as the production site of knowledge. Unlike many interview guides and writers, Kvale declares that the process of interviewing may bring about changes in awareness and changes in meaning for the interviewee and that the researcher must be open and sensitive to these possibilities. And finally, the researcher must work to ensure that the interview process is a positive one for the interviewee. The emphasis on the possibility of change and the importance of the interview being a positive experience for the interviewee reminds me of a student's reaction in a class I taught on social and cultural issues in counseling. As an assignment I had asked the class to interview someone culturally different from themselves. In reporting her interview experience with a middle-aged Eastern European immigrant woman, the student ended her report by telling the class that at the end of the interview the Eastern European woman commented that she had never realized how interesting a life she had led. I told the student that she could have been paid no finer compliment about her interview skills, even as the student expressed doubt about whether a research interview should lead to this kind of change. The memory of the story of the Eastern European woman's powerful positive experience with the student interviewer and her changed and enriched awareness of her own life still delights me many years later. I have no misgivings about the experience of change to which the interview led for this woman.

On the other hand, Parker (2005) warns narrative researchers against believing that their interviewing work is therapeutic for the interviewee and further warns researchers against being too personally intrusive. There is a significant difference between acknowledging that the research interview can function as a catalyst for personal change and holding a position that intensive interviewing is usually therapeutic. The former is a reasonable, theoretically sound constructionist and evidence-based position to hold; the latter is naive and probably dangerous. Parker, however, makes the point: researchers are not therapists and the two roles should not be confused.

Personal and family narratives can be immeasurably enhanced by asking research participants to bring in photographs, drawings, or other special mementos of personal or family life. Creswell (2002) notes that such memorabilia can help participants to remember details that they might not have included in their face-to-face interview. Historical narrative research can be done through the use of such artifacts alone. A dazzling and heart-wrenching example of historical narrative research using only children's drawings and poems is Volavkova's (1993) book *I Never Saw Another Butterfly: Children's Drawings and Poems from Terezin Concentration Camp, 1942–1944*. This book is a collection of art and poems from some of the 15,000 children under 15 years of age who were imprisoned at Terezin outside of Prague. Fewer than 100 of these children survived. The pictures and poems reflect the juxtaposition of the conditions in the concentration camp and the experiences of the children—hope amid horror, sunshine amid darkness and deprivation.

Sources of narrative can be collected from any of the forms of expression that are present in a culture. Music, art, literature, film, advertising, graffiti, dance, theater, letters, Web logs, and everyday conversation are examples of readily available forms of cultural expression and narrative that could be studied through narrative research. For example, rap music represents a collection of personal narratives put to musical beats. Tupac Shakur's 1992 rap song "Brenda's Got a Baby" packs a world of experience, meaning, and story into 42 short lines. This rap song is an in-your-face storied indictment of how the short life of misery of one illiterate girl affects the whole community. An illiterate girl (Brenda) lives in the ghetto and becomes pregnant as a result of being molested by her cousin. Brenda's family is mainly interested in the welfare check that Brenda's baby will provide. When Brenda has the baby alone because no one is really interested and throws the baby in the trash, her family kicks her out, and Brenda ends up as a slain prostitute.

Early rap music especially represents a large collection of stories of marginalization, race, race relations, poverty, violence, neglect, death, and rage.

Researching rap music for the stories of the meaning of everyday experiences jam-packed into them is an example of doing narrative research without interviewing. Creswell (2002) suggests that the researcher's ultimate retelling or restorying of a narrative "is based on the assumption that the story told by the participant will be better understood by the listener and the reader if it is resequenced into a logical order" (p. 534). In the case of doing narrative research of rap music, the researcher's retelling of the stories and meanings of rap could function like a Trojan horse — bringing those stories to an audience or a group of stakeholders, usually identifiable by age, class, and race, who typically refuse to even hear or listen to the stories of rap.

Summary: Narrative Research Data Collection Procedures.

- Conduct face-to-face interviews with the research participant or subject whenever possible.
- Do follow-up interviews to add detail, fill in gaps, and check meanings and interpretations.
- Conduct witness or collateral interviews whenever possible and as appropriate.
- Ask the interviewee to bring in drawings, poems, pictures, photographs, or other mementos and talk about these, as appropriate.
- Examine documentary, historical, or archival material, as appropriate for the particular study.
- Examine forms of expression in the culture, for example, music, art, literature, film, advertising, graffiti, dance, theater, letters, Web logs, and everyday conversation, as appropriate for the particular study.
- Be aware of common interview pitfalls, namely the following,
  - Insufficient attention to developing an atmosphere of trust and goodwill.
  - Not asking more questions about the tone and content of the interviewee's responses when there is little variety in the descriptions.
  - Seeking clarity and specificity when the interviewee consistently describes experiences in ambiguous ways instead of accepting the story or a part of it as uncertain or ambivalent.
  - Not asking for richer, thicker descriptions and meanings when the interviewee's story seems too pat or glossed or structured to please the interviewer.

The narrative researcher would select the appropriate data collection procedures from the preceding list. Of course, not all procedures would be used for every study. The nature of the narrative study, feasibility, time, and budget will determine which procedures are most suitable for a particular study.

Data Analysis Procedures

The narrative researcher has a number of choices to make in determining how to go about analyzing stories and other narrative data that have been collected. A number of options for narrative analysis are outlined and described in the following subsections.

Structural Analysis.   One choice the narrative researcher could make is to analyze stories in terms of their structural elements. Structural analysis of narratives involves coding the narrative according to its structural elements. If Labov's (Labov, 1972; Labov & Waletsky, 1967) schema is used, then narrative data are coded by examining the narrative line by line and identifying the abstract, which introduces and summarizes the story; the orientation, which provides contextual details of character, time, and place; the complication, which describes critical events in the story; the evaluation, which outlines the meaning and implications of the narrative; the result, which provides the outcome or resolution of the story; and the coda, which describes how the storyteller brings the events and meanings of the story back into the present. The researcher then fashions a new story emphasizing the key structural elements of the narrative and how they have come together to form a particular story with a particular meaning pattern.

Burke's (1969) structural analysis could be used in a similar way to analyze a narrative line by line, but with the focus on identifying the act, scene, agent, agency, and purpose of the story. The researcher would then also retell a new story but with the emphasis on analyzing the actor's purpose, motives, and intentionality.

There are many other possibilities for examining narratives structurally. These would involve examining the narrative for the literary elements of a story, namely, plot, time, scene or context, characters, events and actions, outcomes and meanings. As in the two preceding examples of structural analysis, the researcher would then retell a new story, perhaps emphasizing a particular aspect of the original narrative such as character development or the unfolding of events over time or how the plot, characters, and outcomes work together logically or otherwise.

Narrative Analysis from a Psychological Perspective.   Narrative analysis from a psychological perspective reflects a movement away from attempting to understand personality, psychopathology, the self, and intentionality through the lens of scientific theories such as psychoanalysis, behaviorism, humanism, and even systems theory. Such theories carry the weight of the scientific worldview that, apart from quantum science, sees human behavior in Newtonian, mechanistic terms. For example, psychoanalysis refers to drives and impulses, ids, egos, and superegos. Behaviorism talks about contingencies of reinforcement and conditioning. Humanism speaks of self-actualization and unhindered free will. Systems theory refers to feedback loops, homeostasis, and interdependence.

Rather, narrative analysis from a psychological perspective moves us toward examining the meanings people attach to their lives and behaviors, how they use language to talk to themselves and to describe themselves to themselves and to others. Narrative psychological analysis attends to the metaphors of self-description and intentionality that are revealed in people's narratives. The researcher interested in psychological narrative analysis examines narrative for the patterns of metaphors, words, phrases, and speech acts that provide the thread of continuity making up and maintaining the self. This linguistic thread of continuity should be examined for its consistency, coherence, and congruence, not for its factual truth (George et al., 1996; Schafer, 1992; Spence, 1987). Inconsistencies and discontinuities of self-description, evidenced by significant changes of patterns of metaphors, words, phrases, or speech acts, or incoherent self-description are marked as reflecting critical narrative turns in the development and maintenance of the linguistic self. As Bruner (2004) points out, it is this linguistic self that becomes the self that is lived out in daily life.

Narrative Analysis of Identity Development.   Narrative analysis from a psychological perspective tells the story of a life from the inside to the outside, starting with the individual self as the star and then connecting that already-developed individual self to the outside world. Narrative analysis of identity development does just the opposite. It starts with the outside stories of the culture and explores how those outside stories create the inside story of the self. It is a fascinating difference in perspective.

The difference emerges in the juxtaposition of the realist view of the self with the postmodern, social constructionist view of the self. The realist view, upon which almost the entire history of psychology is built, regards the self as a separate, self-contained individual entity generally stable over time. The social constructionist view regards the self as relationally constructed, unstable, evolving, and being constructed or manufactured and deconstructed and reconstructed through engagement in multiple roles and relationships over time within the context of a more encompassing, powerful social discourse. It makes sense, then, that the social constructionist view denies the existence of an essential, real self (Denzin, 2001).

The tool of the narrative researcher interested in identity development is the reflexive interview. Reflexivity technically refers to the bending back on oneself. In the reflexive interview, the narrative researcher poses questions to participants that ask the participants to examine how their way of thinking, feeling, and being in the world has come to be the way that it is. The reflexive interview uses the kinds of questions illustrated earlier in this chapter that relate to authorial voice. These questions invite the participant to examine who they are in relation to the larger cultural discourse and to imagine alternative discourses that would result in the production of alternative identities. Narrative research from this perspective assumes the plasticity of identity and proceeds to examine how a particular identity has been molded under the direction of authorial voice(s).

There is no question that narrative research from an identity development perspective has the potential to affect profound changes in people's stories of themselves. The dialogical inquiry that is characteristic of reflexive interviewing focusing on scripts of identity, although respectful, can also be challenging. It can shake a person's self-story to realize through identity development questions that he or she is living out larger social scripts the person may never have thought about before. For example, a millionaire entrepreneur may find it difficult to realize that he is treating money and his family's use of it as if he were still eking out an existence on the side of a hill in the same way that his father was forced to do in his native country. The authorial voice of this man's view of the use of money is located in the larger scripts of poverty and scarcity that long ago ceased to be useful in his own personal and family life, and that, in fact, were now hurtful.

The narrative researcher's role in conducting analysis from the perspective of identity development is to interrogate the scripts of identity that people have come to believe and perform, to retell the story of the history of those scripts, and to include in the new story the shifts in identity that have occurred as a result of such inquiry and changed awareness. Clearly, in narrative analysis from the perspective of identity development, the researcher must be aware that every question is potentially an agent of change and therefore ethically charged. In this perspective, every action of the narrative researcher has ethical import. Every question asked or unasked, every story retold or left untold, has ethical significance for both the researcher and participant.

Artistic and Aesthetic Narrative Analysis.   Stories are art forms with the language, rhythms, cadences, turns, surprises, and meanings of a narrative bringing a universal form of art — the story — to life. Narrative researchers can be regarded as impresarios encouraging the creation of artistic and aesthetic performances by their research participants through the telling of life stories. As an impresario, the narrative researcher encourages the production and performance of stories by participants and stands in appreciation and awe of the complexity and power of a life story as a form of art. Narrative researchers, in this form of analysis, enter into the emotional and sacred ground of their participants as participants tell their life stories, and the researchers allow themselves to fully and emotionally experience and then record their own emotional responses to these stories. Such emotional experiencing by the narrative researcher completes and fulfills the relationship between artist and audience, who are intimately connected with one another. Often, the participants, too, are surprised by the power of their own artistic performances of their life stories to change the way they think about themselves, others, and their own lives. Thus, the artistic and aesthetic narrative researcher experiences the stories of participants in a holistic and organismic way and retells these stories by including his or her own emotional reactions and reflections. The appreciation of a life story as a form of art and the retelling of it from the standpoint of this appreciation and with the inclusion of the researcher's own emotional responses are the heart and soul of artistic and aesthetic narrative analysis. The reader also becomes involved in artistic and aesthetic narrative research by becoming emotionally affected and moved by the narrative re-storying.

Summary: Narrative Research Data Analysis.

- ◆ Identify the particular method of narrative analysis to be used. For example, structural narrative analysis, psychological narrative analysis, identity development narrative analysis, or artistic and aesthetic narrative analysis.
- ◆ Examine the narrative in terms of the criteria of interest based on the selected method of analysis. For example, elements of literary form and structure; patterns of metaphor and word use, as well as narrative consistency, coherence, and congruence; interrogating the history of persons' scripts of identity and their connection to the larger social discourse; fully emotionally experiencing and appreciating the stories of peoples' lives as art forms and retelling those stories while including the researcher's own emotional reactions in them.
- ◆ Retell the story of the narrative from the perspective of the selected method of analysis, being mindful to keep the literary elements of narrative present in the new story.

TRUSTWORTHINESS AND CREDIBILITY IN NARRATIVE INQUIRY

Trustworthiness and credibility in narrative research refer to the degree to which the participants have been fully included in the research process and have had the opportunity to reflect on and comment on their story as retold by the narrative researcher. Both the researcher and the participant then share the responsibility of the re-storying process. In research that emphasizes collaboration, it seems to me like arrogance to place the entire burden of ensuring the faithfulness of an account on the researcher alone. There are many situations in which the participants' only way of being heard and telling their stories is through participating in research, and the participants therefore have a strong interest in wanting participant stories to reflect the narrative truth of their experiences. The researcher's obligation is to provide meaningful opportunities for the participants to review transcripts and the researcher's retold stories. Any changes, concerns, or objections simply become part of the story of the research and can be included in the narrative, with review again by the participants.

With the increasing trend toward transparency of procedure in qualitative research (Chenail, 1995; Constas, 1992), the narrative researcher has an obligation to explicate all procedures followed in the research process. This transparency includes revealing to the reader the following information about the research process: (1) clearly identifying the research question, (2) disclosing where the research data came from, that is, first-person accounts, witness accounts, documentary, archival data, historical data, and/or samples of a variety of possible cultural forms of expression, (3) identifying and describing the steps in the analysis of the data, and (4) attending to the issues of voice in the re-storying and re-presenting of the narrative by clearly indicating who the narrator is—the researcher, the participant, both in sequential form, both in composite form, or both as interpreted and re-storied by the researcher. A further criterion for assessing the trustworthiness of narrative research is whether the narrative research evokes emotion in the reader. This has been the subject of much discussion in my qualitative research classes. Indeed, we have discussed at length whether the primary function of narrative research should be to move the reader through the evoking of emotion. If it is not the primary function, I believe it is a critical one.

Summary: Trustworthiness and Credibility in Narrative Inquiry.

- ◆ Include the participants fully in the research process.
- ◆ Provide meaningful opportunities for the participants to review transcripts and the researcher's retold story and participant comments and reactions to the story of the research.
- ◆ In the interests of transparency, ensure that all research procedures and steps are fully described.
- ◆ Consider whether the narrative research story evokes emotion.

ETHICS IN NARRATIVE RESEARCH

The storying of a part of one's life and the sharing of that story with a researcher can lead to a number of different emotional reactions. On the one hand, a person can experience catharsis and relief. On the other hand, a person can become distressed and upset. Or the person can express a strong desire to have the story finally heard and told, even if the telling is done anonymously; knowing that one's story will be told can be validating and powerful. Or the person, through examining his or her connection to the beliefs and values of the larger social world, can experience rapid and profound change in the understanding of identity, of whom and how the person is in the world. None of these reactions are neutral.

For many, the telling of the story to a researcher is a dialogical encounter of the kind that Buber (1958) refers to as "I" and "Thou." The "I" and "Thou" encounter is one of mutuality and reciprocity. In the language of social constructionism, it is one of co-construction. In some forms of narrative research, the co-construction is of the very identity of the person. To some extent, this is moving into territory where angels properly fear to tread. The responsibility of the narrative researcher is clear. The narrative researcher must be aware of the potential for profound personal change and intense emotional experiencing that could be generated through the process of narrative interviewing and always must approach the participant with sensitivity and respect. Hearing and gathering the stories of peoples' lives also requires that the researcher be fully present to the participants. In addition, the researcher must be comfortable with hearing stories of lives that can reflect the panoply of possible human experiencing. Some researchers simply are not comfortable with the kind of intimate knowing of the other that occurs in narrative research and therefore should avoid it. These guidelines fall into the category of ethics that McNamee and Gergen (1998) refer to as relational responsibility.

The standard ethical guidelines for any researcher studying human subjects also apply. Consent to participate in the research study should be fully informed, meaning that prospective participants have the opportunity to discuss the study and have any questions fully answered. Prospective participants should have an understanding of the nature and purpose of the study and know that participation is voluntary and that they can discontinue participation at any time without penalty. If Institutional Review Board (IRB) approval is required, the researcher must submit the proposal and obtain approval for the study before beginning. If the researcher is not operating in an institutional context where IRB approval is required, the researcher should still follow the federal guidelines developed for the protection of human subjects in research studies. Issues of identification and confidentiality should be fully discussed and agreed upon prior to the collection of data. Where confidentiality is required, the researcher has an obligation to protect the confidentiality of research participants by using pseudonyms and camouflaging contextual details of the study sufficiently so that readers would not be able to identify the participants. This obligation confers another one on the researcher: the obligation to maintain the integrity of the study by camouflaging identifying information without changing it so much that it no longer reflects the context and experiences of the participants.

Summary: Ethics in Narrative Research.

- ◆ Narrative research requires relational responsibility.
- ◆ The researcher must be sensitive, respectful, and fully present to the participant.
- ◆ The researcher must be mindful that personal change and intense emotional experiencing could result from the interview process.
- ◆ The researcher must be comfortable with the intimacy required of narrative research and hearing stories of lives that include the panoply of human experiences.
- ◆ Standard ethical procedures, including obtaining fully informed consent, protecting participant confidentiality, and obtaining IRB approval, must be followed.
- ◆ The researcher must safeguard the integrity of the study when camouflaging contextual details to protect client confidentiality.

CONCLUSION

Narrative research is about the storied nature of peoples' lives and the nature of how people make sense out of their lives by putting their experiences in story form. Narrative research is not neutral because it sits at the crossroads of individual identity and the culture stories that fashion it. It is not possible to ask people about the stories of their lives without entering into intimate relationships with those people. Intimacy changes people. Asking questions and telling stories change people. It is not possible to tell about a life without talking about the people, the place, the time, and the events that were going on during the time of that life and ordering those elements into something that makes sense—a story. Well-told stories of peoples' lives evoke emotion in those who hear or read the stories, and then the listeners and readers change, too, and become hungry for more stories. And in the betwixt and between of art and human science, narrative research provides a way of gathering stories that, in the end, describe all the ways there are of being human and living life. So, all this means that there are a lot more stories are out there.

REFERENCES

Bruner, J. (2004). Life as narrative. *Social Research, 71,* 691–710.

Buber, M. (1958). *I and thou.* (R. G. Smith, Trans.). New York: Scribner's.

Burke, K. (1969). *A grammar of motives.* Berkeley: University of California Press.

Chenail, R. J. (1995). Presenting qualitative data. *The Qualitative Report* [On-line journal], 2(3). Retrieved August 15, 2005, from http://www.nova.edu/ssss/QR/QR2-3/presenting.html.

Constas, M. A. (1992). Qualitative analysis as a public event: The documentation of category development procedures. *American Educational Research Journal, 29,* 253–266.

Creswell, J. W. (2002). *Educational research: Planning, conducting, and evaluating quantitative and qualitative research.* Upper Saddle River, NJ: Merrill Prentice Hall.

Denzin, N. (2001). The reflexive interview and a performative social science. *Qualitative Research, 1,* 23–46.

Foucault, M. (1970). *The order of things: An archaeology of the human sciences.* New York: Pantheon.

Foucault, M. (1973). *The birth of the clinic: An archaeology of medical perception.* (A. M. Sheridan-Smith, Trans.). New York: Pantheon.

Foucault, M. (1976). *Mental illness and psychology.* (A. Sheridan, Trans.). New York: Harper & Row.

Foucault, M. (1978). *Discipline and punish: The birth of the prison.* (A. Sheridan, Trans.). New York: Pantheon.

Freedman, J., & Combs, G. (1996). *Narrative therapy: The social construction of preferred realities.* New York: W. W. Norton.

George, C., Kaplan, N., & Main, M. (1996). *Adult attachment interview.* Unpublished manuscript (3rd ed.), Department of Psychology, University of California, Berkeley.

Goffman, E. (1959). *The presentation of self in everyday life.* New York: Doubleday Anchor.

Goffman, E. (1963). *Stigma: Notes on the management of spoiled identity.* Englewood Cliffs, NJ: Prentice Hall.

Goffman, E. (1974). *Frame analysis: An essay on the organization of experience.* New York: Harper & Row.

Kvale, S. (1996). *InterViews: An introduction to qualitative research interviewing.* Thousand Oaks, CA: Sage.

Labov, W. (1972). The transformation of experience in narrative syntax. In W. Labov (Ed.), *Language in the inner city* (pp. 352–396). Philadelphia: University of Pennsylvania Press.

Labov, W., & Waletsky, J. (1967). Narrative analysis: Oral versions of personal experience. In J. Helm (Ed.), *Essays on the verbal and visual arts* (pp. 12–44). Seattle, WA: American Ethnological Society.

McNamee, S., & Gergen, K. J. (Eds.). (1998). *Relational responsibility: Resources for sustainable dialogue.* Thousand Oaks, CA: Sage.

Parker, I. (2005). *Qualitative psychology: Introducing radical research.* Buckingham, England: Open University Press.

Phillips, D. C. (1997). Telling the truth about stories. *Teaching and Teacher Education, 13,* 101–109.

Riessman, C. K. (1993). *Narrative analysis.* Newbury Park, CA: Sage.

Schafer, R. (1992). *Retelling a life: Narration and dialogue in psychoanalysis.* New York: Basic Books.

Schwandt, T. A. (1998). Constructivist, interpretivist approaches to human inquiry. In N. K. Denzin & Y. S. Lincoln (Eds.), *The landscape of qualitative research: Theories and issues* (pp. 221–259). Thousand Oaks, CA: Sage.

Somers, A. (2005). Background: Terri Schiavo's right to live or die. Does Terri's husband have the right to end her life? Retrieved August 5, 2005, from http://civilliberty.about.com/cs/humaneuthinasia/a/bgTerry.htm.

Spence, D. P. (1987). *The Freudian metaphor: Toward paradigm change in psychoanalysis.* New York: W. W. Norton.

Volavkova, H. (Ed.). (1993). *I never saw another butterfly: Children's drawings and poems from Terezin concentration camp, 1942–1944* (2nd ed.). New York: Schocken Books.

Weingarten, K. (2000). Witnessing, wonder, and hope. *Family Process, 39,* 389–402.

White, M., & Epston, D. (1990). *Narrative means to therapeutic ends.* New York: W. W. Norton.

17

Exemplar: Four Types of Stories about Family Caregiving

Lioness Ayres

ABSTRACT

Researchers across disciplines have found that sometimes persons in relatively similar caregiving situations demonstrate very different responses to those situations. One reason for this difference lies in the different meanings persons make out of the events in their lives. This chapter describes findings from a study that combined two qualitative strategies, across-case, thematic analysis and within-case, narrative analysis, to investigate meaning in accounts of family caregiving. Themes identified in the across-case analysis were interpreted in the context of patterns identified in the narrative

This research was partially supported by an Individual National Research Service Award, NRO6602, and by a Clinical Scholars Grant from West Suburban Hospital Medical Center. Grateful acknowledgment is made to the University of Illinois at Chicago, and particularly to the College of Nursing, for facilitating this study. Dr. Kathleen Knafl of the College of Nursing and Dr. Suzanne Poirier of the College of Medicine at the University of Illinois at Chicago were tireless and invaluable mentors. This chapter was originally published in *Research in Nursing & Health*.

analysis, as well as in the overall framework of caregivers' process of making meaning. Caregivers in this study told four types of stories: stories of ideal lives, stories of ordinary lives, stories of compromised lives, and ambiguous stories. Characteristics of each story type are described, and an example of one type of story is included as an illustration of the method. Findings suggest a new approach to understanding family caregiving that incorporates the diverse meanings caregivers make of their often similar experiences.

Researchers across disciplines have recognized considerable individual variation among caregivers in their response to the experiences of caregiving (*cf.*, Braithwaite, 1996; Davis, 1992; Haley, Levine, Brown, & Bartolucci, 1987; Magai & Cohen, 1998). According to Hooker, Monahan, Bowman, Frazier, and Shifren (1998), "A consistent theme in caregiving research is the attempt to understand why caregivers under similar circumstances show such great variability in their ability to adapt to the situation" (p. P73). Hooker and colleagues proposed that this variability was a result of personality, that is, that "people assign meaning to a situation through an interactive process in which personality plays a key role . . ." (p. P73). Hooker and colleagues studied the influence of personality variables, including neuroticism and optimism, on caregivers' mental and physical health. According to the researchers, personality is important because it influences the meanings people assign to situations. In addition, meanings may arise from the context of caregiving: from family relationships, sociocultural practices, and, of course, the history of the relationship between caregiver and receiver (Poirier & Ayres, 2002). To date, although the importance of meaning has been acknowledged, little is known about the kinds of meaning caregivers make of their situations or about the ways meaning might influence caregiver outcomes such as burden or depression.

As early as 1966 (Hoenig & Hamilton, 1966), researchers who studied family caregiving recognized the central role of individualized meaning in families' experience. Hoenig and Hamilton urged clinicians to recognize that caregiving "may mean totally different things according to the point of view of the patient and his family or of those outside his kin group" (pp. 106–107), or, as suggested by Archbold and Stewart (1996), according to the point of view of the investigator. Hoenig and Hamilton (1966) continued, "A 'burden' taken on in loving care . . . may not be regarded as such . . ." (p. 107). Subsequent investigators have recognized the contribution of individual caregivers' perceptions of their experience to the development of strain or burden (Archbold & Stewart, 1996; Braithwaite, 1996; Haley et al., 1987; Hooker et al., 1998; Nolan, Grant, & Ellis, 1990; Poulshock & Deimling, 1984). Other investigators have studied beliefs about caregiving (Phillips, Rempusheski, & Morrison, 1989; Phillips et al., 1995) and the influence of beliefs about the caregiving role on the quality of care provided. To date, however, less is known about the meanings caregivers bring to and make from caregiving. Such research would require both a neutral conceptualization of caregiving and a method that allows participants to describe the experience of caregiving in the context of their own lives. The purpose of this chapter is to describe the findings from within- and across-case analyses (Ayres, Kavanaugh, & Knafl, 2003) of interviews with family caregivers. Narrative and thematic analysis identified four types of stories about family caregiving, each of which assigned a different meaning to the experience.

METHOD

Sample

Participants in this mixed-methods study were recruited by nurses from two home health agencies, by two private health care providers, and through snowball sampling. A description of the sample of 36 caregivers and 44 care recipients appears in Table 17–1. This study used the maximum variation sampling strategy described by Patton (1990). Sources of variation included race, gender, length of caregiving, and recipient diagnosis, because caregiving researchers have suggested that meanings for caregiving may be influenced by these characteristics (Barer & Johnson, 1990; Barusch & Spaid, 1989; Connell & Gibson, 1997; Cox, 1995; Davis, 1992; Given et al., 1992; Kuhlman, Wilson, Hutchinson, & Wallhagen, 1991; Miller & Cafasso, 1992; Pruchno, Kleban, Michaels, & Dempsey, 1990; Schultz, O'Brien, Bookwala, & Fleissner, 1995; Silliman & Sternberg, 1988; Vitaliano, Young, & Russo, 1991; Walker, Pratt, & Eddy, 1995; Young & Kahana, 1995). For this study, recruiters identified persons as African American or White, and I did not ask participants to specify their race or ethnicity. During the second half of data collection, I also asked recruiters to identify and recruit persons who were especially distressed or troubled to maximize variation on this characteristic.

Procedure

Participants were interviewed in their homes or other locations of their choosing. Interviews were based on a semistructured interview guide so that

TABLE 17–1 Characteristics of the Sample of 36 Family Caregivers and 44 Recipients of Care

Characteristic	N
Caregiver age group	
< 45 years old	6
45–65 years old	20
> 65 years old	10
Minimum reported age: 39 years	
Maximum reported age: 92 years	
Caregiver gender	
Male	11
Female	25
Ethnicity of caregiving dyad	
African American	9
White	27
Recipient age group	
> 45 years old	6
45–65 years old	12
> 65 years old	26
Minimum reported age: 14 years	
Maximum reported age: 99 years	
Relationship to caregiver of recipient	
Spouse	14
Parent	18
Child	6
In-law	4
Sibling	1
Other	1
Recipient gender	
Male	19
Female	25
Length of caregiving	
1 year or less	8
2–5 years	17
6–10 years	5
11–20 years	2
> 20 years	4
Minimum reported length of caregiving: 6 weeks	
Maximum reported length of caregiving: 50 years	
Recipient diagnoses (some recipients had more than one diagnosis)	
Stroke	9

TABLE 17–1   continued

Characteristic	N
Mental retardation	9
Alzheimer's disease, dementia	5
Perceptual deficit (blindness, deafness)	4
Arthritis, orthopedic problems	4
Cancer	4
Heart disease	3
Insulin-dependent diabetes	2
Spinal cord injury	2
Chronic mental illness	1
Traumatic brain injury	1
Parkinson's disease	1
Multiple sclerosis	1
Circulatory problems, stasis ulcer	1
Renal failure	1
Huntington's disease	1

each participant responded to the same set of questions, although the language of some questions was clarified after participants early in the study found it confusing. The interview guide provided participants with opportunities to talk about variables of interest from previous caregiving research ("What sorts of things does your family member need help with?"). Use of open-ended questions ("How did you come to be the person taking care of your family member?") and neutral probes gave participants the opportunity to illustrate their answers with stories or to provide evidence for particular conclusions they had drawn. All interviews were tape-recorded and transcribed verbatim.

Data Analysis

Interview data were analyzed through an iterative process of comparison called the hermeneutic spiral (Reason & Rowan, 1981; Tesch, 1990), a process in which "the analyst moves back and forth between individual elements of the text and the whole text in many cycles" (Tesch, 1990, p. 68). Each cycle integrated three kinds of analytic comparisons: comparisons across all accounts to identify particular themes, subthemes, categories, and classes; comparisons within each individual account to identify meanings that were implicit rather than explicit in the text; and comparisons of one whole account with another, to identify overall patterns of meaning. The strategy of integrating within-case and across-case approaches to analyze qualitative data has been explained in more detail elsewhere (Ayres, Kavanaugh, & Knafl, 2003).

For across-case comparisons, data were coded using a hierarchical strategy (Richards & Richards, 1995) to identify themes and subthemes. Initial coding categories were reorganized into themes and subthemes through iterative comparisons within and across cases. Themes were then arranged in descending order of complexity into subthemes, categories, and classes; this structure was examined for patterns across cases. A similar analytic procedure was previously described by Knafl, Gallo, Breitmayer, Zoeller, and Ayres (1993). Three general themes were identified: definitions, management activities, and motivations and rewards. Some examples of the hierarchical arrangements of themes, subthemes, categories, and classes of responses are shown in Table 17–2.

Some interviews were difficult to classify on some categories or classes. For example, individual interviews sometimes provided contradictory or conflicting information about a particular classification within a category. A respondent might state explicitly that his or her relationship with the recipient was "good" or "fine" but provide only examples of mutual antagonism. These interviews required a within-case, narrative approach to interpretation. The narrative approach in this study used the "narrative tools" of overreading described by Poirier and Ayres (1996) to refine and contextualize the ways themes varied across cases. Overreading includes attention to characteristics of texts such as repetitions, evasions, omissions, implied endings, and incongruities. When an interview provided strong evidence for two mutually exclusive classes, for example, for definitions of the recipient as both absolved and unworthy, a new class of "ambiguous" was added to the category "Evaluation of the recipient." In addition, narrative tools were used to distinguish between missing data and evasions or omissions. For example, if I failed to ask a respondent about his or her previous relationship with the recipient, this information was coded as missing. If, on the other hand, I asked the question and the respondent changed the subject or remained silent, this information was classified as an evasion or an omission, respectively.

Generally, overreaders interpret repetitions, evasions, omissions, and incongruities as indications of tension within the narrative, what Kermode (1981) refers to as "secrets." The use of narrative methods cannot resolve those secrets; rather, the identification of repetitions, evasions, omissions, or

TABLE 17–2 Examples of Themes, Subthemes, Categories, and Classes of Responses

Theme	Subtheme	Category	Class
Definitions	Oneself and one's own life	Self as caregiver	Active agent Thwarted agent Victim Ambiguous
		Life changed by caregiving	Life better Life the same Life worse Ambiguous
	Recipient and relationship	Evaluation of recipient	Normal and ordinary Absolved Unworthy Ambiguous
		Current relationship	Reciprocal Role reversal Antagonistic Custodial Ambiguous
	Caregiving	Own view	Pleasure Normal responsibility Challenge Identity Burden Ambiguous
Management activities	Managing care	Priorities	Policing Assessing Negotiating Mixed or ambiguous
	Day-to-day care		Learning the ropes Established routines Anticipated crises Perpetual crisis Ambiguous
	Managing own affect	Positive strategies	Avoidance Distraction Reframing Processing Prayer

continues

TABLE 17–2   continued

Theme	Subtheme	Category	Class
		Negative strategies	Losing it Blaming Dwelling
		Ambiguous responses	
Motivations and rewards	Motivations	Duty	Justice Relationship
		Affection	
		Other reasons	Destiny Appeasement Compulsion Ambiguous

incongruities offers an additional kind of data, found "between the lines" of the literal text of the interview. Secrets suggest unresolved conflict or confusion regarding particular areas of experience; however, identification of a secret neither condemns the narrator as unreliable nor privileges the reader to resolve the tension with his or her own explanations. The use of narrative tools to inform the thematic analysis is an example of the cyclical and iterative nature of the hermeneutic spiral, through which findings from each analytic strategy inform the other strategies.

FINDINGS

Categories and classes from the thematic analysis, along with representative quotes from each interview that supported the classification, were displayed in a large, handwritten matrix to facilitate analytic immersion and to identify patterns across cases. The matrix also included representative quotes identifying expectations, explanations, and strategies (Ayres, 2000) and, where present, evidence of the "secrets" described earlier. This integration of findings from within-case and across-case analyses facilitated the development of a typology of stories in the tradition of Frank (1995) and Hawkins (1993). Three story types had identifiable meanings: stories of caregiving as an ideal life (IDEAL), stories of caregiving as a normal or ordinary life, and stories of caregiving as a compromised life. A fourth group of stories was called ambiguous and included components of at least two of the three meanings such that they could not be classified further. Table 17–3 shows the distribution of the

TABLE 17–3 Story Types of 36 Caregivers by Race, Gender, and Length of Caregiving

Story Type	Males	Females	Total Caregivers	African American	White	Length of Caregiving
Stories of ideal lives	2		2	2		< 1 year = 1 > 20 years = 1
Stories of normal or ordinary lives	5	12	17	3	14	< 1 year = 2 2–5 years = 11 6–10 years = 2 10–20 years = 1
Stories of lives compromised by caregiving	2	6	8	1	7	< 1 year = 2 2–5 years = 2 6–10 years = 3 > 20 years = 1
Ambiguous stories	2	7	9	3	6	< 1 year = 4 2–5 years = 5

sample by gender, race, and length of caregiving across the four types of stories.

Stories of Ideal Lives

Only two caregivers in this sample told stories of ideal lives. Both were African-American men, one in his 20s and the other in his 50s. Both men took care of the women who had raised them. One recipient of care had a long history of chronic mental illness, whereas the other had been recently disabled.

The two caregivers who told IDEAL stories had very modest expectations and were satisfied with the way those expectations were realized in caregiving. These narrators explained events in terms of how much better their lives were now than they had been before caregiving. They explained their situation as destiny—something meant to be. One man said, "This is what I was put here for, I guess. This is my calling."

Narrators of IDEAL stories explained their lives as improved, if not saved, by caregiving. Both men described time lived "on the street" before returning home to provide care, and both believed that they would not have survived without changing their ways. As evidence, both alluded to prior acquaintances who had died or were in prison. When asked how he thought other people would describe his life now, one man replied, "Grand."

Rewards in IDEAL stories came from love between caregiver and recipient. In stories of caregiving as an ideal life, narrators interpreted events in a way that emphasized the positives in the recipient's situation while minimizing or ignoring the negatives. Both narrators of IDEAL stories described the importance of the lifelong relationship each had with the recipient of care. Both of these narrators also exonerated the recipient from remarks or behaviors that they would otherwise have found objectionable. For example, one man explained, "You have to be this type of person where you're gonna say 'Well, I can put up with this . . . because this is how this person is feeling right now.'" In both cases, caregivers explained that both their love of the recipient and the recipient's frail health made otherwise unacceptable behaviors tolerable. Consistent with an expectation that sometimes care recipients will not behave as well as they might, and an explanation that these behaviors are a result of ill health and thus not to be taken personally, caregivers negotiated care strategies with the recipient and sometimes chose to omit treatments or medications that the recipient found objectionable. Finally, these caregivers took what appeared to be a short view of the future because they expected their lives to continue to get better. Neither narrator suggested that caregiving might end.

Stories of Normal or Ordinary Lives

Stories of caregiving as a normal or ordinary life made up the largest group in the sample. Stories about ordinariness varied widely in the range of difficulties caregivers encountered, the degree of stress they felt outside of caregiving, and the ways they responded to those stresses. Diagnoses of care recipients included Huntington's disease, traumatic brain injury, Alzheimer's disease, cardiovascular disease, multiple sclerosis, cancer, mental retardation, and stroke.

Narrators of stories of ordinary lives described flexible expectations. If strategies failed to succeed on the first try, these caregivers described either revising their strategies or reframing their expectations. Reframing strategies included both explaining outcomes in new ways so they fulfilled expectations and also modifying expectations to match actual outcomes. In either case, caregivers with ordinary life stories constantly identified, executed, and evaluated strategies to manage both the needs of the recipient and their own emotional responses to care. More than any other respondents, this group of caregivers described utilizing community resources to help them manage care responsibilities, and those who did so were unanimously satisfied with the results.

Although narrators of stories about caregiving as an ordinary life showed considerable flexibility toward the demands of caregiving, such generosity was not always extended to others outside the caregiving dyad. Some of these caregivers held others, for example, family members or health care providers, to stricter standards of accountability and were quick to condemn coldness, selfishness, or carelessness. Thus, in stories of caregiving as an ordinary life, the choice to blame or excuse was a deliberate explanation, not a habit of mind. In these stories, caregivers' motivations all included affection for the recipient, and this affection combined with a strong sense of the recipient's point of view to inspire strategies and decisions in which recipients participated as actively as they were able in making decisions about their care.

Caregivers with stories of ordinary lives rejected the word *burden* when applied to their situations, although they acknowledged that "other people" might think caregiving was burdensome. Narrators of stories of the ordinary type expected change, both positive and negative; they explained change as a normal characteristic of family life. In this context, caregiving was described as routine, and even crises were minimized and managed. For example, an 83-year-old man who took care of his comatose wife said, "People usually say, 'It's pretty bad, isn't it?' I always tell them it's just routine as far as I'm concerned."

Although these caregivers did not worry about the future, they did recognize that there would likely be disappointments ahead and used this possible darker future as a downward comparison to improve their appreciation of the present. In general, caregivers who told stories of the ordinary type deliberately chose not to worry about the future, which they called "dwelling." These caregivers felt that dwelling would undermine their emotional well-being, and so they avoided it, sometimes to the extent that they avoided thinking about the future at all except in the most general terms. One woman explained, "You know, I don't know that you dwell on the long-term part of it. . . . If you begin to sit and think and worry about what's—you don't *know* what's going to happen."

Stories of Caregiving as a Compromised Life

Diagnoses of care recipients in this group included Alzheimer's disease, mental retardation, arthritis, cardiovascular disease, diabetes, spinal cord injury, and cancer. Five of these caregivers were recruited as part of a purposive sampling strategy during the second half of data collection. Stories of caregiving as a compromised life were characterized by predictable patterns of inconsistency. Narrators described unrealistically high expectations both for themselves and for others. When these expectations were unmet, these stories often revealed a second expectation of failure. Common explanations of unmet expectations were, "Nothing that I can do is good enough" or "There isn't anything that will help." Such explanations were usually personalized, and failure was attributed to flaws in either the recipient's character or the caregiver's own. For example, one unhappy caregiver described herself as "mean" and "stupid" and her mother as "vindictive" and "nasty." Explanations in stories of this type did not acknowledge that expectations might be improbable or strategies unworkable. In sharp contrast to stories of caregiving as an ordinary life, caregivers who told stories of lives compromised by caregiving described "dwelling" on both difficulties in the present and also in the anticipated future. In these stories, even when daily life was relatively free of strain, caregivers "borrowed trouble," envisioning and worrying about future difficulties. For example, one caregiver said of her elderly father, "Either he'll break a hip at home, or he'll break a hip in a nursing home. Either way I'll feel guilty."

Stories of caregiving as a compromised life were unbalanced. Sometimes narrators so effaced themselves that only the recipient's version of events seemed to matter; these caregivers saw themselves as victims and sought always to meet the recipient's or other family members' expectations. Other narrators described recipients, other family members, and health care professionals only as illustrations of the multiple ways the narrator's attempts to provide care were thwarted by others. Stories of compromised lives were characterized by evasions, omissions, and misdirections that served to obscure all but one point of view, most often the caregiver's own, but occasionally the recipient's.

Strategies described in these stories were similarly unbalanced and seldom successful, consistent with explanations based on character flaws. Strategies frequently omitted either acknowledgment of the recipient's autonomy or the legitimacy of the caregiver's own well-being. Caregivers who told stories of compromised lives had expectations that seemed impossible to achieve. Some caregivers expected to control all of the recipient's activities and decisions; in other instances caregivers rejected their own judgment in acceding to the recipient's wishes. The two caregivers in this group who had been providing care for less than 1 year were both finding nursing home placement for the care receivers; other caregivers said that they often thought about institutionalization but at the same time were unable to find an explanation that could rationalize their expectations for themselves as caregivers with this decision. One woman, who would have liked to put her disabled parent in a nursing home, said she was "waiting for a fax from God" because she felt unable to make the decision on her own. A more detailed description of one story of caregiving as a compromised life can be found in Ayres and Poirier (2003).

Many caregivers who talked about compromised lives seemed desperate for attention, acknowledgment, and affirmation, perhaps because their stories described so few satisfactions. Yet, consistent with their expectations, they dismissed offers of support by explaining that no one could understand them or their experiences, or by explaining themselves as undeserving. The close relationship between expectation, explanation, and experience in these stories illustrates the difficulty of separating the responsibilities of caregiving from the meaning of caregiving responsibilities, further complicating the measurement task of separating meaning from the caregiver's affective response to those meanings. It was not possible to know, based on evidence in the text, to what degree caregivers' lives were compromised by external circumstances or by the meanings they made of those circumstances.

Ambiguous Stories

The final nine stories in this sample were too ambiguous to classify further. In general, caregivers in this group had been providing care for less time than caregivers in other groups had been. Diagnoses of care recipients in this group included cancer, perceptual deficits, mental retardation, spinal cord injury, renal failure, and cardiovascular disease.

Like stories of compromised lives, ambiguous stories were difficult to read. As stories, they lacked coherence, offered incomplete explanations, and described strategies whose rationales I could never quite understand. They were unsatisfying as stories—they did not fulfill my expectations for "a good story" (Poirier et al., 1992). They held too many secrets, provided too little evidence, made too many unsupported assertions. They were very difficult for me to make sense of. In addition, like stories of lives compromised by caregiving, ambiguous narratives were unbalanced. Narrators of ambiguous stories kept the focus on themselves and minimized or omitted other points of view, including the recipient's.

In ambiguous stories, the expectations, explanations, and strategies didn't fit together. Narrators of ambiguous stories might describe flexible expectations in the context of very controlling strategies, or alternately blame and exonerate recipients of care for the same behaviors. Narrators sometimes described their lives as ideal in one part of a story and as compromised in another. Although literature scholars would describe these narrators as "unreliable," such a description suggests a deliberate deceptiveness that was generally absent from tellers of ambiguous stories. I believe ambiguous stories represent a stage in the process of "getting the story straight," that is, of making meaning in lives that had recently been disrupted by the serious— sometimes terminal—illness of a close family member. Tellers of ambiguous stories seemed to be trying out various combinations of expectations, explanations, and strategies, testing the fit of each version until a story emerged that made sense *to the narrator* of changed circumstances. In ambiguous stories the frequent inconsistencies, omissions, repetitions, and evasions reflect the attempt to master, both narratively and literally, these changes. Ambiguous stories had important secrets, hidden not just from me but from the narrator as well. Because ambiguous stories are the most complex both to describe and to generalize, an example of an ambiguous story is provided here.

The Ambiguous Story of Ms. A and Her Husband

Ms. A and her husband, S, have survived one horrible year, but Ms. A explains her story as coming at what she calls a plateau. The ambiguity of Ms. A's story comes from her attempts to integrate the story of the horrible year, a story about lives compromised by serious, possibly fatal, illness with the ordinary or even ideal life story Ms. A envisions for them now. In the latter version, the As live happily ever after, leaving behind the horror of S's illness. The challenges of integrating the mutually exclusive possibilities of S dying and S surviving, of putting S's illness behind them, and of finding a happy ending produce the ambiguity in this story.

The As had been married for 20 years when S began to have indigestion, which he ignored. Ms. A says S can be "passive resistive in some ways." S's indigestion turned out to be caused by a tumor. S's responses to treatment were not encouraging: he developed respiratory failure and septicemia. Then, as if to add insult to injury, a CAT scan found widespread metastases. The situation was grave; S talked about suicide. Then, remarkably, he rallied. With hospice support, S was able to go home. At the time of the interview, S was sleeping in his own bedroom, eating at his own kitchen table. Life seems to be back to normal, a happy ending to a scary story.

Ms. A's narrative, on the surface, was an heroic story of triumph over great odds. In it, Ms. A is the protagonist and other characters play minor roles as they help or hinder her quest to rescue S both from illness and from despair. Ms. A describes the physicians who, without her persistence, might have abandoned S; the nurses who danced the macarena when S felt low; the neighbor who recommended hospice. In this heroic story, even S himself plays an essentially supporting role, the object of actions and reactions by others. For this story to make sense, it needs to end now with S safe and sound.

Ms. A is an intelligent woman, and a realist, and she recognizes that S's soundness might be temporary. Cancer, the real antagonist, is seldom mentioned. Instead, Ms. A tells the story of epic struggles in which S is delivered safely from a succession of life-threatening complications: respiratory failure, infection, depression. Ms. A offers plenty of evidence for the kind of happy ending she would prefer, and hopes to have found, in which she and S enjoy normal and ordinary lives. She describes her pleasure in the meal she served to S on the night of the interview: "turkey and mashed potatoes and gravy and creamed cauliflower and a salad that was mango and cantaloupe and cranberries on it and for dessert later he'll have strawberry pie with a little whipped cream. I mean, it's a wonderful diet." A few months ago, such a dinner seemed forever beyond S's reach; until recently, S's nutrients dripped into his stomach through a gastrostomy tube, and frequently came right back out of his mouth, although this last detail was omitted in Ms. A's account, as I will shortly explain. Ms. A, with a little self-mockery, refers to an article she found in a medical journal that has raised her hopes. In this case report, a patient somewhat like S was found not to have metastases at all; the CAT scan was proved wrong. Ms. A tells a story of hope and provides ample evidence for optimism.

There are signs that perhaps S's expectations are less positive. S has steadfastly refused to dress in the clothes he wore before his illness, although she has urged him to do so. In addition, although S has returned to the marital bedroom, Ms. A sleeps alone in the couple's king-sized bed. S keeps to his hospital bed, where his suction machine and infusion pump wait nearby, unused reminders of the bad time. The suction machine and infusion pump, like the wheelchair collapsed in the hall, play a very small role in Ms. A's account. Of the wheelchair she says only that they no longer need it but . . . Here her explanation trails off. Another artifact of the bad time is S's antidepressant medication. S doesn't think he necessarily needs it, but Ms. A insists. It is very important to Ms. A that S not get depressed again.

Before S was discharged to home, Ms. A managed her negative affect in part by redecorating. In their beautiful modern bedroom, S's little corner is visually astonishing, a grim souvenir of the recent past that Ms. A might prefer, at least for now, to forget. Although I did not usually talk to recipients of care, Ms. A insisted that I meet S, to hear firsthand about the good life they now share. S's story did not fulfill Ms. A's expectation; it fit the hospital bed and suction pump, not the beautiful room. When I entered the bedroom, S was sitting up in his hospital bed watching television. He gestured to the suction machine. "I used to throw up horrible black stuff," he said without preamble. "It used to clog up the tube. I just stuck this in my mouth to suck it up." Part of the complexity of Ms. A's narrative comes from these divergent stories. Ms. A's story is about their current normal, perhaps even ideal life. S's story is about the horrible black stuff. Additional ambiguity is introduced by the uncertainty of S's future.

The narrative ambiguity in this story can be seen in the incongruity between the literal text, in which everything is fine and getting better all the time, and the story "between the lines," in which the As' current happiness is only a respite between horror and loss, a story in which their lives have unquestionably been compromised, not by caregiving but by illness. At the same time she is telling her heroic rescue story, Ms. A told bits of a story that ends further into the future, in which she lives on alone. "We're riding the plateau," she says of S's current well-being, in a comment inconsistent with her hope for a mistake in the CAT scan:

> You know, it is a lot of responsibility, and because S has leveled off and I just try to look at him and think—for the day when this is maybe gonna change and it's gonna be downhill—we're riding on the plateau. And we're enjoying that very much. But I try and think when these are gonna be dark days, how is it going to be? And I guess I'll go back to where I'm feeling anxious and apprehensive and hope that I'll still be able to make all the right decisions that are gonna be important for him. You know, I was a grown woman when I married S, and I knew then that I would be probably a

widow for a long time, and so I—I never deluded myself into thinking that he was gonna be there. I had lived an independent life, I paid all my bills—and that is very different than the person who's never had that experience, so, you know, I think that if S starts to decline, I think I'll be able to make those kinds of decisions for him.

Ms. A has already begun to plan for S's decline. She describes her contingency plan to hire a live-in caregiver to supplant S's home health aide, who now provides all of S's personal care. Although she never explicitly acknowledges it, Ms. A herself does none of S's physical care. She will gladly make him wonderful dinners, entertain his friends when they come to visit, search the medical literature for advances in cancer care, chase a team of physicians into the elevator for a straight answer about a CAT scan, but as for that horrible black stuff, Ms. A is silent. Whether this is not her expectation for herself, or whether she had expected it of herself and been disappointed, remains a secret. If S had expectations for her, these, too, remain undisclosed.

Ms. A's story is ambiguous because it is a work in progress. The ambiguity arises from confusion about the end and helps to illustrate the force endings exert over meaning. Ms. A's two stories are both about survival, but one story is about her rescue of her husband and the other story is about her relentless agency on his behalf and then her ability, afterward, to go on without him. For either story to be meaningful, S must fulfill his role: to prosper, both physically and psychologically, until the end. Such a story cannot accommodate S suffering or afraid, which may explain Ms. A's insistence on the antidepressants. In addition, Ms. A's story is incompatible with the more terrible story S might choose to tell about his recent experiences and uncertain future. Ms. A's two stories make meanings that sustain her, but this sustenance might come at the expense of S's story to which, as a nurse, I found my sympathies most drawn.

For these reasons, Ms. A made me angry at first, and that anger made it harder for me to interpret her narrative. In addition, as previously noted, ambiguous stories do not lend themselves to definitive interpretations; they are works in progress. Neither Ms. A nor I know yet what taking care of S will mean in Ms. A's life. It is clear that Ms. A's collection of meanings sustains her, and perhaps S as well, in a situation that might easily defeat a less resourceful narrator. Furthermore, the strategies she has chosen are necessary to her well-being, which in turn is necessary to S. Ms. A never describes S as having chosen to come home, one of many omissions and evasions in this, as in all of the ambiguous narratives; nevertheless, if home is where S wants to be, then Ms. A is doing all she can to keep him there. And if only Ms. A will remain at the end of this story, she is also doing all she can to have a story that will make sense to her afterward.

DISCUSSION

Caregivers who told ideal, ordinary, compromised, and ambiguous story types were not strikingly different from one another in age, gender, race, or in the relationship of the caregiver to the care recipient, as shown in Table 17–3. The two tellers of ideal stories, both of whom were African American, might represent a unique perspective on caregiving. Connell and Gibson (1997) describe African-American caregivers as feeling more satisfied with caregiving, expressing more mastery, and experiencing less burden than White caregivers did; this description suits the two tellers of ideal stories in this study. Contrariwise, Connell and Gibson (1997) also describe African-American caregivers as typically female, older, and widowed, unlike the two caregivers in this study who told stories of ideal lives. Cox (1995) describes African-American caregivers as expressing less of a sense of competence than White caregivers do, perhaps because African-American caregivers set higher standards for themselves than their White counterparts do. This, too, differed from the men in this sample who told stories of ideal lives. Thus, there is still more to be learned about the experience of African-American caregivers. In addition, there is a need for additional narrative research with other ethnic populations conducted by researchers who are highly competent in the narrative and meaning-making traditions in those populations.

More than half (19 out of 36) of the caregivers in this study told stories in which caregiving was described in a positive way, either as an ideal life or as a normal or ordinary life. It may be that at least until recently "the disproportionate emphasis in the literature on burden and depression has deflected our attention from significant positive outcomes" (Walter, Acock, Bowman, & Li, 1996). It appears that caregivers often see caregiving as part of normal family life, as suggested by Brody (1985). Even among caregivers for whom the disabling event was sudden or unexpected, as in the case of traumatic brain injury, cancer, or multiple sclerosis, many respondents did not describe caregiving responsibilities as threatening or extraordinary. Rather, as described by family researchers such as Thorne (1985), Knafl, Breitmayer, Gallo, and Zoeller (1996), and Knafl and Deatrick (1986), many caregivers worked hard to view themselves and their lives as normal. Research would be helpful to extend the concept of normalization, if applicable, to family caregivers.

For those caregivers whose stories were less positive, the group who told stories of caregiving as a compromised life most closely resembled a model of caregiving characterized by burden, depression, and strain. In this study, 8 caregivers out of 36 told stories of compromised lives, although this number should be interpreted with caution because more than half of these (5) were recruited purposively to expand and clarify the developing analytic framework. Caregivers in this group had expectations and explanations that were consistent with poor quality caregiving strategies as described by Phillips et al. (Phillips et al., 1995; Phillips, Rempusheski, & Morrison, 1989). In particular, caregivers who told stories of compromised lives used reasoning similar to Phillips et al.'s construct of Caregiving Dogmatism, in which caregivers' reasoning was based on "a priori truth or assumptions rather than empirical evidence" (1989, p. 208). In addition, Phillips et al.'s (1989) description of a monitoring role definition, in which caregivers perceive their dominant role as "to control behavior by whatever means necessary" (p. 208), was very similar to the class of management strategies called "policing" in this study, which were most commonly described by caregivers who told stories of compromised lives. Dogmatism and monitoring care priorities were all associated with potentially poor quality care (Phillips et al., 1989). Unfortunately, the present study lacked a measure of the quality of caregiving. Further research is urgently needed to measure caregiving quality and explore links between the meaning of care and the quality of the care provided.

Ambiguous stories of caregiving have not previously been reported in the literature; this group of stories provides the most scope for further research and, potentially, for nursing intervention. It may be that all caregivers go through a process of "getting their stories straight," moving at variable speed toward an integration of definitions, management strategies, motives, beliefs, reasoning, and expectations. If these ambiguous stories represent a stage in a process that ends in the development of the story of an ideal, an ordinary, or a compromised life, it is in the interest of nurses to encourage the development of stories of ordinary lives and avert, if possible, stories of lives compromised by caregiving. Thus, further research is indicated to increase knowledge about these ambiguous stories. Such research may need for a time to use qualitative or observational methods because the inherent contradictions in ambiguous stories undermine the usefulness of structured self-report measures with these caregivers. At the same time, a better understanding of stories of normal or ordinary lives may provide nurses with the tools to help caregivers who are engaged in getting their stories straight to develop meanings that are both inherently satisfying and consistent with high-quality care.

Narrative methods have particular strengths and weaknesses. Because narrative is always a moral undertaking (Fisher, 1987), researchers and clinicians who use narrative methods run particular risks of bias. As an interpretive researcher, I struggled with some of the stories in this sample, and I sometimes found myself using the evidence in them to condemn or exonerate certain narrators based less on their circumstances than on the quality of the stories they told. The notion that interpretation of meaning gives investigators or clinicians license to turn literary judgments into moral judgments is a troubling one and demands considerable reflexivity from readers or listeners. For this study, I used strategies recommended by Poirier and Ayres (1996) as appropriate to reader-response theory, including an exhaustive audit trail and consultation with content and methods experts, to identify bias and to ensure internal consistency of interpretation.

The narrative method used in this study, and in particular the development of both story types and exemplar stories, has implications for research utilization. Hunter (1991) has found that, among physicians, medical knowledge is often transmitted through stories. If this is also the case for nursing, the use of stories could enhance information exchange among researchers and clinicians. Because one of the barriers to research utilization is the language used by researchers (Phillips, 1986; Sandelowski, 1998), the use of stories, told in ordinary language, may help to bridge this gap.

In conclusion, this study used a combination of across-case, thematic analysis and within-case, narrative analysis to develop a typology of stories for family caregivers. Four story types were described: stories of caregiving as an ideal life, stories of caregiving as a normal or ordinary life, stories of caregiving as a compromised life, and ambiguous stories. Both researchers and clinicians can benefit from interpretive methods that offer access into the processes and products of making meaning through stories. Often, it is easier to see the possibilities for reinterpretation from outside a story than it is from within it. Because nurses are uniquely privileged to hear so many stories, it may be that nurses will also be uniquely able to help clients who are in the process of "getting the story straight" to find new, more sustaining meanings and even to live more happily ever after.

References

Archbold, P. G., & Stewart, B. (1996). The nature of the caregiving role and nursing interventions for caregiving families. In E. A. Swanson & T. Tripp-Reimer (Eds.), *Advances in gerontological nursing* (pp. 133–157). New York: Springer.

Ayres, L. (2000). Narratives of family caregiving: The process of making meaning. *Research in Nursing and Health, 23,* 424–434.

Ayres, L., Kavanaugh, K., & Knafl, K. A. (2003). Within-case and across-case approaches to qualitative data analysis. *Qualitative Health Research, 13*, 871–883.

Ayres, L., & Poirier, S. (2003). Rational solutions and unreliable narrators: Content, structure, and voice in narrative research. In J. Latimer (Ed.), *Advanced qualitative research for nursing* (pp. 115–134). Oxford, England: Blackwell Science.

Barer, B. M., & Johnson, C. J. (1990). A critique of the caregiving literature. *Gerontologist, 30*, 26–29.

Barusch, A. S., & Spaid, W. M. (1989). Gender differences in caregiving: Why do wives report greater burden? *Gerontologist, 29*(5), 667–676.

Braithwaite, V. (1996). Between stressors and outcomes: Can we simplify caregiving process variables? *Gerontologist, 36*, 42–53.

Brody, E. M. (1985). Parent care as a normative family stress. *Gerontologist, 25*, 19–29.

Connell, C. M., & Gibson, G. D. (1997). Racial, ethnic, and cultural differences in dementia caregiving: Review and analysis. *Gerontologist, 37*, 355–364.

Cox, C. (1995). Comparing the experiences of black and white caregivers of dementia patients. *Social Work, 44*, 343–349.

Davis, L. L. (1992). Building a science of caring for caregivers. *Family and Community Health, 15*(2), 1–9.

Farran, C. J., Keane-Hagerty, E., Salloway, S., Kupferer, S., & Wilkin, C. S. (1991). Finding meaning: An alternative paradigm for Alzheimer's disease family caregivers. *Gerontologist, 31*, 175–183.

Fisher, W. R. (1987). *Human communication as narration: Toward a philosophy of reason, value, and action*. Columbia: University of South Carolina Press.

Frank, A. W. (1995). *The wounded storyteller*. Chicago: University of Chicago Press.

Given, C., Given B., Stommel, M., Collins, C., King, S., & Franklin, S. (1992). The Caregiver Reaction Assessment for caregivers to persons with chronic physical and mental impairments. *Research in Nursing Health, 15*(4), 271–283.

Given, B. A., & Given, C. W. (1991). Family caregiving for the elderly. In J. J. Fitzpatrick, R. L. Taunton, & A. K. Jacox (Eds.), *Annual review of nursing research*. New York: Springer.

Haley, W., Levine, E., Brown, S., & Bartolucci, A. (1987). Stress, appraisal, coping, and social support as predictors of adaptational outcome among dementia caregivers. *Psychology and Aging, 2*, 323–330.

Hawkins, A. H. (1993). *Reconstructing illness: Studies in pathography*. West Lafayette, IN: Purdue University Press.

Hoenig, J., & Hamilton, M. (1966). Elderly psychiatric patients and the burden on the household. *Psychiatric Neurology (Basel), 152*(5), 281–294.

Hooker, K., Monahan, D. J., Bowman, S. R., Frazier, L. D., & Shifren, K. (1998). Personality counts for a lot: Predictors of mental and physical health of spouse caregivers in two disease groups. *Journals of Gerontology: Psychological Sciences, 2*, P73–P85.

Hunter, K. M. (1991). *Doctor's stories: The narrative structure of medical knowledge*. Princeton, NJ: Princeton University Press.

Kermode, F. (1981). Secrets and narrative sequence. In W. J. T. Mitchell (Ed.), *On narrative* (pp. 79–98). Chicago: University of Chicago Press.

Knafl, K. A., Breitmayer, B. J., Gallo, A. M., & Zoeller, L. H. (1996). Family response to childhood chronic illness: Description of management styles. *Journal of Pediatric Nursing, 11,* 315–326.

Knafl, K. A., & Deatrick, J. A. (1986). How families manage chronic conditions: An analysis of the concept of normalization. *Research in Nursing and Health, 9,* 215–222.

Knafl, K., Gallo, A., Breitmayer, B., Zoeller, L., & Ayres, L. (1993). One approach to conceptualizing family response to illness. In S. Feetham, J. Bell, S. Meister, & K. Gilliss (Eds.), *The cutting edge of family nursing* (Vol. 2). Newbury Park, CA: Sage.

Kuhlman, G. J., Wilson, H. S., Hutchinson, S. A., & Wallhagen, M. (1991). Alzheimer's disease and family caregiving: Critical synthesis of the literature and research agenda. *Nursing Research, 6,* 331–337.

Magai, C., & Cohen, C. I. (1998). Attachment style and emotional regulation in dementia patients and their relation to caregiver burden. *Journals of Gerontology: Psychological Sciences, 53B,* P147–P154.

Miller, B., & Cafasso, L. (1992). Gender differences in caregiving: Fact or artifact? *Gerontologist, 32,* 498–507.

Nolan, M. R., Grant, G., & Ellis, N. C. (1990). Stress is in the eye of the beholder: Reconceptualizing the measurement of caregiver burden. *Journal of Advanced Nursing, 15,* 544–555.

Patton, M. Q. (1990). *Qualitative evaluation and research methods.* Newbury Park, CA: Sage.

Phillips, L. R. (1986). *A clinician's guide to the critique and utilization of nursing research.* Norwalk, CT: Appleton-Century-Crofts.

Phillips, L. R., Morrison, E., Steffl, B., Young, M. C., Cromwell, S. L., & Russell, C. K. (1995). Effects of situational context and interactional process on the quality of family caregiving. *Research in Nursing and Health, 18,* 205–216.

Phillips, L. R., Rempusheski, V., & Morrison, E. (1989). Developing and testing the Beliefs about Caregiving Scale. *Research in Nursing and Health, 12,* 207–220.

Poirier, S., & Ayres, L. (1996). Endings, secrets, and silences: Overreading in narrative inquiry. *Research in Nursing and Health, 20,* 551–557.

Poirier, S., & Ayres, L. (2002). *Stories of family caregiving: Reconsiderations of theory, literature, and life.* Indianapolis, IN: Nursing Center Press.

Poirier, S., Rosenblum, L., Ayres, L., Brauner, D., Scharf, B., & Stanford, A. F. (1992). Charting the chart. *Journal of Literature and Medicine, 1,* 1–22.

Poulshock, S., & Deimling, G. (1984). Families caring for elders in residence: Issues in the measurement of burden. *Journal of Gerontology, 39,* 230–239.

Pruchno, R. A., Kleban, M. H., Michaels, J. E., & Dempsey, N. P. (1990). Mental and physical health of caregiving spouses: Development of a causal model. *Journal of Gerontology: Psychological Sciences, 45,* P192–P199.

Reason, P., & Rowan, J. (1981). *Human inquiry: A sourcebook of new paradigm research.* Chichester, NY: Wiley.

Richards, T., & Richards, L. (1995). Using hierarchical categories in qualitative data analysis. In U. Kelle (Ed.), *Computer aided qualitative data analysis* (pp. 81–95). Thousand Oaks, CA: Sage.

Sandelowski, M. (1999). Writing a good read: Strategies for re-presenting qualitative data. *Research in Nursing and Health, 21,* 375–382.

Schultz, R., O'Brien, A. T., Bookwala, J., & Fleissner, K. (1995). Psychiatric and physical morbidity effects of dementia caregiving: Prevalence, correlates, and causes. *Gerontologist, 35,* 771–791.

Silliman, R. A., & Sternberg, I. (1988). Family caregiving: Impact of patient functioning and underlying causes of dependency. *Gerontologist, 28,* 377–382.

Tesch, R. (1990). *Qualitative research.* New York: Falmer Press.

Thorne, S. (1985). The family cancer experience. *Cancer Nursing, 8, 285–291.*

Vitaliano, P. P., Young, H. M., & Russo, J. (1991). Burden: A review of measures used among caregivers of individuals with dementia. *Gerontologist, 31,* 67–75.

Walker, A. J., Pratt, C. C., & Eddy, L. (1995). Informal caregiving to family members: A critical review. *Family Relations, 44,* 402–411.

Walter, A. J., Acock, A. C., Bowman, S. R., & Li, F. (1996). Amount of care given and caregiving satisfaction: A latent growth curve analysis. *Journals of Gerontology: Psychological Sciences, 51B,* P130–142.

Young, R. F., & Kahana, E. (1995). The context of caregiving and well-being outcomes among African and Caucasian Americans. *Gerontologist, 35,* 225–232.

18

Action Research: The Methodologies

Ron Chenail, Sally St. George, and Dan Wulff

INTRODUCTION

Action research has a unique place among the many varieties of research methodologies. It is at once a type of formal academic methodology while also being a social enterprise that is, in various and significant ways, conducted by the people affected by the issues. Action research involves the joining of those who recognize and respond to a need for changes in life or work conditions through a systematic inquiry/praxis.

The democratic or participatory nature of action research (process) is coupled with its focus on action or change (outcome). The focal problem and the associated means utilized to make significant changes are integrated such that change is embedded within the steps/phases of the inquiry. The researchers/inquirers are those people intimately invested in the situation undergoing review and change. Action researchers are not dispassionate outsiders—they are insiders who are intent on reforming aspects of their world (Waterman, Tillen, Dickson, & de Koning, 2001).

The term *action research* has been used by many authors in differing ways. To illustrate this, in Reason and Bradbury's (2001) *Handbook of Action Research*, note a sampling of chapter titles: "participatory (action) research," "participatory research," "emancipatory action research," "pragmatic action research," "action science," "co-operative inquiry," "appreciative inquiry," "community action research," "action inquiry," "educational action research," "transpersonal co-operative inquiry," and "collaborative inquiry." Although these various terms describe characteristics of action research that have the potential to uniquely shape inquiries, they also inadvertently contribute to the confusion of classifying and labeling within the field of action research (Holter & Schwartz-Barcott, 1993). These terms may represent nuanced differences or may be different terms (reflective of personal preferences) used for the same idea or conceptualization. Thus, action research is not a single methodology but rather a family of research approaches, each in some way distinct from the others.

The family of action research methodologies has found a home in the field of nursing for a number of important reasons. Hart and Anthrop (1996) see action research as a professionalizing strategy as nursing seeks to achieve the status of a research-based profession, as a vehicle for developing reflective practitioners, and as a means for producing knowledge for practice. They also note that the humanistic qualities of these methodologies appeal to nurses who embrace action research as an emancipatory strategy and as a form of collaborative inquiry rooted in reflective practice. In addition, Robinson (1995) suggests that action research offers nurses the potential to develop transformative shifts in nursing culture. Many nursing researchers point to action research's potential to introduce innovation and facilitate change in practice and to generate and test theory relevant to their world of practice (Titchen & Binnie, 1993; Waterman, Webb, & Williams, 1995). Last, Walters and East (2001) suggest that action research approaches are appealing mainly because they allow nurse practitioners and researchers to work *with* and *for* (rather than on) patients.

The variety of professional areas in which nurses have employed the family of action research approaches to generate new knowledge and to produce new change is remarkable. These projects include research (1) defining the evolving nursing profession (e.g., Kelly, Simpson, & Brown, 2002; Walsgrove & Fulbrook, 2005); (2) connecting with communities to produce local change (Parsons & Warner-Robbins, 2002; Walters & East, 2001); (3) producing change in hospitals, clinics, and other practice locations (e.g., Reed, Pearson, Douglas, Swinburne, & Wilding, 2002; Staff of Mountbatten Ward, Wright, & Baker, 2005); (4) assessing and improving education and training (e.g., Chien, Chan, & Morrissey, 2002; Walker, Bailey, Brasell-Brian, & Gould, 2001); (5) improving practice based upon patients' insights and experiences (e.g., Lauri & Sainio, 1998; Olshansky et al., 2005); and (6) improving practice based upon nurses and other health care providers' feedback (e.g., Coetzee, Britton, & Clow, 2005; Mitchell, Conlon, Armstrong, & Ryan, 2005).

In this chapter, we discuss *action research (basic)*, *participatory action research*, and *appreciative inquiry*. These three varieties of action research are not the only types, but are selected for two reasons. First, as shown earlier, they possess utility for the advancement of the nursing profession and practices, and their usage reflects a large segment of the extant action research found in contemporary nursing research. Second, they allow us to show how specific methodologies within the family of action research approaches can vary along several key dimensions, specifically the *change/mobilization process, theoretical grounding, leadership, decision making, specific strategies*, and *beneficiaries*. It is also important to remember that even *within* each of the three approaches to action research discussed in this chapter there exists variation in how researchers concentrate on problems, improvements, or level of involvement as well as how experimental, organizational, professionalizing, and/or empowering a particular study may be (Hart & Bond, 1996).

THE FAMILY OF ACTION RESEARCH METHODOLOGIES

Action research (basic) is used to target and solve an identified dilemma or problem. Stringer (1999) states that action research (AR) enables "people (a) to investigate systematically their problems and issues, (b) to formulate powerful and sophisticated accounts of their situations, and (c) to devise plans to deal with the problems at hand" (p. 17). In AR, people adversely affected by some circumstance carefully examine the problem, form a picture of the problem, and develop actions designed to remediate or eliminate the problem. This whole process is referred to as AR.

As an illustration, some parents of children who attended an elementary school joined with the teachers and administrators of that school to employ AR to solve a child safety issue. The problem was that many children needed to cross a very busy and dangerous one-way thoroughfare to get to their school and then to return to their homes after school. These parents along with some school personnel met to discuss the problem and developed some strategies on how they could show city leaders the seriousness of the situation and enlist their help in altering the traffic pattern. The parents did their "homework" and made the case to the city council, and a traffic light was installed.

Participatory action research (PAR) is generally used to counteract oppressive conditions experienced by a particular segment of society (Schwandt,

2001). The PAR project is used to challenge the social customs and assumptions that keep those persons marginalized and oppressed. In an example of a PAR project, a group of mentally retarded adults joined with one of their residential caretakers to discuss the ways in which they were treated (Valade, 2004). Their discussions led to a consensus that the public transportation system provided by the city failed to meet their needs in many ways. The primary problem they were encountering was that the reservation system for the vans provided by the city was not dependable and these adults were completely dependent upon this transportation to attend their daily programs, medical appointments, and social outings. They approached this issue with the knowledge that they had little power to exact any change — they faced this issue with full awareness of the power differential and subsequent risk that speaking out might pose. In this study, the group invited the transportation company officials for a conversation that resulted in some policy changes. A byproduct of this project was that the group's level of confidence in taking a public stance grew through this experience. This, perhaps more than the procedural changes, was the most significant development resulting from this study.

Appreciative inquiry (AI) is generally used to join the members of an organization to make internal changes by focusing on what is already working. More elaborately, AI refers to both a search for knowledge and a theory of intentional collective action that are designed to help evolve the normative vision and will of a group, organization, or society as a whole. It is an inquiry process that affirms our symbolic choice and cultural evolution (Cooperrider & Srivastva, 2000, pp. 85–86). For example, one company was experiencing difficulties with numerous incidences of sexual harassment of female employees by some of the male employees. Numerous previous attempts to solve this problem had been unsuccessful. *Appreciative inquiry* was utilized to transform the issue from one of simply reducing or eradicating harassment events to inquiring into examples of good cross-gender relations within the organization and ways to build upon these positive events and interactions. The organization moved its thinking from trying to reduce some unwanted behaviors to reenvisioning what it could become (Cooperrider & Whitney, 1999).

WORKING INSIDE AND OUTSIDE OF TRADITIONAL QUALITATIVE PARAMETERS

AR is located within the qualitative research tradition because it is grounded in understanding specific and local phenomena in context, privileging the words/language used by participants, and proceeding thoroughly and systematically. Value is placed on the complexities of factors that contribute to real-world "messiness" of problems to promote increased understanding of the issues in need of change. The language of participants is privileged over researcher interpretations. Such interpretations are carefully acknowledged and explicitly connected to the words and descriptions offered by the participants. Staying so close to the data (the participants' words and ideas) helps to develop a more textured picture of the experiences and issues from which to generate new understandings and possible action steps (Waterman et al., 2001).

The research process is intentional, but at the same time is fluid. Although deliberate plans are made, there is receptivity to altering the method to suit the ongoing needs of the project and the participants. In the best qualitative tradition, action researchers are intent on attending to the current/local situation rather than creating generalizable findings. Finally, action researchers work systematically to conceptualize and understand the situation-of-interest and consistently to reflect upon the decisions made and the steps taken. A researcher practice of transparency, that is, explaining positions and research decisions, builds confidence in those who come to know the researchers' work.

Although AR is akin to qualitative methods in general, we have identified some procedures and processes in conducting AR that differ somewhat. One difference is that change is both the outcome and the process. Initiating the inquiry itself is an intervention that begins the change process. The act of studying something that is problematic by the people who experience the problem enhances the chances that people significantly invest in the effort to bring about change. Change is not constrained by a linear process of data collection, analysis, and final report of the study, but it is rather begun and continued throughout the steps/phases of the project (and beyond). A second difference is that there is a collectivity of persons involved in the inquiry process who all hold responsibility for the actions taken because they are the stakeholders and have voice in the decisions made about study procedures. At the same time the participants are the intended beneficiaries because the change that is effected will be to their advantage. A third major difference is that the methodology is more described by the process of change rather than the form of analysis employed (a wide range of analytical procedures, including quantified data and statistics, may be combined and used in AR). The fourth distinction is that AR is research carried out in public—this publicness builds relationships, both internally and externally. The steps or phases in the research context are public knowledge and made known as they occur—therefore, knowledge and action are revealed before the project is completed (Hope & Waterman, 2003).

PHASES OF ACTION RESEARCH

The phases of AR have similarities across the three types we discuss. Action researchers operate from the value base that there is a need for some change or correction to a problem or dilemma (Brown & Tandon, 1983). The process is mobilized by this problem and the search for a solution and/or difference. In addition, the process is cyclical with multiple iterations of the questions and the analysis of the data; as noted earlier, the common "result" is that change is activated by the introduction and beginning of the inquiry process itself.

There are also differences among the various action research methodologies. According to Brown and Tandon (1983), the differences are primarily located in (1) the values and ideologies of the inquiry, and (2) the political economy of the inquiry. The values are the "preferences for courses of action and outcomes" (p. 280), and the ideologies are the "sets of beliefs that explain the world, bind together their adherents, and suggest desirable activities and outcomes" (p. 280). The political economy of inquiry refers to questions such as: "What actors have interests in the decision? What authority and resources are relevant to the decision? How will decisions affect actor interests and distributions of authority and resources?" (p. 284).

We, too, think it is useful to illustrate commonalities and uniquenesses among AR, PAR, and AI. To do so we compare each using the following dimensions of inquiry that we have thematically derived from the literature and from our experiences of editing qualitative research. The dimensions are change/mobilization, theoretical orientation, leadership, decision making, methods/strategies, and beneficiaries (see Table 18–1).

Action Research (Basic)

Action research (basic) is initiated with a very practical problem within a context. For example, communication between different staff members in a hospital setting, workload issues, or specification of roles and tasks might be a problematic area that is in need of change to maximize efficiency and quality care as well as to improve the work environment for health workers (Holter & Schwartz-Barcott, 1993). Some personnel in this context would agree that these issues are interfering with the work and that a systematic proposal for change is warranted. In this case, an outside research consultant may be invited to help by working closely with each of the affected groups (e.g., floor nurses, administrators, supervisors) to develop actions "that are purposeful and aim at creating desired outcomes" (Greenwood & Levin, 2005). The guiding theory would be that of pragmatism (Greenwood &

TABLE 18–1 Comparisons and Contrast Among AR, PAR, and AI

Type	Change/ Mobilization Process	Theoretical Grounding	Leadership	Decision Making	Methods/Strategies	Beneficiaries
Action research (basic)	Using praxis to solve a specific problem while not threatening the existing structures of the system or organization	Pragmatism Consensus social theory	Usually an outsider assists the internal group working on the problem	Cooperation among the various groups involved	Quantitative and/or qualitative methods of data gathering and analysis	All parties affected by the problem
Participatory action research	To solve a problem of inequality or unfairness by challenging and changing oppressive practices/rules	Conflict theory Critical theory Marxism	Leadership usually arises from within the oppressed group	Cooperative and collaborative within the group seeking change, but conflictual with the larger organization or society	Quantitative and/or qualitative methods of data gathering and analysis Education	The group seeking change
Appreciative inquiry	To create change in an organization by using the momentum already present	Social constructionism	An external consultant is usually brought in to organize the work groups that represent a microcosm of the organization	Consultant enlists members of the organization to examine what the organization is doing well	Unconditional positive questioning (Ludema, Cooperrider, & Barrett, 2001) 4-D cycle: discovery, dream, design, destiny (Ludema, Cooperrider, & Barrett, 2001; Whitney & Trosten-Bloom, 2003)	All parties

Levin, 2005) and consensus social theory (Brown & Tandon, 1983). The consultant would facilitate the data collection and analysis of the data information. The data could be collected through a variety of means such as surveys and interviews and could be analyzed statistically and/or qualitatively. Based on the information gleaned, a solution will be developed that improves the conditions for those groups who were experiencing difficulty. It is important to note that such praxis is not intended to dramatically change the current rules or structure of operation—rather, it seeks to improve the functioning of the current overall system.

Walsgrove and Fulbrook's (2005) project, designed to develop the nurse practitioner role in an acute care hospital, exemplifies the usefulness of AR to improve care at a hospital by bringing affected parties together to increase awareness and to enact new strategies leading to change. At the advent of their study, Walsgrove and Fulbrook found there was a limited understanding of and minimal support for the development of the nurse practitioner role in an English hospital. To address this concern they combined practice development theory with four overlapping AR cycles to collect nurse practitioner practice information from hospital personnel by using questionnaires, semistructured interviews, meetings, and discussions as well as their own field notes. Their concurrent analysis of this stakeholder-provided information led to a grounded understanding of the nurse practitioner value from a knowledge perspective based on insiders' input, which led to greater support for nurse practitioners within the hospital system. This project illustrates how practice development (i.e., the role of nurse practitioners) and AR can be combined in a systematic process to not only develop and support professional roles of nurses, but also to improve the quality of patient care and the effectiveness of health care services.

Participatory Action Research (PAR)

The goal of engaging in PAR, like action research (basic), is practical change. However, there is the additional objective of changing the larger rules and structures that keep the problem in place. Coming from traditions of conflict theory, critical theory, and Marxism, PAR is a "social and education process [in which] the 'subjects' of participatory action research undertake their research as social practice [and] the 'object' of participatory action research is social" (Kemmis & McTaggart, 2005, p. 563).

In the nursing context, hierarchies that determine work conditions, salaries, or status may pose problems that go beyond the "problem–solution" remedies of AR. The issue may center on basic inequalities, marginalization, or oppression of groups that have become part of the status quo in the organization or profession-at-large. PAR is used to challenge those basic inequities, even if such efforts would bring conflict with those groups in power. PAR serves the mission of changing the status quo for the benefit of the oppressed group (Kelly, 2005). According to Kemmis and McTaggart (2005),

> At its best, then, participatory action research is a social process of collaborative learning realized by groups of people who join together in changing the practices through which they interact in a shared social world in which, for better or worse, we live with the consequences of one another's actions. (p. 563)

PAR is characterized by the collaboration with which projects are planned and conducted. The whole group decides the best ways to gather information and to make sense of it. The entire process is marked by demystification (as all work is made transparent) as well as reflection in which each research decision and interpretation is subjected to a critical review for increased understanding (Patton, 2002).

When faced with a professional development challenge after problems arose regarding the moving and handling of patients in a British stroke unit, Mitchell and colleagues (2005), instead of relying on traditional top-down training from unit management, used PAR to facilitate the nurses taking ownership of their moving and handling practices. The researchers accomplished this goal by providing a context in which nurses could share their insights and real-world experiences in moving and handling patients following stroke, identifying facilitators of safer moving and handling practice, and empowering themselves in collaboration with physiotherapists to direct changes in their practice. Mitchell and colleagues' insider PAR approach featured data generated from focus group meetings, brainstorming sessions, observational studies, and from written reflective accounts, which led nurses to identify equipment, environment, communication, and teamwork strategies that would facilitate their use of rehabilitative moving and handling practices. Besides producing this new knowledge and practice wisdom about moving and handling stroke patients, the PAR project helped its participants to feel a greater degree of involvement and value along with improved teamwork.

Appreciative Inquiry (AI)

AI fits into the AR family because of its focus on change. However, although what is problematic is acknowledged, the focus of change begins with what is already going well (no matter how small) toward the desired change. Operating from a social constructionist stance, AI begins with an affirmative topic choice. The objective is to have people talk about those issues that describe the "life-giving" forces and practices that those involved would like to have in place (Cooperrider, Whitney, & Stavros, 2003). For example, if in nursing, communication patterns or interactions among personnel were expressed as problematic areas in the workplace, the AI researcher would begin to focus on incidents, behaviors, conditions, and times that communication patterns and respectful interaction were already occurring, regardless of how infrequent or seemingly insignificant (Keefe & Pesut, 2004). AI researchers proceed through the 4-D cycle in which members of the organization answer four questions. The first question is "What gives life?" This is called the discovery phase. Second, the members of the organization are asked to enter the dream phase by considering the question, "What might be?" This is followed with the question, "How can it be?" which is identified as the design phase. The process concludes with the destiny phase in which the question, "What will be?" is posed (Ludema, Cooperrider, & Barrett, 2001; Whitney & Trosten-Bloom, 2003).

In conducting AI, a consultant enlists a variety of the members creating a microcosm in the organization wanting change to decide what data to collect and the best ways to collect them (Cooperrider et al., 2003). The inclusion of many participants who are talking with each other about successful events begins the change process (creating greater understanding and possibilities for action) and ensures investment in both the method and information obtained.

At a U.S. college of nursing, Farrell, Douglas, and Siltanen (2003) used AI to explore and develop the college's community of interest and to create a collective and shared vision of excellence. To accomplish this goal, they collected data from inside and outside stakeholders through one-on-one interviews and focus groups and analyzed the data using quantitative and qualitative methods. Their findings suggested that the community shared values of preserving the college's past and of its vision for the college's future, but the participants also differed in the means of putting this newly cocreated vision into practice. Their study also helps to show that AI, like other forms of AR, can produce new questions and can help the organization identify challenges heretofore unknown or invisible to the organization itself.

EVALUATING ACTION RESEARCH

Evaluating AR must include assessing the degree of success in achieving the twin purposes of AR methodologies, which are to stimulate change and to involve stakeholders in the process of change. Both are vital, so no rank order of the two is possible. Achieving set goals without maintaining the participatory nature diminishes AR's success; maintaining participation but not reaching the goals of the effort is similarly discouraging (Livesey & Challender, 2002).

Another criterion by which to evaluate AR is the occurrence of unexpected positive events or outcomes. These serendipitous events add to the overall value of the AR effort, even though they cannot be fully anticipated.

These occurrences are likely a result of the fact that action researchers are setting constructive processes into motion and their outcomes cannot be wholly predicted (e.g., Farrell et al., 2003).

Having stated earlier the importance of achieving outcomes along with developing and maintaining participation, some believe that the participatory nature of AR can stimulate persons to generate additional efforts for future projects that add to the value/importance of the current AR project. Particularly with PAR, the development of confidence in producing change can transform individuals and groups into activists who may develop new change programs (e.g., Lindsey & McGuinness, 1998).

Action researchers who see their work as primarily affecting change in their local setting may not develop scholarly works from the research, seeing such products as tangential to the committed focus of their work. But making the project known (in some form) is inevitable because of the multiple persons involved in the project itself and the performance of the research in the natural setting, whether it be a school, a hospital, or the community-at-large.

In addition to this presentation "as you go," making clear the process and the results of the project is important. Included in these decisions would be the intended audience and the form of presentation. To an academic audience, written scholarly works or presentations as professional conferences/meetings would be necessary. To lay audiences, brochures or informal discussions/presentations may well suffice. To politicians or other policymakers, information from the project regarding potential impact on certain groups or identifying financial resources required to affect specific changes may be necessary for decisions to be made.

The issue of theory generation that is a component of most research efforts is also an issue within the field of AR. Greenwood and Levin (2005) see AR as a "disciplined way of developing valid knowledge and theory while promoting positive social change" (p. 55), whereas Cooperrider and Srivastva (2000) ask, "Why is there this lack of generative theorizing in action-research?" (p. 76). The role or importance of generating useful knowledge and theory is widely supported, but the degree to which AR lives up to this goal is debated (Badger, 2000).

CHALLENGES

In our effort in this chapter to delineate a set of AR methodologies, we have drawn distinctions and highlighted commonalities. This is done for the purpose of reviewing the large contours of the field of AR. The blending of research and action poses some challenging questions regarding whether research/inquiry can or should be so intimately connected with action. What is taught about scientific rigor would have us see such connections with action steps to be a source of contamination, while others lament the current lack of usefulness of research that is compartmentalized from implementation (Rolfe, 1996).

Besides concerns regarding the scientific validity as raised earlier, AR presents other significant hurdles. Along these lines Coghlan and Casey (2001) highlight the management challenges for nurses when conducting AR in their own professional settings. For example nurse researchers often need to combine their AR role with their regular organizational roles, and this role duality can create the potential for role ambiguity and conflict. Williamson and Prosser (2002) argue that because AR approaches rely on a close collaborative working relationship between researcher and participants, this close relationship can also be the source of political and ethical problems for the researchers and participants. They suggest that these close relationships can jeopardize some of the usual ethical guarantees concerning confidentiality and anonymity, informed consent, and protection from harm that might not arise with the use of quantitative and other qualitative methodologies. Both Coghlan and Casey (2001) and Williamson and Prosser (2002) underscore the importance for nursing action researchers to be aware of the political conditions of their respective organizations and to be prepared to manage the political and ethical dynamics as they inevitably arise through the course of an AR project.

Despite these challenges practitioners and researchers alike find AR particularly appealing and useful given the synchronicity between the practices/procedures of AR and the practices/procedures of practitioners. One could use the steps or phases of AR to outline the essential components of competent practice or to develop new policy and procedures.

In our work reviewing and editing AR projects from around the world for many years, we are heartened by the creativity and willingness to experiment with AR, often stretching the parameters of what we have come to understand as "legitimate" or "true" AR. With the growing variety within this family of methodologies, AR continues to present nursing with a vehicle to explore many interesting questions and to suggest new and generative ways of thinking about how to positively impact our worlds.

REFERENCES

Badger, T. G. (2000). Action research, change and methodological rigour. *Journal of Nursing Management*, 8(4), 201–207.

Brown, L. D., & Tandon, R. (1983). Ideology and political economy in inquiry: Action research and participatory research. *Journal of Applied Behavioral Science*, 19(3), 277–294.

Chien, W. T., Chan, S. W., & Morrissey, J. (2002). The use of learning contracts in mental health nursing clinical placement: An action research. *International Journal of Nursing Studies, 39*(7), 685–694.

Coetzee, M., Britton, M., & Clow, S. E. (2005). Finding the voice of clinical experience: Participatory action research with registered nurses in developing a child critical care nursing curriculum. *Intensive and Critical Care Nursing, 21*(2), 110–118.

Coghlan, D., & Casey, M. (2001). Action research from the inside: Issues and challenges in doing action research in your own hospital. *Journal of Advanced Nursing, 35*(5), 674–682.

Cooperrider, D. L., & Srivastva, S. (2000). Appreciative inquiry in organizational life. In D. L. Cooperrider, P. F. Sorensen, Jr., D. Whitney, & T. F. Yeager (Eds.), *Appreciative inquiry: Rethinking human organization toward a positive theory of change* (pp. 55–97). Champaign, IL: Stipes.

Cooperrider, D. L., & Whitney, D. (1999). *Appreciative inquiry.* San Francisco: Berrett-Koehler.

Cooperrider, D. L., Whitney, D., & Stavros, J. M. (2003). *Appreciative inquiry handbook: The first in a series of AI workbooks for leaders of change.* Bedford Heights, OH: Lakeshore Communications.

Farrell, M., Douglas, D., & Siltanen, S. (2003). Exploring and developing a college's community of interest: An appreciative inquiry. *Journal of Professional Nursing, 19*(6), 364–371.

Greenwood, D. J., & Levin, M. (2005). Reform of the social sciences and of universities through action research. In N. K. Denzin & Y. S. Lincoln (Eds.), *The Sage handbook of qualitative research* (3rd ed., pp. 43–64). Thousand Oaks, CA: Sage.

Hart, E., & Anthrop, C. (1996). Action research as a professionalizing strategy: Issues and dilemmas. *Journal of Advanced Nursing, 23*(3), 454–461.

Hart, E., & Bond, M. (1996). Making sense of action research through the use of a typology. *Journal of Advanced Nursing, 23*(1), 152–159.

Holter, I. M., & Schwartz-Barcott, D. (1993). Action research: What is it? How has it been used and how can it be used in nursing? *Journal of Advanced Nursing, 18*(2), 298–304.

Hope, K. W., & Waterman, H. A. (2003). Praiseworthy pragmatism? Validity and action research. *Journal of Advanced Nursing, 44*(2), 120–127.

Keefe, M. R., & Pesut, D. (2004). Appreciative inquiry and leadership transitions. *Journal of Professional Nursing, 20*(2), 103–109.

Kelly, D., Simpson, S., & Brown, P. (2002). An action research project to evaluate the clinical practice facilitator role for junior nurses in an acute hospital setting. *Journal of Clinical Nursing, 11*(1), 90–98.

Kelly, P. J. (2005). Practical suggestions for community interventions using participatory action research. *Public Health Nursing, 22*(1), 65–73.

Kemmis, S., & McTaggart, R. (2005). Participatory action research: Communicative action in the public sphere. In N. K. Denzin & Y. S. Lincoln (Eds.), *The Sage handbook of qualitative research* (3rd ed., pp. 559–603). Thousand Oaks, CA: Sage.

Lauri, S., & Sainio, C. (1998). Developing the nursing care of breast cancer patients: An action research approach. *Journal of Clinical Nursing, 7*(5), 424–432.

Lindsey, E., & McGuinness, L. (1998). Significant elements of community involvement in participatory action research: Evidence from a community project. *Journal of Advanced Nursing, 28*(5), 1106–1114.

Livesey, H., & Challender, S. (2002). Supporting organizational learning: A comparative approach to evaluation in action research. *Journal of Nursing Management, 10*(3), 167–176.

Ludema, J. D., Cooperrider, D. L., & Barrett, F. J. (2001). Appreciative inquiry: The power of the unconditional positive question. In P. Reason & H. Bradbury (Eds.), *Handbook of action research: Participative inquiry and practice* (pp. 189–199). London: Sage.

Mitchell, E. A., Conlon, A.-M., Armstrong, M., & Ryan, A. A. (2005). Towards rehabilitative handling in caring for patients following stroke: A participatory action research project. *Journal of Clinical Nursing, 14*, 3–12.

Olshansky, E., Sacco, D., Braxter, B., Dodge, P., Hughes, E., Ondeck, M., Stubbs, M. L., & Upvall, M. J. (2005). Participatory action research to understand and reduce health disparities. *Nursing Outlook, 53*(3), 121–126.

Parsons, M. L., & Warner-Robbins, C. (2002). Formerly incarcerated women create healthy lives through participatory action research. *Holistic Nursing Practice, 16*(2), 40–49.

Patton, M. Q. (2002). *Qualitative research and evaluation methods* (3rd ed.). Thousand Oaks, CA: Sage.

Reason, P., & Bradbury, H. (Eds.). (2001). *Handbook of action research: Participative inquiry and practice.* London: Sage.

Reed, J., Pearson, P., Douglas, B., Swinburne, S., & Wilding, H. (2002). Going home from hospital: An appreciative inquiry study. *Health and Social Care and the Community, 10*, 36–45.

Robinson, A. (1995). Transformative 'cultural shifts' in nursing: Participatory action research and the 'project of possibility.' *Nursing Inquiry, 2*(2), 65–74.

Rolfe, G. (1996). Going to extremes: Action research, grounded practice and the theory-practice gap in nursing. *Journal of Advanced Nursing, 24*(6), 1315–1320.

Schwandt, T. A. (2001). *Dictionary of qualitative inquiry* (2nd ed.). Thousand Oaks, CA: Sage.

Staff of Mountbatten Ward, Wright, M., & Baker, A. (2005). The effects of appreciative inquiry interviews on staff in the U.K. National Health Service. *International Journal of Health Care Quality Assurance, 18*(1), 41–61.

Stringer, E. T. (1999). *Action research* (2nd ed.). Thousand Oaks, CA: Sage.

Titchen, A., & Binnie, A. (1993). Research partnerships: Collaborative action research in nursing. *Journal of Advanced Nursing, 18*(6), 858–865.

Valade, R. (2004). *Participatory action research with adults with mental retardation: "Oh my God. Look out world."* (AAT 3134205). Retrieved August 27, 2005, from http://www.lib.umi.com/dissertations, ProQuest Dissertations and Theses database.

Walker, J., Bailey, S., Brasell-Brian, R., & Gould, S. (2001). Evaluating a problem based learning course: An action research study. *Contemporary Nurse, 10*(1–2), 30–38.

Walsgrove, H., & Fulbrook, P. (2005). Advancing the clinical perspective: A practice development project to develop the nurse practitioner role in an acute hospital trust. *Journal of Clinical Nursing, 14*(4), 444–455.

Walters, S., & East, L. (2001). The cycle of homelessness in the lives of young mothers: The diagnostic phase of an action research project. *Journal of Clinical Nursing, 10*(2), 171–179.

Waterman, H., Tillen, D., Dickson, R., & de Koning, K. (2001). Action research: A systematic review and guidance for assessment. *Health Technology Assessment, 5*(23). Retrieved August 25, 2005, from http://www.ncchta.org/execsumm/summ523.htm.

Waterman, H., Webb, C., & Williams, A. (1995). Parallels and contradictions in the theory and practice of action research and nursing. *Journal of Advanced Nursing, 22*(4), 779–784.

Whitney, D., & Trosten-Bloom, A. (2003). *The power of appreciative inquiry: A practical guide to positive change.* San Francisco, CA: Berrett-Koehler.

Williamson, G. R., & Prosser, S. (2002). Action research: Politics, ethics and participation. *Journal of Advanced Nursing, 40*(5), 587–593.

19

Exemplar: Practical Discourse as Action Research: Inquiry into Post-Myocardial Behavioral Coaching

Edward M. Freeman

INTRODUCTION

This chapter presents action research as a method of inquiry that liberates the prescribing subject (clinician) from the partnered "patient." Liberation may be conceived in both a *limited* and *expanded* view.

On the one hand, a limited view of liberation can be conceived as removing or disentangling the two participants—clinician and partnered patient—from the interaction. Thus, the limited view of liberation purges the subject and partner of distorted meanings that the clinician and "patient" bring to the interactions. However, after the manner of Habermas (1988), liberation is not defined as reducing distorted meanings in communication between clinician and patient. Liberation, so defined by the limited view, tries to remove distorted meanings, but has disengaged clinicians from their real enterprise in encounters with patients. Instead, an expanded view of liberation turns both clinician and patient into reflective partners.

Reflective partners are engaged in communicative feedback so that shared meanings are evoked and discussed inside a clinical encounter. Such communicative feedback minimizes subtle harm that may befall patients as a result of curtailing self-determination and reducing the "patient's" input in clinical decisions.

It is necessary to identify ways to talk about caregivers and recipients of care, not to remove distorted meanings, but to level the playing field between caregiver and recipients of care. Therefore, this chapter identifies the provider of care and participant of care by name or title because multiple meanings have contributed to confusion about some words, such as *clinician* and *patient*, and narrative is favored over "white-coat" language. Therefore, the clinician who provides care is called *nurse practitioner* or *NP*, and the recipient of care is called by his first name.

GOALS OF INQUIRY

The first goal of inquiry in this chapter is to present a case study that exemplifies action research. The case study involves a middle-aged man, named Hal, who recently experienced a heart attack. After initial hospitalization and stabilization of his coronary arteries and heart muscle, Hal experiences problems with returning to work. He turns to an NP for care.

The second goal of inquiry is to discuss the applications of multiple concepts derived from a German philosopher named Habermas. Particular emphasis is focused on concepts of practical discourse, moral intuition, an expanded view of liberation, intersubjectivity, and ideal roles. Each concept is defined in the discussion and applied to the case. Narrative segments, also called dialogue clips, are dispersed throughout the text so that a feedback loop vis-à-vis action research occurs immediately following each clip.

A third and final goal is to influence deliberative action by and among action researchers. Because the method of reflection upon action research employed herein is philosophical in nature, the goal is to stimulate debate concerning these philosophical concepts and to search for expanded ways to debate action research in light of insights derived from Habermas. The goal of influencing others to adopt a philosophical method for action research is the subject of the final part of the chapter.

DEFINITION OF ACTION RESEARCH FOR USE IN THIS CHAPTER

Elsewhere in this volume, comprehensive definitions of action research have been presented. For the purposes of this chapter, action research ". . . is an intentional, systematic method of inquiry used by a group of practitioner-researchers who reflect and act on the real-life problems encountered in their own practice" (Ziegler, 1996). Key elements of this definition include the intentionality of action research, which is to say that there are goals or aims to action research that might not be associated with other qualitative designs, such as grounded theory. In addition, the definition associates practitioners with their practices and keeps inquiry in actual practice situations. The case study of this chapter illustrates each of these points in Ziegler's definition. Certain assumptions underscore Ziegler's definition. Three assumptions include (1) practice is the foundation for action research; (2) researchers are partnered with their "subjects"; and (3) action research necessitates the application of a system to inquiry.

ACTION RESEARCH EXEMPLAR

A 58-year-old man named Hal experienced a heart attack 4 weeks ago. By his own admission, he had been in good health most of his life except for the occasional colds and flu. Hal tells the NP that everything just "fell apart" after his heart attack. Inquiry into the meaning of "fell apart" uncovered important questions that were on Hal's mind.

Questions centered on what the future might bring. Father of three adult children and husband of Susan, to whom he has been married 32 years, Hal felt anxious that his resources would not sustain more time off from work. He took 3 weeks sick time immediately after the heart attack, but fatigue and depression after the heart attack sapped his energy, making return to work a daily grind.

Hal reported his fatigue and depression to his primary care physician 3 weeks after the heart attack. The physician diagnosed situational depression and directed Hal to begin treatment with an antidepressant called paroxetine (Paxil). Hal started taking Paxil at a dose of 10 mg every day and returned to the physician 2 weeks later. The fatigue and depression were not improved, and the physician asked Hal to double the dose of Paxil.

Back when the heart attack happened, the cardiologist identified an elevated level of total cholesterol and low-density lipoprotein, which prompted the cardiologist to prescribe a low-cholesterol diet and a statin-type anticholesterol medication called atorvastatin (Lipitor). The cardiologist discussed side effects, untoward effects, and intended therapeutic effects of Lipitor with Hal when he prescribed Lipitor. Hal expressed concerns about Lipitor, but knew that he never wanted to go through a heart attack again and believed the cardiologist when the cardiologist said that Lipitor might help prevent cholesterol buildup in his coronary arteries. Hal and the cardiologist did not discuss Hal's concerns at the time.

Immediately after the heart attack, in addition to Lipitor, the cardiologist directed Hal to start taking clopidogrel (Plavix) and aspirin. In combination with two stents that another cardiologist placed in Hal's coronary arteries after the heart attack, Plavix and aspirin were intended to keep the blood platelets from sticking to the walls of the arteries and thereby prevent clots from attaching to the arteries.

Therefore, a month after the heart attack, Hal was taking not one but four new medications. Previous to the heart attack, Hal took only a multivitamin once per day, if he remembered to do so. According to the primary care physician and cardiologist, Hal must continue taking Lipitor, Plavix, and aspirin for the rest of his life. Hal tells the NP that "the rest of his life" could mean that he must take medications for 40 years, which is "an eternity."

Hal complains that four new medications have diminished his quality of life, making him feel crippled not only by the heart attack but also by the pill burden of four pills. Pill burden is an interpretive outcome of chronic disease that is treated by conventional Western medicine, which often adds medications to a treatment plan. It is common and well documented that persons living with chronic disease interpret pills as burdensome to them in terms of remembering to take (Clay, 2004), cost of the medications (Cahn, 2003; Hussey, Hardin, & Blanchette, 2002; Parish, 2004), limitations created by side effects (Cahn, 2003; Dyck, Deschamps, & Taylor, 2005; McCarter-Bayer, Bayer, & Hall, 2005), monitoring laboratory tests (Medvedeff, 2003), and being reminded by the pills that the illness is ever present and might possibly become worse (Bowers, 2004). Bowers (2004) offers the view that younger women after heart attack must learn to live with the fear of matters becoming worse along with challenges to their self-image and psychosocial development.

The Trouble with a Medical Plan: The Subject Plays Expert and the Object Must Receive

There is trouble in implementing a medical plan. Assuming that a medical plan must start with a combination of expert judgment and consensual decision making, problems arise when expert judgment supercedes consensual discourse.

One notes that Hal's medical plan promises recovery and stabilization based upon expert medical judgment, but Hal's adaptation to the plan hangs in the balance between regrets over how he might have better cared for himself in the past and hopelessness concerning the future. Professional encounters with cardiologists and the primary care physician gave Hal the expert medical judgment that contributed to recovery and stabilization of cardiac disease. But these encounters and resulting expert judgment played only a part in Hal's recovery and stabilization.

The encounter with the NP occurs after expert medical judgment and resulting recommendations are established, and Hal has returned to work full time. Full-time work for Hal means that coworkers have assumed some of his tasks temporarily, which Hal admits contributes to his guilt feelings. But Hal's energy level will not support performance of some tasks. Others now perform what he could do in half the time prior to the heart attack because they must learn the routine.

Not only is Hal anticipating 40 years of pill burden, but also he regrets the weight he accumulated on his waist after reaching middle age. He regrets reducing his activity level 10 years ago and not curtailing poor nutritional choices. The medical plan might become assimilated into Hal's life in the future, but, for now, the plan reminds Hal of everything that he did wrong. He recites his regrets internally and foresees further decline in health as age increases.

The NP must identify how to help Hal liberate himself from regrets and hopelessness, which is his state of mind after the heart attack. Part of the liberation is to integrate the heart attack and changes resulting from the same into Hal's life through discourse. The process of discourse creates shared ethical space between Hal and the NP, thus arguably balancing expert medical judgment and shared decision making with Hal.

Ethical space is conceived as a discursive method and mode of communication, whereby the practitioner and Hal engage in free and equal dialogue about Hal's overall health and treatment plan. Ethical space, so conceived, is practical in the sense of practical discourse employed by Habermas (1990).

First, let us set the stage of practical discourse by briefly treating Habermas's position. Habermas portrays practical discourse as a "communicative process *simultaneously* exhorting *all* participants to ideal role taking" (1990, p. 198). Simultaneity in participation is defined as an act of communication that occurs between or among participants without the benefits afforded one or the other by planning. Without the benefit of a plan, each meets the other in a shared or simultaneous moment in time. The lack of a plan equalizes the practical discourse, thereby freeing discourse from a lopsided expertise attributed to some clinicians in white coats. Elsewhere in this text, simultaneity has been identified with serendipity, whereby "action researchers are setting constructive processes into motion and their outcomes cannot be wholly predicted" (see Chapter 18).

Second, application to Hal's experience, first with medical treatment and later with his responses of regrets and hopelessness, calls for more information about what happens next in the encounter with the NP.

After the Medical Plan: Achieving Practical Discourse with Hal

The NP and Hal began discourse after a medical plan was established. Initiating practical discourse after implementing a medical plan is not ideal in terms of Hal's adaptation to components of the plan, but practical discourse as Habermas presents it seldom occurs in the days immediately following a heart attack. Right after a heart attack, physicians apply medical expertise to *keeping the organism alive,* which is a phrase, reminiscent of Maslow's hierarchy of needs, intentionally used to distinguish the objectivity of the medical plan from the subjectivity of practical discourse.

The subjective sense that Hal brings to the first encounter with the NP is far different from whether he adheres to the medical plan as prescribed by the physicians. Again, there are reasons that Hal feels regrets and hopelessness, and until these reasons are identified in practical discourse, the outcome of the medical plan hangs in the balance. It was Hal's resolve to do what the doctors told him right after the heart attack, but time passed. Will Hal keep doing what he was told? Indeed, a month after the heart attack, Hal felt remorse over not having cared well for himself, which might have contributed to the heart attack, and hopeless over a future of pill burden by following the medical plan.

A first step for the NP is to engage Hal in discussion about the changes in his life and ask Hal about the medical plan first enacted following the heart attack. By asking Hal about the medical plan, the NP hopes to remove the barriers to communication and full participation, which might have been created when the plan was first implemented in the moment of crisis following the heart attack. Hoping to remove the barriers to communication, the NP builds the intention *with Hal* that the goals of therapy are mutually derived in discourse. Therefore, the NP asks Hal open-ended questions with no purpose other than to be attentive to communication in the moment of discourse.

Attentiveness to communication in the moment of discourse further clarifies what Habermas suggested in the previous quote. Namely, Habermas (1990) calls for practical discourse that exhorts "*all* participants to ideal role taking" (p. 198). Ideal role taking is a public affair, which is to say that subjective roles, such as Hal's and the NP's roles, are enacted in the discourse in a way that is public or transparent to both of them. They see themselves in the discourse as subjects who create the story(ies) of Hal's responses to his heart attack. If both the NP and Hal create stories of Hal's responses, then both have a stake in the outcomes of the stories.

Identifying Hal's responses as stories underscores the narrative nature of inquiry that the NP and Hal share. Together they narrate arguments favoring components of the plan that they create. Of course, the two will not always agree on the merits of arguments, nor should they agree because that is the nature of free and unrestricted inquiry, which is the very foundation of Hal's recovery from this point forward and cements the bond of action inquiry between Hal and the NP. The NP must bring nursing and medical expertise to employ an "ideal role," and, for Hal to play an ideal role, he must express his knowledge, opinions, and preferences. Together, Hal and the NP stand a chance of creating a balanced plan for recovery after the heart attack.

Creating a Balanced Plan for Recovery: Hal in the Months That Follow after Practical Discourse Has Begun

Action research searches for solutions to problems. Hal brings the problems of regrets and hopelessness to the initial contact with the NP a month after his heart attack. The NP agrees with Hal, during their first encounter, that regrets and hopelessness can lead to problems later on. That is why the NP asks, "How is it going with taking the medications that the doctors have prescribed?"

Hal answers that he cannot see himself taking "pills for the rest of my life." The practitioner responds, "The rest of your life is a long time." The practical discourse continues:

Hal:	*You're right about that. I never used to take pills.*
NP:	*Taking pills cannot be the focus of the day; otherwise, taking pills might be the only thing that you do each day or at least the only thing that you think about.*
Hal:	*Yeah. I want to think about something other than being sick.*
NP:	*You're thinking that taking pills makes you think that you're sick.*
Hal:	*Don't you think that everybody thinks about being sick when they take pills?*
NP:	*Yes, I think that some people believe that they're sick when they take pills.*
Hal:	*(Silence for several seconds . . . then . . .) I guess that's what I think. I am sick and I am not going to get back to where I used to be . . . (voice trails off)*

Several elements of practical discourse are identifiable in the preceding dialogue. First, an overall theme of searching for a solution to the problem of pill burden is apparent in the dialogue. The NP begins the dialogue with an open-ended question, but the question is really not the beginning of this discourse because Hal and the NP have already established that regrets and hopelessness are problems that require their shared attention. Instead, the question is an implied argument, bearing in mind the NP's expertise in nursing and medicine. The implied argument is that Hal's regrets and hopelessness are connected with changes added to Hal's daily life created by taking medications. An implied argument provides direction to the discourse, performing what Habermas (1990) calls the "cooperative search for truth" (p. 198). Cooperation is apparent in Hal's response to "The rest of your life is a long time." Hal agrees with the argument, thus confirming a common base, and adding that the past did not involve taking medications.

A second example of argumentation follows when the NP asserts that taking medication should not become the focus of living. Hal brings his opinion to the argument by saying that taking medication is an expression of being sick. Two ideas are implied in the NP's response. First, in the vein of action research, the NP portrays an ideal role, which is practitioner expertise, by distinguishing taking medication from the sick role. Second, also in line with action research, Hal and the NP honestly disagree, which is evidence that they test their ideas with one another.

What follows provides evidence that Hal and the NP do not agree. Tersely stated, Hal questions whether it is not common knowledge that everyone who must take medications daily is not sick. Hal's question might rebuff either a novice or one who does not agree with or conceive practical discourse in the way of Habermas. However, because the NP believes that the discourse is public, and that together they create the story of recovery, it is possible to make an important distinction in response. The distinction to be made is that not *all* people who take medications think of themselves as sick.

The NP's response draws Hal into thoughtful silence. Hal clarifies his point of view. Maybe it was not that all people who take medications think of themselves as sick, but as long as Hal takes medications, he cannot get back to where he used to be.

The practical discourse between the NP and Hal continues:

NP: *Where you used to be must have been better than where you think [emphasis] that you are now.*

Hal: *Huh? That's too complicated for me. I don't know what's better. You've gotta play the cards you're dealt.*

NP: *I agree that there are some things you just cannot change. I'd like to talk about what we can change together.*

Hal: *Like what?*

NP:	*Like your pills. You're taking Lipitor, for example. Right now you're taking 20 mg. Maybe with tweaking your diet and adding some exercise, you can drop some pounds and reduce the Lipitor dose over time. Who knows? Maybe you'll get your cholesterol problem under control.*
Hal:	*You're telling me that I might come off Lipitor one day?*
NP:	*I don't see the future. I think about others like you. Maybe you can think about the possibility of stopping Lipitor as one way of sticking to a low-fat diet.*

Several themes repeat themselves in this dialogue clip, such as argumentation, disputes in points of view, and the intersubjectivity of discourse. In reference to the intersubjectivity of discourse, which is a point not well developed in this chapter thus far, Hal and the NP fail to understand one another as but one example. The NP emphasizes "you think," which complicates the sentence structure, especially in many clinical settings where there are time constraints.

By intersubjectivity we refer to the collective way that language exchanges meaning. Most important to intersubjectivity is how well the lack of clarity, or admitted lack of clarity on the NP's part, distinguishes one subject from the other in the dialogue clip. Hal tells the NP that the first statement is too complicated, thus leading him to posit a fatalistic view that he holds about himself. The NP's tenor in discourse is hopefulness, but not so Hal's. Hal uses the metaphor of a game of chance to distinguish himself and his point of view from the NP's.

A second example of intersubjectivity emerges and would seem to disentangle the NP from the expert's hopefulness toward the future. In the last line of the clip, the NP replies to Hal, "I don't see the future." Further exploration of the last NP response underscores an attitude inherent in action research that Habermas captures in the term *"moral intuitions."*

Moral intuitions for Habermas (1990) are insights that make us adapt our behaviors to perceived vulnerabilities in others. For example, the NP might perceive that Hal is vulnerable in reference to his fatalistic view about his health after a heart attack. Hal's point of view toward his future is fragile, just as his "sick" self could break apart with changes in behavior after the heart attack. The "sick" self is constructed by Hal and his caregivers, which could lead to reconstructions of the self or even deconstructions as time and circumstances demand. Here we suggest that the NP behaves as if an intuition came in reference to predicting the future. Instead of the NP arguing the point about whether the future could be bright or not, the NP admits that the future is unknown and that it is possible that Lipitor could be reduced or, even, canceled. According to the view of moral intuition, the NP turns the tables on future outcomes, possibly motivating Hal to lose weight. And weight reduction is the point, not what the future might hold. If Hal were to lose weight and keep it off, he might need to deconstruct his "sick" self with the assistance of the NP.

The moral intuition about Hal is a critical moment in this action research dialogue clip. It is the NP who admits that the future is fuzzy, thus exposing mutual vulnerability and connectedness with Hal. Not only is the future uncertain for Hal but for the NP, as well. Such action in the moral intuition directs the dialogue to further conditions that could return control to Hal and reestablish that former sense of self that Hal claims to have lost. The NP suggests: *"Maybe you can think about the possibility of stopping Lipitor as one way of sticking to a low-fat diet."* Could Hal write a new chapter in his life?

A New Story Emerges: Hal Asks for Help

Consider a paraphrase of one of three questions that Nussbaum (1986) explores about luck in ancient Greek literature: Why are the good times in life so vulnerable? Raising this question exposes a fault line in the preceding dialogue shared by Hal the NP. On one side of the fault is the NP's knowledge, which we have called judgment and expertise. On the other side of the fault is Hal's own knowledge about himself, his life, and the imagined course of his own destiny. The overall aim of practical discourse has been to span the fault, thus introducing balance by employing practical discourse as an example of action research.

Nussbaum (1986) answers her own question by exploring ancient Greek poetry, particularly Aescalus' tragedies, in combination with Plato's dialogues. Nussbaum's method exemplifies the participatory manner that action research is rendered in this chapter. In particular, action research is viewed herein as a philosophical reflection on narrative text, but not just the words themselves as the intended meanings embedded in the words and the context, such that the intended meanings in the text point to the fragile consciousness that links the researcher and participant.

Fragility in consciousness is nowhere more pronounced than in the vistas where the dialogue last left off. The NP makes a suggestion about sticking to a diet, and Hal answers:

Hal: *I have trouble sticking to anything except this beer-belly* [points to his waist]. *My waist has been around for 10 years or so.* [Laughs . . .]

NP:	*I know what you mean, my daughter called me everyday for 3 weeks to remind me not to eat chocolate . . . a lot of good that did, I just found ways to eat more chocolate; (we) just gave up!*
Hal:	*Chocolate is good for your health. [Laughs] . . . But seriously, could I actually get off Lipitor?*
NP:	*I don't know. Right now your cholesterol numbers are still high. . . . Time will tell if we can get these numbers down. What have you and your wife, Susan, discussed about the low-fat diet?*
Hal:	*Not much. Susan's still scared, you know, after the heart attack. She and I both need to lower cholesterol. Maybe we two can do something together.*
NP:	*You know what they say . . . two heads are always better than one. Could be a smart idea. What's the chance that we can meet together with your wife to talk about a low-fat diet plan?*
Hal:	*Chances are good, I think. I dunno. . . . Susan's bought a book with recipes that lower fat in the cooking. Got any advice about that?*

The trouble with diets is that they seldom last. The NP concludes that diets seldom last by drawing upon a rich body of literature pertaining to weight-loss plans, identifying the social context of eating in the approach of educating Hal and his wife in the same session. It remains unknown whether Hal and his wife do anything together—much is to be uncovered in time—but changes introduced with both family members present might produce incremental but lasting results.

If there is tragedy to be read in Hal's story, in that his right to a serene retirement is impeded by changes so onerous as pill burden and uncertainty, then something must be said by action research about the common bond forged in discourse between Hal and the NP. In the preceding dialogue clip, Hal and the NP laugh over shared mistakes with food. To be exact, Hal cannot follow a diet, at least not thus far, and the NP fails to resist chocolates. Reason alone does not control or predict human behavior. If reason prevailed, Hal might not ever have had a heart attack. Bad genes cannot account for the entire mess that Hal got in.

Reason does not prevail when it comes to enacting healthy behaviors; otherwise, no one would still smoke tobacco. What prevails is a need to share a story, even to re-create a story with one's partner. In this action research example, Hal is partner to an NP. The NP joins Hal in making the story about diets, which frees Hal from the burden of carrying resistance to temptations alone. This is what could be meant by the context of story making, pointing attention toward the context of shared meanings that two partners create.

But the meaning is also purely contextual because Hal must decide between at least two situations: on the one hand, Hal could reverse 10 years of cheating on diets by making lasting changes, and on the other hand, Hal could not change anything. Each decision bears sacrifice and tragic loss because the situations are particular to Hal's story and universal to us all. Hence, the NP's compassion is identifiable in her laugh with Hal. They are deciding together whether they will live well or might not live at all.

More important, we do not know whether any change will result in a desired outcome. Too many unknowns are at play, which leave Hal and the NP with what Nussbaum (1986) calls serious claims upon their "practical attention" (p. 17). Choosing one situation, Hal might be left with "some regret that he did not do the other thing" (p. 17).

So we arrive at the conundrum of action research as far as discourse ethics is concerned. Ethical discourse can do no more nor any less than remain grounded in dialogue, which we have viewed as narrative in this chapter. Groundedness implies that ethical discourse in the case of Hal and the NP must address the questions that arise *in situ* without extrapolating to moral claims that permit global applications.

Yet global are the claims of grounded dialogues such as shared between Hal and the NP. The claims can be at once global and particular because the condition that they share is called human. Therefore, global and particular claims can be drawn from action research as shared in ethical discourse between Hal and his NP.

Conclusion

This chapter presents action research through a philosophical and practice lens. A case involving Hal and his NP illustrates the dilemmas or problems encountered in Hal's care after a heart attack. Philosophical reflections upon liberation, as a goal of action research, are considered from a larger view by discussing liberation through practical discourse.

Hal was not liberated from erroneous conclusions or distorted meanings, but instead the NP and Hal formed a partnership to explore in real time what each considered solid arguments. The discourse that involved arguments is presented as a search for truth embedded in a practice situation. Each argument first appears inside dialogue clips followed by philosophical elaborations derived from Habermas's primary texts.

Further Implications for Practice: Philosophical Reflection as Action Research

The action researchers of this chapter have been identified as NP and Hal—perhaps also Susan, Hal's wife, by extension of the definition that action researchers are coparticipants. Viewed as coparticipants in creating meaning, the NP, Hal, and Susan have performed what Kirk (2004) calls "co-meaning making," which Kirk considers "a central part . . . of healing."

The question remains how to educate nurses or NPs to become coparticipants in action research. Answers to the educational question are varied. Troublesome among answers is a jaundiced eye, which reads "coparticipant" as unessential to understanding disease outcomes in populations or aggregates.

Many textbook editors, who make the judgment that knowledge about disease outcomes in populations and aggregates is essential for graduate-level nurses, have raised the importance of some topics, such as pharmacotherapeutics, while dimming the light on other topics such as the therapeutic use of self. For example, a critical reading of many current nursing textbooks elevates an understating of populations above grasping the concept of the individual, arguably because nursing and medicine must share similar bases of knowledge, even though application to clinical learning in nursing or medicine clear the way for significant differences. In short, a term like *coparticipant* eludes significance to the textbook editor. Nevertheless, an understanding of "coparticipant" is foundational to a comprehensive articulation of the advanced practice nursing role and practice-based research as discussed in this chapter.

Graduate education for the NP can teach the technical information associated with medications that were addressed in this chapter. Graduate education can also address ways to reflect upon practice through action research. Notwithstanding, technical knowledge and action research are just two components of graduate-level curricula in nursing. But graduate education, on the whole, inhibits students from philosophical reflections upon primary texts because, even at this higher level of academic inquiry, graduate nursing students have not laid a firm foundation in reading and interpreting primary philosophical literature. One might dare say that social work, psychology, occupational therapy, nutritional sciences, physical therapy, medicine, and a host of other graduate-level helping professions, along with nursing, share similar flaws.

Laying a firm foundation for dialogue with primary philosophical texts by and among nurses, however, resembles the story of the Hydra, a mythological serpent. Hercules needed help killing the Hydra, just as nurses will need help to dialogue with primary philosophical texts. According to the ancient narrator Apollodorus (1921), Hercules slew the nine-headed Hydra in Lerna but not without receiving help. Hercules cut off each of the nine heads of the Hydra, and Hercules' nephew, Iolaus, seared the tissue at the neck with a torch to prevent regrowth of the heads. The analogy to nursing focuses on the help that Iolaus gave Hercules. The story of help came because Hercules could not complete his task alone. His foot was stuck in one of the serpent's coils, limiting Hercules' movements, and every decapitated head grew back before Iolaus burned the tendons of the serpent's neck. Without Iolaus' help, Hercules was sure to have been defeated.

The Herculean task is to produce philosophical inquiry in graduate-level education. Help for the task will come from action researchers in graduate schools who teach students how to dialogue with primary texts. But where are the action researchers who teach philosophical inquiry using primary texts? Without a critical mass of published findings from other action researchers employing philosophy as analysis, the aid that Iolaus gave Hercules will not arrive. Therefore, Iolaus' torch, in this analogy, is a critical mass of published results from action research that utilizes philosophical inquiry.

Of course, there are philosophers whose inquiry is to explicate the ethical, epistemological, and metaphysical veins of practical discourse. Such interested philosophers have already become partners in the enterprise. However, meaning that is cocreated by the NP and Hal, to use the example of this chapter, cannot come from outside the interactions that the NP and Hal shared or might share. In other words, the action research example of this chapter offers the view that the NP and Hal are hermeneutic partners. As partners, they must live with Hal's pill burden and hopelessness, and if these experiences are transformed by the partnership, then healing might occur. Time will tell.

REFERENCES

Apollodorus. (1921). *Apollodorus, the library.* [Trans. Sir James George Frazer]. Cambridge, MA: Harvard University Press.

Bowers, M. J. (2004). Beckoning the heart: A guided autobiographical approach to understanding women's recovery following myocardial infarction (Doctoral dissertation, University of British Columbia, 2004). *Dissertation Abstracts International*, DAI-A, 65/08, p. 2905, Feb 2005.

Cahn, P. (2003). What to start with, and when? *Advanced Studies in Medicine*, 3(9B), S903-7, S931-3.

Clay, P. G. (2004). Actual medication pill burden and dosing frequency in HIV-infected patients with undetectable viral loads. *Journal of the International Association of Physicians in AIDS Care*, 3(2), 49–55.

Dyck, A., Deschamps, M., & Taylor, J. (2005). Pharmacist's discussions of medication side effects: A descriptive study. *Patient Education and Counseling, 56*(1), 21–27.

Habermas, J. (1988). *On the logic of the social sciences.* Cambridge, MA: MIT Press.

Habermas, J. (1990). *Moral consciousness and communicative action.* Cambridge, MA: MIT Press.

Hussey, L. C., Hardin, S., & Blanchette, C. (2002). Outpatient costs of medications for patients with chronic heart failure. *American Journal of Critical Care, 11*(5), 474–478.

Kirk, T. W. (2004). Nursing ethics is not professional ethics: Philosophical problems with the boundary paradigm in nursing. *Abstracts: Introduction to the Philosophy of Nursing Conference,* Wales, Swansea, U.K.

McCarter-Bayer, A., Bayer, F., & Hall, K. (2005). Preventing falls in acute care: An innovative approach. *Journal of Gerontological Nursing, 31*(3), 25–33.

Medvedeff, D. (2003). Early experiences in e-prescribing; the state of Florida deploys handhelds and prescription management software to Medicaid phyisicans, to drive down the cost of medications and to provide point-of-care decision support for doctors. *Health Management Technology, 24*(12), 34–36.

Nussbaum, M. C. (1986). *The fragility of goodness: Luck and ethics in Greek tragedy and philosophy.* New York: Cambridge University Press.

Parish, T. G. (2004). Financing smoke-related illness and smoking cessation in the United States: Can it be done? *Internet Journal of Allied Health Sciences and Practice, 2*(1), 1–8.

Ziegler, M. (1996). *Improving practices synthesizing the cases.* Cambridge, NY: Cambridge University Press.

PART III

Internal and External Considerations in Qualitative Research

The following chapters, which comprise Part III, are designed to address a variety of essential considerations to attain the highest level of research science quality. This section answers questions and concerns frequently expressed not only by students of nursing science, but also by faculty, consultants, and reviewers of qualitative research. Many of these questions may be on your mind as you contemplate doing your own qualitative research studies.

Part III of this edition has also been expanded and is now even more helpful than ever! You will find new authors here as well and chapters concerning Evidenced Based Practice and Qualitative Research, ethical considerations, institutional review, strategies for intra-project sampling, combining qualitative and quantitative methods for mixed-method designs, evaluation of qualitative research, on-line and Internet resources, and an invitation to re-imagine qualitative research. I think the final chapter is a wonderful way to end a text of this nature, with its invitation to you to re-imagine from your perspective this exciting and rewarding way of *doing research*.

These eight chapters do not intend to provide the *only answers or interpretations* to these questions and concerns, and the reader is encouraged to study the references for additional perspectives. For example, the question of combination of methods is a subject that has provoked heated discussions. If the reader is to be truly informed about these critiques, additional reading is necessary. Another example is evaluation. There are many systems developed for evaluating qualitative research. Most are a difference in language, but it is a good idea to become familiar with those authors' perceptions, as well.

This is the last section before some summary remarks. Enjoy and be stimulated!

PLM

20

Evidence-Based Nursing and Qualitative Research: A Partnership Imperative for Real-World Practice

Patti R. Zuzelo

Evidence-based practice (EBP) discussion has reached the "tipping point" (Gladwell, 2002) within and between nursing and medical professional organizations. The "tipping point" refers to the name popularized by Gladwell that describes the contagiousness, big effects, and dramatic changes associated with an epidemic, in this case, an EBP "epidemic," when everything changes all at once.

EBP popularity is astonishing given the fact that nursing research utilization of the 1970s and 1980s called for similar practice changes and, yet, was generally regarded noncommittally by nurses providing direct care. The term *evidence-based nursing* (EBN) is relatively new and has already become central to professional nursing discussions. A quick search on Microsoft Network's popular search engine revealed 1,253,386 results containing "evidence based nursing." Journals, conferences, academic centers, books, and practice guidelines offer opportunities to develop EBN expertise. EBN is a phenomenon that appears to have staying power given its emphasis on best practices and the appealing belief that scientific credibility underlies many or most practice decisions. EBN is particularly attractive given the concurrent emphasis on evidence-based medicine (EBM). It is important for nurses to have a firm grasp of EBN characteristics and processes to appraise its potential benefit to patient outcomes and to make informed decisions as to the application of EBN practice recommendations. It is also important for nurses to have a clear appreciation of EBN and EBM characteristics so as to ensure that the unique contributions of nursing practice are not subsumed within the positivistic worldview of medical science. Qualitative research has a critical role to play in EBN and, yet, it is often overlooked because quantitative approaches receive preferential consideration. This chapter addresses the importance of qualitative research to EBN and explores the barriers, opportunities, and contributions of qualitative research methodologies to EBN.

EBN AND QUALITATIVE RESEARCH: FUNDAMENTAL ISSUES AND CONCERNS

What Is EBN?

EBN is the integration of solid research evidence, patient preference, and clinician expertise (Figure 20–1) (DiCenso, Guyatt, & Ciliska, 2005). In general, nurses are advised to (1) make certain to take practice recommendations from good research only; (2) solicit patient preferences and actions; and (3) evaluate these recommendations, preferences, and actions within the context of clinical expertise and resources. These steps seem simple and clear. In reality, challenges are associated with EBN, including concerns that EBN is research utilization with a new name and disagreement as to what constitutes "good" research and "evidence." These questions are important and provide the foundation for this chapter.

Ciliska, Pinelli, DeCenso, and Cullum (2001) note that *EBN* is a fairly recent term that evolved from the initial concept of EBM. Stetler (2001) asserts that the research utilization movement of the 1970s in nursing was actually the forerunner to EBN and that some EBN models are entrenched in prior research utilization work. DiCenso et al. (2005) describe EBN as "much broader than research utilization" (p. 6) because it incorporates clinical expertise, patient values, and clinical resources. Although this definition is widely acknowledged in the published literature, it is also important to note that there is variation in the emphasis on the breadth of this definition. Some authors emphasize "evidence" and the hierarchical value of evidentiary types without much mention of clinician judgment and patient input (Moore et al., 1995). This inconsistency is of concern and may be part of the

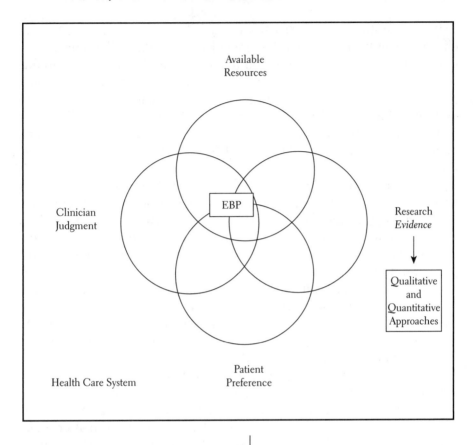

Figure 20–1 EBP and Outcomes Improvement
Source: Adapted from A. DiCenso & N. Cullum. (1998). Implementation forum. *Evidence-Based Nursing, 1*(2), 38–40.

reason why some nurses find it difficult to understand the difference between EBN and research utilization. When EBN or EBP is described without attending to clinical expertise and patient values, it is similar to basic research utilization and may be more consistent with a medical model of disease-based, positivistic, clinical decision making.

It is interesting to note that the terms *EBN* and *EBP* are used interchangeably in the literature with shared ideas from *EBM*. The variations in terms may be important and should be explored as they contribute to the confusion experienced by nurses as they navigate the literature. For the purpose of this chapter, *EBP* is used to generically refer to the overarching focus on using evidence to identify best practices and improve patient/client outcomes. What constitutes "best" practices and "best evidence" is dependent upon the circumstances at the time. *EBN* refers to EBP activities that are unique to nursing.

Liberati and Vineis (2004) note that the real failure of medical practice prior to EBM was not that people did not use evidence but that no framework and no set of rules for using evidence in a systematic way existed. The authors identify that acquiring critical appraisal skills is one of the most important tenets of the EBM movement. This point may be relevant to nursing practice as well.

The ability to appraise the quality and relevance of both quantitative and qualitative research studies within the context of real-world practice challenges is vitally important to nursing and difficult to consistently achieve given the widely divergent educational backgrounds of practicing nurses. Why is defining "evidence" so important to nursing?

It is important to have a balanced appraisal of the benefits of EBN. Avoiding the hype of EBN and the resultant tendency to jump on board without careful consideration is critical. What is the "evidence" of EBN (French, 2002)? Nursing, as both a science *and* an art, needs to actively make certain that qualitative research is as much a part of the considered evidence as quantitative research is. Nurses need to appreciate the complexity of EBP and cannot assume that EBP in its current form is compatible with nursing values and practice (Dale, 2005).

French (2002) conducted a frequency analysis on the key words "evidence-based medicine," "evidence-based practice," "evidence-based nursing," "evidence-based healthcare," and "evidence-based decision making." Findings revealed a cumulative total of 6,194 papers, most of which have a publication date of 1995 or later. French asserts that EBP is commonly a euphemism for information management, clinical judgment, professional practice development, or managed care.

There is little evidence that EBP has added value to quality assurance and research-based practice. The paradox of EBP is likened to the intense enthusiasm followed by disenchantment that occurred with the Problem Oriented Medical Record, Nursing Process, Primary Nursing, and Reflective Practitioner (French, 2002). French examines the utility of EBP within the context of symbolic interactionism. French provides a selective review of the definitions of EBP and points out that these varied definitions have important inconsistencies and reveal two issues: What is the meaning of the word *evidence*, and what is the process of EBP?

Dale (2005) suggests that there is a range of evidentiary sources, including personal reflection, journal articles, policies, guidelines, professional consensus, research, and audit. *Relevance* and *best* are value-laden terms and need to be explored fully within the context of nursing practice—a practice that is inherently different from medical practice. Dale notes that current forms of EBP may be incompatible with nursing because nursing requires a pluralistic approach. Questions drive methods, and some questions are best answered using qualitative methods, particularly those questions that are often of great interest to practicing nurses.

Why Use Qualitative Methods for Evidenced-Based Practice?

Carper (1978) identifies four patterns of knowing that provide the foundation for nursing. These patterns include empirics, aesthetics, personal knowledge, and ethics. Quantitative research methodologies are applicable to better understanding the science, or empirics, of nursing. The other three patterns are not amenable to "hard" science or positivism. Understanding the whole patient, knowing the patient as a unique individual, engaging with the patient in an authentic relationship, and addressing ethical conflicts relate to qualitative ways of knowing that are vitally important to nursing.

Building on Carper's (1978) knowledge typology, Edwards (2002) notes that aesthetic knowledge relates to expert nursing practice and caring. Aesthetics affirms the artistic nature of nursing by recognizing that the small "tasks" of nursing are truly complicated and important. Empirical knowledge is usually recognized as positivistic and rational but has been broadened to include qualitative methodologies. Personal knowledge is coupled with self-awareness and is connected to experiential knowledge and intuition. Ethical knowledge relates to moral knowledge. Appreciating the various types of knowledge is important because it affirms the duality of nursing research: quantitative *and* qualitative approaches. Edwards (2002) suggests that in quantitative research people are "reducible and measurable objects independent of historical, cultural and social contexts" (p. 41).

Qualitative methodologies are often less valued by medical professionals, and hold lower stature in funding requests, and yet, embrace the traditional values of nursing that emphasize personal, connected, holistic caring. Qualitative research questions seek a higher level of intimacy with participants. It is about knowing people and valuing differences. Qualitative research uses the written word to describe feelings and life experiences. This approach shares information in a way that makes patient stories readily accessible to nurses and relevant to their care experiences (Cohen, Kahn, & Steeves, 2002).

Dale (2005) suggests that EBP may potentiate interprofessional conflicts given its particular relevance to medicine with its focus on disease-driven science. Dale notes that the range of research design necessary for generating the evidence base required in medicine is very narrow. Medicine is well suited to quantitative research, and published evidential tiers are very relevant. Quantitative studies require control and measurement. These needs create an artificial experience that can make it difficult for health care practitioners to apply research findings to clinical practice. Nursing practice is inherently broader than is medical practice and is built upon the premise that experiences are individual and unique. "Control" and "measurement" may be appropriate concerns in some nursing contexts or situations but certainly not all. As a result, nursing requires a pluralistic, multimethod approach to its knowledge-building endeavors. When nurses apply a positivistic model to nursing practice, qualitative research methodologies become less valuable — despite their relevance and importance to all four patterns of knowing.

Nurses' ways of knowing may include collecting patient stories, learning through experiencing during clinical practice, or generating evidence (Dale, 2005). These knowledge-building activities do not signify that "nursing evidence is less rigorously obtained than that of medicine. It is indicative of the fundamental differences between the two forms of practice and the extent of development of each specific knowledge base" (Dale, p. 51). It is imperative for nurse researchers to generate knowledge in all forms because all forms are relevant to nursing practice and patterns of knowing. The best evidence promotes the most clinically effective practice (Dale). To determine what is "best," nurses must know the patient from a holistic perspective. Qualitative approaches tend to best answer questions that relate to "knowing" patients' preferences, experiences, concerns, and priorities.

The Shortcomings of EBP: Lack of Standardization and a Positivistic Stance

There is no single, agreed-upon process for EBP. The lack of a unifying definition contributes to the confusing array of EBP models that may or may not recognize nursing's unique contributions and perspectives. Nursing discussions tend to recognize a combination of concerns that include research findings, clinician expertise, and patient preference; however, these priorities are not consistently included in EBN and EBM literature. Authors also vary in their delineation of strong to weak research study designs (Figure 20–2).

Oncology Nursing Society (2005)	Moore et al. (1995)
1. Meta-analysis of multiple controlled clinical trials 2. Individual trials or experiments 3. Integrative reviews of all types of research 4. Nonexperimental multiple studies, including descriptive, correlation, and qualitative research 5. Program evaluation, quality improvement data, or case reports 6. Opinions of experts—standards of practice, practice guidelines	I. Strong evidence from at least one systematic review of multiple well-designed randomized controlled trials II. Strong evidence from at least one properly designed randomized controlled trial of appropriate size III. Evidence from well-designed trials without randomization, single group pre-post, cohort, time series, or matched case-controlled studies IV. Evidence from well-designed nonexperimental studies from more than one center or research group V. Opinions of respected authorities, based on clinical evidence, descriptive studies, or reports of expert committees

Figure 20–2 Exemplars of Evidentiary Hierarchies

Randomized clinical trials (RCTs) are viewed as the evidentiary EBP gold standard by many written accounts. RCTs are quantitative studies that involve randomization with a control group, manipulation of a variable, a double-blind study design, and, ideally, a large sample size. The Moore Hierarchy of Strength of Evidence (Moore et al., 1995) illustrates the importance of quantitative studies by ranking the systematic review of several tightly designed RCTs well above descriptive studies. In fact, this hierarchy groups "descriptive studies" with the opinions of respected authorities and reports of expert committees. It is important to note that this hierarchy is written from an EBM perspective rather than an EBN one. This particular hierarchy is referred to throughout the medical literature (Akobeng, 2005; Chung & Reid, 2001).

Akobeng (2005) asserts that the ability to track down and critically appraise evidence and then to incorporate this evidence into daily practice are key tools of EBM. The discussion centers on evidence and includes such terms as *sound* and *scientific*. Akobeng uses a patient or problem, intervention, comparison, outcomes or patient or problem, intervention, outcome(s) format for structuring clinical questions. This structure is only relevant within a positivist paradigm. Recommendations for evidence examination include appraising the evidence for validity and its importance and applicability to the patient or patients of interest. Tools are available to appraise randomized controlled trials, systematic reviews, case-control studies, and cohort studies. There is no mention of the need to consider qualitative studies, although it is true that many clinical exemplars in medicine do address topics that are more appropriately investigated using quantitative approaches. This makes sense given the narrow but deep specialization of medicine. It also points out why it is so important for nurses to appraise EBM models and to select the aspects that enhance nursing practice and to disregard or alter the processes that do not enhance practice.

Another example of a positivistic persuasion to EBP is exemplified by Flemming (1998), who offers strategies for asking answerable questions. The examples that are offered suggest that there are three elements to questions: situation, intervention, and outcome. Although this perspective is true in some cases, it provides a narrow view of a researchable question. Questions are not always asked out of a need to "do" or "intervene." At times, important questions address concerns such as "what is it like for people when. . . ?" and "what is important to people" and "what does it mean when people experience, think, believe. . . ?" These questions relate to the art of nursing, the experiential knowing that influences intuition and caring. An additional concern with the situation, intervention, and outcome model is that it presumes that the situation is well understood and that concepts/constructs are measurable with one particular interpretation or meaning. For example, grief, pain, anxiety, loss, mourning, love, caring, or knowing hold different meanings and are associated with different possibilities. Flemming addresses strategies for developing questions without first acknowledging that there are questions underlying the questions. This area of research question formulation highlights the unique contributions of a qualitative approach.

The current emphasis on positivistic approaches affects other health care disciplines interested in EBP and causes concern. Henderson and Rheault (2004), writing from a physical therapy perspective, note that qualitative research methods are needed if EBP is truly about *best* evidence. They offer four decision rules for determining the inclusion of qualitative research studies in EBP decisions. These rules pertain to assumptions, qualitative screens, levels of evidence, and grades of recommendation. Several models are offered for appraising the quality of qualitative studies; however, there is no established hierarchy for ranking the evidentiary value of different types of qualitative studies. Given the varied philosophical underpinnings of the major qualitative approaches, phenomenology, ethnography, and grounded theory, such a hierarchy would not be meaningful.

EBN may differ from EBM in ways that have not been unequivocally addressed. Ciliska et al. (2001) identify five steps of EBN: (1) formulate an answerable question related to a patient problem or situation; (2) search for research evidence to answer the question; (3) appraise the validity, relevance, and applicability of the evidence; (4) make a decision as to whether or not to change practice; and (5) evaluate the decision's outcome. Flemming (1998) offers a slightly different approach to EBN by suggesting that, when making a decision about changing practice, the best available evidence should be used, as well as clinical expertise and the patient's perspective. In addition, Flemming offers that performance should be evaluated using self-reflection, audit, or peer assessment.

Similar to EBN, the steps of EBM are identified as follows: (1) converting information needs into answerable questions; (2) finding the best evidence with which to answer the questions; (3) critically appraising the evidence for its validity and usefulness; (4) applying the results of the appraisal into clinical practice; and (5) evaluating performance (Akobeng, 2005). The major difference between the steps of EBN and EBM appear to be in the meaning of the term *evidence*. This is a critical difference that cannot be taken lightly. Evidence for nursing needs to be drawn from the entire range of quantitative and qualitative methods. Otherwise, nursing runs the risk of excluding large areas of nursing knowledge from its practice base. In fact, the qualitative area of understanding and knowledge may be exactly why nursing is highly valued and trusted—its continued emphasis on what is human and immeasurable—the qualities that many patients believe is missing from modern health care.

How Does the Evidence Debate Affect Real-World Practice?

One problem area directly related to the rationalism versus empiricism debate is funding priorities. Researchers are pressured to demonstrate measurable effectiveness, an outcome that may be narrowly defined and quantified (Gilgun, 2004). The pressure to demonstrate effectiveness in as short an amount of time as possible is related to the need to keep down costs (Gilgun). In other words, increased effectiveness relates to efficiency, which influences health care costs. The potential for cost savings is an appealing aspect of quantitatively determined outcomes.

In addition to the appeal of potentially impacting health care costs, quantitatively designed studies are attractive to funding agencies because of their congruency with established hierarchies of evidence. Most practitioners recognize the difference in status afforded to researchers well versed in the hard sciences as compared to those skilled in qualitative methodologies. Although experienced researchers realize that the research question drives the method, in the real world of competitive funding, nurse researchers may be persuaded to select studies based on the method rather than the value of the particular question to nursing practice. Edwards (2002) concurs and argues that those with power determine what counts as knowledge. Power is equated to financial means, and those questions that are deemed worthy of funding shape nursing practice and affect nursing's definition of itself. Edwards suggests that there should be a much broader perspective of nursing knowledge to include quantitative research findings, qualitative approaches, and other forms using intuitive understanding. Each knowledge form should be regarded equally. Edwards calls for a postmodern view of nursing in which "anything that enhances or informs practice" (p. 44) is justified given nursing's unique practice discipline.

In summary, critical points to consider when examining the idea of evidence in its relationship to nursing practice include (1) the metaparadigm of nursing with its emphasis on holism demands a pluralistic approach to research; (2) nursing's broad discipline requires an evidence-based approach that may differ from medicine or other health professions; (3) defining the nature of evidence is important to EBN; (4) research utilization is connected to EBN, and nursing should credit itself with these early evidence-based endeavors; and (5) once fundamental issues are resolved, there is a need to examine strategies for standardizing EBN practices within the education and practice of nursing, particularly given the various levels of entry into the profession.

THE BARRIERS TO INCLUDING QUALITATIVE STUDY FINDINGS IN EBN EFFORTS

The Challenge of Systematically Reviewing Qualitative Studies

Practitioners are increasingly comfortable with accessing systematic reviews to provide practice recommendations. One popular resource for EBP decision-making based upon systematic review is the Cochrane Collaboration. Chung and Reid (2001) identify that the systematic review is a process involving the application of scientific strategies to the assembly, critical appraisal, and synthesis of the studies relevant to a specific clinical question. Cochrane review groups are reluctant to accept studies based on qualitative data and prefer to include papers that are either randomized controlled trials or clinical trials (French, 2002). Ciliska et al. (2001) note that systematic reviews are quantitatively based and tend to have little relevance to qualitative research studies; however, a popular abstraction journal, *Evidence-Based Nursing*, does address both quantitative and qualitative studies.

Sandelowski and Barroso (2002) observe that there are challenges associated with "finding the findings in qualitative studies" (p. 213). The researchers analyzed reports ($N = 99$) of studies that used a qualitative approach to study women with HIV infection. The goal of the project was to design a systematic, practical, comprehensive, and communicable research protocol for conducting qualitative metasyntheses. Qualitative investigators use a variety of reporting formats and tend to use inconsistent and individually determined styles. The lack of standardization makes it difficult to synthesize findings from multiple studies that explore similar questions. The greatest barrier to integrating qualitative study findings is the difficulty of finding them in published works (Barroso et al., 2003; Sandelowski & Barroso, 2002).

Sandelowski and Barroso (2002) also identified challenges with the misrepresentation of data and analysis as findings, misuse of quotes and incidents, inconsistent use across studies with the use of the terms *theme* and *pattern*, and theoretical confusion. The researchers challenge qualitative investigators to make certain that findings are clearly evident to readers. Jones (2004) concurs with the urgency of this challenge and notes that identification of qualitative studies relevant to a research question is far more time-consuming than the identification of RCTs for a quantitative systematic review. In addition, Jones notes that the paperwork load is much greater when reviewing qualitative studies, sometimes because abstracts and titles are unclear, compelling the investigator to retrieve whole articles for review. The difficulty in clearly identifying research findings as well as the problem with inconsistencies that may diminish the quality of the findings are significant barriers to incorporating qualitative studies into EBN practice guidelines.

Misperceptions of Scientific Inadequacies

Russell and Gregory (2003) offer guiding questions to assist with appraising the potential value of qualitative studies (Table 20–1). They suggest that whereas quantitative researchers have specific guidelines and strategies for determining sample size adequacy, qualitative researchers have only general principles, primarily based on judgment. Data saturation determines sample size rather than the power analyses associated with quantitative studies. Quantitative researchers unfamiliar with the different yet appropriate sampling plans of qualitative research studies may be skeptical of the smaller sample sizes. In fact, qualitative researchers also identify the need for larger samples without offering explanations as to the rationale for needing a greater number of participants (Cohen et al., 2002). The general critiques related to sample size offered by qualitative researchers when

---

TABLE 20–1   Qualitative Research Appraisal Questions

Questions to Help Critically Appraise Qualitative Research

Are the findings valid?
- ◆ Is the research question clear and adequately substantiated?
- ◆ Is the design appropriate for the research question?
- ◆ Was the method of sampling appropriate for the research question and design?
- ◆ Were data collected and managed systematically?
- ◆ Were the data analyzed appropriately?

What are the findings?
- ◆ Is the description of findings thorough?

How can I apply the findings to patient care?
- ◆ What meaning and relevance does the study have for my practice?
- ◆ Does the study help me understand the context of my practice?
- ◆ Does the study enhance my knowledge about my practice?

Source: C. Russell & D. Gregory. (2003). Evaluation of qualitative research studies. *Evidence-Based Nursing, 6,* 36. Reproduced with permission from the BMJ Publishing Group.

---

identifying potential limitations to study findings may reinforce the impression that qualitative and quantitative methodologies are best served with large samples.

Terminology Dissonance

Morse, Barrett, Mayan, Olson, and Spiers (2002) identify the challenges associated with establishing reliability and validity in qualitative research. One of these concerns relates to the different terminology used by qualitative researchers when describing processes developed to ensure rigor. The authors argue that returning to validity as a process for rigor while using verification techniques enables researchers to be consistent with quantitative scientists while remaining true to the different philosophical perspectives innate to qualitative approaches. The different terms used by qualitative researchers, including *trustworthiness* and *confirmability*, exacerbate the perception that qualitative research is "soft" compared to positivistic approaches that emphasize validity and reliability.

Other researchers assert that it is important for researchers to feel confident in the value of using auditability, confirmability, and fittingness as measures of quality (Goding & Edwards, 2002). This dilemma represents more than a debate of semantics. It represents a belief that there is a need to avoid conformity to a positivist, reductionist worldview. This issue requires resolution to facilitate standardization of appraisal guidelines.

THE CONTRIBUTIONS OF QUALITATIVE APPROACHES TO EBN

Studies exploring human behavior, thoughts, emotions, relationships, human experiences, or complex occurrences are best explored using qualitative methods. Quantitative studies emphasize causal relationships. The qualitative approach should be used if it is appropriate to the research question that is being asked. Goding and Edwards (2002) assert that the positivistic approach to EBP suggests that there is one "truth" waiting to be discovered rather than many "truths" to be interpreted. If quantitative research is treated as the best way to approach evidence, how do nurses account for the important, but less tangible aspects of practice such as nursing interactions, interpersonal skills, and intuition?

Thompson, Cullum, McCaughan, Sheldon, and Raynor (2004) suggest that nurses are expected to be active decision makers in health care. This active decision making requires an active command of appraising research evidence. "Evidence-based decision making—like all decision making—involves choosing from a discrete range of options, which may include doing nothing or a wait and see strategy" (p. 68). Nurses deal with differing decision types requiring a variety of research methods and questions. These differing decision types require different questions and different methods. Thompson et al. (2004) offer several examples of decision types. Whereas some, for example, prevention, intervention/effectiveness, or assessment, may be best suited to a quantitative approach, others seem better addressed using an empirical approach. For example, decisions related to communication or experience and meaning relate best to qualitative considerations.

Describing Patient Needs and Experiences: A Phenomenological Exemplar

One example of a qualitative approach to ascertaining patient needs to provide appropriate, targeted nursing care is exemplified by a research study examining the lived experience of having a neobladder (Beitz & Zuzelo, 2003). Neobladder construction is a relatively new surgical intervention that has become standard therapy for *in situ* bladder cancer. Neobladder involves the use of small intestine or small bowel/large bowel combinations to create a low-pressure reservoir that attaches to the person's urinary sphincter following cystectomy (Beitz & Zuzelo). Many nurses are unfamiliar with this surgical procedure, and, because it is relatively uncommon, patients presented with the opportunity for neobladder construction usually lack basic familiarity with the procedure, unlike more common procedures such as cholecystectomy or coronary artery bypass grafting.

This phenomenological study describes the lived experience and the meanings and essences of the experience of people who chose neobladder construction in response to a diagnosis of bladder cancer. Findings reveal many concerns and worries that should be included in routine neobladder teaching. Participants were very affected by changed sexuality, and this concern was often not manifested until long into the recovery period. Support groups were important to participants and provided them with long-term friendships and companionship as they struggled with the physical changes in voiding and sex while dealing with the potential threat of recurrent cancer.

Beitz and Zuzelo (2003) discovered that the bladder cancer experience profoundly affected the survivors. Thematic analysis uncovered a relationship between time and major themes (Figure 20–3). Participants' stories were richly detailed and suggested that areas of patient teaching and counseling required improvement. The study question could have been addressed using a quantitative approach, including survey methodology. However, no published studies explored the neobladder experience from the patient's perspective. Clinicians may have had expertise with the neobladder procedure and familiarity with the typical postoperative trajectory. However, familiarity as an outsider or etic perspective is potentially flawed. Surveys developed from a clinician perspective would have potentially missed the critical importance of support groups; the need for better counseling specific to sexual functioning and sexual loss; the postoperative challenges associated with bladder catheterization and voiding in the day-to-day physical environment in which many people live their lives and work their jobs. This study provided a voice to the many people living with a neobladder. Future questions may be answered using quantitative methods; however, this descriptive study provides important information that would have been missed had a quantitative approach been used. These data may improve the relevance and specificity of future studies concerning neobladder.

Instrument Development and Evaluation: An Exemplar

Qualitative methods are appropriate for instrument evaluation and capture the nuances of instrument use that are not amenable to quantitative discovery. Gilgun (2004) developed the Clinical Assessment Package for Risks and Strengths (CASPARS) for families and children and the 4-D for adolescents who have experienced adversities. Concepts were identified based on Gilgun's long-term qualitative research with adults who had experienced adversities during childhood and adolescence. The qualitative work was necessary for the concept identification important to the instruments' development. Gilgun identified that psychometric testing revealed high instrument reliability.

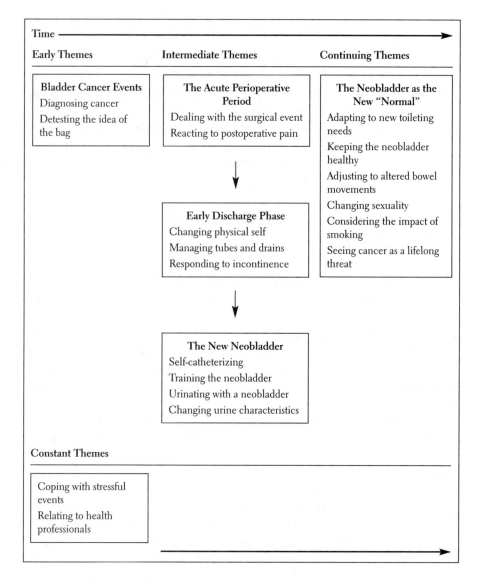

Figure 20–3 Major Themes of Living with a Neobladder
Source: J. Beitz & P. Zuzclo. (2003). The lived experience of having a neobladder. *Western Journal of Nursing Research*, 25(3), 299. Copyright 2003 by Sage Publications, Inc. Reprinted by permission of Sage Publications, Inc.

Alpha coefficient, interrater reliabilities, and construct validities were impressive. Gilgun credits the initial qualitative life history research as providing the theoretical underpinnings critical to the integrity and theoretical consistency of the instruments. Qualitative evaluation of the CASPARS reveals that users found the instrument useful and easy to score and interpret.

This evaluation, partnered with the quantitative data, reinforced the value of the CASPARS.

Gilgun (2004) also used qualitative evaluation strategies for the 4-D and discovered that the 4-D was not as ideal as the psychometric data suggested. Qualitative evaluation of the 4-D provided the impetus to establishing systems changes that were not revealed as necessary through quantitative evaluation approaches. In addition, practitioner feedback led to modification of instrument scoring. Gilgun concludes by asserting that qualitative research provides information that is at the level of specificity that is required for effective clinical assessment tools.

Theory Development: A Grounded Theory Exemplar

In Chapter 9, Beck adds to the Teetering on the Edge theory of postpartum depression. This grounded theory provides an excellent example of the impact that qualitative research has on theory development. In turn, theories provide a context and framework for subsequent research studies, utilizing qualitative, quantitative, and mixed methodologies, to explore phenomena and conditions of interest to establish evidence that may be used to enhance outcomes and improve nursing practice. Teetering on the edge was the basic social process identified in this study. Findings suggest that practitioners should focus their efforts on assisting women experiencing postpartum depression with interventions targeted to the women's particular stage of the recovery process. The *evidence* to support these targeted interventions is provided within the context of the grounded theory. This grounded theory assists practitioners in making resource allocation decisions and facilitates the development of individualized plans of care rather than a one-size-fits-all approach to women diagnosed with postpartum depression. A positivistic approach would not have answered the research questions and would not have provided the detail necessary to understanding postpartum depression within and between diverse cultural orientations.

Developing Definitions to Better Understand Medical Errors in Primary Care: An Exemplar

Kuzel et al. (2003) provide an excellent example of the critical contribution of qualitative research to health care practice in a study exploring medical errors in primary care. The authors' proposal was funded by the Agency for Healthcare Research and Quality (AHRQ), thereby demonstrating that funding opportunities are available, although not plentiful, for well-constructed qualitative studies. The study objectives were to develop a patient-targeted typology of medical errors and injuries; understand patients' perceptions of the most common and most injurious medical errors; obtain primary care physician descriptions of medical errors and contrast these with patient descriptions; and provide a basis for other research that will use the study findings to correct medication use systems. This study is an excellent example of the need to use a qualitative approach to develop clear case definitions to gather further data and develop effective, targeted interventions.

CONCLUSION

Qualitative research is an important contributor to both EBN and professional practice. Qualitative research reports humanize health care. Written research reports put nurses in touch with patient and caregiver experiences in meaningful ways that are rich with detail, in contrast to the reductionist data of quantitatively designed studies. Qualitative studies also lay the foundation for instrument development and evaluation. Qualitative approaches play an important role in the elucidation of concepts and the definitions of key terms that facilitate the meaningfulness of subsequent quantitative studies. EBN is presumed to be important to the science of nursing in a broader sense than its predecessor, research utilization. The combined challenges and opportunities of EBP, outcome indicators, AHRQ (2004) and American Nurses Association (1999) quality indicators, and the Translating Research into Practice program (AHRQ, 2001) emphasize the importance of quantitative studies to improved health care systems. As a result, nurses may be inclined to ignore or minimize the contributions of qualitative approaches to research. It is imperative that nurses keep in mind the aspects of nursing practice that are unique and different from medical practice. These aspects tend to be related to the art of nursing, best approached through qualitative examination.

REFERENCES

Agency for Healthcare Research and Quality. (2001). *Translating research into practice (TRIP)-II.* [Fact sheet. AHRQ Publication No. 01-P017]. Retrieved August 20, 2005, from http://www.ahrq.gov/research/trip2fac.htm.

Agency for Healthcare Research and Quality. (2004). *General questions about the AHRQ QI: AHRQ quality indicators.* Retrieved August 20, 2005, from http://www.qualityindicators.ahrq.gov/general_faq.htm.

Akobeng, A. (2005). Principles of evidence based medicine. *Archives of Disease in Childhood, 90,* 837–840.

American Nurses Association. (1999). *Nursing facts: Nursing sensitive quality indicators for acute care settings and ANA's safety and quality initiative.* Retrieved August 20, 2005, from http://nursingworld.org/readroom/fssafety.htm.

Barroso, J., Gollop, C., Sandelowski, M., Meynell, J., Pearce, P., & Collins, L. (2003). The challenges of searching for and retrieving qualitative studies. *Western Journal of Nursing Research, 25*(2), 153–178.

Beitz, J., & Zuzelo, P. (2003). The lived experience of having a neobladder . . . including commentary by Artinian BM and Watson LA with author response. *Western Journal of Nursing Research, 25,* 294–321.

Carper, B. (1978). Fundamental patterns of knowing in nursing. *Advances in Nursing Science, 1*(1), 13–23.

Chung, F., & Reid, D. (2001). Evidence-based practice: Assessing the quality of evidence, Part II: Grading the evidence. *Cardiopulmonary Physical Therapy, 12*(4), 117–122.

Ciliska, D., Pinelli, J., DiCenso, A., & Cullum, N. (2001). Resources to enhance evidence-based nursing practice. *AACN Clinical Issues, 12*(4), 520–528.

Cohen, M., Kahn, D., & Steeves, R. (2002). Making use of qualitative research. *Western Journal of Nursing Research, 24*(4), 454–471.

Dale, A. (2005). Evidence-based practice: Compatibility with nursing. *Nursing Standard, 19*(40), 48–53.

DiCenso, A., & Cullum, N. (1998). Implementation forum. *Evidence-Based Nursing, 1*(2), 38–40.

DiCenso, A., Guyatt, G., & Ciliska, D. (2005). *Evidence-based nursing: A guide to clinical practice.* St. Louis, MO: Elsevier Mosby.

Edwards, S. (2002). Nursing knowledge: Defining new boundaries. *Nursing Standard, 17*(2), 40–44.

Flemming, K. (1998). EBN notebook: Asking answerable questions. *Evidence-Based Nursing, 1,* 36–37. Retrieved August 9, 2005, from http://ebn.bmjjournals.com/cgi/content/full/1/2/36.

French, P. (2002). What is the evidence on evidence-based nursing? An epistemological concern. *Journal of Advanced Nursing, 37*(3), 250–257.

Gilgun, J. (2004). Qualitative methods and the development of clinical assessment tools. *Qualitative Health Research, 14*(7), 1008–1019.

Gladwell, M. (2002). *The tipping point: How little things can make a big difference.* Boston, MA: Back Bay Books.

Goding, L., & Edwards, K. (2002). Evidence-based practice. *Nurse Researcher, 9*(4), 45–57.

Henderson, R., & Rheault, W. (2004). Appraising and incorporating qualitative research in evidence-based practice. *Journal of Physical Therapy Education, 18*(3), 35–40.

Jones, M. (2004). Application of systematic review methods to qualitative research: Practical issues. *Journal of Advanced Nursing, 48*(3), 271–278.

Kuzel, A., Woolf, S., Engel, J., Gilchrist, V., Frankel, R., LaVeist, T., & Vincent, C. (2003). Making the case for a qualitative study of medical errors in primary care. *Qualitative Health Research, 13*(6), 743–780.

Liberati, A., & Vineis, P. (2004). Introduction to the symposium: What evidence based medicine is and what it is not. *Journal of Medical Ethics, 30,* 120–121. Retrieved August 2, 2005, from www.jme.bmjjournals.com.

Moore, A., et al. (Eds.). (1995). Evidence based everything. *Bandolier, 1*(12), 1. Retrieved July 26, 2005, from http://www.jr2.ox.ac.uk/bandolier/band12/b12-1.html.

Morse, J., Barrett, M., Mayan, M., Olson, K., & Spiers, J. (2002). Verification strategies for establishing reliability and validity in qualitative research. *International Journal of Qualitative Methods, 1*(2), Article 2. Retrieved August 2, 2005, from http://www.ualberta.ca/~ijqm/.

Oncology Nursing Society. (2005). *Evidence-based practice resource center: Critique.* Retrieved August 6, 2005, from http://onsopcontent.ons.org/toolkits/ebp/process_model/critique/critique.htm.

Russell, C., & Gregory, D. (2003). Evaluation of qualitative research studies. *Evidence-Based Nursing, 6*, 36–40. Retrieved August 9, 2005, from http://www.ebn.bmjjournals.com.

Sandelowski, M., & Barroso, J. (2002). Finding the findings in qualitative studies. *Journal of Nursing Scholarship, 34*(3), 213–219.

Stetler, C. (2001). Updating the Stetler Model of Research Utilization to facilitate evidence-based practice. *Nursing Outlook, 49*(6), 272–279.

Thompson, C., Cullum, N., McCaughan, D., Sheldon, T., & Raynor, P. (2004). Nurses, information use, and clinical decision making—the real world potential for evidence-based decisions in nursing. *Evidence-Based Nursing, 7*, 68–72. Retrieved August 9, 2005, http://www.ebn.bmjjournals.com.

21

*Ethical Considerations in Qualitative Research**

Patricia L. Munhall

As members of the scientific community, nurse researchers have become adept at identifying and applying criteria for evaluating the various aspects of quantitative research. We may have even surpassed our colleagues in other disciplines in the level of rigor we apply when evaluating the design, method, and protection of human subjects of a study. With regard to the protection of human subjects, I like to think that rigor is founded on a profound reverence for human beings and their experiences. As nurse researchers, we have become increasingly sophisticated in our qualitative research endeavors and have begun to identify distinct considerations and criteria for viewing the ethical dimensions of qualitative research.

Naturalistic, direct involvement and participation with people necessitate acknowledging the subjective nature and activity of the researcher as the main "tool" of research. Qualitatively oriented nurse researchers prize this direct involvement yet, contextually, are faced with the canonization of objectivity and the resulting detachment of most prevailing conventions. In contrast, qualitative nurse researchers face the nitty-gritty, the serendipitous,

This chapter is used with permission. Originally published as P. L. Munhall. (1988). Ethical considerations in qualitative research. *Western Journal of Nursing Research, 10*(2), 150–162.

the passions, the complexity of subjectivity and attachment to people and their vicissitudes.

The purpose of this chapter is to provide one of the steppingstones needed to differentiate criteria that are essential and appropriate for ethical considerations for qualitative research methods in nursing. This discussion focuses on selected ethical considerations with the following themes interwoven throughout: ethical means and ends, collaborators as means, conflict methodology, models of fieldwork, and process consent. Potential for role conflict within the investigator is discussed from the perspective of the therapeutic imperative and the research imperative.

UNDERLYING ASSUMPTIONS AND DILEMMAS

In the tradition of qualitative research methods, I would like to state, or bracket, here my own beliefs and values and their implications for ethical considerations when doing qualitative nursing research:

1. The therapeutic imperative of nursing (advocacy) takes precedence over the research imperative (advancing knowledge) if conflict develops.
2. Nursing reflects a deontological ethical system (people are not to be treated as means). However, if individuals consent to be part of our research, they have, in essence, joined the research enterprise. Instead of being called *subjects* or *objects*, they are now collaborators (Punch, 1986).
3. Informed consent is a static, past-tense concept. Qualitative research is an ongoing, dynamic, changing process. Because of unforeseeable events and consequences, a past-tense consent is not appropriate. We need to facilitate negotiation and renegotiation to protect our collaborators' human rights. Therefore, a verb like *consent* seems necessary, and the concept of process consenting reflects the ongoing dynamic nature of qualitative research.

ETHICAL MEANS AND ENDS

Bellah (1981) sets our stage for ethical dialogue with the premise that all inquiry has normative commitments. Arguing that all social inquiry is linked to ethical reflection, he uses the expression "moral sciences" interchangeably with "social sciences." He states: "Social science must consider ends as well as means as objects of rational reflection" (p. 2). Laudan (1977) also focuses on the consequence side of science when he states: "Science is essentially a problem-solving activity" (p. 66). Wilson and Fitzpatrick (1984) state that the purpose of nursing science is "to render reality intelligible as it relates to human health and development" (p. 41). The question to be asked from an ethical perspective is: Toward what goal and for what end? For our purposes here, let us suggest that, for the most part, nurse researchers are very much interested in problem-solving or problem-preventing research and that our motives are to produce an end that is in some way considered "good." In this way, research assumes a normative commitment, something that "ought" to be. The most apparent example of this commitment is that many of our research endeavors focus on facilitating health. The search for a means to produce a desired health outcome requires critical ethical reflection.

Other aims that we have in addition or in conjunction to the attainment of health are assisting people to reach their potential, to self-actualize, and to reach their maximum well-being. Actually, many of these ends are equivalent to or similes of the concept of health.

Acknowledgment that our aims have normative commitments is critical because we then move on to ways (means) of achieving our decided good. In essence, our aims become prescriptive. An example may serve to illustrate this point.

ETHICAL AIMS

One of our normative commitments is to help individuals achieve their maximum potential. In this pursuit, we do a qualitative study of a group of "underachievers" who are not attaining full intellectual potential or physical health potential. The ethical questions that arise include whether the ethical aim is to assist the subjects we study or future generations. What do the underachievers we study have to gain from our studying them? Further, is it a given that our mission is to help people reach their maximum potential if unrequested?

Although our society has accepted and promoted some goods, we need to reflect on them. Some may actually be in opposition to others. For example, a steady state or some form of equilibrium may indeed be in opposition to an achievement ethic. In qualitative research, knowledge of our collaborators' aims and normative commitments is an intrinsic component of the research process. We need to reflect on our own and, perhaps more important, their normative commitments.

ETHICAL MEANS

In *The Prince*, Machiavelli proclaims his aim of a free, independent Italy, free from outside governance, as an end that was readily proclaimed as good. However, his means to that end illustrated moral vacuity. Machiavelli believed that corruption is natural to humankind. However, by generalizing a behavior to all "men," he justifies his means to obtain an end. Human experimentation is based on the ends justifying the means principle. Changing people's behaviors, often an aim in the helping professions, contrasts sharply with understanding different behaviors and accepting and supporting those differences. Perhaps not all people need or want to reach their maximum potential. Some philosophers, such as Immanuel Kant, believe human beings have a moral obligation to reach their maximum potential. The question then becomes, Do nurses have a moral obligation to help others attain a moral obligation? This is an example of an ethical consideration that needs in-depth exploration by nurse researchers.

AIMS VERSUS MEANS

Ethical consideration in qualitative research (and quantitative as well, though it is not spelled out) entails knowing explicitly and implicitly what our ethical means and aims are. Entering into a collaboration and participating with our collaborators seem precious experiences that call on us to reflect, know, and critically evaluate our ethical means and ends. A negotiated view requires such reflection.

Perhaps the most critical ethical obligation that qualitative nurse researchers have is to describe the experiences of others in the most faithful way possible. This ethical obligation is to describe and report in the most authentic manner possible the experience that unfolds, even if it is contrary to your aims. Perhaps it might appear wonderful not to strive to reach maximum achievement of your potential! Not having to achieve a numerical level of significance to accomplish your aim may be the highest degree of freedom possible when doing research.

THERAPEUTIC VERSUS RESEARCH IMPERATIVE

Ethics is a tangled web of principles where one can usually see the position of the opposition as having some legitimacy. That is why ethical dilemmas are thorny, at best. In the instance of the therapeutic imperative and the research imperative, the ethical systems of deontology and utilitarianism potentially conflict. The nurse who is doing research needs to acknowledge what her therapeutic imperative is. Is it deontological, where the individual is not a means to an end but an end as such? Is it advocacy for human beings? Is it based on justice, beneficence, and respect for patients' rights? The researcher also needs to reflect on the research imperative. Is it utilitarian, where people are used as means to further knowledge? Is the researcher imposing possibly uncomfortable conditions on participants? Is the researcher working under a utilitarian posture where the ends may justify the means? In qualitative research, some conflicts that present dilemmas for researchers are the following:

Means	Possible ends
Entry	Departure
Confidence	Disappointment
Elation	Despondency
Commitment	Perceived betrayal
Friendship	Desertion

From a utilitarian perspective, the listed results may seem unavoidable in fieldwork. From the deontological perspective, they are ethically problematic. Role conflict evolves from behavioral expectations in the nurse's therapeutic imperative that may differ from those in the researcher's imperative. Given the potential for harm in fieldwork, consideration must be given to these dilemmas so as to minimize them or prevent them from occurring. Communication is an essential process, as is a team or joint approach to research. Perhaps even the term *participant observer* could be abandoned, and instead we could simply title all those taking part *participants* or, as already mentioned, *collaborators*. It may be helpful to understand, from a human perspective, that, if there is to be a departure, all who take part are prepared and that the researcher, too, often does feel sad. In essence, there is a real "joining" of feelings and understandings.

IS BEING A COLLABORATOR A MEANS TO AN END?

Suppose a nurse-anthropologist-researcher asked you to participate in her study titled "Contemporary Women's Hassles: An Exploratory Study," and she asked whether she could visit you in your home at various times when you were available to "sort of" observe and interview you. In addition, she asks, "Would it be all right to visit you in your office?" Rock (1979) states: "No sociologist I know would himself agree to become a subject of observational research" (p. 261).

Well, what is at stake here? When I think of this, very much is at stake, and we need to walk in our collaborators' shoes. Sure, there are hassles for the contemporary woman, but having this researcher come into my home seems not only another hassle, but perhaps a crisis! One needs to be concerned about the usual ethical considerations of fieldwork: privacy, confidentiality, achieving accurate portrayal, and inclusion and exclusion of information. In this instance, however, as in many others, the psychological burden and threat that an outsider might pose need serious consideration. Regardless of all of our efforts to act in the collaborators' best interest, some invasion, as it were, occurs to the person or people involved. The end that we hope to accomplish may be laudable, but we are fooling ourselves, I think, if we are not aware that there is some inconvenience or discomfort in the process of being observed. The unknown consequences of the observation could contribute to a pervasive state of anxiety for the participants, whether consciously or unconsciously. Rather than the casual "Within 2 to 3 weeks the person seemed comfortable with my presence" or "I was virtually unnoticed after 2 or 3 weeks," we need, as advocates, to attend to other possibilities that occur with observations. We can ask ourselves, "Would we be comfortable until the results were in?" Empathizing with and attending to the process of being an observee must be ongoing on the researcher's part. We may feel blended into a culture, but that does not mean that the observees are experientially where we are.

As already mentioned, nursing seems to espouse the deontological principle that human beings are to be treated as ends and not means. In contrast with that system is utilitarianism, which argues that the ends justify the means. From that perspective, one can use another person for the good of others and to advance further knowledge. Technically, the research enterprise turns people into means, and—though one could argue that this occurs far less with qualitative research—the potential still remains. We have come to some peace with this issue through the process of informed consent, where, in effect, the individual joins the research enterprise. Joining the effort accords individuals the opportunities of contributing to society, of being of service, and perhaps of advancing a cause of their own. We may not have thought of informed consent from that perspective, but ethically it helps to resolve the means–end dilemma and makes the term *collaborator* much more accurate.

INFORMED CONSENT IN QUALITATIVE RESEARCH

Fieldwork that is existential and authentic requires the negotiation of trust between the researcher and the participants. Entering into fields in the various roles of participant–observer is a privilege. We are "allowed" into someone else's world with its customs, practices, and events, which we promise to describe faithfully and without bias. While we are negotiating entry into this world, we invite the participants to become part of the research enterprise and validate that agreement with an informed consent. Informed consent has been defined as:

> knowing consent of an individual or the individual's legally author-
> ized representative, so situated as to be able to exercise free power of
> choice without undue inducement or any element of force, fraud,
> deceit, duress, or other forms of constraint or coercion. (Annas,
> Glantz, & Katz, 1977, p. 291)

Typically, informed consents include the title, purpose, and explanation of the research and the procedures to be followed. Risks and benefits are to be spelled out clearly. A statement that the participant has had an opportunity to ask questions and that the participant is free to withdraw at any time also is included (Field & Morse, 1985). This model of informed consent evolved out of experimental research; some of it is applicable to qualitative research, but to resolve some of the aforementioned dilemmas more is needed.

PROCESS CONSENT

Because qualitative research is conducted in an ever-changing field, informed consent should be an ongoing process. Over time, consent needs to be renegotiated as unexpected events or consequences arise. For example, I may, in a weak moment, sign a consent form for the previously mentioned researcher to observe me in my home, but without the full realization of what the consequences might be. To be ethical in this situation, the researcher needs to assess the effects of involvement in the field and continually acquire new permissions. Maybe children will react negatively to an outsider in their home, and perhaps the contemporary woman will find that keeping some semblance of cleanliness of her home on a daily basis is just the hassle that will take her over the edge.

Common sense plays a large part in renegotiating informed consent. If our focus should change, we need to ask participants for permission to change the first agreement. This is important from the perspective of sensitivity to our collaborators as well. They may wonder why you "lost" interest in a particular part of the field and chose something that you obviously have found "special." Continually informing and asking permission establish the needed trust to go further in an ethical manner.

SECRETS

Another area that needs ethical consideration in fieldwork is confidentiality of the exchanges between the researcher and the participants. Both informed and process consent should carefully delineate the data to be included in the study. Role conflict can be generated when the participant wants to tell you a secret or an off-the-record remark. The "nurse" listens to this, and in fact, knows that a valuable bond has been established. However, the "nurse researcher" and participants will probably be better off if the researcher gently reminds the participant of the purpose of the study and that all communication is supposed to be part of the study (Field & Morse, 1985). If it is possible, as may be the case in a health care facility, the participant can be referred to an appropriate person with any information not relevant to the study. The idea here is to discourage participants from telling secrets unless these secrets can be part of the study. This, of course, needs to be done with the utmost care, because secrets are treasures, but, more important, they imply promises to keep them. Most often these problems can be discussed quite openly with collaborators.

Witnessing unethical or illegal conduct can pose another ethical dilemma. If we are nurses and, as such, the clients' advocates, we cannot place the research imperative above the therapeutic imperative. Some (Estroff & Churchill, 1984) suggest that clear procedures be established prior to the start of the study that spell out the channels the researcher will go through if unethical or illegal practices are witnessed. Researchers are morally obliged from the therapeutic imperative to report such violations. The ethical response of whistle-blowing helps us to understand this particular problem.

FINDINGS AND PUBLICATION

Anonymity of subjects individually or as a group is often a requisite of qualitative research. However, sometimes individuals and cultures allow themselves to be identified. An understanding about anonymity is part of informed and process consent. What is often not mentioned or planned for is publication and dissemination of findings. With all research, what the researcher intends to do with the findings needs to be explained as part of the consent. A longitudinal view from point of entry to publication needs to be agreed upon with the collaborators. The experience of being observed can be quite different from reading a description of yourself or of your culture or hearing from someone who has such information. To prevent misunderstandings, all taking part need to agree on the various stages and activities of the entire project. What will happen to the descriptions? Will they be presented at a conference? Will they be published, and where, and for what purpose? All collaborators need to agree to dissemination of findings, from an ethical perspective of deontology, because they are part of the entire project. Because we may not foresee the consequences of publication, it is wise in this litigious society to protect not only our collaborators but also ourselves.

CONFLICT METHODOLOGY

Conflict methodology in fieldwork is built on the interactionist and eth- nomethodological perspective, adding the belief that ordinary social life is characterized by deceit and impression management (Douglas, 1979). Op- ponents of this method maintain that the researcher is justified in using sim- ilar techniques because it is the explicit purpose of research to expose the powerful and that deception is "legitimate" (Punch, 1986, p. 32).

The argument is based on an end that may in itself be highly moral (re- call Machiavelli); yet the means are acknowledgedly unethical but, within the conflict methodological view, justified. Ethical arguments are advanced for conflict methodology, but, if civilization hangs on to the Kantian princi- ple, certainly this is a most dangerous practice. The counterargument to jus- tifying deceit is nicely summed up by Warwick (1982):

> Social scientists have not only a right but an obligation to study con- troversial and politically sensitive subjects . . . but this obligation does not carry with it the right to deceive, exploit or manipulate people. My concern with backlash centers primarily on the alien- ation of ordinary individuals by research methods which leave them feeling that they have been cheated, deceived, or used. (p. 55)

In nursing research, deception, exploitation, or manipulation of people would be ethically antithetical to all that we philosophically stand for pro- fessionally. Our concept of client advocacy precludes the use of conflict methodology. In addition, we need to be alert to nuances in our research that could cause individuals to feel cheated, deceived, or used. I have often heard collaborators comment that they were supposed to receive a copy of the re- search report but never did; thus, they feel cheated. In some of our methods and consents, the collaborators actually see the report or description before its finalization to elicit their response and agreement on whether the por- trayal is accurate. This may also assist in validation. From an ethical per- spective, we need to determine which models of fieldwork seem consistent with our belief system.

MODELS OF FIELDWORK

The extent to which invasion into a social setting is ethical is often a matter of common sense. The researcher needs to be aware of what is not being told, as well as what is being said. The extent to which the research is a covert or overt operation also is open to ethical evaluation. Here, again, the ethical aim needs to be clear. There is a fine line between doing anthropological research and an investigation in the journalistic or "FBI" sense. Punch (1986) conceives of three models of fieldwork and relates them to ethical features of trust and deceit:

1. *The hypothetical "problemless" project:* For instance, a graduate student gains entry into a commune, shares daily life, is accepted, departs to write a description, and allows the culture under study to read and validate what has been written. There is no high trauma, drama, or problems, and, as Punch (1986) points out, this type of study is like the classical ethnography when the investigator could be sure that the Ashanti and Nuer would not be scouring the anthropological journals with their lawyers for negative references to tribal life. Today, I am not sure that we can even say that!

2. *The "knotty" project:* The institution erects barriers against outsiders and gaining access becomes difficult. An example might be a state mental institution where those associated with certain practices fear publication in the interest of preserving the institution's and their own reputation.

3. *The "ripping and running" project:* There is deliberate concealment, which, in addition to being ethically indefensible, is illegal. This model depends on an unrevealed person posing as a member of the group. This practice has the connotations of spying and undercover investigating and certainly violates civil liberties.

Many of us doing fieldwork like to believe that, as moral agents, we may come to identify problems and abuses within cultures or institutions. Because of that ethical aim, we may be tempted to justify unethical means, such as bending the truth, to gain entry to obtain an accurate portrayal. Such practices again constitute conflict methodology and have serious consequences for collaborators and researchers in the field. The second and third models of fieldwork hold the potential for moral, social, and political change. However, in the long run, using these two models will have the effect of closed doors in the field because of loss of trust, credibility, and confidence in nurse researchers. The last model of fieldwork violates the very foundation of our nursing practice. Whistle-blowing again is the topic that needs to be addressed and certainly is not limited to practices witnessed by researchers. For instance, in any type of health care facility where unethical practices exist, the moral obligation of reporting such practices belongs to all involved. However, as was mentioned earlier, preplanning for such events, should they occur, is one way of ensuring that your course of action is known and has been agreed on prior to the commencement of the study.

Summary Remarks

There is much more to be discussed within the topic of ethical consideration of qualitative research. There is much still to be discussed about qualitative research methods in nursing. So these remarks are not concluding but contribute to the dialogue centered on the developed interest in these methods. One facet is clear: one cannot adopt criteria for quantitative research and apply them to qualitative research. The static, past tense of informed consent does not adequately protect human subjects in qualitative studies. For that matter, it may not always do so for quantitative methods.

The most glaring difference, however, springs from the dynamic, process-oriented qualities of qualitative research. Qualitative research could be thought of as a verb, a process, with the ethical components constantly being scrutinized. "Process consenting" might be a way to remind ourselves of the ongoing nature of discussing with our collaborators the means and the aims of our study. In addition, our therapeutic imperative and research imperative need to be made as clear as possible. From an ethical perspective, the therapeutic imperative undergirds the research imperative so that efforts to avoid any difficulties for or disadvantages of the collaborator need our constant vigilance if the research is to proceed ethically. Because we, as nurses, have the ethical theme of deontology threaded throughout our philosophies, I think we are humanistically ahead of many other disciplines in considering the ethics of our research enterprise. Our egos are not split. We are patient–client advocates, and trust, compassion, and empathy encompass all our nursing endeavors, including research.

References

Annas, D. J., Glantz, L. H., & Katz, B. J. (1977). *Informed consent to human experimentation: The subject's dilemma.* Boston: Ballinger.

Bellah, R. (1981). The ethical aims of social inquiry. *Teachers College Record, 83*(1), 1–18.

Douglas, J. D. (1979). Living morality versus bureaucratic fist. In C. B. Klockars & F. W. O'Connor (Eds.), *Deviance and decency.* Beverly Hills, CA: Sage.

Estroff, S. E., & Churchill, L. R. (1984). Comment (Ethical dilemmas). *Anthropology Newsletter, 25*(7).

Field, P., & Morse, J. (1985). *Nursing research: The application of qualitative approaches.* Rockville, MD: Aspen.

Laudan, L. (1977). *Progress and its problems: Towards a theory of scientific growth.* Berkeley: University of California Press.

Punch, M. (1986). *The politics and ethics of fieldwork.* Beverly Hills, CA: Sage.

Rock, P. (1979). *The making of symbolic interactionism.* London: Macmillan.

Warwick, D. P. (1982). Tearsome trade: Means and ends in social research. In M. Bulmer (Ed.), *Social research ethics*. London: Macmillan.

Wilson, L., & Fitzpatrick, J. (1984). Dialectic thinking as a means of understanding systems in development: Relevance to Roger's principles. *Advances in Nursing Service, 6*(2), 41.

ADDITIONAL REFERENCES

Aamodt, A. (1983). Problems in doing nursing research: Developing criteria for evaluating qualitative research. *Western Journal of Nursing Research, 5,* 398–402.

Amason, J. P. (1990). Cultural critique and cultural presuppositions: Hermeneutics and critical theory. *Philosophy and Social Criticism, 15*(1), 125–150.

Cutliffe, J. R., & Ramcharan, P. (2002). Leveling the playing field? Exploring the merits of the ethics-as-process approach for judging qualitative research proposals. *Qualitative Health Research, 12*(7), 1000–1010.

Denzin, N., & Lincoln, Y. (1994). *Handbook of qualitative research*. Thousand Oaks, CA: Sage.

Ensign, J. (2003). Ethical issues in qualitative health research with homeless youths. *Journal of Advanced Nursing, 43*(1), 43–50.

Erlandson, D. A., Harris, E., Skipper, B. L., & Allen, S. D. (1993). *Doing naturalistic inquiry: A guide to methods*. Newbury Park, CA: Sage.

Ferguson, L., Yonge, O., & Myrick, F. (2004). Students' involvement in faculty research: Ethical and methodological issues. *International Journal of Qualitative Methods, 3*(4), article 5.

Flicker, S., Haans, D., & Skinner, H. (2004). Ethical dilemmas in research on Internet communities. *Qualitative Health Research, 14*(1), 124–134.

Hofman, N. G. (2004). Toward critical research ethics: Transforming ethical conduct in qualitative health care research. *Health Care for Women International, 25*(7), 647–662.

Kayser-Jones, J. (2003). Continuing to conduct research in nursing homes despite controversial findings: Reflections by a research scientist. *Qualitative Health Research, 13*(1), 114–128.

Lemmens, T., & Singer, P. (1998). Bioethics for clinicians: Conflicts of interest in research, education, and patient care. *Canadian Medical Association Journal, 159*(8), 960–965.

Morse, J. (2005). Ethical issues in institutional research. *Qualitative Health Research, 15*(4), 435–437.

Lincoln, Y., & Guba, E. (1985). *Naturalistic inquiry*. Beverly Hills, CA: Sage.

Orb, A., Eisenhauer, L., & Wynaden, D. (2001). Ethics in qualitative research. *Journal of Nursing Scholarship, 33*(1), 93–96.

Patterson, D., & Brogden, L. (2004). Living spaces for talk within the academy. *International Journal of Qualitative Methods, 3*(3), article 2.

Richards, H. M., & Schwartz, L. J. (2002). Ethics of qualitative research: Are there special issues for health services research? *Family Practice, 19*(2), 135–139.

Sandelowski, M. (1986). The problem of rigor in qualitative research. *Advances in Nursing Research, 8,* 27–37.

Schutz, S. (1994). Exploring the benefits of a subjective approach in qualitative nursing research. *Journal of Advanced Nursing, 20*(3), 412–417.

Shenton, A. K. (2004). Strategies for ensuring trustworthiness in qualitative research projects. *Education for Information, 22*(2), 63–75.

Ulrich, C., & Grady, C. (2004). Editorial: Financial incentives and response rates in nursing research. *Nursing Research, 53*(2), 73–74.

Van-Amburg, R. (1997). A Copernican revolution in clinical ethics: Engagement versus disengagement. *American Journal of Occupational Therapy, 51*(3), 186–190.

Van den Hoonarrd, W. C. (Ed.). (2002). *Walking the tightrope: Ethical issues for qualitative researchers*. Toronto: University of Toronto Press.

Watson, J. (1990). Caring knowledge and informed moral passion. *Advances in Nursing Science, 13*, 15–24.

Watson, J. (1995). Postmodernism and knowledge development in nursing. *Nursing Science Quarterly, 8*(2), 60–64.

Watson, L., & Girard, F. (2004). Establishing integrity and avoiding methodological misunderstanding. *Qualitative Health Research, 14*(6), 875–881.

Wilde, V. (1992). Controversial hypothesis on the relationship between researcher and informant in qualitative research. *Journal of Advanced Nursing, 17*, 234–242.

Zeni, J. (Ed.). (2001). *Ethical issues in practitioner research*. New York: Teachers College Press.

22

Institutional Review of Qualitative Research Proposals: A Task of No Small Consequence

Patricia L. Munhall

PLACING THE TASK IN CONTEXT

A colleague of mine sent her research proposal to a large university hospital where the sample for her study was to be derived. She followed the format precisely and was somewhat surprised when she was asked to appear before the institutional review board (IRB) of the hospital. When she arrived, she was astonished to find 26 members of the board present. They discussed the project with her for 2 hours and engaged in what appeared to be an internal struggle over the design and conceptual framework of the study before granting her permission to conduct the study.

My colleague's study was a traditional *quantitative* research project. Ironically, the study was not to be conducted within the institution itself; rather, the nurse researcher wanted to do a follow-up mailing to all patients who had

Reprinted with permission from Sage Publications; *Qualitative Nursing Research: A Contemporary Dialogue*, J. Morse (Ed.), 1989, 1991, pp. 258–271.

had hip replacement surgery. My purpose in this chapter is to place the review of qualitative research proposals in a perspective from which this context can be understood.

The foregoing example is given to demonstrate the institutional review of your proposal, whether qualitative or quantitative, can be a challenging task at best. According to Noble (1985), institutional reviews often pose problems for researchers, *regardless* of the research method: "A frequent solution . . . is to engage in minimally clinical projects, such as research involving healthy, intelligent, middle-class clients" (p. 293). Using this solution, many researchers have looked for subjects outside institutions, which is one alternative. However, because many nurse researchers are committed to research within institutions, the aim of this chapter is to facilitate the IRB process, specifically with qualitative research proposals.

THE SETTING

In this chapter, the presentation of qualitative research methods to IRBs in institutional settings is addressed. Similarities of IRB requirements for qualitative and quantitative research designs are discussed. Departures and additions specific to qualitative research methods are analyzed, with emphasis on the educational aspect of research proposals. The idea of process consent also is examined, and the appearance of qualitative researchers before IRBs with research proposals is discussed.

IRBs are the conscience of an institution. They are deeply concerned with human rights and human dignity. The principles of patient autonomy and rights of privacy, confidentiality, anonymity, self-determination, and safety are critical components of the philosophical statements of IRBs.

The most important aspect of any research proposal is the education of our colleagues about qualitative methods and the assurance that we have the same concerns for the dignity and rights of our human subjects. A psychological principle pervades this need for education because most people are generally invested in the status quo, that is, the familiar. Individual members of IRBs are, for the most part, accustomed to the traditional quantitative research design and thus feel a certain amount of confidence when reviewing these proposals. Qualitative research designs within the traditional medical science setting present problems for these IRB members and raise questions simply because the reviewers are unfamiliar with the more unstructured qualitative research methods. This leaves the qualitative nurse researcher with a task of no small consequence.

THE CHALLENGES

Qualitative research in institutional settings presents challenges different from those of more traditional research methods. The three main challenges in receiving permission to conduct qualitative research in institutions are as follows:

1. The IRB's possible unfamiliarity with the methods, language, and legitimacy of qualitative research
2. The structural-functionalist perspective that pervades most institutions
3. The conscious or unconscious perception of the similarity of qualitative research methods to investigative-type activities

Although these challenges are interrelated, each one is addressed separately.

Unfamiliarity with Qualitative Research Methods

Most IRBs (and, in fact, many grant review panels) have members who are unfamiliar with the aims and outcomes of qualitative research. At present, many IRBs are developing guidelines and are uncertain about the role that the boards play in their institutions. Their task is complex—so complex that a request for the release of names to do a follow-up mailing to former patients (as previously described) can result in a major meeting of the IRB. The receipt of a proposal with a method called "phenomenology" also may result in an invitation to provide further information. Phenomenological studies aim at understanding a phenomenon by studying the essences of a life experience with thoughtful attention, and they search for what it means to be human in the attempt to discover plausible insight. Many members of IRBs are not familiar with such language in a research proposal. They will ask, "What is phenomenology?" or "What is grounded theory?" Although these questions do not spell disaster for proposed qualitative research projects, they do complicate matters because these important questions are asked from the structural-functional perspective of institutions.

The Structural-Functional Approach of Institutions

The structural-functional perspective is often viewed as the sacrosanct way of organizing a bureaucratic institution. Roles are prescribed, functions are distributed, behavior and outcomes are predictable, and all should go well according to fixed rules and procedures. The values in our health care institutions seem removed from or, at best, unrelated to qualitative research aims.

For the most part, within our health care institutions, pragmatic goals prevail. There should be an action, an intervention, and a concrete observable task with a measurable outcome. Pragmatism in research is narrowly perceived—for example, the idea of testing something to solve some problem. The idea that understanding preceding experience or any lived experience has pragmatic value is not self-evident from the highly structured functional perspective. From this perspective, the search for meaning appears irrelevant. It is this search for meaning that creates confusion in some minds about the difference between qualitative research and investigative journalism.

Similarity of Qualitative Methods to Investigative Journalism

All research methods are essentially investigations, but perhaps they are more threatening to individuals when unstructured interviews and the possibility of a participant observation technique are part of the research design. Quantitative research designs are by nature more specific, the variables are already known, and the researcher searches for relations between variables. On the other hand, discovery, the finding out about something otherwise not fully understood, is often the aim of qualitative research designs.

Within institutions, such studies may be perceived as threatening. Interviewing patients may cause staff to worry about negative information that the patient may give—for example, complaints, reporting incidents, and so forth. If there is to be observation, who does not experience some anxiety about the idea of being observed? Fear, then, is an important feeling to consider, and one that cannot be summarily dismissed: What if you do "discover" some "negative" findings that do not reflect well on the institution or staff?

These challenges must be addressed in any proposal presented to an IRB. The strategies for meeting these challenges include education and translation, the establishment of compatible values, and the generation of trust.

MEETING THE CHALLENGES

Education and Translation

Becoming sympathetic to the concerns and psychological dynamics of the members of IRBs is the best place to start. In many cases, qualitative research proposals may not be understood by these people, may be contrary to the way that they think, and may be threatening to them. In addressing these challenges, one should realize that the normal human response to change is resistance. Many qualitative nurse researchers in institutions have reported that "resistance" was the only response to their research proposals and that they have had to change their proposals or move out of the institution. Although this situation is unfortunate, it can be prevented if qualitative nurse researchers will educate their colleagues who sit on IRBs about the nature and philosophy of qualitative methods.

Most board members are thoroughly familiar with the methods associated with the Western mind-set of objectivity, control, prediction, and so forth. No one needs to explain ex post facto correlation, experimental design, or statistical test, but phenomenology, grounded theory, ethnography, or whatever qualitative research method is going to be used must be explained. Not only must it be explained, but it must be presented in language that can be understood by people familiar with deductive, pragmatic, numerical ideologies. There is a need to explain in concrete terms the primacy of perception, embodiment, and the philosophical concepts. All these ideas should be clearly stated in language that the reader will understand. For example, in submitting a proposal for a qualitative research project that will examine the needs of patients who have had a mastectomy so that appropriate nursing interventions can be developed, language such as "the lived experience" of having a mastectomy, "consciousness," and "essences" may be used but need to be explained. Is this a capitulation, a compromising of our principles? On the contrary, it is the recognition that it can take years to understand these concepts and that, in a proposal, there is a limited amount of time and space for explanation. So, instead of a capitulation, it is actually a pragmatic action for a pragmatic setting. If the institution uses a structural-functionalist approach, it is unrealistic to think that this perspective will not also be reflected in the process of an IRB review.

Compatible Values

In structural-functional bureaucracies, the reality is that the search for meaning, the apprehension of essential relations among essences, the thematic analysis of cultures, the perception of another's world, and the discovery of core variables are at odds with the predominant problem-task orientation. Helping patients find meaning does not rank high among institutional objectives. So this objective must be stated in the proposal in pragmatic terms—such as, this study will result in improved nursing care, or this study will act as the basis for developing nursing intervention. The qualitative method must also appear structured, even if the design allows for fluidity and some flexibility. As far as possible, research aims should be compatible with the aims of the institution. The members of the IRB must not think that they are making an exception by accepting a qualitative research proposal because it appears different from their value orientation. It is best, from any point of view, to demonstrate the convergence of values between the institution and the qualitative study by stating how the study's quest for discovery is laying the groundwork for nursing intervention.

Generating Trust

Developing trust and alleviating fear or anxiety or both within the institution are critical to a successful qualitative research proposal, and they are also two of the more awkward challenges. This awkwardness arises from the perplexing situation in which the staff worry about the researcher having access to potentially damaging information or observing poor nursing care. They wonder what the researcher is going to do with possible "negative" findings. The difficulty can be dealt with by pointing out that quantitative researchers in institutions may witness and be part of the same environmental activities as qualitative researchers and that the staff are probably aware of whatever problems exist. Ideally, ethics committees or quality assurance programs address these problems, yet there is always the possibility that qualitative research may uncover some problems, and consequently, the staff may feel threatened.

The first step in dealing with this problem is to include a category for "unexpected findings" in the proposal and to carefully spell out what channels the nurse researcher will use to share such findings. If the members of the IRB understand that the discovery of findings that indicate problems is important so that they can then be solved, members and staff might be more assured. Again, education is important for achieving this perceptual shift.

Traditionally, IRBs are familiar with research that attempts to solve problems. The value of research that may identify problems so that they, too, may be addressed needs to be stressed, and stressed, and stressed. Indeed, it is critical to identify the right problem before testing solutions. Sometimes this is difficult to do, such as when patients complain during interviews about poor nursing care. A good qualitative researcher looks at the larger context (before reporting such a result, ethics demands that the lens of the study must be widened) and finds that there is inadequate staffing. Although the administration may not be happy with that finding, the nurses on the unit will be glad to have such an important need substantiated. At other times, the problem is thornier. Perhaps the poor nursing care is the result of an incompetent nurse. Although the nurse researcher cannot be the only one to know of this, he or she is ethically obligated to report such a finding through the channels that are established prior to starting the project.

Although this is essentially whistle-blowing, with its attendant conse-quences, sometimes good, sometimes bad, *this action embodies the belief that the therapeutic imperative of nursing (advocacy) takes precedence over the research imperative (advancing knowledge) if conflict develops* (Chapter 21 herein). These problems have fewer ramifications for researchers not re-searching in their home institutions, and, if possible, it may be wise not to conduct research in one's home institution. Additionally, IRBs have mem-bers who wish to protect their institutions or their own reputations or both. This difficult problem should be addressed in qualitative research proposals in positive, helpful terms and fully discussed with staff. They, too, need to be fully informed about the research project.

SIMILARITIES BETWEEN QUALITATIVE AND QUANTITATIVE PROPOSALS

Many similar areas in qualitative and quantitative proposals are of concern to IRBs. More than likely, the same form will be used for both types of meth-ods, and the researcher will be asked to address the following areas:

1. Objective of study
2. Research methodology
3. Characteristics of group(s)
4. Special groups (e.g., children of compromised adults)
5. Type of content
6. Confidentiality of data
7. Possible risks

Although there may be other variables, ensuring that individual rights and human dignity are protected needs to be demonstrated and documented. Of-ten, IRBs have more elaborate requests than those listed here, and qualita-tive research proposals are often evaluated on the basis of adherence to traditional scientific method. Scientific legitimacy, then, is being evaluated rather than human subjects' protection. This may not be a problem 10 years from now, but, today, proposals come back from IRBs with questions that in-dicate reluctance of the IRB to approve the proposal because the board does not understand the method and its concomitant language. As previously sug-gested, educating members of IRBs about the scientific legitimacy of quali-tative studies is an additional task for qualitative nurse researchers. What follows are some distinguishing characteristics of qualitative research that need to be addressed in IRB proposals.

Departure and Additions for Qualitative Research Proposals

A brief overview of the aim and purpose of qualitative research methodology may precede the proposal or, perhaps, be the introductory paragraph, depending on the institution. This overview does not have to be a highly sophisticated discourse about worldviews and paradigms, with quotations from Husserl, Erasmus, or Speigelberg; rather, a simple paragraph explaining how qualitative research methodology seeks to discover new knowledge, uses narrative descriptions in the findings, includes interviews with individual participants, and so forth, is all that is necessary. Stating that these aspects of the methodology can be used to build on one another may be important. Nurse researchers often get into difficulty by discussing intersubjectivity, going "to the things themselves," living the question, and so on. Understandable language is critical.

Objective of the Study.   As previously discussed, the objective of the study should be ultimately stated in pragmatic language. Often the aim of qualitative research is stated in existential terms. Remember the setting and take the existential purpose one step further by showing how the study might, for example, (1) improve staff performance, and (2) assist the patient in recovery. This approach is appropriate because it is the qualitative research baseline that enables quantitative researchers to develop hypotheses for nursing intervention, staff performance, and assisting patients in their recovery. Stress the importance of the study in pragmatic terms.

Research Method.   Perhaps the most important part of the proposal, the research method offers the best opportunity for educating members of IRBs. Introduce the method, the rationale for choosing the method, and the outcome of this method. Take the reader through a step-by-step narrative in language that is familiar. This may mean taking the proposal that was written for nursing colleagues of a similar bent and translating it for persons who may be puzzled by the use of the word *phenomenon*. For example, instead of saying "lived experience," just say "experience." In fact, someone once asked me "what other kind of experience is there?" Perhaps replacing the phrase "ontological commitment" with "it is my belief that" also would be helpful. Although it may be human to want to impress one's colleagues with a high level of abstraction, it will probably be counterproductive. In any case, it seems paradoxical when qualitative research is actually very interested in the concrete. No one wants to feel inadequate, and it seems unwise to send out proposals loaded with unfamiliar language. Again, to achieve IRB approval, members must be able to read qualitative research proposals without a dictionary!

So, qualitative researchers need to be clear and emphatic about their research methods. They need to teach about the method and its pragmatic usefulness to nursing sciences in language that will not distract the readers but keep them focused on the substance.

Consequence.   There is a debate in the literature about whether informed consent is necessary when observations and discourse take place in the course of a nurse's routine work (Noble, 1985; Oberst, 1985). Interviews have often been exempt from formal informed consent procedures if individual verbal consent is given. However, I fear we will be on a slippery slope if too many of these exceptions to the written consent process are allowed. Common sense must prevail.

Within institutions, qualitative researchers need to anticipate a request for informed consent. If more than one interview or observation is going to take place, the idea of a process consent seems to exemplify a negotiated view of not only the phenomenon but also the study itself (Chapter 21). All consents need to take into consideration the capacity of the person consenting, full disclosure of the research activity, and the freedom of participants to voluntarily enter and withdraw.

A proposal for process consent is suggested because an informed consent represents a past-tense concept. Qualitative research is often an ongoing, dynamic, changing process. A process consent offers researchers and participants opportunities to actualize a negotiated view and to change arrangements if necessary. A process consent encourages mutual participation and, perhaps, mutual affirmation for the participants and the researcher.

A process consent for qualitative nursing research should be developed with the research participants' input, ideas, and suggestions and should be reviewed at specific times if necessary. This approach is appropriate if the researcher is going to be doing observations or participant observations over a period of time. In addition to the informed consent, a process consent should address some of the processes listed in Table 22–1.

It is probably wise to have information about self-disclosed secrets in the process consent. It should be stated that all data obtained will be part of the study. In other words, secrets should be discouraged if they cannot be included in the study. It is best to explain to the participants that some secrets pose a dilemma for researchers who are also concerned about patient well-being. The question of secrets and patients' confidentiality needs to be planned, and ethical dilemmas need to be considered before the proposal is written (see Chapter 21).

Confidentiality and Anonymity.   The same guarantee of confidentiality of data and anonymity of participants that quantitative researchers give must be made a general principle of qualitative research. This is a general principle

---

TABLE 22-1 Process Consent

Researcher and participants as collaborators come to agree on the following:
- How you will enter the field
- How often, for how long
- How you will leave the field
- How you will prepare to leave
- How you will share the information
- How you will keep the information anonymous and confidential
- How you will ensure an accurate portrayal
- What you will do if focus changes
- What you will do with "unanticipated findings"
- What you will do with secrets and confidential material
- What you will do with inclusion and exclusion of information
- Where the findings are to go

Comments by participant

Comments by researcher

Dates reviewed and changes made

Signatures

Note: Each study would require a specific process consent, depending on the substance of the study. This process consent is in addition to the usual components of informed consent.

because some institutions allow participant identities to be known, especially if the study is going to reflect positively on them. In addition, some participants enjoy being identified in certain kinds of interviews or studies. However, the general principle is to maintain confidentiality and anonymity.

In qualitative research, can we promise confidentiality when we include precise quotations from the transcripts in our publications? The answer is no, but we can provide anonymity by protecting the identity of the participant. Consequently, individuals and institutions will want assurances that only the researcher(s) will have access to the data and that there will be no identifying evidence, such as names on cassettes, names on computer printouts, and so forth. They will also want information about how and where the data will be stored. In this section of the proposal, it might be helpful to identify the lines of communication that have been established for reporting findings. Information concerning the plans for disseminating the findings (i.e., publication, presentation, and who will receive final reports) should be included and mutually agreed on.

Possible Risks. Qualitative research is considered noninvasive, but, in a sense, that is a limited perception of the word. Although it is true that qualitative researchers do not physically alter the participants with interventions, there are invasions of their space and psyches. Although such invasion is often therapeutic, it can pose possible risks if certain precautions are not taken.

It is well substantiated that talking has therapeutic benefits. Patients in institutions, or staff for that matter, often find relief just "getting it out of their system" or "off their chest." Nursing intervention often provides opportunities for patients to ventilate their feelings, and interviews provide such opportunities. Attention is usually viewed as a positive experience, and being important enough to study can be viewed positively. That someone's experience is worth studying can have a validating effect.

Are there risks in qualitative research? One reviewer from an IRB asked about "triggering" an emotional response within an informant. This possibility cannot be lightly dismissed if the experiences under study are highly charged. Because of their training, nurse researchers are usually able to intervene appropriately and make good assessments about how a patient is responding. It may be normal if a patient becomes upset in the course of an interview, and the nurse researcher must be supportive and manage the interview with good clinical judgment. Arrangements also should be made with the patient's primary caretaker to support the patient after leaving the field. Aamodt (1986), still very relevant today, writes:

> In the Human Subject Consent Forms we had said there were no
> psychological or social risks. Because communication in response
> to client feelings is an expected nursing intervention, to ignore
> such a need could be classified as irresponsible. We planned that
> interviewers would not be the primary caretaker of the child, and
> when the situation demanded it, the child and parent were referred
> to the primary caretaker. (p. 167)

An inaccurate portrayal of participants or situations can also cause harm. A statement of how you intend to ensure the accurate description of participants and situations should be included in this section of the proposal. Validation by the participants is respectful and necessary for authentic representation. The harm/benefit question is succinctly placed in context by Morse (1988) when she states:

> Are the risks to the participant any greater than the everyday risk
> from confiding in a friend? And the "friend" in this context is a reg-
> istered nurse who is accustomed to handling confidential informa-
> tion, counseling the dying and the distressed, observing and
> listening. Yet, suddenly, because the information is obtained under
> the auspices of "research" (rather than practice), the activities of
> the nurse may be considered by the IRB as potentially harmful. We
> must learn to trust our colleagues. (p. 214)

PRESENTING TO THE IRB

When presenting to an IRB panel, anticipate as many questions as possible. Consider the presentation a wonderful opportunity to discuss your study. However, educating IRB members about your research methods and translating them into clear, concrete, pragmatic terms should also be done in the verbal presentation. Know who the board members are and avoid answering questions in a philosophical or existential style. If there is a member of the clergy on the board, he or she might understand your answer, but the lawyer, the physician, the two laypeople, the banker, and the accountant might not, so keep your discussion clear and precise. Remember, the intentions of the IRB are the same as yours: to protect the patient.

In summary, writing clearly (especially philosophical translation), suggesting compatible values between the institution's goals and the research goals, developing trust, and establishing clear lines of communication are important areas to consider when submitting a qualitative research proposal to an IRB.

CONCLUSION

What I would like to stress again when writing a proposal for the IRB are the parts of this chapter that suggest keeping the language of your proposal as close as possible to understandable, everyday language. Examples have been provided in this chapter. The language of qualitative research is often philosophical and calls for an understanding, for example, of the philosophical underpinnings of phenomenology. Those concepts need to be translated into everyday language and terms.

The rule here is to simplify, simplify, simplify. This is not the time to sound as knowledgeable as you are, when you know that most members of IRBs do not have knowledge of, or familiarity with, the language of qualitative methods.

IRBs and granting organizations are making a concerted effort to include qualitative researchers on their panels, which is encouraging. Look at who is on your IRB to ascertain who your audience is and then you can adjust your proposal accordingly.

REFERENCES

Aamodt, A. (1986). Discovering the child's view of alopecia: Doing ethnography. In P. Munhall & C. Oiler (Eds.), *Nursing research: A qualitative perspective* (pp. 163–171). Norwalk, CT: Appleton-Century-Crofts.

Morse, J. (1988). Commentaries on special issues. *Western Journal of Nursing Research,* *10*(2), 213–216.

Noble, M. (1985). Written informed consent: Closing the door to clinical research. *Nursing Outlook, 33*(6), 292–293.

Oberst, M. (1985). Another look at informed consent. *Nursing Outlook, 33*(6), 294–295.

ADDITIONAL REFERENCES

Burns, R. (1989). Standards for qualitative research. *Nursing Science Quarterly, 2,* 44–52.

Byrne, M. (2001). Disseminating and presenting qualitative research findings. *AORN Journal, 74*(5), 731–732.

Denzin, N., & Lincoln, Y. (1994). *Handbook of qualitative research.* Thousand Oaks, CA: Sage.

Dixon-Woods, M., Shaw, R. L., Agarwal, S., & Smith, J. A. (2004). The problem of appraising qualitative research. *Quality and Safety in Health Care, 13*(3), 223–225.

Erlandson, D. A., Harris, E., Skipper, B. L., & Allen, S. D. (1993). *Doing naturalistic inquiry: A guide to methods.* Newbury Park, CA: Sage.

Field, P., & Morse, J. (1985). *Nursing research: The application of qualitative approaches.* London: Croom Helm.

Jones, M. L. (2004). Application of systematic review methods to qualitative research: Practical issues. *Journal of Advanced Nursing, 48*(3), 271–278.

Lincoln, Y. S., & Tierney, W. G. (2004). Qualitative research and institutional review boards. *Qualitative Inquiry, 10*(2), 219–234.

Miller, S., & Fredericks, M. (2003). The nature of "evidence" in qualitative research. *International Journal of Qualitative Methods, 2*(1), article 4.

Morse, J. M. (2003). A review committee's guide for evaluating qualitative proposals. *Qualitative Health Research, 13*(6), 833–851.

Munhall, P. (1988). Ethical considerations in qualitative research. *Western Journal of Nursing Research, 10*(2), 150–162.

Munhall, P., & Oiler, C. (1986). *Nursing research: A qualitative perspective.* Norwalk, CT: Appleton-Century-Crofts.

Powell, A. E. (2001). Reading and assessing qualitative research. *Hospital Medicine, 62*(6), 360–363.

Richards, H. M., & Schwartz, L. J. (2002). Ethics of qualitative research: Are there special issues for health services research? *Family Practice, 19*(2), 135–139.

Sandelowski, M., & Barosso, J. (2002). Reading qualitative studies. *International Journal of Qualitative Methods, 1*(1), article 5.

Thorne, S., Joachim, G., Paterson, B., & Canam, C. (2002). Influence of the research frame on qualitatively derived health science knowledge. *International Journal of Qualitative Methods, 1*(1), article 1.

23

Strategies of
Intraproject Sampling

Janice M. Morse

Sampling, that is, deciding whom to interview or to observe, is a significant issue in qualitative inquiry. The participants selected to participate in the study and the interviewing or observational skills of the researcher invariably influence the nature of the data, the scope of the study, the depth of meaning, the complexity of the interpretation obtained, and the rate at which saturation is obtained. Although much has been written about strategies for, and types of, sampling to be used at the beginning of a project, sampling strategies to be used once analysis is developing have been relatively ignored. Researchers are advised to scope the domain by sampling for variation, to theoretically sample (according to the needs of the developing theory [Glaser, 1978]), and to continue sampling until saturation occurs.

   In this chapter, I briefly review strategies for sampling used at the beginning of a project, to ensure familiarity with all the terms and approaches to and conditions for sampling. The major focus of the chapter, however, is on

An earlier version of this chapter was published as Morse, J. M. (2001). Types of talk: Modes of responses and data-led analytic strategies. In P. Munhall (Ed.), *Nursing research: A qualitative perspective* (3rd ed., pp. 565–578). Boston: Jones and Bartlett Publishers.

strategies of intraproject sampling—mechanisms of sampling used once the analysis is underway and the theoretical scheme is developing—and one of the most difficult problems of all, how to recognize that saturation has been reached and when to stop sampling.

REVIEW OF SAMPLING STRATEGIES USED AT THE BEGINNING OF A PROJECT

Qualitative researchers sample for *meaning*, rather than frequency. We are not interested in how much, or how many, but in *what*. For this reason, as well as the fact that qualitative data are clumsy, time-consuming, and expensive to analyze, we deliberately seek participants according to two criteria: first, the fit between their experience and our research question, and second, the presence of the characteristics of a "good informant."

1. *Experiential fit*: We deliberately select participants who may be considered experts in the same phenomenon that we are exploring. The participants will have either lived through the experience (for a retrospective account), are presently undergoing the experience, or have observed someone going through the experience. All of these perspectives differ and have important ramifications for the design of the study. The quality of the data is determined in part by the content, the information, and the type of description, detail, and range of experience offered by the participant.

   I have argued that qualitative inquiry is deliberately biased. We deliberately select the best case and the participants who are maximally experienced rather than those having "average" experiences. When we purposefully select according to the best example, the characteristics of whatever we are studying are easier to identify than in situations that are muted with contextual factors.

2. *Qualities of a good informant*: The second set of characteristics to be considered involves the personal qualities of the participant. Obviously, a researcher would be wasting time to interview a participant who was not willing to talk, or who did not have time to participate. Because the *quality of the data* is determined by the willingness of the participant to talk, to reflect, and to describe, and his or her ability to share the experience with the researcher, the researcher must consider the personal traits of participants when inviting them into the study. The researcher should take time to develop trust with the par-

ticipant, and, of course, the interview is largely facilitated by both the ability to listen and the skills of the researcher as an interviewer.

Qualitative researchers deliberately select their sample using these two criteria—a process called a *purposive sampling*. Often, however, the qualitative researcher is unable to obtain adequate information about participants before the interview is scheduled. Participants are usually obtained by using a convenience sample: they volunteer, are self-identified by advertising, or are recruited by a third person. If they are recruited by some criterion that ensures variation in the sample, such as gender, age groups, or even scores on some test, it is called a *quota* sample. Occasionally, the researcher is studying a topic that makes it difficult to break into a social group (for instance, the researcher may be studying a stigmatizing topic or illegal behavior); when the first participant is requested to solicit another participant, it is called a *snowball* or *nominated sample*.

Random samples are never used in qualitative inquiry because characteristics in a population are distributed according to some form of a normal curve. This means that the qualitative researchers can oversample in the center of the distribution and undersample in the tails. This is problematic because qualitative researchers consider the experience to be equally important anywhere along the baseline, and if we use random sampling, we will have excessive data about common experiences, which wastes our funds during analysis. Moreover, these data overwhelm and dominate the analysis (perhaps by lulling the investigator into premature closure), and because too few data are obtained at the tails of the distribution, data are inadequate for analysis or for saturation. Worse, these data may even be ignored. For these reasons, the distribution of a qualitative study should resemble a rectangle rather than a curve. In actual fact, data analysis part way through the project is not that neat, but is uneven, resembling "pumpkin denture work," with ample data obtained on some aspects and inadequate data in others. Once this is recognized, sampling may be targeted to the deficient areas. I discuss this later in the chapter.

Other factors influence the quality of the initial sample. People volunteer to be in a study for many reasons—perhaps volunteering means they can get away from work and sit down; perhaps they are curious about what is being asked or what goes on in the interview room. When nonpurposeful sampling is used, often the researcher may not discover until the interview is underway that the participant is not a good fit for the project. What to do? I recommend *secondary sampling*. Complete the interview, politely thank the participant, label and make comments on the tape, but do not enter the tape into the data set. Do not spend funds to have it transcribed or spend time analyzing it, but also do not discard it. Later in the study when you understand what is going on, this interview may be invaluable as an excellent example of thus-and-so—or maybe not.

In summary, sampling is initially guided by the availability of participants and is continued until the researcher has a feel for the topic and has often begun coding and categorizing. At this point, data collection is not a matter of simple perseverance, a "hit or miss" process of collecting yet more data, but rather a thoughtful and deliberate process.

STAGES OF INTRAPROJECT SAMPLING

The form and strategies of sampling change as the project progresses. In this section, I discuss sampling for *scope*, sampling to *determine variation*, sampling for *saturation*, and sampling for *verification*. Each of these strategies is used according to the level of development of the project, entails different techniques, and must be separately attended to and evaluated.

Sampling for Scope

Scoping is the process of identifying the boundaries of the phenomenon. It enables the researcher to determine what is and what is not an example of the phenomenon, what is included or excluded, and why. Scoping is attended to early in the study because if the researcher decides to define the phenomenon very tightly and narrowly, the sample (and the study itself) will be much smaller than if the project were more broadly defined. Narrow projects saturate much more rapidly than do more expansive projects and are easier to conduct because they are less complex, but they are also less useful and less generalizable. Narrow projects often are conducted by students, and many use a sample size of less than 10 participants.

Scope is invariably determined by the participants. One method is to use Spradley's (1979) method of unstructured interviews, asking one "grand tour" question, and then providing the participants with space to "tell their story" with minimal interruption, at their own pace, starting wherever they wish to start. An excellent example of determining the scope of a project was provided once by a doctoral student. Her topic was the bereavement experiences of spouses with partners who had died of Alzheimer's disease. This student settled down with her tape recorder and her first participant, explained what the interview was about, and obtained consent. To her surprise, the participant started the interview by telling her all about her marriage, what happened when her spouse became ill, and then when he died. Because the student was conducting the project without a grant and did not have research funding (or spare tapes), she turned the tape recorder off at the beginning of the story. Only when the participant reached the "relevant" part of the story (i.e., the bereavement process after the death of the spouse), did she begin to record the interview.

When she conducted the second interview, the same thing happened. That widow also began her story by describing her marriage, the illness, and her husband's death; again, the student turned off the tape recorder, not wanting to waste tapes on extraneous details. In fact, it was not until the fourth interview that the student realized that her participants were telling her that unless she understood the nature of their relationship during their marriage and the impact of the illness on their relationship, she could not understand the bereavement process. Thereafter, she turned her recorder on at the beginning of each narrative.

The researcher becomes an active listener in an unstructured interview, tracking the story as it is told, and stacks questions about additional details to be asked at a later time. The interviewer must remember critical junctures so that at the end of the interview the researcher can take the participant back to those points and ask about alternative storylines. Questions that the researcher may ask during the interview must be done without interrupting the flow of the narrative and are asked at the end of the interview, or in subsequent interviews: "You told me that when you received news about the positive biopsy you resisted your husband's pleas to seek alternative therapy. Can you tell me about that?"

The form of unstructured interviews varies. The researcher may decide to interview participants prospectively as they are going through the experience. In this case the interviews could be conducted at various points during the experience. Alternatively, the interviews could be retrospective, conducted after the event, with the participant being asked to relate "the whole story." Participants usually define the parameters of the events themselves so that, as the researcher increases the number of participants in the study, there is some variation not only in how the event was experienced, but there may also be differences in focus (including how the self or others are presented), differences in levels of generality, and differences in perspectives. For instance, the researcher may be interested in identifying dimensions of scope (best case/worst case). In this example, the scope or parameters of an area are elicited by expanding from the generalized case to the worst case:

Interviewer: Do you have any memories of some very unpleasant situations?

Subject: Yup. Yeah, there was one incident. It was just after I had moved into Edmonton and by then, things had—the colitis had become what I call just a minor inconvenience for the most part I thought. But there was one day. I lived in a suburb of Ottawa, so I used to take the bus to work. It was about a 40-minute trip. This one day I was back in Ottawa on business. But we hadn't moved so I was staying at home. Got on the bus and was fine but got within about 10 minutes of the office and the cramps got really severe, really bad. Literally walking up to the building feeling so bad that I thought I was going to have to . . .

Sampling to Determine Variation

Variation in a qualitative sample is usually the number of groups to be interviewed. Again, these are identified by the participants. These groups may be the groups that are usually compared in research (such as demographic comparison of old with young, male with female, etc.), or the groups may be completely unanticipated at the beginning of the study and identified by the participants themselves as the research progresses.

Less discussed, however, is what I call *shadowed data* (Morse, 2001b). During the process of the interview, participants may speak for themselves or for others like, or not like, themselves. In doing so, participants are sorting the world for the analyst. Participants do this also by defining parameters, reporting the frequency of occurrence, sorting the commonplace from the exceptional (thus defining norms), and reporting on best and worst cases (thus defining extremes). In this way, awareness of the structure of the phenomenon develops *while the interview is occurring*, enhancing understanding of variation in those being studied, and thus facilitating analysis. In the following example, the participant is using "you" and "you're" to indicate the *generalized self*, in this case a class of people who use wheelchairs:

At first, *you* don't want to go back in the world; *you* don't want to face people. *You* don't want to go to malls; *you* don't want to go to restaurants, but—at first I found it really, really hard. Especially in the wheelchair. Everybody, it doesn't matter, *you're* at everybody's mercy.

How participants partition their world into "us" and "them" using linguistic indexes is important. Participants' use of *you* and *your* and *you're* (*the generalized self*) is an attempt to normalize incomprehensible changes to the self.

The *generalized other* refers to a group of persons who behave in a particular way or who have characteristics that are not shared by the participant. In the next example, the participant is sorting his world into those who are not like him; they are the *objectified other*—those like *that*. Let's look at some data, to see how these indexes can be used analytically:

> A little kid came up and asked me, "What happened?"—you know, "Where's your hand?" . . . And, you can't say, "Look, kid, beat it," you know . . . 'cos they're innocent—they don't understand what is going on. I just told him, "Well," I said, "I really—I had a bad accident, and I, uh—lost my hand." And he says "Well, were you awake when you lost it?" And I said, "No, no, I—I was asleep. The—the doctor took it off, you know." And he was just dumbfounded. He couldn't—couldn't see how you could lose your hand. It's just something you didn't lose, you know, like—he thought—I'd lost it. It just happened to—fall off.

Notice the first "you know" is an example of the *generalized self*. The next "they're" and "they" is an example of the *generalized other:* "Cos *they're* innocent" and "*they* don't understand." For the purposes of sampling variation, this group—the generalized other—identified by the participant may be a group that should be sampled as a means to enrich the data set. Thus, identifying how participants sort the world, rather than adding confusion, adds the necessary information required for sampling and, eventually, saturation.

Sampling for Saturation

There are two types of saturation, and the researcher may be seeking to meet the criteria of one or both types. The first type of saturation is to sample until no new information occurs. As new participants are added to the study, and their narratives are added to the database, nothing new is learned by the investigator. However, when ongoing analysis reveals no new information appearing and no new categories emerging, sampling may cease. Margaret Mead used investigator boredom during analysis to indicate when saturation had occurred.

It is important to note that at one level, no two participants report with exactly the same story. People have different living conditions, different family types and levels of support, different levels of resilience, and abilities to cope with whatever you are studying. To achieve saturation, the researcher must decontextualize the major processes from such contextual (or context-bound) variables. This is achieved once the researcher learns to tell a generalized story, synthesizing all of the interviews: "These people do *thus and so* . . ." and "Some do *this* and some do *that*." Recall this is pertinent to methods that are seeking to develop theory, such as ethnography and grounded theory. Those who are working with phenomenology work to keep the individual differences, from which phenomenological meaning is identified.

Earlier I discussed the *distribution* of qualitative data and noted that qualitative researchers need adequate data to determine infrequent events or experiences and must be careful to control the collection of common events and experiences. Midway through the data collection, researchers should deliberately assess the amount of information obtained in each category, and further sampling in those categories in which data are inadequate or *thin*, disregarding extraneous data that continue to accrue, should be gathered. The process of building up data in thin areas is *sampling for saturation*. Data replicate, verifying earlier insights, making the project solid and rigorous.

The second type of saturation occurs when researchers examine incidents representative of some feature important to analysis. In this case, all of the instances used to identify saturation differ from one another, and theoretically one could go on sampling indefinitely. However, data collection continues until the analyst is confident that his or her hunch is correct. For instance, when trying to determine the strength of the modesty taboo in the Fijian East Indian culture and make a case that the modesty taboo interfered with health, I observed that the taboo was strong enough to cause bodily harm. The following are examples used to verify the relationship between the modesty taboo and health:

♦ Infants were breast-fed in the hospital at a regular time, rather than on demand. At infant feeding times, a sign was placed in the hallway announcing that infants were being fed, warning males to stay away. Modesty had priority over infant hunger.

♦ It was reported in the paper that a public health nurse went into an Indian village to give contraceptive information to women. The nurse was stoned and driven away by the elderly women, who said, "Their mothers did not need that information!"

♦ During development, Indian women were not given information about intercourse. Brides running away on their wedding night was considered a problem.

♦ Fiji Indian women did not know the signs and symptoms of pregnancy. Young married women might not know they were pregnant until their mothers-in-law observed the increasing abdominal size. Therefore there was no alteration in the mothers' work role, diet, or early prenatal care.

♦ Neither did these women know the signs of labor. Mothers either came to the hospital very early or very late in labor.

♦ Primigravidae Fiji Indian women in labor did not know how the baby was going to get out. This information was withheld culturally from mothers even during pregnancy. In one case, a husband brought his wife to the emergency room in the middle of the night and told the nurses that his wife was waiting in the car with a stomach pain. When the nurses went to lift the woman, they realized she had given birth and had not even removed her underwear. They were upset, especially when they could not resuscitate the infant. When they asked the husband why he did not tell them she had given birth, he replied, "I was too embarrassed." (Morse, 1989)

Note that these events are not identical, but are interrelated. At some level of abstraction, they confirm the significance of the value of modesty and its effect on health.

Saturation occurs when the researcher is convinced that the conjecture is probably correct. This confirming type of saturation is also a type of verification.

Sampling for Verification

Verification may be considered a deductive process, seeking instances in collected or in new data that further confirm emerging hunches or relationships. Thus, sampling for verification occurs when *linkages are made between categories and/or concepts in the developing analysis.* In other words, as theory emerges, data collection continues. Theory linkages are not made devoid of data, no matter how abstract. Sometimes the necessary examples are present in the database, but take on a new meaning once the implications of the theory are realized. Occasionally, new data need to be collected because the original focus and significance of some aspects of data were not recognized. One way to collect such data is to conduct *theoretical group interviews.* I do this by recalling my best participants (i.e., most informative) in pairs. Note that when inviting these participants, they must know that they will be sharing their story with others; without this additional consent, a breach of confidence and anonymity will occur. I give them lunch, so they can become acquainted and share their story with each other (these data will already be in the data set). Then I present the emerging theoretical schemata. If this is theoretically abstract, they will not be able to recognize their individual stories. As a process of verification, I ask them "how they managed to . . . ", or "What strategies did you use to . . ." or whatever it is I need to know to verify and to build the theory.

For example, I used theoretical group interview to increase and verify data about strategies for enduring hospitalization. I invited groups of two (I quickly found that three participants "crowded the conversation") to share their story over lunch. I then presented the theoretical information about enduring and emotional suffering (Morse, 2001a, 2005) and asked them to give me examples of how they were enduring illness and hospitalization. Specific strategies and examples were offered that verified and saturated the theory. While presenting the theory deductively, we are working within a scaffold (Morse & Mitcham, 2002) and are not therefore violating principles of induction. Data collection was continuing. Note that this strategy differs profoundly from those researchers who bring participants back to confirm their theory.

CONCLUSION

Although many authors have written about the concurrent process of data collection and data analysis in qualitative inquiry, the reciprocal interaction has not been explicated. In this chapter, I have presented four modes in intraproject sampling that are guided by the interviews of the participants and the emerging analysis. Each sampling strategy is used at a different stage and for a different purpose in the emerging analysis. Elsewhere, Meadows and Morse (2001) argue that if qualitative inquiry is conducted with care and deliberation, the research process is valid and self-correcting in the process of inquiry. It is therefore unnecessary, even blasphemous, to consider quantitative verification of qualitative theory. If quantification is used following the development of a qualitative theory, it must be for the purpose of determining the distribution of the characteristics within a population, thereby extending the usefulness of the qualitatively derived theory, as in sequential QUAL → quan designs (see Morse & Niehaus, Chapter 24 in this volume).

REFERENCES

Glaser, B. (1978). *Theoretical sensitivity*. Mill Valley, CA: Sociology Press.

Meadows, L., & Morse, J. M. (2001). Constructing evidence within the qualitative project. In J. M. Morse, J. Swanson, & A. Kuzel (Eds.), *The nature of evidence in qualitative inquiry* (pp. 187–200). Newbury Park, CA: Sage.

Morse, J. M. (1989). Cultural responses to parturition: Childbirth in Fiji. *Medical Anthropology, 12*(1), 35–44.

Morse, J. M. (2001a). Types of talk: Modes of responses and data-led analytic strategies. In P. Munhall (Ed.), *Nursing research: A qualitative perspective* (3rd ed., pp. 565–578). Boston: Jones and Bartlett.

Morse, J. M. (2001b). Using shadowed data [editorial]. *Qualitative Health Research, 11*(3), 291.

Morse, J. M., & Mitcham, C. (2002). Exploring qualitatively derived concepts: Inductive-deductive pitfalls. In J. M. Morse, J. E. Hupcey, J. Penrod, J. A. Spiers, C. Pooler, & C. Mitcham (Eds.), Issues in validity: Behavioral concepts, their derivation and interpretation. *International Journal of Qualitative Methods, 1*(4), article 3. Retrieved December 15, 2002, from http://www.ualberta.ca/~ijqm.

Spradley, J. (1979). *The ethnographic interview.* New York: Mosby.

24

Combining Qualitative and Quantitative Methods for Mixed-Method Designs

Janice M. Morse
and
Linda Niehaus

Nurses are interested in the whole person—that is, the psychosocial, the physiological, and the spiritual. Nurses are interested in the individual, the family, and the community; in sick persons, those recovering and healthy; in elderly persons, adults, children, those newly born, and those as yet unborn. Nurses are interested in the cellular and behavioral; in the environmental, and in the institutional; in health and in illness; in emotions and the unconscious. Given these interests, we need the skills to describe minutely and globally in research designs that allow us to understand mechanisms, associations, and risks. Thus, because of its very broad focus and its encompassing

We acknowledge the contributions of Ruth Wolfe and Seanne Wilkins in preliminary work for this chapter. Reprinted and extensively revised from Morse, J. M., Niehaus, L., & Wolfe, R. R. (2005). The utilization of mixed-method design in nursing research. *International Nursing Review (Japanese)*, 28(2), 61–66. Copyright © 2005 Janice M. Morse perspectives, nursing research is by its very nature eclectic. Nurse researchers must be versatile and adept at many types of research, both qualitative and quantitative. To grasp nursing phenomena, nursing research often demands that more than one method be used at once and that a mixed- or multi-method research design be used. The purpose of this chapter is to explicate the processes of conducting mixed-method research, both for simultaneous and sequential designs.

Mixed-method research is defined as a research design consisting of one complete method with additional supplementary strategies drawn from a second, different method. It often involves the use of both qualitative and quantitative methods. For instance, a qualitative method with an additional quantitative strategy could be used to allow for measurement of some dimension of the phenomenon under investigation. Alternatively, a quantitative method with an additional qualitative strategy could be employed to allow for description of an aspect or component of the phenomenon that cannot be measured. Qualitative and quantitative research have been described as belonging to different and incompatible paradigms, so *how* the researcher combines the qualitative and the quantitative components in a single project is essential if rigor is to be maintained.

TERMINOLOGY AND CONSIDERATIONS FOR CONDUCTING MIXED-METHOD RESEARCH

Before we begin to describe the process of mixed-method design, we review the definitions of all the necessary terms (see Box 24–1). The *core* compo-

Component	*A phase of the research, driven by the overall direction of the inquiry, during which one or more methodological strategies are used as research tools to address the research question.*
Core component of the project	*The primary (main) study in which the primary or core method is used to address the research ion. This phase of the research is complete or scientifically rigorous and can therefore stand alone.*
Method	*A cohesive combination of methodological strategies or set of research tools that is inductively or deductively used in conducting qualitative or quantitative inquiry.*
Mixed-method design	*A plan for a scientifically rigorous research project, driven by the inductive or deductive theoretical drive, and comprised of a qualitative or quantitative*

	core component with qualitative or quantitative supplementary component(s). These supplementary components of the research fit together to enhance description, understanding, or explanation and can either be conducted simultaneously or sequentially with the core component. Mixed-method design can also take place as internal transformation of a single data set.
Multi-method design	A plan for a scientifically rigorous research program comprised of a series of related qualitative and/or quantitative research projects over time, driven by the theoretical thrust of the program. The theoretical drive of an individual project may on occasion counter but not change the overall inductive or deductive direction of the entire program.
Strategy	A methodological research tool, drawn from a qualitative or quantitative method, for addressing the research question by either collecting or analyzing data.
Supplementary component of the project	In this phase of the research, one or more supplementary methodological strategies are used to obtain an enhanced description, understanding, or explanation of the phenomenon under investigation. This component of the project can either be conducted at the same time as the core component (simultaneous) or it could follow the core component (sequential). The supplementary component is incomplete in itself or lacks some aspect of scientific rigor, cannot stand alone, and is regarded as complementary to the core component.
Theoretical drive	The direction of the inquiry (Morse, 2003) that guides the use of the appropriate qualitative and/or quantitative methodological core. The nature of the research question determines the theoretical drive of a project.
Theoretical thrust	The overall inductive or deductive direction of a research program. The theoretical drive of an individual project may on occasion counter but not change the theoretical thrust of the research program.

Revised from Morse, J.M., Wolfe, R.R., & Niehaus, L. (2005). Principles and procedures for maintaining validity for mixed-method design. In L. Curry, R. Shield, & T. Wetle (Eds.), *Qualitative methods in research and public health: Aging and other special populations.* Washington, DC: GSA and APHA.

Box 24-1   A List of Terms for Types of Mixed-Method Design nent of the project is the primary or main study in which the core method is used to address the research question. The *supplementary* component fits into the core component and consists of strategies added to obtain the necessary supplemental information. The core component is therefore always dominant, complete (i.e., scientifically rigorous), and can stand (and even be published) alone, whereas the supplemental component is conducted only until the researcher is certain the additional supplemental findings are adequate to provide the necessary information. We therefore refer to the methodological research tool used to obtain supplementary information as a *strategy* rather than a *method*. Nomenclature for different types of mixed-method designs is presented in Box 24–2. Uppercase letters are used to denote the core component of the project, and the supplemental component is indicated with lowercase letters.

Recognize the Role of the Theoretical Drive

Research projects are conducted either inductively (usually using a qualitative method) or deductively (usually using a quantitative method). In mixed-method design, the overall inductive or deductive direction of the inquiry is referred to as the *theoretical drive*, and this encompasses *both* the core and the supplementary components with the data or findings of the supplemental component contributing to the findings of the core component (Morse, 2003; Morse, Wolfe, & Niehaus, 2005). Further, the theoretical drive of the core component overrides the drive of supplemental components (see Figure 24–1). For example, if the project is QUAL–quan, the theoretical drive is inductive and qualitative, regardless of whether the minor component is deductive and quantitatively driven. If a research program involves a series of interrelated mixed-method projects over time (as in multimethod design), the overall *theoretical thrust* of the program is maintained, irrespective of the theoretical drive of individual projects (Morse, Wolfe, & Niehaus, 2005). The nature of the programmatic research question determines the overall inductive or deductive direction (thrust) of the research program (see Figure 24–1). Note that a multimethod research program may also include projects using different single methods.

Other aspects that must be attended to when conducting mixed-method design are sampling issues and the pacing of the project.

Sampling Issues

When the mixed-method design involves qualitative and quantitative components, sampling becomes difficult. In a QUAN–qual study, the quantita-

QUAL + quan:	Qualitative core component of the project (inductive theoretical drive) with a *simultaneous* quantitative supplementary component.
QUAL → quan:	Qualitative core component of the project (inductive theoretical drive) with a *sequential* quantitative supplementary component.
QUAL + qual:	Qualitative core component of the project (inductive theoretical drive) with a *simultaneous* qualitative supplementary component.
QUAL → qual:	Qualitative core component of the project (inductive theoretical drive) with a *sequential* qualitative supplementary component.
QUAN + qual:	Quantitative core component of the project (deductive theoretical drive) with a *simultaneous* qualitative supplementary component.
QUAN → qual:	Quantitative core component of the project (deductive theoretical drive) with a *sequential* qualitative supplementary component.
QUAN + *quan:*	Quantitative core component of the project (deductive theoretical drive) with a *simultaneous* quantitative supplementary component.
QUAN → *quan:*	Quantitative core component of the project (deductive theoretical drive) with a *sequential* quantitative supplementary component.
QUAN ↓ *qual*	Researchers using experimental design with qualitative data as documentation to describe differences between groups.
QUAL ↓ *qual*	A quantitative descriptive design using numerical data in the process of description.

Box 24-2   Nomenclature for Types of Mixed-Method Design

tive sample (which is too large and randomly selected) is unsuitable for use with the qualitative component, and in a QUAL–quan study, the qualitative sample (which is too small and purposefully selected) violates the needs of the quantitative component. In the next section, we discuss specific ways to overcome these limitations and processes of conducting mixed-method research.

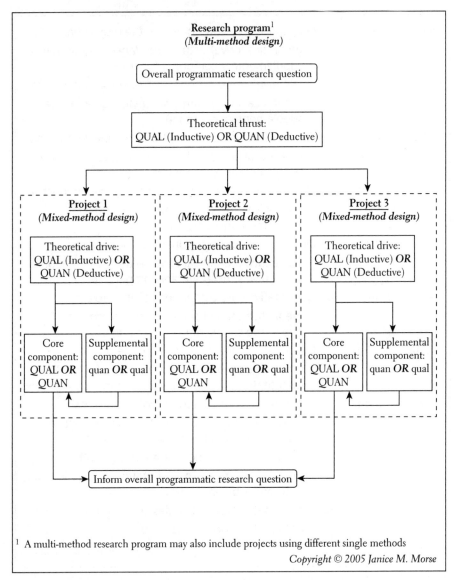

Figure 24–1   Mixed-method design versus multi-method design.

The Pacing of the Project

If the supplementary component is conducted at the same time as the core component, we describe it as *simultaneous mixed-method design*, and it is indicated with a plus (+) sign; if the supplementary component follows the core component, perhaps because the results are interesting and additional information is required, the mixed-method design is *sequential* and is indicated with an arrow ($\rightarrow$) symbol.

Consider an example for a mixed-method project. Suppose we are conducting a qualitatively driven study in the relatives' waiting room to explore relatives' experiences of waiting for news of the condition of an injured person in the emergency room. The theoretical drive of this study would be inductive, and the core (main) method used may be grounded theory. But, if in the course of conducting the study we noticed that the relatives were anxious, we may decide to measure their anxiety using a quantitative standardized anxiety scale. In this example, the *core* component would be qualitative (QUAL) using grounded theory, and the *supplemental component* would be quantitative (quan) using the anxiety scale. Given that the supplementary component is conducted at the same time as the core component, we would describe the design as a QUAL+quan study.

Conversely, we could decide to conduct the same project using a theoretical framework stating that waiting for news of an injured relative was anxiety-producing, and this anxiety could be reduced if relatives could receive social support by waiting together. This would be a quantitatively driven study, using a battery of tests such as an anxiety scale and a social support measure. But during the pilot study we observe that the use of television is another variable that eases anxiety, and so we decide to document the nature and use of television by those who are waiting and watching. However, because we cannot find or develop a more suitable instrument to rate this variable, we decide to describe this aspect of the phenomenon qualitatively. This second project has a deductive theoretical drive, is quantitatively driven (QUAN), and has a qualitative supplementary component (qual). We would describe the design as QUAN+qual. To be even more complex, we may decide then to transpose these qualitative data to form a quantitative variable(s), and our design would be QUAN+qual$\rightarrow$quan.

PROCESSES OF CONDUCTING MIXED-METHOD RESEARCH

The inductive or deductive theoretical drive of a project is determined by the nature of the researcher's question, and the nature of the question in turn determines the selection of the research method and, subsequently, the research design and procedures. Figure 24–2 shows the process of conducting a mixed-method research design. Important to note is that, although the

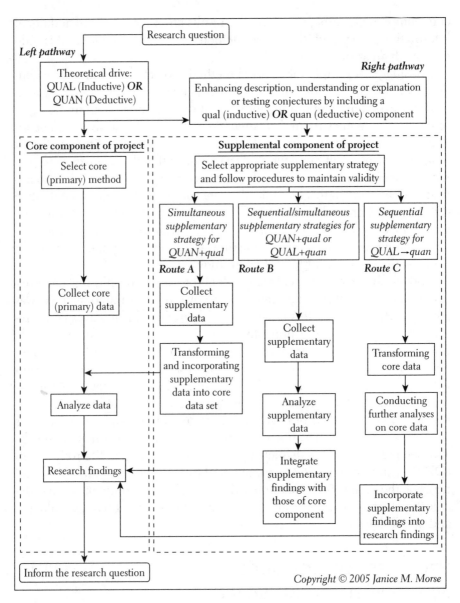

Figure 24–2 An overview of the process of Mixed-method design.

theoretical drive and the pacing of the procedures (for sequential or simultaneous designs) alter the design of the project, the actual procedures can be represented on the same chart. There are two basic pathways: the core component is described in the left pathway, and the supplementary component in the right pathway.

The Core Component

With both sequential and simultaneous designs, the core component (the left pathway in Figure 24–2) is conducted according to standard procedures for the methods selected until the data have been collected. The core component must always be conducted according to the principles of the selected method and will meet qualitative standards for reliability, validity, and rigor and may be publishable without the supplementary component. Of most importance, the researcher must remember that the supplementary findings are not methodologically complete and cannot be published alone. Their role is to contribute "missing pieces" to the results of the core component, which are stronger and more comprehensive with the contribution than without it.

The Supplementary Component

Maintaining validity of the supplementary component (the right pathway in Figure 24–2) is the most difficult task. *If* the supplementary component is conducted simultaneously and supplementary data have been collected, these data are analyzed with the core data; *if* the supplementary data are collected sequentially, they are integrated into the findings after the core analysis is completed; *if* the supplemental analysis is conducted on the primary data following the core analysis, the results contribute to the overall research findings (see Figure 24–2). Also, the researcher must attend to issues in sampling and the type of data used because these problems are exacerbated when the supplementary component is from the opposite paradigm (quantitative with a qualitative study or vice versa).

In this chapter, we describe and illustrate only *two qualitatively driven* and *two quantitatively driven* mixed-method research designs because these four designs have the greatest potential for error and threats to validity.

QUAL–quan: Qualitatively Driven Mixed-Method Designs

In both types of QUAL–quan designs, the theoretical drive of the project is inductive and qualitative. The primary role of the supplemental component (quan) is to enhance description of aspects of the phenomenon being studied or to test conjectures by using quantification (see Figure 24–2). This can be done by quantifying qualitative characteristics of the sample that appear to be important during analysis (a supplementary data transformation analysis strategy) or by collecting quantitative data about characteristics of the sample participants (a supplementary data collection strategy). The supplementary strategy is drawn from quantitative methods either during the core component of the project so that qualitative and quantitative methods are carried out simultaneously (QUAL+quan) or following the core component so that qualitative and quantitative methods are carried out sequentially (QUAL→quan). These types of mixed-method designs are illustrated here:

♦ *QUAL+quan (Figure 24–2, Route B):* When the core project is qualitative, and the supplementary strategy is quantitative, the qualitative sample (purposefully selected and small) does not meet the quantitative criteria of size (large) and randomization. For a simultaneous design, if the quantitative data are used to enhance description (as in the example of measuring how anxious the relatives were in the earlier example), the quantitative instrument used must have external norms. The scores obtained for the participants in the small qualitative sample may then be interpreted with the normative populations, because the researcher can draw conclusions about *how anxious* the sample is, and add this to the description. These scores for the qualitative participants are not averaged and presented as group scores unless the sample size meets the minimum requirement of $n = 30$, the minimum number required to estimate a mean score (Pett, 1997).

♦ *QUAL→quan (Figure 24–2, Route C):* Quantitative data may be used to enhance a qualitative study by transposing the qualitative data collected in the core component and conducting further analyses on the primary data. For this technique, first the nature of the qualitative interviews used must be examined because data transformation can be conducted only if all of the participants have been asked the same questions (as in semistructured, open-ended interviews) or if the answers can be inferred from the interviews (for instance, the same five or six guiding questions have been used for all interviews). Data cannot be transformed if the researcher has used interviews that have evolved as the study has progressed, as is often used in ethnography (Spradley, 1979). Procedures for quantifying qualitative data are well described elsewhere (Bernard, 2000). Briefly, the researchers must develop categories within the qualitative data, code responses numerically, develop definitions for the codes, establish interrater reliability, code the transcripts, analyze the resulting numerical data, and incorporate the supplementary findings into the qualitative results to enhance conclusions and implications. For instance, in our example of the anxiety of relatives waiting, we may observe that those who appear to meditate have less need for the support provided by relatives. In the interviews with these relatives, those who are spiritual have spoken of their use of meditation. This information may be coded and the nonparametric statistical analysis could be conducted to determine whether there are significant associations between relevant variables. Note that this data analysis strategy is sequential because the transformation of the qualitative data cannot be performed until the qualitative analysis is completed, and these results inform the research findings rather than build the findings per se.

QUAN–qual: Quantitatively Driven Mixed-Method Designs

In QUAN–qual mixed-method designs, the overall direction of the inquiry is deductive and quantitative. The primary role of the supplemental component (qual) in these designs is to enhance description, understanding, or explanation about the phenomenon that the core method cannot access (see Figure 24–2). This can be done either by collecting qualitative data using open-ended questions within an otherwise structured instrument (QUAN+qual) or by collecting and analyzing qualitative data separately to explain puzzling findings (QUAN→qual). These mixed-method designs are discussed in this section with specific attention to issues associated with simultaneous or sequential designs. A decision flowchart for the selection of a sample for a qualitative supplementary component while conducting a quantitatively driven core component is shown in Figure 24–3. The decisions for simultaneously driven research are on the left, and those for sequential are on the right pathway.

♦ *QUAN+qual (Figure 24–2, Route A):* Simultaneously deductively driven components of a project provide a problem for the qualitative supplemental component: the quantitative sample is too large and randomly selected for the supplementary qualitative component. *If* the study involves a quantitative questionnaire with several open-ended questions at the end, although these open-ended questions may be analyzed qualitatively, it is a stronger design to transpose the qualitative data to quantitative data and incorporate these data into the quantitative analysis (for instructions, see Bernard, 2000). An example of this design is a quantitatively driven survey that had 10% of the items written as semistructured open-ended questions used to obtain evidence regarding the incidence and severity of untoward effects on participants of unstructured interviews. The sample size of 500 respondents was not extraordinarily large for the management of the textual data, the transposition of these qualitative data to enable their incorporation into the statistical analysis was not prohibitive, and the

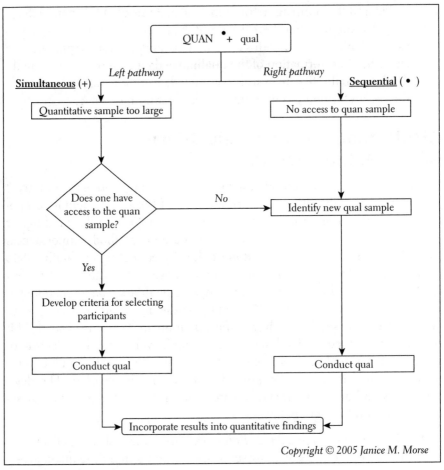

Figure 24–3   QUAN-qual mixed-method designs.

inductive qualitative component greatly added to the validity of the overall project.

♦ QUAN→qual *(Figure 24–2, Route B):* The greater challenge is the project in which the qualitative supplementary component follows the quantitative core component. *If* the role of the supplemental component is to collect additional data to add description to the quantitative component, *if* the researcher has access to the quantitative sample, criteria for the purposeful selection of participants should be developed. This should be according to the criteria of a "good informant": the ability to articulate, have knowledge about the interview

topic, be willing to reflect on the topic, and have the time to participate (see Spradley, 1979). *If* the researcher has access to the quantitative participants (for instance, research assistants who are collecting
the quantitative data may be able to make referrals), the principles of
qualitative sampling should be followed. If the researcher has no access to the quantitative participants (for instance, they cannot be
traced or recalled), the researcher has no alternative but to draw another sample, according to the needs of the qualitative supplementary
component. Participants may be selected by scores achieved on the
quantitative component. Obviously, this design is only slightly weaker
than is a multiple-method design in which the sample is that of a
complete study and the results are rigorous enough to be published
separately. An example of this mixed-method design is a quantitative
survey of a neighborhood that reveals no correlation between working
mothers of toddlers and the use of day care facilities. Follow-up qualitative interviews reveal that many of the fathers in these areas were
students with flexible schedules, and the fathers organized their
schedules to assume care of their children during the day and elected
to do their studies in the hours their wives were able to be home. This
flexible arrangement for child care had not been anticipated by the
researchers, and the subsequent qualitative component was necessary
to provide explanation for the unexpected findings.

Discussion

Mixed-method design may allow for more complete understanding than can
be obtained by a single method used alone. However, combining a core
method with a supplementary strategy, in particular qualitative and quantitative strategies, requires expert understanding of the principles of both qualitative and quantitative methods and knowledge of sampling strategies and
data transformation to maintain validity.

Is conducting a mixed-method design rather than a multiple-method design cutting corners? Should not all designs that explore complex phenomena use multiple methods in which all components employ complete
methods as in multiple-method design? The answer is that there is a role for
mixed-method design and for the completion of the project more expedi-
tiously than for the conduct of a multiple-methods design. In fact, ethnography may be considered a qualitatively driven mixed-method design that has
become so institutionalized and eclectic that its very flexibility has become
institutionalized as a complete method.

Mixed-method design, if conducted rigorously, is a stronger design than a design in which a single method is used alone because the supplemental component enhances validity of the project per se (see, for example, Locke, Silverman, & Spirduso, 1998, p. 117). Further, with mixed-method design all components are published as a whole, although Morgan (2004) notes that on occasions the supplemental component may be criticized by reviewers as being weak or unscientific and often can be the cause for the rejection of the article. However, the strongest design—multiple-method design—is often weakened at the point of publication if the researcher is tempted to publish each method separately.

REFERENCES

Bernard, H. R. (2000). *Social research methods: Qualitative and quantitative approaches.* Thousand Oaks, CA: Sage.

Locke, L. F., Silverman, S. J., & Spirduso, W. W. (1998). *Reading and understanding research.* Thousand Oaks, CA: Sage.

Morgan, D. (2004, September). *Mixed-method design.* Keynote address at the 5th Qualitative Research Conference in Health and Social Care, Bournemouthe University, England.

Morse, J. M. (2003). Principles of mixed methods and multi-method research design. In A. Tashakkori & C. Teddlie (Eds.), *Handbook of mixed methods in social and behavioral research* (pp. 189–208). Thousand Oaks, CA: Sage.

Morse, J. M., Wolfe, R. R., & Niehaus, L. (2005). Principles and procedures for maintaining validity for mixed-method design. In L. Curry, R. Shield, & T. Wetle (Eds.), *Qualitative methods in research and public health: Aging and other special populations.* Washington, DC: GSA and APHA.

Pett, M. A. (1997). *Nonparametric statistics for health care research: Statistics for small samples and unusual distributions.* Thousand Oaks, CA: Sage.

Spradley, J. P. (1979). *The ethnographic interview.* New York: Holt, Rinehart & Winston.

25

Evaluation of
Qualitative Research

Marlene C. Mackey

The intent of this chapter is *not* to tell you the best way to evaluate qualitative research. Rather the purpose of this chapter is to present an overview of current thinking about evaluating qualitative research. Unlike with quantitative research for which evaluation criteria are relatively clear and generally accepted, there is no one set of criteria one can use to evaluate a qualitative research report. The literature is replete with recommendations, analyses, debates, concerns, and challenges about standards and evaluation criteria for qualitative research. Engel and Kuzel (1992) argue that standards for judging qualitative research may vary according to the discipline of the creators and users of research findings and that one set of criteria may not be appropriate for all types of qualitative research.

When nurses first started to conduct qualitative research, they frequently studied with sociologists, anthropologists, psychologists, or philosophers who taught them the qualitative methods that were developed in those fields. Little was written on the quality of qualitative research—you knew it when you saw it. However, as nurses used these methods to study nursing problems, they began to write about criteria to evaluate qualitative research or sought criteria from other disciplines.

EARLY EVALUATION CRITERIA

Aamodt (1983) was one of the first nurses to introduce the need for specific criteria for evaluating qualitative research. She proposed that the criteria should include something about discovery/development of constructs, domains of time and space to bracket a territory for study, the reflex activity of the researcher and the phenomenon of study, detailed descriptions of the context of the study, and the contributions of the substantive or theoretical data to nursing practice, research, or theory. The implication is that a reader of qualitative research should expect information about these components of the research process.

Burns (1989) was one of the first nurse researchers to propose specific criteria to evaluate qualitative research. After describing skills needed to critique qualitative studies and elements of a qualitative research report, Burns listed five steps to critique a research report, whether qualitative or quantitative. The reviewer needs to understand the report, compare the elements of the report to an ideal version (or standard), judge the adequacy of the logic within the study, evaluate the usefulness of the study for clinical practice, and compare the findings of the study to previous scientific knowledge. She then described five standards (and threats to the standards) by which the reader could evaluate qualitative studies: (1) descriptive vividness, (2) methodological congruence (rigor in documentation, procedural rigor, ethical rigor, and auditability), (3) analytic preciseness, (4) theoretical connectedness, and (5) heuristic relevance (intuitive recognition, relationship to existing body of knowledge, and applicability). These standards can be found in the latest edition of the Burns and Grove (2005) research textbook and have been useful to many reviewers of qualitative reports.

With the publication of the Lincoln and Guba book (1985), nurses and others quickly embraced the guidelines they proposed for conducting qualitative research. The evaluation criteria that Lincoln and Guba described for the naturalistic (or constructivist) paradigm became extremely popular and continue to be used by qualitative researchers today (Denzin & Lincoln, 2005). Lincoln and Guba used the term *trustworthiness* to refer to a quality research report. Trustworthiness consists of four criteria — "credibility" (truth value, replaces internal validity), "transferability" (applicability, replaces external validity), "dependability" (consistency, replaces reliability), and "confirmability" (neutrality, replaces objectivity). A reader/reviewer looks for the following evidence of credibility: prolonged engagement, persistent observation, triangulation, peer debriefing, negative case analysis, referential adequacy, and member checks. An audit trail of methods and decisions from a reflexive journal provides evidence of confirmability.

Drawing from Lincoln and Guba (1985), Leininger (1994) argued for the need to develop and use criteria that fit a qualitative paradigm and criticized reviewers for using quantitative criteria. She presented six criteria to use to evaluate qualitative studies; however, her citations suggest she developed these criteria specifically for her ethnomethod. Her criteria include "credibility" (truth established through prolonged engagement), "confirmability" (repeated and direct evidence from participants and documents), "meaning-in-context" (data became understandable within holistic context), "recurrent patterning" (instances, sequence of events, experiences, or lifeways), "saturation" (redundancy, no new information), and "transferability" (whether findings can be transferred to another similar context) (pp. 105–106).

Later, nurse researchers questioned the appropriateness of the Lincoln and Guba (1985) criteria for evaluating the validity of a qualitative study. The rigid following of procedures in attempts to ensure the trustworthiness of the study may actually threaten validity (Sandelowski, 1993). Research participants do not have the credentials to validate qualitative research findings (Morse, 1998, 1999a; Sandelowski, 1993). Even qualitative research experts do not have the depth of understanding of another's research to be qualified to validate research findings (Sandelowski, 1998).

"Validity is not an inherent property of a particular method, but pertains to the data, accounts, or conclusions reached by using that method in a particular context for a particular purpose" (Maxwell, 1992, p. 284). Using this realist conception of validity, Maxwell described five types of validity used in qualitative research. "Descriptive validity" refers to an accurate, factual description of everything the researcher saw, heard, felt, or smelled. "Interpretive validity" refers to an accurate presentation of the "meaning" that objects, events, and behaviors had to the people engaged in and with them. "Meaning" encompasses intention, cognition, affect, belief, evaluation, and other kinds of "participants' perspectives." "Theoretical validity" refers to the theory the researcher developed, including the concepts and their relationship. "Generalization" is the extent to which the findings (typically the theory) can apply to other people and other settings. "Evaluative validity," applying an evaluative framework to the study's findings, is typically not a central concern in qualitative research.

LATER EVALUATION CRITERIA

When Janice Morse launched *Qualitative Health Research* in 1991 and later the *International Journal of Qualitative Methods*, nurses and other health-related researchers had a forum for a dialogue about evaluating qualitative research. Scholars could test their thinking and share their concerns and ideas about what is good qualitative research.

Morse (1991) described the four broad guidelines reviewers use to evaluate manuscripts for possible publication in *Qualitative Health Research*. Reviewers assess the importance or "significance" of the study in terms of the development of new knowledge or theory. The article should excite, impress, or at least interest the reader. A "theoretical evaluation" is done by determining whether the results extend beyond description to some level of abstraction and whether the theory is logical, clear, complete, and intuitively makes sense. Implications of the theory for use in extending knowledge and for praxis and linkages to the literature are clearly described. Reviewers conduct a "methodological assessment" to determine whether an inductive approach was used and whether the clearly presented research problem or question was studied using an appropriate research method and data analysis technique. Selection of the sample is evaluated for appropriateness and adequacy and data collection for saturation. Reviewers also evaluate "adherence to ethical standards" in the conduct and reporting of the study.

As editor of *Qualitative Health Research*, Morse (1999b) has witnessed the disagreement among experienced qualitative researchers in their reviews of manuscripts for the journal. Some reviewers accept descriptive reporting of "raw" data, whereas others believe this to be inadequate. "Qualitative research must, in my view, add something more to the participants' words for it to be considered a research contribution, whether it be synthesis, interpretation, or development of a concept, model, or theory" (p. 163). Other manuscripts may report complex theory but fail to link the theory to data from which it was derived, troubling some reviewers but not others. Reviewers also disagree on the type of results that should be published—common sense vs. innovative, intriguing, and surprising findings. Journal reviewers in the process of reviewing are indirectly shaping criteria that may be used to evaluate qualitative research. Morse (2003), however, cautioned us about the trend to use standards to evaluate qualitative studies that focus on the techniques of doing the study rather than on the findings or the contributions to theory.

REVISING/EMERGING EVALUATION CRITERIA

Lincoln (1995) suggested additional criteria to evaluate the quality of qualitative research. Lincoln urges a dialogue about the following emerging criteria: positionality or standpoint judgments (all texts are partial, incomplete, and never represent any complete truth), community as arbiter of quality (research serves the community), voice (extent to which alternative voices are heard), critical subjectivity or reflexivity (awareness and understanding of subtle differences in the personal and psychological states of others), reciprocity (intense sharing of observer and others), sacredness (create relationships based on mutual respect, granting of dignity, and appreciation of the human condition), and sharing the perquisites of privilege with those we study (sharing financial and other benefits the researcher gains).

Thorne (1997) described four principles of evaluation (epistemological integrity, representative credibility, analytic logic, and interpretive authority) and five principles of critique (moral defensibility, disciplinary relevance, pragmatic obligation, contextual awareness, and probable truth) in qualitative research. The intent and meaning of these principles are presented elsewhere (Fossey, Harvey, McDermott, & Davidson, 2002; Popay, Rogers, & Williams, 1998). The one exception is pragmatic obligation in which the researcher must consider that research findings may be applied in practice and therefore must be presented in such a way as to avoid harm.

Stiles (1999) proposed criteria to evaluate the research method and the validity of data interpretation. The reviewer should examine the research report for clarity and justification of the study questions, selection of participants, and methods of gathering and analyzing data. In evaluating data analysis, the reader considers *engagement with the material* (intense, persistent, prolonged), *iteration* (cycle between interpretation and observation), *grounding* (systematically linking interpretations and observations), and *asking "what," not "why"* (participant interviews). The reader of a research report needs information about the investigator's forestructure (preconceptions, values), the social and cultural context, and the investigator's internal processes (personal experiences, relationship with participants). Stiles suggested validity criteria; that is, readers, participants, and investigators evaluate the impact of data interpretations on their own preconceptions or bias and determine whether the findings are either a fit/an agreement or represent real change or growth in understanding.

Patton (2002) proposed criteria to evaluate a number of approaches to qualitative research, including artistic and evocative criteria and critical change criteria. His "social construction and constructivist criteria" most closely address the types of research nurses typically conduct: subjectivity acknowledged (discusses and takes into account biases), trustworthiness (Lincoln & Guba, 1985), authenticity, triangulation (capturing and respecting multiple perspectives), reflexivity, praxis, particularity (doing justice to the integrity of unique cases), enhanced and deepened understanding (*Verstehen*), and contributions to dialogue (p. 544).

Drawing heavily on the work of Lincoln (1995), Popay, Rogers, and Williams (1998), and Stiles (1999), Fossey and colleagues (2002) organized and discussed the previously mentioned scholars' work under the steps of the research process. The "research design and questions" should be clearly and explicitly presented to meet two essential criteria for quality research: (1) the reader can evaluate the congruence (fit) between the purpose of the study and subsequent sampling, data collection, and analysis, and (2) the reader can determine whether something was learned from the participants that goes beyond initial assumptions, understanding, and interpretations (i.e., the views of the participants were authentically presented). "Sampling strategies" (both purposive and theoretical) should be clearly presented for the reader to evaluate their appropriateness and adequacy to provide the information needed to meet the study's aims. The reader should have enough information about the "data collection methods" to evaluate whether the researcher could adequately explore the subjective meaning, actions, and social context of the participants. An adequate report of "data analysis" includes a description of conceptual processes used to explore the meanings, patterns, or connections among data and how the researcher's own thought, reflection, and intuition were used. Quality research reports reflect transparency (openness and honesty) of data collection, analysis, and presentation.

> Qualitative research findings are presented as textual descriptions that should illuminate the subjective meanings of the phenomena, or social world, being studied, but which should also place the findings in context, so as to represent the real world of those studied and in which their lived experiences are embedded. However, the extent to which anyone is able to represent the experiences and intentional meanings of others depends on interpretations that are necessarily personal, experiential, and political, making qualitative findings at once both descriptive and interpretive. Principle issues related to their trustworthiness are related to the representation of views (authenticity); how the findings are presented (coherence); claims about their typicality; and the contribution of the researcher's perspective to the interpretation (permeability). (Fossey et al., 2002, p. 730)

Morse and colleagues (2002) expressed concern about the rejection of the terms *reliability* and *validity* by qualitative researchers and an emphasis on strategies for evaluating trustworthiness and utility after the research is completed. They argued that reliability and validity are appropriate concepts as indicators of rigor in qualitative research. They urged qualitative researchers to reclaim responsibility for reliability and validity by implementing verification strategies while conducting research. "*Verification* is the process of checking, confirming, making sure, and being certain . . . the mechanisms used during the process of research to incrementally contribute to ensuring reliability and validity and, thus, the rigor of the study" (p. 9). These verification strategies are *methodological coherence* (congruence between research question and methods), *appropriate sample* (adequacy evidenced by saturation and replication), *collecting and analyzing data concurrently*, *thinking theoretically* (ideas from data reconfirmed with new data), and *theory development* (as an outcome of the research process).

Drawing on the work of Beach (1993), Eisner (1985), and Shapin (1984), among others, Sandelowski and Barroso (2002) challenged readers of qualitative research to reconceptualize the "research report as a dynamic vehicle that mediates between researcher/writer and reviewer/reader, rather than as a factual account of events after the fact" (p. 3). Instead of using rigid standards and criteria to evaluate these research reports, the reader's task should be to read to understand the meaning being communicated.

> Although useful, existing guides for evaluating qualitative studies (variously comprised of checklists and/or narrative summaries of criteria or standards) tend to confuse the research report with the research it represents. They also do not ask the reviewer to differentiate between understanding the nature of a study-as-reported and estimating the value of a study-as-reported, nor do they allow that any one criterion might be more or less relevant for any one study and to any one reviewer. We prefer the word *appraisal* as opposed to evaluation, as appraisal more explicitly encompasses understanding in addition to estimating value. Any work of art—including the research report—must be understood, or appreciated, for what it is before it can be judged as a good or bad example of its kind. Appreciated here means the exercise of wise judgment and keen insight in recognizing the nature and merits of a work. (pp. 9–10)

Reviewers/readers of qualitative reports may have difficulty in evaluating the studies if they are unfamiliar with the various "forms" (Sandelowski & Barroso, 2002, p. 12), that is, structure or "reconstruction of a research study" (p. 10) the report comes in. They need to know what they are looking for and at and where to find it. Reviewers also must be able to distinguish between "reporting adequacy versus procedural or interpretive appropriateness" (p. 12) and "actual versus virtual presence or absence" (p. 13) of information about the study. Therefore, Sandelowski and Barroso developed a reading guide to assist the reader in the health-related practice disciplines to find information in the report—research problem, research purpose(s)/

question(s), literature review, orientation to the target phenomenon, method, sampling, sample, data collection, data management, validity, findings, discussion, ethics, and form. The guide includes a comprehensive definition of each category and asks the reader to determine the presence and the relevance of each of the appraisal parameters. The reading guide is readily available online (see reference list). The authors invite feedback from readers/reviewers to enhance the quality and utility of the guide.

EVALUATION CRITERIA FOR PHENOMENOLOGICAL RESEARCH

Munhall (1994) proposes *One P, Ten Rs* as evaluation criteria to evaluate phenomenological research for rigor and merit (pp. 189–193). The *Phenomenological Nod* (i.e., nodding in agreement when reading or listening to the study's findings) indicates recognition of the findings and agreement that the researcher has captured, at least partially, the meaning of the experience to the participants. To evaluate the *Rigor* of the study, the reviewer can consider additional *Rs*:

Resonancy: The interpretation of the meaning of the experience is familiar, sounds correct, "resonates" with past experiences.

Reasonableness: All activities of the study, including the interpretation of the meaning of the experience, sound "reasonable"; the researcher presented carefully reasoned rationale for all aspects of the study.

Representativeness: The findings represent the many dimensions of the lived experience; this is evident because of the multiple data sources examined.

Recognizability: The reader becomes more aware of an experience by recognizing some aspects of that experience, which leads to the next criterion.

Raised consciousness: The reader focuses on and gains understanding of an experience, a new insight not thought of before.

Readability: Writing should be concrete, readable, interesting, and understandable.

Relevance: Research findings "should bring us close to our humaness, increase our consciousness, enable understanding, give us possible interpretations, offer us possible meaning, and guide us in our lives, personally and professionally" (p. 192).

Revelations: As the reader gains a deeper understanding, "behind or underneath what is revealed to us, we have considered what is being concealed or what wishes to be concealed" (p. 192).

Responsibility: Ethical considerations are evident, including process consent, sensitivity to content of conversations, and authentic representation of meanings.

Munhall (1994) challenged scholars to add to the list of criteria for evaluating phenomenological research. She added to her own list by suggesting *Richness* ("a full embodied, multifaceted, multilayered, thoughtful, sensitive, impassioned description of a human experience" [p. 193]) and *Responsiveness* (people are moved to rethink preconceptions or to act in some way in response to the study) as additional *R*s for evaluating phenomenology.

EVALUATION CRITERIA FOR GROUNDED THEORY RESEARCH

Nurses have conducted grounded theory research for many years. The originators of the method, Glaser and Strauss (1967), proposed criteria to evaluate the quality of grounded theory.

"If a reader becomes sufficiently caught up in the description so that he feels vicariously that he was in the field" (p. 230), the credibility of the grounded theory is judged favorably. The reader also judges credibility by assessing the methods the researcher used to develop the theory. Additionally, before using the grounded theory, the reader evaluates the "fit" of the theory to the area to which it will be applied. The theory should be easily "understandable" to a lay person and be "general" enough to fit a variety of changing situations. The theory's concepts can be "controlled" by the user to fit ongoing variation and change.

More recently, Strauss and Corbin (1998) presented six criteria (questions to ask about the adequacy of the research process) for use in evaluating a grounded theory study, such as questions about sampling, identifying major categories, and verifying categories. They also propose eight additional criteria (questions about concepts, conceptual linkages, conditions for variation, process, and significance) with which to evaluate the empirical grounding of the research.

Most recently, Charmaz (2005) offered the following criteria to evaluate grounded theory studies:

Credibility

1. Has the researcher achieved intimate familiarity with the setting or topic?

2. Are the data sufficient to merit the researcher's claims? Consider the range, number, and depth of observations contained in the data.

3. Has the researcher made systematic comparisons between observations and between categories?

4. Do the categories cover a wide range of empirical observations?

5. Are there strong logical links between the gathered data and the researcher's argument and analysis?

6. Has the researcher provided enough evidence for his or her claims to allow the reader to form an independent assessment—and *agree* with the researcher's claims?

Originality

1. Are the categories fresh? Do they offer new insights?
2. Does the analysis provide a new conceptual rendering of the data?
3. What is the social and theoretical significance of the work?
4. How does the work challenge, extend, or refine current ideas, concepts, and practices?

Resonance

1. Do the categories portray the fullness of the studied experience?
2. Has the researcher revealed liminal and taken-for-granted meanings?
3. Has the researcher drawn links between larger collectivities and individual lives when the data so indicate?
4. Do the analytic interpretations make sense to members and offer them deeper insights about their lives and worlds?

Usefulness

1. Does the analysis offer interpretations that people can use in their everyday worlds?
2. Do the analytic categories speak to generic processes?
3. Have these generic processes been examined for hidden social justice implications?
4. Can the analysis spark further research in other substantive areas?
5. How does the work contribute to making a better society? (p. 528)

APPLICATION OF QUALITATIVE HEALTH RESEARCH

Swanson, Durham, and Albright (1997) posed 16 questions that practitioners could ask in evaluating theory, or findings, from a qualitative study for use in practice:

1. What is this study about? What is the "story line" (theory about why something occurs)?

2. Does the "story line"/theory fit with my experience in my practice, or do I feel I have to force a fit?
3. Can I understand what the investigator(s) is trying to say? Is there jargon, or is it understandable to me or a lay person?
4. Is the theory general enough to apply to situations I encounter in practice on a daily basis?
5. Does the story line account for the wide range of behaviors seen in my practice over time?
6. What are the concepts presented in the findings? Are they just named or are they supported by their characteristics (properties) and the range and variation of those characteristics (dimensions)? Are the concepts supported by anecdotal data? Are any of the concepts linked to one another? Do any of the concepts give me an "ah-ha" reaction? Have I seen this or experienced it?
7. Are there conditions that show how the theory varies? Are these sufficiently broad to encompass my practice experience?
8. Can I expand on the theory by thinking of other conditions under which the theory would be applicable?
9. Do the investigators state how the theory can be applied in practice? Can I refute their claim(s) or add to their list of applications?
10. Does the theory (e.g., findings) increase awareness of sociological, psychological, moral, ethical, or organizational aspects of practice?
11. Does the theory suggest accountability for sociological, psychological, moral, ethical, or organizational aspects of practice rather than for technical aspects of practice only?
12. Does the theory suggest application/use, including pre- and postinstitutionalization?
13. Does the theory suggest application/use such as "trajectory" or "biography"?
14. Are issues presented from the research that can be raised among the general public?
15. Does the research address empowerment issues for consumers, families, and/or communities?
16. Does the research address the role of the social system (such as the health care system or the educational system) in addressing the social problem?

Popay, Rogers, and Williams (1998) argued that qualitative research is needed in health services research to provide "evidence on appropriateness (i.e., the extent to which care can be said to meet the self-perceived needs of the person to whom it is being offered) and evidence of the factors that affect decision making among policy makers, clinicians, and patients (i.e., why people, both lay and professional, behave as they do when they do)" (p. 342).

To assess the quality of a qualitative research report, they presented a list of questions the evaluator should ask to determine the usefulness of the research findings. The questions are as follows:

1. Does the research, as reported, illuminate the subjective meaning, actions, and context of those being researched?
2. Is there evidence of the adaption [sic] and responsiveness of the research design to the circumstances and issues of real-life social settings met during the course of the study?
3. Does the sample produce the type of knowledge necessary to understand the structures and processes within which the individuals or situations are located?
4. Is the description provided detailed enough to allow the researcher or reader to interpret the meaning and context of what is being researched?
5. How are different sources of knowledge about the same issue compared and contrasted?
6. Are subjective perceptions and experiences treated as knowledge in their own right?
7. How does the research move from a description of the data, through quotation or examples, to an analysis and interpretation of the meaning and significance of it?
8. What claims are being made for the generalization of the findings to either other bodies of knowledge or to other populations or groups? (pp. 345–348)

Popay and colleagues argued that the primary standard for qualitative research is "lay accounts and the privileging of subjective meaning" (p. 344). The evaluator then looks for evidence of responsiveness to social context and flexibility of design, theoretical or purposeful sampling, adequate description, data quality, theoretical and conceptual adequacy, and potential for assessing typicality.

CONCLUSION

The search for criteria or standards with which to evaluate qualitative research continues. The review of the literature demonstrates that reviewers are concerned with the adequacy and appropriateness of the research methods employed and with the validity and usefulness of the research findings. This literature review presents a number of different frameworks that the reader could use when evaluating qualitative research reports. This chapter is intended to give the reader an overview of these frameworks to help the reader understand the complexity of evaluating qualitative research and to help identify criteria to explore in more depth. The reader is urged to consult the original sources of the material presented in this chapter.

REFERENCES

Aamodt, A. M. (1983). Problems in doing nursing research: Developing a criteria for evaluating qualitative research. *Western Journal of Nursing Research, 5,* 398–402.

Beach, R. (1993). *A teacher's introduction to reader-response theories.* Urbana, IL: National Council of Teachers of English.

Burns, N. (1989). Standards for qualitative research. *Nursing Science Quarterly, 2,* 44–52.

Burns, N., & Grove, S. F. (2005). *The practice of nursing research: Conduct, critique, and utilization* (5th ed.). St. Louis: Elsevier Saunders.

Charmaz, K. (2005). Grounded theory in the 21st century: Applications for advancing social justice studies. In N. K. Denzin & Y. S. Lincoln (Eds), *The Sage handbook of qualitative research* (3rd ed., pp. 507–535). Thousand Oaks, CA: Sage.

Denzin, N. K., & Lincoln, Y. S. (2005). The discipline and practice of qualitative research. In N. K. Denzin & Y. S. Lincoln (Eds.), *The Sage handbook of qualitative research* (3rd ed., pp. 1–32). Thousand Oaks, CA: Sage.

Eisner, E. (1985). Aesthetic modes of knowing. In E. Eisner (Ed.), *Learning and teaching the ways of knowing: Eighty-fourth yearbook of the National Society for the Study of Education, Part II* (pp. 23–36). Chicago: National Society for the Study of Education.

Engel, J. D., & Kuzel, J. D. (1992). On the idea of what constitutes good qualitative inquiry. *Qualitative Health Research, 2,* 504–510.

Fossey, E., Harvey, C., McDermott, F., & Davidson, L. (2002). Understanding and evaluating qualitative research. *Australian and New Zealand Journal of Psychiatry, 36,* 717–732.

Glaser, B. G., & Strauss, A. L. (1967). *The discovery of grounded theory: Strategies for qualitative research.* Chicago: Aldine.

Leininger, M. (1994). Evaluation criteria and critique of qualitative research studies. In J. Morse (Ed.), *Critical issues in qualitative research methods* (pp. 95–115). Thousand Oaks, CA: Sage.

Lincoln, Y. S. (1995). Emerging criteria for quality in qualitative and interpretative research. *Qualitative Inquiry, 1,* 275–289.

Lincoln, Y. S., & Guba, E. G. (1985). *Naturalistic inquiry.* Beverly Hills, CA: Sage.

Maxwell, J. A. (1992). Understanding and validity in qualitative research. *Harvard Educational Review, 62,* 279–299.

Morse, J. M. (1991). Evaluating qualitative research. *Qualitative Health Research, 1,* 283–286.

Morse, J. M. (1998). Validity by committee. *Qualitative Health Research, 8,* 443–445.

Morse, J. M. (1999a). Myth #93: Reliability and validity are not relevant to qualitative inquiry. *Qualitative Health Research, 9,* 717–718.

Morse, J. M. (1999b). Silent debates in qualitative inquiry. *Qualitative Health Research, 9,* 163–165.

Morse, J. M. (2003). The significance of standards. *Qualitative Health Research, 13,* 1187–1188.

Morse, J. M., Barrett, M., Mayan, M., Olsen, K., & Spiers, J. (2002). Verification strategies for establishing reliability and validity in qualitative research. *International Journal of Qualitative Methods, 1*(2), article 2. Retrieved August 2, 2005, from http://www.ualberta.ca/~ijqm/.

Munhall, P. L. (1994). *Revisioning phenomenology: Nursing and health science research.* New York: National League for Nursing Press.

Patton, M. Q. (2002). *Qualitative research and evaluation methods* (3rd ed.). Thousand Oaks, CA: Sage.

Popay, J., Rogers, A., & Williams, G. (1998). Rationale and standards for the systematic review of qualitative literature in health services research. *Qualitative Health Research, 8,* 341–351.

Sandelowski, M. (1993). Rigor or rigor mortis: The problem of rigor in qualitative research. *Advances in Nursing Science, 16*(2), 1–8.

Sandelowski, M. (1998). The call to experts in qualitative research. *Research in Nursing and Health, 21,* 467–471.

Sandelowski, M., & Barroso, J. (2002). Reading qualitative studies. *International Journal of Qualitative Methods, 1*(1), article 5. Retrieved August 2, 2005, from http://www.ualberta.ca/~ijqm/.

Shapin, S. (1984). Pump and circumstances: Robert Boyle's literary technology. *Social Studies of Science, 14,* 481–520.

Stiles, W. B. (1999). Evaluating qualitative research. *Evidence-Based Mental Health, 2,* 99–101.

Strauss, A., & Corbin, J. (1998). *Basics of qualitative research: Techniques and procedures for developing grounded theory* (2nd ed.). Thousand Oaks, CA: Sage.

Swanson, J. M., Durham, R. F., & Albright, J. (1997). Clinical utilization/application of qualitative research. In J. M. Morse (Ed.), *Completing a qualitative project: Details and dialogue* (pp. 253–281). Thousand Oaks, CA: Sage.

Thorne, S. (1997). The art (and science) of critiquing qualitative research. In J. M. Morse (Ed.), *Completing a qualitative project: Details and dialogue* (pp. 117–132). Thousand Oaks, CA: Sage.

26

Locating Qualitative Research Resources Online

Ronald Chenail and Maureen Duffy

For graduate students contemplating their first piece of research, the idea of designing, implementing, and analyzing a research project can be daunting. Beginning researchers and students find it helpful to see what more experienced researchers are thinking and doing. For the more experienced researcher, it is fascinating to see what others are doing and to see the proliferation of serious qualitative studies in the social and health sciences. There is no better place to get a bird's-eye view of what is going on in the qualitative landscape than on the Internet.

It can take anywhere from 6 to 18 months for a refereed article to appear in print in an academic journal. The publication of a book can take the same amount of time or longer. Ideas, works-in-progress, and finished articles can be placed on the Internet in a matter of minutes, making the Internet what Marshall McLuhan would have called a "hot" medium. The Internet as an indispensable information resource is becoming even more of a fact as a majority of scholarly journals now provide some open access to the papers they publish (Bailey, 2005). All of these factors should encourage researchers to take the opportunity to keep up-to-date with the growing amount of information and inspiration about qualitative research that the Internet provides, especially because there is an abundance of high-quality material related to qualitative research on the Internet.

Surfing the Net for qualitative research stuff can be fun and productive. It can seem a lot more like play than does sitting down and poring over a research text, however interestingly written the text may be. Many individual people and groups have spent an incredible amount of time pulling together some of the most helpful ideas about qualitative research and posting them on the Web, often on impressively organized Web sites. It would be a shame not to take advantage of the fruits of their work.

This chapter provides directions to some of our favorite qualitative research Web sites. Our hope is that you also will find these resources helpful as you develop your research projects and programs. The chapter is not intended to be a comprehensive list of qualitative research sites, but rather a welcoming invitation to visit some Internet resources we enjoy.

COMPREHENSIVE QUALITATIVE RESEARCH WEB SITES

A few Web sites provide a comprehensive array of all kinds of information about qualitative research. These omnibus Web sites are excellent jumping-off points for beginning and then narrowing your own search. They include a focus on multiple issues in qualitative research and have links to other quality resources.

International Institute for Qualitative Methodology
http://www.uofaweb.ualberta.ca/iiqm/

Under the auspices the University of Alberta's Faculty of Nursing, Jan Morse and her talented interdisciplinary group of colleagues worldwide manage the International Institute for Qualitative Methodology (IIQM), which has as its primary goal the facilitation of the development of qualitative research methods across a wide variety of academic disciplines. Importantly, the IIQM is an international network, housed at the University of Alberta, Canada, and linking seven international sites. These sites are situated in University of Johannesburg (South Africa), Ben Gurion University (Israel), University of Utrecht (Netherlands), University of Sao Paulo (Brazil), Ewah Women's University (Korea), University of Guadalajara (Mexico), and the University of Newcastle (Australia). Each of these regional sites is linked in turn to additional universities and research organizations—at present numbering 108 cooperating sites. The IIQM does not charge fees, and each cooperating site is responsible for setting its own program in support of qualitative inquiry.

The IIQM Web site contains information about the institute: its two annual conferences (Qualitative Health Research and Advances in Qualitative Methods) and workshops, its summer program, and EQUIPP—its pre- and postdoctoral program, Enhancing Qualitative Understanding in Illness Processes and Prevention, funded by the Canadian Institutes for Health and visiting scholar program. Thinking Qualitatively is a one-week conference of workshops held each summer in which participants can mix and match sessions to meet their own needs. The site also contains information about the institute's annual dissertation award for the best English-language dissertation in monograph format. The Qual Press is the publications arm of the institute and is responsible for *The International Journal for Qualitative Methodology* and the publication of monographs—excellent dissertations reconfigured as monographs. If you are interested, you can read the first chapter of each online before buying one. *Qualitative Health Research* is a print journal published 10 times per year by Sage Publications. And, of course, the site features a very useful qualitative research resource page.

Qualitative Research Resources on the Internet
http://www.nova.edu/ssss/QR/qualres.html

Ron Chenail has been building a wonderful qualitative research Web site for more than a decade at Nova Southeastern University in Fort Lauderdale, Florida. Ron's Web site has an extensive list of links to qualitative research resources worldwide. He also has a collection of abstracts, posters, and full-text articles in qualitative research by a wide range of authors. Included in this collection of textual sources are articles about qualitative research in nursing, a review of qualitative research in psychotherapy, and many reports of specific research as well as contributions about methodological issues. Ron has also gathered a variety of qualitative research course syllabi from around the world that teachers of qualitative research will undoubtedly find very helpful. His Web site also houses *The Qualitative Report (TQR)*, an online journal dedicated to qualitative research and critical inquiry. *TQR* accepts submissions from students and professional researchers alike.

Kerlins.net Qualitative Research Page
http://kerlins.net/bobbi/research/qualresearch/

Bobbi Kerlin's award-winning Web site, Kerlins.net, also known as Bobbi's Place, includes an excellent qualitative research section. She provides an outstanding bibliography on qualitative research topics ranging from action research to photoethnography to journaling to oral history and narrative. She has bibliographies for validity and paradigms and case study and more. An endless source of lateral reading recommendations is available to the serious researcher here.

A somewhat unique feature of Kerlins.net Qualitative Research site is the section dealing with qualitative research software. Web site visitors can learn about a whole array of software for voice transcription and for qualitative research data management. She also provides references and links to articles discussing the positives and negatives of using computer-based programs for data management and analysis and articles comparing the widely used data management systems. For those researchers interested in computer-assisted management of data and analysis, these resources are invaluable.

For those interested in theory, this Web site is a treasure trove. Postmodernism, critical theory, phenomenology, educational theory, sociological theory, and the theory of theory are all included, along with other theoretical perspectives and accompanying links, references, and resources. Bobbi's list of philosophers who have influenced educational, psychological, and postmodern thought is superb. She provides a biography of each thinker, an overview of his or her major ideas and work, fascinating miscellaneous information, references, and links to further information. Each time we visit Bobbi's Web site, we are filled with awe and gratitude for her amazing work and for her willingness to share so much.

The International Institute of Human Understanding
http://www.iihu.org/

This institute, headed by Tricia Munhall, first started as the International Institute for Phenomenological Inquiry in 1994. In a twofold effort to become more inclusive, the name was changed to welcome all methods of inquiry that assist in human understanding and to become more interdisciplinary. All members of disciplines that focus on coming to understand being human are invited to join. The institute sponsors an annual international conference, as well as workshops, and offers consultation and workshops on request.

SPECIALIZED QUALITATIVE RESEARCH WEB SITES

A number of specialized sites focus on some particular aspect of qualitative research that a persistent Web surfer can find. The comprehensive sites described in the preceding section have links to hundreds of them. We are going to give you a preview of some of our personal favorites here.

ENQuIRE: East of Scotland Network for Qualitative Inquiry, Research and Education, University of Dundee
http://www.dundee.ac.uk/generalpractice/research/qualitat.htm

This site describes the work of a group of qualitative researchers in the area of health care research. The group offers advice and support, both formal and informal, to other researchers and is committed "to raising the profile of Qualitative Health Research by promoting excellence in design, process and reporting."

An interesting qualitative research course syllabus that contains simple, clear goals for the qualitative learning experience is posted on the Web site. Most interesting, though, are the abstracts and summaries of the research publications of group members. A grounded-theory study on medication-taking behavior in primary care is summarized. In another study, an action research design was used to find ways of incorporating adult and reflective learning methods into the general practice training year for physicians. The site also contains an advocacy statement for utilizing qualitative research methods in health care settings.

Narrative Psychology Internet and Resource Guide
http://web.lemoyne.edu/~hevern/narpsych.html

Father Vincent Hevern of Lemoyne College in Syracuse, New York, is the editor and manager of this sophisticated site about narrative theory and narrative psychology. Narrative perspectives in the humanities and social sciences focus attention on how people understand and make sense of the experiences of their lives. Exploring "meaning" is central to the process of narrative psychology, and qualitative methods are used to gather the meanings that people assign to events and situations. Narrative perspectives attend to the stories that people tell about themselves and others and to how human experience is embodied in story. Both personal and cultural stories are considered important and are regarded as interdependent.

Here, again, there are wonderful bibliographies that offer a lifetime of reading and learning. Resources about narrative in multiple disciplines, including medicine, nursing, health care, and Holocaust studies, are provided. Resources for qualitative methods also are plentiful, in particular for interviewing techniques, case study, and oral history. The interested Web visitor can find information and resources about somewhat esoteric disciplines and techniques such as psychobiography or biographical psychology (these terms are used interchangeably).

Gary Shank: Privateer of the Semiotic Seas!
http://www.geocities.com/Athens/5260

We have not met Gary Shank, but we think we would probably like him a lot. When we see his e-mail address on qualitative research discussion lists such as QUALRS-L (more details are discussed later), we approach his contributions with more interest and excitement than we do when some others contribute to a thread. In the midst of some really good ideas, some even brilliant, there is an honesty and vulnerability in Gary's writing that is very attractive. You can see this for yourself in Gary's writings that are posted on his Web site and in his recently published textbook (Shank, 2005). Among many other things, Gary is passionate about semiotics and the philosophy of Charles Sanders Peirce. You will find many resources for both at his Web site.

Gary's Web site is a little more randomly put together than are the others on which we have commented here. But remember, where there is no randomness, there is no creativity. At Gary's Web site, there is plenty of randomness and plenty of creativity. As well as articles and resources on qualitative research, semiotics, and C. S. Peirce, you can also find Grateful Dead stuff and information about medievalists. Gary says that he's a closet one, whatever it is.

Computer Assisted Qualitative Data Analysis
Software (CAQDAS) Networking Project Page
http://caqdas.soc.surrey.ac.uk/

The best site on the Web for information on the vast array of software programs researchers can use to organize and analyze qualitative data is the Computer Assisted Qualitative Data Analysis Software (CAQDAS) Networking Project led by Ann Lewins. Because the University of Surrey's CAQDAS has no commercial links with any software manufacturers, the information presented among its many pages tends to be unbiased and fair. Besides including links to all of the major qualitative date analysis software developer home pages, CAQDAS also hosts Qual-software, the leading online discussion group dedicated to all issues pertaining to the use of these specialized software packages.

Arguably, joining Qual-software along with the University of Georgia's QUALRS-L (http://www.coe.uga.edu/quig/list.html), the fine virtual community moderated by Judith Preissle, will keep qualitative researchers up-to-date with the latest developments and major issues facing qualitative researchers today. Both online groups are also home to some wonderfully helpful researchers, faculty, students, and general aficionados of qualitative inquiry who always seem to provide the necessary guidance, wisdom, and resources when their fellow community members are in need.

Cochrane Qualitative Research Methods Group and Campbell Process Implementation Methods Group
http://mysite.wanadoo-members.co.uk/ Cochrane_Qual_Method/index.htm

Over the last decade the importance of evidence-based practice and systematic reviews of effectiveness in health care research have risen dramatically. Networks within two leading groups in the preparation, maintenance, and dissemination of these systematic reviews, the International Cochrane Collaboration and the Campbell Collaboration, have established a worldwide community dedicated to developing methods for the inclusion of findings from qualitative research into systematic reviews. Their Web site presents the latest developments in these important efforts along with a comprehensive bibliography.

THE FUTURE IS ALREADY HERE

One of the many challenges in writing about information technology is the speed at which today's groundbreaking headlines quickly become yesterday's old news. This trend seems to be especially true when it comes to the leading search engines on the Internet, although Google (http://www.google.com) is doing its best to be the exception that proves the rule.

In 2005, Google introduced Google Scholar (http://scholar.google.com), an easy-to-use search engine that allows users to search for scholarly materials across multiple disciplines and sources. Instead of jumping from index to index such as Medline, CINAHL, or PsychInfo to find papers in medicine, nursing, or psychology, Google Scholar provides a simple way to search smartly for scholarly literature regardless of the field, discipline, or source. This search tool is also a marked improvement over the regular Google search engine, which returns Web pages as well as Web-based documents. In contrast, Google Scholar returns only papers, chapters, books, and other textual presentations of scholarly information. In addition, Google Scholar is an excellent tool for locating full-text qualitative research papers online, especially from open-access (i.e., scholarly journals providing total access to their content at no cost to readers) qualitative research journals: *The International Journal of Qualitative Methods* (http://www.ualberta.ca/~ijqm/), *Forum: Qualitative Social Research* (http://www.qualitative-research.net/fqs/fqs-eng.htm), *Social Research Update* (http://www.soc.surrey.ac.uk/sru/), and *The Qualitative Report* (http://www.nova.edu/ssss/QR/index.html). Last, if this search strategy does not quite fit your needs, you can always access the University of Missouri–St. Louis's Ward E. Barnes Library's Qualitative Research Subject Guide for Health, Education, Social and Behavioral Sciences Journals (http://www.umsl.edu/services/scampus/ERSubGqualresjour.html) to find a comprehensive list of journals that have published and/or may publish qualitative research with special notations included to indicate the publication type or review process.

As the science fiction writer William Gibson ("There's no future in sci-fi," 2000) once said, "The future is already here and it is very unevenly distributed and it arrives in bits and pieces constantly." Fortunately for qualitative researchers with tools like Google Scholar and the aforementioned Web sites, even the most unevenly distributed qualitative research Web gem is now just a click away.

REFERENCES

Bailey, C. W., Jr. (2005). *Open access bibliography: Liberating scholarly literature with e-prints and open access journals.* Washington, DC: Association of Research Libraries.

Shank, G. D. (2005). *Qualitative research: A personal skills approach* (2nd ed.). Upper Saddle River, NJ: Prentice Hall.

There's no future in sci-fi [Electronic version]. (2000, April 2). *London Sunday Express.* Retrieved November 3, 2005, from LexisNexis database.

27

Opening Doors to Reimagining Qualitative Research

David M. Callejo Pérez

INTRODUCTION

The topic of this chapter is how to reimagine qualitative research for begin-ning researchers and graduate students. I did not think of myself as a person who could address this question like other thinkers who have pushed the boundaries of what counts as qualitative research (Barone, 2001b; Eisner & Peshkin, 1991; Lather, 1986; & Wolcott, 1973, 1990). In this chapter, I hope to touch on several issues that beginning researchers have to examine when they conduct qualitative research. I have questioned tenets of research in the past 5 years, especially the notion of what counts as qualitative research. This piece is not a literature review but a philosophical argument meant to illicit thought and responses by qualitative researchers involved in research. I do not so much address strategies to conduct research as raise questions that should be asked before, during, and after conducting qualitative research.

In 10th grade I discovered my white whale (five-paragraph essay), which would haunt my intellectual life through different permutations, whether the five- chapter dissertation or the scientific method. I wrote my first five-paragraph expository essay in Ms. Rinehart's English class on angst and identity after reading *A Catcher in the Rye*. I chose to write a fictional account on how Holden Caulfield would survive in our middle-class public high school in Miami, Florida. I had to do a great deal of research to find out what conditions were actually like. I combined fiction with nonfiction. I actually conducted research through story-telling. Good research has always been the ability to tell a good story. The undergirding principle of this idea is viewing research (see Heaton, 2000; Macintyre Latta, 2001) as a search. You first must search, an act of curiosity; then search again. Thus, research is an act of seeing and seeing again and making connections (Albers, 1965; Dewey, 1934). What I have described was not traditional research, but nonetheless research. I went to the library, studied people in the hallways, asked questions, triangulated data, and interpreted it to see if Holden Caulfield would actually survive in our school. I wrote an essay (good enough for a B+) explaining Holden's inability to deal with women, lack of adult figures, and a sense of alienation toward life. The foray into Holden Caulfield was the beginning of a question that I discovered in much more detail later in life when studying angst and fiction as measures of identity in schools (Callejo Pérez, 2003, 2005a, 2005b; Callejo Pérez & Toral, 2002). Experimentation at an early stage of the research process was important for me later on in my research career. As researchers we should strive to get our students to experiment and manipulate research methods to achieve a methodology that they are comfortable using. It is very uncomfortable for persons trained in the scientific method to let go and trust human inquisitiveness and curiosity. However, what is research? Is it not the result of curiosity? Researchers need to remember that their work needs to be driven by curiosity, not methods.

For years I did not understand that there were rules to research. Although I do not recommend this for everyone, it worked for me. This experience allowed me to experiment and break the rules of qualitative research. I was unintentionally allowed to take my research methods outside my discipline. I sat in on research methods courses in sociology, anthropology, history, and political science. My experiences benefited my dissertation research, which became my first book (Callejo Pérez, 2001). The ethnographic and historical study followed the form of the subject (civil rights and identity in Mississippi). I tried writing the dissertation as a movie; writing in terms of scenes instead of chapters. I used *Midnight in the Garden of Good and Evil* as a stylistic framework, intertwining critical theory and oral histories to describe a suspenseful story to paint a 10-chapter historical picture that I believed was accurate. In the end, it was still my interpretation—and possessed a sense of innocence of seeing research as virgin ground—seeking to ignore but not forget the rules of qualitative research.

QUALITATIVE RESEARCH AS A SUBJECTIVE KNOWLEDGE

In this short chapter, I reexamine the idea of what counts as qualitative research. The first step in carrying out conversations and reinterpretations of research is to look at what qualitative research should be. I want to outline several steps that "good qualitative research" should contain. All qualitative research should seek to describe, in other words, reconstruct what has been observed. Reconstruction requires that the researcher interprets what was seen. Interpretation dictates researcher reflection. In qualitative research, reflection needs to be inward. This means understanding where you stand philosophically. In this process, subjectivity is extremely important—knowing yourself is crucial—and as close as a person gets to objectivity. Objectivity and subjectivity have long been debated in qualitative research (Babbie, 1998; Denzin & Lincoln, 2000, 2003; Eisner & Peshkin, 1991). What is objectivity and where does it belong in qualitative research? For our case, objectivity has had to bear the burden of Max Weber's (1925/1946) "value free sociology" that called for the elimination of personal values from sociology. This is an almost impossible task and, as critics of the sciences (Babbie 1998; Kuhn 1969) have demonstrated, it is impossible for researchers to divorce themselves from their interpretation. In recent years, research influenced by critical feminist researchers (Behar, 1993; Brantlinger, 2004; Ellsworth, 1984, 1989) and the work of Cherryholmes (1988) and Wolcott (1973) have questioned the role of objectivity by stating that objectivity is in fact understanding relationships between the subject, yourself, and your point of view. I return to this discussion later, positioning objectivity within the context of the rise to prominence of the social sciences and the scientific method in the late 1800s emboldened and celebrated by the birth and rise of research institutions such as Johns Hopkins and the University of Chicago (Kliebard, 2003; Rippa, 2000).

Earlier I emphasized the importance of researcher reflection, which also underscores that the researcher and the knowledge driving the work need to be symbiotic. It allows us to examine and look at data through two lenses: personal reflection and historiography or canonic knowledge. Ultimately, good qualitative research is political. And good qualitative researchers understand that their work is political (whether within their own field or in the public domain). At this time, I want to spend the rest of the chapter explaining the importance of politics of research, including the significance of reclaiming the research language, reevaluating the omnipotence of quantitative research, moving beyond the scientific method, and moving beyond research as methods by focusing on interpretation.

RECLAIMING THE LANGUAGE OF RESEARCH

Research, moreover, qualitative research, needs to revisit its discourse. Using Jacques Derrida's (1979) notion of deconstruction in grammar, I put the discourse on research through a set of rigorous tests meant to understand power relations within the field. I examine the sign (word), its signifier (meanings), and the signified (lived experience) as tools to open doors to reimagining research. Let us first begin with the word *research* itself. Research assumes certain perceptions (Albers, 1965; Craig, 2003). First, as taught to graduate students, research signifies certain assertions; it is rigorous, logical, reflective; and it seeks truth. Thus, its discourse creeps into our language through powerful and absolute statements such as "research-based," "research-driven," and the "research shows." These ostentatious statements assume the infallibility research has assumed as unquestioned if it follows a methodology. Questioning this certainty, qualitative researchers made an erroneous assumption in the 1980s and 1990s (Janesick, 1998; Landson-Billings, 2000; Tierney, 2000).

They challenged the infallibility of research and reenvisioned qualitative research as inquiry; a process of constant searching. However, in questioning what counted as research, they created a vertical relationship between research and inquiry, where research remained the axis point or the reference (I) and inquiry the referent (Other). Thus, inquiry could not stand alone; it was simply what research was not. If research is rigorous, then inquiry is not. If research is scientific, then inquiry is not. On a side note, gender-specific terms surfaced to describe each (masculine for research, feminine for inquiry). As a researcher, I am on a mission to erase the word *inquiry* from qualitative research. It is research, it is not inquiry (inquiry is what you do when you drive to work in the morning); and as feminist researchers have repeatedly asserted, power lies within language. In recent years, Thomas Barone (2001b) has attempted to reclaim power by asserting that all work of inquiry is research and should be referred to as research, not inquiry.

QUESTIONING QUANTITATIVE RESEARCH

A second relational discourse exists between quantitative and qualitative research. Quantitative research in most research handbooks is taught as "experimental" and qualitative has become "descriptive." The most popular qualitative research books such as those of John Creswell (1997, 2002) or those used in basic research courses (Babbie, 1988; Gay, 2004) seek to quantify and objectify qualitative research methods by simplifying what counts as arts-based research, phenomenological or hermeneutic, ethnography, historical research, and so forth. Although, it is more complex a debate than what I have asserted, research (especially in education, nursing, and social work) does not value the problematic debate of research text and the discourse it spawns. In conversations about dissertations, qualitative research becomes what quantitative is not. It is not experimental (scientific), rigorous (triangulation), logical (statistical), valid (constructs), or generalizable ($n = 1$). This simplistic view of research affects qualitative research because most doctoral students usually take a statistics course, a basic qualitative and quantitative course, and then do a five-chapter dissertation. There is little time to delve into the complexities of research. For the purpose of our conversation, let us deconstruct this relationship and see how false idols become divine in graduate work.

Validity, for example, is a synonym for *objectivity*, and *objectivity* is a synonym for *scientific*, and *scientific* is the mantra of American psychology, specifically turn-of-the-century behaviorism whose roots came from the explanation of humans and how they learn by application of the scientific method (Alvesson & Skoldberg, 2000). The reality is that researchers spend too much time validating results and little time examining the construct validity (Cherryholmes, 1988) of their research questions (especially true in quantitative research); they heavily rely on the infallibility of statistics and statistical analysis, and do not question the generalizability of quantitative research. Research then becomes a narrow view of inquiry (as a sense of questioning). In the narrow definition of quantitative research learned in graduate school, the goal is to construct an experimental approach (reviewed by piloting), testing before applying, and eliminating any factors or variables that affect the results. In other words, questions in quantitative research serve to limit rather than expand knowledge by placing limits of what the research is searching. The sad aspect is that this position has been validated by the passage and acceptance of the No Child Left Behind Act (NCLB; U.S. Department of Education, 2001) in education and in medicine with the Health Insurance Portability and Accountability Act (HIPAA; 1996) and the narrow research agendas they spawned. We once again see the polemics of research: it is victim to funding, publishing, and other outside influences that violate the sanctity of objectivity. Funded research is a reality of academia and public entities. Funding agencies are reluctant to fund alternative grants and projects, and journals only publish articles that strengthen the paradigm. How can research expand our knowledge base if we seek only to re-create what has been researched? Research should not seek to be safe; it should be curious and adventurous, while understanding the rules that exist as guides and not dogma.

Another important factor to question is the relationship between research and policy. Quantitative researchers have wrongly assumed that their research causes changes in policy. The reality is that policy is altered on the basis of anecdote; pointing to disconnection between researchers and what guides practice in education and nursing. For example, Howard Gardner's (1983) conceptual leaps or stories about how we learn have greatly influenced practice in the classroom and increased the importance of felt experiences in nursing. There is no research basis in the conventional sense for multiple intelligences. A second example is the perceived panacea of reducing educational gaps between learners can one day lead to reduced socioeconomic gaps in society. NCLB assumes that if all kids can learn at the same level, we will miraculously end poverty and social inequalities. Finally, there is the emphasis on patient autonomy. In working with several medical educators at the Robert Byrd Health Sciences School at West Virginia University, I learned how governmental agendas have influenced what they teach. Many wonder how to instruct patient autonomy when dealing with comatose patients.

THE SCIENTIFIC METHOD AND RESEARCH

Do we actually use research in our own teaching or in policy? I believe we rarely turn to research to make decisions. Look at major policy changes made in the last 20 years and see how little influence research has had on policy and teaching. In reality, teaching methods have changed very little in the last 100 years (Cuban, 1993). We still have desks, most instruction from kindergarten to graduate school is teacher centered, students still sit in rows, and the textbook still drives knowledge transfer. The research on teaching is voluminous, but teaching is still driven by tradition and dictated by folklore. Politicians change policy based on constituency or advice from assistants rather than by searching out the latest research in refereed journals. A novel like Upton Sinclair's (1981) *The Jungle*—not the work of Jacob Riis or unions or doctors researching the dangers of improper food handling—caused the government to monitor meat packing. Research many times is the result of policy change—whether the government is trying to eradicate yellow fever or bring water to California and Arizona in the West.

Research, generally the hegemony of experimental quantitative research, has retreated from interpretation and analysis (artistic/human) and moved toward methodology (technique/scientific). Like Hannah Arendt (1958), we need to focus on research as a relation of nature, focusing on the basic human concept of creation or labor contrasted with the inhuman concept of technique or work (seeking to erase human error or interpretations from research). In the end, what we lose is our ability to be human. We must strike a balance between methodology as a tool (guide) and interpretation (curiosity) as a driving force.

Dewey (1934) states:

> I do not think that the dancing and singing of even little children can be explained wholly on the basis of unlearned and unformed responses to then existing objective occasions. Clearly there must be something in the present to evoke happiness. But the act is expressive only as there is in it a unison of something stored from past experience, something therefore generalized, with present conditions. (p. 71)

Researchers, like the children described by Dewey, have lost their sense of self and play. In focusing on methods and not interpretation, we lose the essence of what research is: the search for knowledge. Elliot Eisner (1979, 1991) views qualitative research as the aesthetic assessment of an educational quality that is more appropriate for our needs in studying people. For Eisner, an educational expert or connoisseur sees and writes like an art critic when examining subjects and situations because of his or her extensive professional experiences. Eisner is not concerned with methods or approach but with the notion of seeing. His notion of the educational encompasses any situation that involves interactions between groups of people where learning leads to changes in one's outlook.

Many qualitative researchers, especially doctoral students, believe that Eisner's notion of connoisseurship is simply enough. Research is more than description. As Dewey (1934) states, power lies in connecting what one sees to its uses in society. However, one major error qualitative researchers make is to stop at this juncture. We do not take the next step, the critical and rigorous construction of our point of view or method. Thus, I value the idea of literature or fiction as research to speak to new audiences or novels as dissertations (Barone, 2001b; Hostetler, 2005). Implications for this type of research are the eradication of methods sections from dissertations and the death of my white whale—the five-chapter dissertation.

INTERPRETATION

When we engage in human inquiry, we must seek to enhance meanings. When we engage in research, we want to complicate meanings and values under which research has occurred. I, like Hannah Arendt (Passerin d'Entreves, 1993), espouse the idea of fragmentary historiography, one that seeks to identify the moments of rupture, displacement, and dislocation in history. Such fragmentary historiography enables one to recover lost potentials of the past in the hope that they may find actualization in the present (p. 4). For Arendt, "It is necessary to redeem from those past moments worth preserving, to save fragments from past treasures that are significant for us" (p. 4). Only against the grain of traditionalism and the claims of conventional historiography can the past be made meaningful again, provide sources of illumination for the present, and yield its treasures to those who search for them with "new thoughts" and saving acts of remembrance (p. 5). It is important that I demonstrate how to adapt Dewey's and Arendt's philosophies to conducting research. One great example is using novels (Barone, 1995a, 1995b; Rosengarten, 1974) as research. As I stated in the introduction, when I wrote my paper on Holden Caulfield, I was conducting research. How then does research reflect Dewey's notion of aesthetic balance and Arendt's possibilities for recovering and retelling the past?

Politicizing Research and Interpreting the Past

An example of this research approach is found through the short story "*Hacia La Tierra del Fin del Mundo* (Toward the Land at the End of the World)," where Joel James (1980) writes a description of war and resistance in Africa similar to George Orwell's description of Burma. In his work, James takes up the Angolan Civil War after independence. "*Hacia la Tierra*," is a nine-month odyssey beginning in 1975, where Cuban troops along with the *MPLA* fight *UNITA* forces in eastern Angola. The description of travel and countryside is magnificent, while there are important connections to the role of rivers in both characters and the journey. James, as a historian, uses and incorporates the local language and culture into his words. For the author, the war in Angola is an extension of the 10 Years' War (1868–1878) and *Playa Giron*, or Bay of Pigs (1961) for Cuba; nothing more than colonialism and its evils. Cuba exists not in the real but in the creation of the soldiers' lives through memories and letters, where it is explored as a mythical place, a reality that was not present. The discussions of Cuba always revolve around the political history of the nation, including the purposeful use of the mulatto *Madruga* to recount the history after 1960. James also revisits the idea of women as leaders and their importance in the liberation role, as well as the *pionero*, the child warrior, who contributed to the war/liberation effort. James contends that revolutionary ideals should be unquestioned, even if there are flaws. Even if individual issues exist as to one's rights and freedoms, the ideology of the movement must remain intact. In James's novel, he demonstrates that community is most important, along with creating places (Angola) that encompass the struggle of postcolonial life and characters (Madruga) who serve as entrée into social history. In this piece, James uses the novel to tell the politicized story of African war and its relationship to colonial struggles and the effects on people. James's novel is not really about Africa or even Cuba; it is an attempt to capture the effects of war, colonialism, and ideology on humans. The idea I portrayed in this short vignette is that political nature of research is best seen in works like *Omeros* by Derek Wolcott (1990), *Things Fall Apart* by Chinua Achebe (1994), *The Wretched of the Earth* by Franz Fanon (1963), *Imagined Communities* by Benedict Anderson (1991), or *Orientalism* by Edward Said (1979), rather than traditional peer-reviewed journals.

Representation and Interpretation

Playing with words, terms, and constructs allows us to ponder human conditions in research. Limiting them by methods leads us to live within what Jurgen Habermas (McCarthy, 1996) calls "negative metaphysics," which rely on the "perspective of the radical outsider, mad, isolated, or aesthetically enraptured, he who distances himself from the life world as a whole, and to no longer have a language, no speech based on reasons, for spreading the message of that which they have seen. Speechlessness finds words only in the empty negation of everything that metaphysics once affirmed (Habermas, 1991, p. 51). If research is political, researchers have to become involved in policy.

Another approach used to manipulate words, terms, and constructs is through Baudrillard's *Simulations*. Jean Baudrillard (1983) compares simulation to representation. Both are cognitive modes, both define reality, and both turn to specific visual portraits that "capture reality." Reality may be seen as an experience, the daily world evaluated in adulterated perceptions. It is ideal, where body and stimuli are unaltered in their interactions. Simulacra are interpretations of reality that become reality (at-risk children are labeled to address a perceived need, and those who are labeled begin to take on the characteristics of the label). Representation in turn captures reality through social devices from reason to religion to reading. Semiotics, for example, studies signs, assumes that linguistic signification is the product of an existing link between a sound and a specific concept. Simulation is radically opposed to representation. According to Baudrillard, it is no longer possible to distinguish between good and bad representations and correct or erroneous interpretations.

CONCLUSION: POSSIBILITIES AND APPROACHES FOR QUALITATIVE RESEARCH

Why do I mention this to you? Because what I want to do is use the preceding as a road toward critical examination of qualitative research and research agendas. If we apply Habermas and Baudrillard to other forms of qualitative research, we can make several assumptions about all research, including qualitative research. Qualitative research (especially action research) has become a popular approach to research in recent years because of its accessibility for first-time researchers. Alex Sidorkin (2002) passionately writes, "Education is but an enterprise dedicated to the production of useless things" (p. 12), which for our purpose is an excellent metaphor for the products of most qualitative research. Let's revisit what good research has to contain: (1) description, (2) reconstruction/retelling, (3) interpretation guided by inward reflection, (4) relationship between researcher and knowledge, and (5) political implications of research for knowledge and policy. These become meaningful only when the researcher has to understand the limitations of how research is taught in most graduate programs.

In "Power of the Powerless," Vaclav Havel (1986) ponders about the state of mind of the store owner in a totalitarian state who places the sign "Workers of the World Unite!" on his storefront window. Havel asks: Why does he do it? Is he making a statement about unity of all workers? Does he understand its meaning? Or has it been lost in years of ritualism. What the store owner understands is that not placing the sign in his window is risking the state's wrath. His consolidated view of society is far from the actual reality. In much of the qualitative research written in graduate work (many times simply action research), the researcher focuses on "action," action for what? Where does this action fit in the larger scheme of life? If we examine the store owner, we see he is just concerned with the action (the outward expression) and cares little about the hidden meanings of the action. Research at its core is meant to uncover meanings that are hidden, as Arendt states, by fragmented memories (Passerin d'Entreves, 1993). Instead, by failing to see the polemics of the action, its consequences, or why the sign exists, we forget what good research is. It becomes in Sidorkin's words, production of useless things. It is labor. Research should be an "eternal dialogue" between I—Thou (Bakhtin, 1986). Reflection and interpretation within research need to contextualize one's reality. Breaking the rules in qualitative research requires that we reclaim language and discourse, reevaluate what research is, question quantitative research, move beyond the scientific method, focus on interpretation and not methods, and treat qualitative research as more than description of action. To do this I offer several tips to new researchers conducting research.

Trust yourself: Research is a daunting undertaking. For many students the dissertation is the first large-scale research they conduct. Uncertainty and fear cloud judgment and force students to worry only about methods instead of their question. In the end, many students quit the dissertation or take years collecting data or reading. They do not trust their ability to make decisions and know when to finish researching. The reality is that research methods as taught are so dogmatic and unwavering that students spend much of their time subjugating their thinking, data, and literature to match methods rather than manipulating methods to fit their question and research literature. Trust your experiences. While working with nurses and social workers at Boys Town, Omaha, Nebraska, I heard them speak of knowing and feeling (or, as they defined it, caring) influencing their decisions. Yet, when it came time to create a dissertation question, they subjugated the power of caring (Noddings, 1992, 2003) to whether they were "doing a qualitative or quantitative dissertation."

Begin with broad problems, not specific questions: Throughout research courses, students are held to unreal and specific choices that do not make sense in real-life research. For example, you are told to choose quantitative or qualitative research, and then everything else should fit. The reality of this inane choice is that it serves to limit what research is truly about: curiosity. In choosing methods first, researchers are forced to create contrived and specific questions that become simplistic and limit the literature review, data collection, and interpretation. The best way to begin research is to start with broad issues or problems. Qualitative research is not about experimental designs. It is about people and should address real problems and issues. For example, in my own dissertation I asked, "What was the role of schools in black identity formation during the Civil Rights Movement?" Many students would be asked to be more specific, give dates, define terms in the questions, and so forth. What is the dissertation for? It is not a question-writing exercise; it is an argument espousing a point of view through evidence found in the literature and field. As such, then operationalization of terms and specifics should be left for the body of the dissertation. In fact, when you write for publication, journals and book publishers ask that you simplify your titles and remove dissertation-like language from the manuscript. If the goal of the dissertation is to demonstrate your ability to write publishable work, it should resemble actual work that will be published. It should be a meaningful exercise and not production of "useless things" (Sidorkin, 2002).

Read the research literature: Technology has allowed researchers to browse and download abstracts from databases through online searches. This has opened many new avenues for research, but it has not helped the students work in research. You still need to read the piece, go to the archive or library, search the text, use bibliographies, know the field you work within, understand philosophical approaches, and so on. Abstracts are one of the most important aspects of research. It is what most people will read. However, we spend very little time writing them; and, therefore, many times we do not disseminate the research project well. You need to read the text to extract the philosophical argument, the data collection, and interpretations. Reading the research literature means physically reading and scanning; in other words it is more than a search, it is re-search (Albers, 1965).

Expand your notion of research literature: As part of researching literature, students need to expand their notion of what counts as research. It is more than refereed articles, reports, academic books, or archived work. Researchers need to look at and accept fiction, art, music, poetry, unpublished works, newspapers, and even other dissertations as research literature. *Omeros* by Derek Wolcott is a poetic saga resembling Homer's *Odyssey*, and one of the best phenomenological descriptions of colonialism. In reading this work, a researcher can glean more about colonialism, Caribbean identity, and race than by studying and scanning hundreds of refereed articles. What has better ability to be generalized or cause policy change— Derek Wolcott or a refereed article in some journal?

There is no right or wrong: This idea is related to the first two suggestions about carrying out research. The scientific method and modernism have been inculcated in students since they entered school. As such, we are taught that there always is a right and wrong answer. In research, especially qualitative research, there is no such thing as wrong or right. It is about interpretation. Studying your question in a rigorous manner, following your methodology, and interpreting data still might not provide "the right answer" for your research. It is okay. My dissertation question about schools and identity formation was "wrong." It was actually a combination of community institutions that did not include schools that caused change in black identity during the Civil Rights Movement. What I learned from that experience is that schools are not as important in influencing children's identity, and that it is extremely important to understand that the current presidential administration wrongly assumes that schools can be used to change how people think.

Research is the ability to argue a point of view: Research is not a five-chapter dissertation, separated with transitional headings. It is an argument made up of interrelated parts. When you write, you need to keep that in mind. The argument should unite your research literature, data, questions, and interpretations. Bonita Sawatzky's (2001–2002; Alvarez et. al., 2004) work using Botox to help children with clubfoot caused a stir in the Canadian medical community. She continued to pursue her work and successfully argued (backed by results) that in her experiences in orthopedic surgery the drug would help reconstruct the foot. It did not have widespread backing until the government read interviews with Sawatzky in the popular press. Eisner (1998) asks us to incorporate our life experiences into qualitative research, focusing on what we know and what we see. Sawatzky was able to do this by challenging the male-dominated field of orthopedic surgery through a different view, dominated by her own experiences.

Be rigorous, record accurately, report fully: Qualitative research is not easy. In fact, without the absolutes of statistics, research rigor becomes much more important. Your job to record accurately what is witnessed and report fully what you have learned is magnified in qualitative research. And because you do not need to worry about right or wrong, it is crucial you tell the readers everything.

Trust readers: Researchers assume that readers are not educated in the research area and will not understand what researchers write. Trust the readers by guiding them through your argument without telling them what to see. Let the readers form their own conclusions. Remember that when it is on paper you lose ownership of the discourse and text. In the end, trusting the readers allows you to follow the preceding suggestions.

Write, rewrite, and seek feedback: Write and rewrite early in the process. Seek feedback often and rewrite constantly. Seek feedback from people outside your area; they will give you different feedback because they do not see what persons in your area assume.

Remember that all research is political: I have tried to show how important research can be if it is political. Your job is to seek change within the context of society. Questions asked have to serve the purpose of addressing important and broad issues, or research does not serve the purpose of causing policy change in and outside your field (Kuhn, 1969).

REFERENCES

Achebe, C. (1994). *Things fall apart.* Garden City, NY: Anchor Press.

Albers, J. (1965). *Search versus re-search.* Hartford, CT: Trinity College Press.

Alvarez, C. M., Tredwell, S. J., Beauchamp, R. D., Keenan S., Choit R., Sawatzky, B. J., & DeVera, M. (2004, April). Treatment of idiopathic clubfoot utilizing Botulinum A toxin: A new method and its short term outcome. *Journal of Paediatric Orthopaedics.*

Alvesson, M., & Skoldberg, K. (2000). *Reflexive methodology.* Thousand Oaks, CA: Sage.

Anderson, B. (1991). *Imagined communities.* London: Verso.

Arendt, H. (1958). *The human condition.* Chicago: University of Chicago Press.

Babbie, E. (1998). *The practice of social research* (8th ed.). Belmont, CA: Wadsworth.

Bakhtin, M. (1986). *Speech genres and other late essays.* Austin: University of Texas Press.

Barone, T. (1995a). Introduction: The uses of educational research. *International Journal of Educational Research, 23*(2), 109–112.

Barone, T. (1995b). Persuasive writings, vigilant readings, reconstructed characters: The paradox of trust in educational storysharing. *International Journal of Qualitative Studies in Education, 8*(1), 63–74.

Barone, T. (2001a, October). Science, art, and the predispositions of educational researchers. *Educational Researcher, 30*(7), 24–26.

Barone, T. (2001b). *Touching eternity: The enduring outcomes of teaching.* New York: Teachers College Press.

Baudrillard, J. (1983). *Simulations.* New York: Semiotext(e).

Behar, R. (1993). *Translated woman.* Boston: Beacon Press.

Brantlinger, E. (2004). *Dividing classes: How the middle class negotiates and rationalizes school advantage.* New York: Routledge.

Callejo Pérez, D. (2001). *Southern hospitality: Black identity and the civil rights movement in the South.* New York: Peter Lang.

Callejo Pérez, D. (2003). Identity, literature, schools and race: Southern writers and literature as a metaphor for place. In D. Callejo Pérez, S. M. Fain, & J. J. Slater. (Eds.), *Pedagogy of place: Understanding place as a social aspect of education.* New York: Peter Lang.

Callejo Pérez, D. (2005a, Spring). A school story: Integrating Belvedere school. *Scholarly Practitioner Quarterly, 2*(3), 53–70.

Callejo Pérez, D. (2005b, Summer). The spirituality of curriculum reform: Reclaiming teacher education. *Taboo: A Journal of Cultural Studies in Education,* 73–80.

Callejo Pérez, D., & Toral, P. (2002). Comparative study of cultural conversation in educational policy among two ethnic minority groups of Spanish origins: Basques in Spain and Cubans in the United States. *The International Journal of Social Education, 17*(2), 1–30.

Cherryholmes, C. (1988). *Power and criticism: Poststructural investigations in education.* New York: Teachers College Press.

Craig, C. (2003). *Narrative inquiries of school reform: Storied lives, storied landscapes, storied metaphors.* Greenwich, CT: Information Age Publishing.

Creswell, J. (1997). *Qualitative inquiry and research design: Choosing among five traditions.* Thousand Oaks, CA: Sage.

Creswell, J. (2002). *Research design: Qualitative, quantitative, and mixed methods approaches.* Thousand Oaks, CA: Sage.

Cuban, L. (1993). *How teachers taught: Constancy and change in American classrooms, 1890–1980.* New York: Longman.

Denzin, N., & Lincoln, Y. (Eds.). (2000). *Handbook of qualitative research.* Thousand Oaks, CA: Sage.

Denzin, N., & Lincoln, Y. (Eds.). (2003). *The landscape of qualitative research.* Thousand Oaks, CA: Sage.

Derrida, J. (1979). *Of grammatology.* Baltimore, MD: Johns Hopkins University Press.

Dewey, J. (1934). *Art as experience.* New York: Pedigree.

Eisner, E. (1979). *The educational imagination: On the design and evaluation of school programs.* Upper Saddle River, NJ: Prentice Hall.

Eisner, E. (1998). *The enlightened eye: Qualitative inquiry and the enhancement of educational practice.* Upper Saddle River, NJ: Prentice Hall.

Eisner, E., & Peshkin, A. (Eds.). (1991). *Qualitative inquiry in education.* New York: Teachers College Press.

Ellsworth, E. (1984). Incorporation of feminist meanings in media texts. *Humanities in Society, 7*(1&2), 65–75.

Ellsworth, E. (1989). Why doesn't this feel empowering? Working through the repressive myths of critical pedagogy. *Harvard Educational Review, 59*(3), 297–324.

Fanon, F. (1963). *The wretched of the earth* (C. Farrington, Trans.). New York: Grove Press.

Gardner, H. (1983). *Frames of mind: The theory of multiple intelligences.* New York: Basic Books.

Gay, L. R. (2004). *Educational research: Competencies for analysis and applications.* Upper Saddle River, NJ: Prentice Hall.

Habermas, J. (1991). *The structural transformation of the public sphere* (T. Burger, Trans.). Boston, MA: MIT Press.

Havel, V. (1986). Power of the powerless. In J. Vladislav (Ed.), *Vaclav Havel or living in truth* (pp. 36–122). London: Farber & Farber.

Health Insurance Portability and Accountability Act of 1996, 42 U.S.C. §201 et seq. (1996).

Heaton, R. (2000). *Teaching mathematics to the new standards: Relearning the dance.* New York: Teachers College Press.

Hostetler, K. (2005, August/September). What is "good" education research? *Educational Researcher, 34*(6), 16–21.

James, J. (1980). Hacia la tierra del fin del mundo. In J. James (Ed.), *Un episodio de la lucha cubana contra la anexión en el año 1900.* Santiago, Cuba: Editorial Oriente.

Janesick, V. (1998). *"Stretching" exercises for qualitative researchers.* Thousand Oaks, CA: Sage.

Kliebard, H. (2003). *The struggle for the American curriculum, 1893–1958.* New York: Routledge.

Kuhn, T. (1969). *The structure of scientific revolutions.* Chicago: University of Chicago Press.

Landson-Billings, G. (2000). Racialized discourses and ethnic epistemologies. In N. Denzin & Y. Lincoln (Eds.), *Handbook of qualitative research* (pp. 537–554). Thousand Oaks, CA: Sage.

Lather, P. (1986). Issues of validity in openly ideological research: Between a rock and a hard place. *Interchange, 17*(4), 63–84.

Macintyre Latta, M. (2001). *The aesthetics of play in the classroom.* New York: Peter Lang.

McCarthy, T. (1996). *The critical theory of Jurgen Habermas.* Boston, MA: MIT Press.

Noddings, N. (1992). *The challenge to care in schools: An alternative approach to education.* New York: Teachers College Press.

Passerin d'Entreves, M. (1993). *The political philosophy of Hannah Arendt.* London, England: Routledge.

Rippa, S. A. (2000). *Education in a free society: An American history.* New York: Longman.

Rosengarten, T. (1974). *All God's dangers: The life of Nate Shaw.* Chicago: University of Chicago Press.

Said, E. (1979). *Orientalism.* New York: Vintage.

Sawatzky, B. (2001–2002). Botox in children with clubfoot's preliminary study. Grant from the Canadian Foundation for Innovation.

Sidorkin, A. (2002). *Learning relations.* New York: Peter Lang.

Sinclair, U. (1981). *The jungle.* New York: Bantam Books.

Tierney, W. (2000). Undaunted courage: Life history and the postmodern challenge. In N. Denzin & Y. Lincoln (Eds.), *Handbook of qualitative research* (pp. 537–554). Thousand Oaks, CA: Sage.

U.S. Department of Education. (2001). *No Child Left Behind Act; Re-Issuance of the Elementary and Secondary Education Act.* Retrieved from http://www.ed.gov/nclb/landing.jhtml.

Wolcott, D. (1990). *Omeros.* New York: Farrar, Straus, & Giroux.

Wolcott, H. (1973). *The man in the principal's office: Ethnography.* New York: Holt, Rinehart & Winston.

Wolcott, H. (1990). On seeking—and rejecting—validity in qualitative research. In E. Eisner & A. Peshkin (Eds.), *Qualitative inquiry in education.* New York: Teachers College Press.

ADDITIONAL REFERENCES

Berendt, J. (1999). *Midnight in the garden of good and evil.* New York: Vintage Books.

Lather, P. (1990). *Getting smart: Feminist research and pedagogy with/in the postmodern.* London: Routledge.

Noddings, N. (2003). *Caring: A feminine approach to ethics and moral education* (2nd ed.). Berkeley: University of California Press.

Salinger, J. D. (1951). *Catcher in the rye.* Toronto, Ontario: Bantam Books.

Weber, M. (1946). Science as a vocation. In H. Gerth & C. W. Mills (Eds.), *From Max Weber: Essays in sociology.* New York: Oxford University Press. (Original work published 1925)

EPILOGUE

In Coming to an Open Closing

Patricia L. Munhall

It is my hope that in reading this volume or parts of it you have come to understand how critical qualitative research is to our nursing practice. Our philosophies of nursing seem to be concerned with the uniqueness of each human being and *the* being taking place in an individual situated context. We profess in our philosophies a respect for autonomy and self-determination of people, which is to say we honor people's perceptions of the world and their decisions, whatever they may be.

If their perception puts them in harm's way, we are in a role to reflect back to them a different way of viewing the world, but we do not discount their perceptions or make assumptions that individuals should see the world the same way we do. As nurses we have different kinds of perceptions from one another, not only the people we serve.

Perceptions originate from an individual's situated context, which we profess we also take into account when we approach individuals from a perspective of holism. Other beliefs we find in our philosophies give voice to humanism, open systems, multiple realities, and the overarching embrace of these beliefs with caring, compassion, and empathy.

Our philosophies of nursing are highly ideal in nature, and often we find the everyday realities impinging on our implementing those beliefs. We want *to live them,* but the world is often "too much with us," in its limited human resources, a very broken health care system, and where health care disparities and shortages make our philosophies sometimes look like *"pie in the sky."* However, we must strive to actualize those beliefs to the extent that we are able. One way to accomplish that is through the pursuit of qualitative research.

You read in Chapter 2 the compatibility of nursing philosophies and the philosophical underpinnings of qualitative research. Those underpinnings speak to each belief cited here as part of a philosophy of nursing. They are very much one and the same. To actualize the core beliefs of nursing, one needs the understanding that qualitative research enables us to have, to provide direction for practice and to give meaning to practice.

This journey of learning about qualitative research methods, if you started with this text, is just the first part. Perhaps a qualitative researcher is about to be born and this volume will represent your gestation.

I wish you a very successful birth. If this turns out to be your research "home" because of the way you are in the world, I think you and the recipients of your research will indeed be fortunate. You will turn to them and their lives, their individual being in the world and in different situated contexts, giving them authentic voice. You, as a nurse researcher, will have the opportunity *to feel* and *learn* things that are inaccessible by other methods. You will gain insights and discover knowledge that comes from listening to another and often hearing interpretations you would never have thought of from your own context. How could you? We really are different!

To paraphrase what was said in this book, qualitative research has the power to liberate us from presuppositions, preconceptions, assumptions, and biases and allows us to see what is real, not what was constructed by others with little or no evidence. This is critical to freeing people and/or emancipating groups from stereotypes that often prevent their acceptance and opportunities to develop.

For us to truly understand the other we must come to know who we are, what we believe, our subjective world. In encounters with others, we enter another world, another subjective space, and we interact in an intersubjective space. Qualitative researchers celebrate subjectivity as the way to knowing: the subjectivity *of the other* speaks to us, and then we come in contact with that world and we can empathize from a place of understanding.

I once heard that *what people want most is to be understood.* Think—isn't that what you want? It is a normal human desire. Often I think it is wondrous to watch *qualitative researchers when they are not doing research,* per se. They are instead *being* qualitative. I watch them either as faculty or practitioners, and I see that they often interact and listen differently to people from the way their colleagues who come from the positivistic paradigm do. They carry over their research practices to their professional and also their personal worlds.

Not everyone who reads this volume will become a qualitative researcher. That certainly would be a remarkable feat, and I am not sure we would want to convert all to qualitative research; however, *I would like to see more realization through funding* as to the potential of qualitative research. But that is not the main point I want to make here.

You may or may not become a qualitative nurse researcher, but even if you do not, I do hope that you will take some of the understandings that you may have gleaned from this perspective into your practice. The foundations through concepts or beliefs of qualitative research when applied to practice, not just research, offer one of the best perspectives in our hope to have our practice characterized by our concern with the individual, the individual's unique circumstances in the world, and our real desire to want to understand from the individual's subjective perspective.

For example, you do not have to do qualitative research to practice *unknowing* as was discussed in Chapter 6. Nor do you have to be a qualitative researcher to take into account a person's *situated context* as the most potent influence on the way that person is in this world. Neither do you have to do qualitative research to reach into the *subjective world* of *the other*.

However, if you have indeed found *an affinity and appreciation* for what qualitative research offers to us as human beings and want to pursue this kind of research, I do welcome you to this most meaningful world of research. With its intense focus on meaning, understanding, and interpretation of experience, it is my hope that this book will be a good foundation for you. You will be entering a world that is very intertwined, in that your professional understandings will become much more philosophical, and it will also become more apparent that the separation between the professional and the personal is quite arbitrary.

This method of research embraces subjectivity and, as such, embraces feelings and emotions. I am not sure you can do this kind of research and not sometimes want to cry or laugh with your participants. That is why it does take a special kind of individual to do good qualitative research. Entering into others' experiences is an *altruistic act* if done for an *altruistic reason*, and a qualitative researcher must be sincere, authentic, and caring. Participants can tell!

In this *open-closing* (there is really no closure), I want to remind us that *we are always in experience*, our *patients are always in experience*, and so it is incumbent upon us to understand and appreciate their life-worlds as well as our own with all the variations and complexities therein. We enter into another's experience, and thus we are both privileged and also indebted— indebted to produce the best quality research, with the most meaning and the most direction for improving practice in its many domains.

To me it is this complicatedness, sometimes called the *messiness* of our human lives, the interconnectedness of phenomena, and the appreciation of intersubjectivity that gives qualitative research the authenticity and existential humanness that has the potential to enrich our lives. The knowledge and insight gleaned are essential to compassion, care, liberation, and finding meaning in our everyday experience. The findings provide authentic groundings to develop theory, to critique practice, to understand why different ways of doing something might be more beneficial, to develop new practices based on understanding the meaning of a phenomenon to individuals, and to shed ourselves as "the knower" who can figure out what is best for people from our own perspectives. Qualitative researchers acknowledge that the experts of experience are those that are in or have been in the experience. To think otherwise is quite presumptuous.

To those of you who say, "Yes, this is what I want to do, this is me, I have found a home," I wish you success in your research endeavors. For those of you who will continue along the positivistic avenue, I also wish you success in your research endeavors. What I do hope is that all of you will have found something in this volume that has touched your heart, soul, and mind and that encourages you to reach out in a more *authentic* way to others, to *listen differently*, to care more about *subjectivity*, *to shed the knowing* of the professional, and to once again come in touch with why you became a nurse in the first place: to help people in a *caring, compassionate,* and *empathic* way.

General Format for Research Proposals and Research Reports

Patricia L. Munhall

Many method chapters and exemplar chapters provide suggested formats for their specific method. What is offered here are some general formats you could follow and tailor to your specific study.

A more detailed explanation and format information can be found in *Qualitative Research Proposals and Reports: A Guide,* last published by NLN and Jones and Bartlett in 2000 and updated for this fourth edition of *Nursing Research: A Qualitative Perspective.*

FORMATS FOR THE RESEARCH PROPOSAL AND RESEARCH REPORTS

In view of the interest in qualitative methodology and the discipline's rela- tively novice status in the use of qualitative designs, the final research report will be of interest not only for the research product but also for the research process. This observation does not distinguish qualitative research reports from those that spring from the dominant positivist paradigm, but it does suggest that the labor of explaining and defending the qualitative choice is meaningful.

Tables I and II provide outlines for a formal research proposal. Overall, the first four sections of the proposal (Introduction: Aim of the study; Evolution of the study; Method of Inquiry: General; and Method of Inquiry: Applied) are usually consistent with dissertation requirements. Both sections on method require considerable expansion, first about the method itself to provide the background that is still necessary for readers to understand your qualitative approach. The applied-method section will be in accord with what actually happened in the research process. Specific illustrations of various features of the research process should be included to substantiate generalities. Literature that was reviewed in data gathering should be cited in the Research Method section, and its use in the research process should be described. In those studies that postpone a formal review of scientific literature until the Discussion section, the literature review should be placed in that section. The Findings of the Inquiry and Reflections on the Findings sections are reported separately, with the material as indicated in the outline. The form of the Findings section is usually narrative, peppered with supportive "raw" data that might include quotations from participants, poems, or field note entries, for example. The aim of meaningful qualitative description should guide the researcher's choices among data-reporting forms and might include graphics as complementary to the narrative. In the Reflections section, the researcher delves deeply into the findings for meanings and understandings, as well as integrating the study's significance, substance, and importance to nursing. Appendices and references are modified as indicated by what actually transpired in the conduct of the research project.

TABLE I Proposal for Qualitative Research Studies

1. Introduction: Aim of the Study
    (a) Phenomenon of interest
    (b) Perceived justification for studying the phenomenon
    (c) Phenomenon discussed within specific context (e.g., a lived experience, a culture, a human response)
    (d) Assumptions, biases, experiences, intuitions, perceptions related to belief that inquiry into phenomenon is important
    (e) Qualitative research method chosen with justification of its potential
    (f) Relevance to nursing
2. Evolution of the Study
    (a) Rationale
    (b) Historical context
    (c) Experiential context

TABLE I   Proposal for Qualitative Research Studies (CONTINUED)

3. Method of Inquiry: General
    (a) Introduction to specific method
    (b) Rationale for choosing method: philosophical and theoretical substantiation projected
    (c) Background of method
    (d) Outcome of method
    (e) Sources (individuals) whose methods will be followed
    (f) General steps or procedures of the method
    (g) Translation of concepts and terms
4. Method of Inquiry: Applied
    (a) Aim
    (b) Sample
    (c) Setting
    (d) Gaining access
    (e) General steps
    (f) Human subject considerations: informed consent, entry, departure, confidentiality, secrets, process consent-if and when situation should change
    (g) Strengths and limitations
    (h) Expected timetable
    (i) Actual feasibility of study-Is access cost possible?
5. Appendices
    (a) Supporting documents
    (b) Consent forms
    (c) Communication
6. References

TABLE II   Outline for Reporting Qualitative Research Studies

1. Aim of the Study
    (a) Same as the proposal but with more breadth.
    (b) Include new outline of remaining report.
2. Evolution of the Study
    (a) Same as proposal.
    (b) More breadth and depth.
3. Method of Inquiry: General
    (a) Same as proposal but more specific.
4. Method of Inquiry: Applied
    (a) As it happened.

TABLE II   Outline for Reporting Qualitative Research Studies (CONTINUED)

5. Findings of the Inquiry
   (a) Findings are discussed according to the method. Example: In grounded-theory method, the aim is generation of theoretical constructs. In this section, then, the researcher would have findings from the process of
      ♦ memoing
      ♦ theoretical sampling
      ♦ sorting
      ♦ saturation
      ♦ review of literature
      ♦ the theory
   (b) With the ethnographic method, the findings may be reported in a smooth, flowing descriptive narrative. The aim of the narrative is to portray the full context, to the extent possible, that was discovered by exploring pieces of reality or experience or both. Review of other sources (literature, art, films) is a plus.
   (c) With phenomenology guiding the method, the findings will be reported differently. An example might include:
      ♦ description of experiential themes
      ♦ essences of experience
      ♦ description of relations among essences
      ♦ review of other sources (literature, art, films)

6. Reflections on the Findings:
   With preconceptions and ideas as discussed in the introduction;
   With existing literature and practice in the area of study;
   With the utilization of the method
   (a) Meanings and understandings
   (b) Implications of the study (for whom)
   (c) Relevance of the study (for whom)
   (d) *Critique* the relevance with furthering the implications and recommendations for political, social, cultural, health care, nursing, family and other social systems.
   Integrate:
   (e) Significance and substance
   (f) Importance to nursing and health care
   (g) Suggestion for future inquiries

7. Appendices
   (a) Dissertation proposals and reports would include all necessary appendices (e.g., consent letters, tables, etc.).

8. References

THE ABSTRACT

Abstracts are commonly required for dissertations, by journals, and by research conference planners. Traditional formats are again troublesome for the qualitative researcher. Rather than sacrifice substance to form, we suggest that formats be modified to accommodate the nature of the qualitative paradigm. Table III presents an alternative that is consistent with the outlines for the proposals and reports and enables clear communication of the study for abstract form.

TABLE III Outline for Qualitative Research Studies

---

1. Aim of the Study
   (a) Phenomenon of interest
   (b) Relevance for nursing
2. Evolution of the Study
   (a) Rational, experiential, and historical contents
3. Method of Inquiry: General
   (a) Brief overview of purpose of method
   (b) Basic steps
   (c) Suggestion for future inquiries
4. Method of Inquiry: Applied
   (a) Brief overview of specific steps: sample, interviews, setting, procedures, consent, and data analysis
5. Findings of the Study
   (a) Brief synopsis of findings of study
6. Reflection on the Findings
   (a) Brief synopsis of the meaning, understandings, and possible implications of the study
   (b) Significance and substance briefly discussed

INDEX